Covid-19 and Cardiovascular Disease: From Basic Mechanisms to Clinical Perspectives

Covid-19 and Cardiovascular Disease: From Basic Mechanisms to Clinical Perspectives

Editor: Robin Davidson

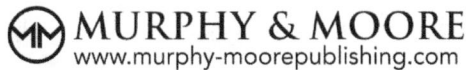
MURPHY & MOORE
www.murphy-moorepublishing.com

www.murphy-moorepublishing.com

⊕ MURPHY & MOORE

Cataloging-in-Publication Data

Covid-19 and cardiovascular disease : from basic mechanisms to clinical perspectives / edited by Robin Davidson.
    p. cm.
Includes bibliographical references and index.
ISBN 978-1-63987-772-0
1. Cardiovascular system--Diseases. 2. COVID-19 (Disease). 3. Cardiovascular system--Diseases--Treatment.
4. Heart--Diseases. I. Davidson, Robin.
RC667 .C68 2023
616.1--dc23

Murphy & Moore Publishing
1 Rockefeller Plaza,
New York City,
NY 10020, USA

ISBN: 978-1-63987-772-0

Contents

Permissions

List of Contributors

Index

Preface

This book has been a concerted effort by a group of academicians, researchers and scientists, who have contributed their research works for the realization of the book. This book has materialized in the wake of emerging advancements and innovations in this field. Therefore, the need of the hour was to compile all the required researches and disseminate the knowledge to a broad spectrum of people comprising of students, researchers and specialists of the field.

Coronavirus disease (Covid-19) refers to a type of an infectious disease caused by the SARS-CoV-2 virus. Symptoms of Covid 19 can vary but frequently include headache, loss of smell, exhaustion, fever, loss of taste, cough and breathing difficulties. Cardiovascular diseases (CVDs) are a group of diseases that affect the blood vessels or heart. Covid-19 has various interactions with the cardiovascular system causing myocardial dysfunction and damage as well as increasing morbidity in patients with underlying cardiovascular conditions. Covid-19 can also lead to cardiovascular diseases such as acute coronary syndrome, myocardial damage, venous thromboembolism and arrhythmias. Medications including angiotensin II receptor blockers (ARBs) and angiotensin-converting enzyme (ACE) inhibitors, which are designed to lower cardiovascular risk have a variety of side effects that may impact the severity or susceptibility of Covid-19. This book provides significant information to help develop a good understanding of links between Covid-19 and cardiovascular diseases. It aims to shed light on some of the unexplored aspects of these diseases. This book will serve as a reference to a broad spectrum of readers.

At the end of the preface, I would like to thank the authors for their brilliant chapters and the publisher for guiding us all-through the making of the book till its final stage. Also, I would like to thank my family for providing the support and encouragement throughout my academic career and research projects.

Editor

Right Ventricular Damage in COVID-19: Association between Myocardial Injury and COVID-19

Yonghao Lan [1,2], Wei Liu [2,3*] and Yujie Zhou [2,3]

[1] Department of Cardiology, Beijing Jishuitan Hospital, Peking University Fourth Hospital, Beijing, China, [2] Department of Cardiology, Beijing Anzhen Hospital, Capital Medical University, Beijing, China, [3] Beijing Key Laboratory of Precision Medicine of Coronary Atherosclerotic Disease, Clinical Center for Coronary Heart Disease, Beijing Institute of Heart Lung and Blood Vessel Disease, Capital Medical University, Beijing, China

*Correspondence:
Wei Liu
liuwei@ccmu.edu.cn

Coronavirus disease 2019 (COVID-19), caused by severe acute respiratory syndrome coronavirus 2, is a global pandemic. It has resulted in considerable morbidity and mortality around the world. The respiratory system is the main system invaded by the virus involved in COVID-19. In addition to typical respiratory manifestations, a certain proportion of severe COVID-19 cases present with evidence of myocardial injury, which is associated with excessive mortality. With availability of an increasing amount of imaging data, right ventricular (RV) damage is prevalent in patients with COVID-19 and myocardial injury, while left ventricular damage is relatively rare and lacks specificity. The mechanisms of RV damage may be due to increased RV afterload and decreased RV contractility caused by various factors, such as acute respiratory distress syndrome, pulmonary thrombosis, direct viral injury, hypoxia, inflammatory response and autoimmune injury. RV dysfunction usually indicates a poor clinical outcome in patients with COVID-19. Timely and effective treatment is of vital importance to save patients' lives as well as improve prognosis. By use of echocardiography or cardiovascular magnetic resonance, doctors can find RV dilatation and dysfunction early. By illustrating the phenomenon of RV damage and its potential pathophysiological mechanisms, we will guide doctors to give timely medical treatments (e.g., anticoagulants, diuretics, cardiotonic), and device-assisted therapy (e.g., mechanical ventilation, extracorporeal membrane oxygenation) when necessary for these patients. In the paper, we examined the latest relevant studies to investigate the imaging features, potential mechanisms, and treatments of myocardial damage caused by COVID-19. RV damage may be an association between myocardial damage and lung injury in COVID-19. Early assessment of RV geometry and function will be helpful in aetiological determination and adjustment of treatment options.

Keywords: COVID-19, right ventricular damage, myocardial injury, cardiovascular magnetic resonance, echocardiography, ARDS

INTRODUCTION

Coronavirus disease 2019 (COVID-19) has spread rapidly and triggered a terrible global pandemic that involves more than 200 countries/regions. On 6 December 2020, there were more than 66.9 million confirmed cases and 1,534,954 deaths internationally (1). Although respiratory symptoms are usually predominant in COVID-19, elevated troponin levels have been found at the early stage in some cases, indicating that COVID-19 also affects the heart. In particular, there is an increased prevalence of cardiovascular complications, including new or worsening heart failure, arrhythmia, acute myocarditis, and myocardial infarction, in severe and critically ill patients with COVID-19. Recent studies have shown that the incidence of acute myocardial injury in hospitalized patients with COVID-19 is ~20–28% (2–4). With an increase in imaging evidence, such as echocardiography and magnetic resonance imaging (MRI), right ventricular (RV) involvement has been observed more commonly than left ventricular (LV) involvement in patients with COVID-19, with ~40% of patients experiencing RV dilatation and RV dysfunction (5, 6). RV damage is associated with a higher incidence of myocardial damage in COVID-19 and generally predicts a worse prognosis (7). This review aims to describe involvement of RV damage in patients with COVID-19, to determine the association of RV damage with COVID-19 and its plausible mechanisms, and to summarize the existing appropriate treatment strategies to improve patients' prognosis.

MYOCARDIAL INJURY IN COVID-19 IS COMMON

Previous influenza-related studies have shown that elevated cardiac enzymes are relatively uncommon (8). Cardiac abnormalities associated with influenza are usually subclinical and/or transient (9). However, COVID-9-related cardiac injury is significantly different from influenza. In a review of 26 studies that included 11,685 patients, the overall prevalence of COVID-19-related acute myocardial injury ranged from 5 to 38% (10). N-terminal pro-brain natriuretic peptide and cardiac troponin-I levels were shown to be significantly higher in critically ill patients with COVID-19 than in non-critically ill patients (2). These findings suggest that the magnitude of elevated cardiac troponin levels may be related to the severity and prognosis of the disease (11). Monitoring cardiac troponin-I levels is important for judging the status of COVID-19, while understanding myocardial injury in patients with COVID-19. Chinese guidelines recommend myocardial enzyme monitoring in patients who are admitted for COVID-19 (12). Troponins are often associated with LV ischaemia and infarction. However, previous studies have shown that the most common mechanism of elevated troponin levels in patients with COVID-19 is

acute RV damage rather than LV functional impairment (5). Specific manifestations of myocardial structural damage require assessment of cardiac imaging. Early retrospective analysis did not show any specificity between electrocardiography and echocardiography (13). However, with publication of more imaging study results, there are particularities in cardiac structural changes. Therefore, imaging assessment of cardiac injury in COVID-19 is important and helpful for differential diagnosis of cardiac events.

RV INVOLVEMENT FROM CARDIAC IMAGES IN PATIENTS WITH COVID-19

With the discovery of COVID-19-related myocardial damage, cardiac imaging is becoming more common, and it can help to better understand the structural characteristics of COVID-19-related myocardial damage. Imaging studies can not only detect lesions, but also guide further treatment. We searched PubMed, EMBASE, and Web of Science until August 2020 for RV clinical research. "Snowball sampling" by searching reference lists and citation tracking was performed in each retrieved article. No language restrictions were applied. Following search terms were used: ("magnetic resonance imaging" OR "echocardiography" OR "myocardial injury" OR "cardiac manifestations" OR "cardiac function" OR "right ventricular damage/injury" OR "right ventricular dysfunction" OR "right ventricular dilatation") AND ("coronavirus" OR "SARS-COV-2" OR "COVID-19"). Recent findings on imaging assessment of cardiac injury in COVID-19 were summarized in **Tables 1, 2**.

MRI Findings

MRI can be used to quantitatively assess myocardial fibrosis and oedema (28, 29). This technique is currently the gold standard for evaluating cardiac morphology and function (30). MRI analysis includes conventional sequences and quantitative mapping sequences. Conventional sequences include short-axis and long-axis cine, T2-weighted imaging (T2WI), and late gadolinium-enhanced scanning (LGE). Quantitative mapping sequences include native T1/T2 mapping and post-contrast T1 mapping. T1 mapping is mainly applied to quantitatively assess diffuse fibrosis, while T2 mapping enables the quantification of edema. Post-contrast T1 mapping can better obtain extracellular volume fraction, which can be used as the most sensitive biomarker of myocardial fibrosis and is highly consistent with histopathological findings (31). Myocardial oedema is assessed on T2WI images, and LV and RV functional parameters are calculated by changes in endocardial and epicardial contours (14). A study of competitive athletes recovered from COVID-19 found that cardiac MRI (CMR) was more sensitive to identify myocarditis, helping to identify the high-risk population. CMR has a negative predictive value for exclusion of myocarditis (16). Two other studies, analyzing of patients who had already recovered from COVID-19 when undergoing MRI, showed increased T1 and T2 signals, positive LGE and/or pericardial enhancement in 58–78% of the population (14, 15). In Huang's study, 26 patients without previous cardiac diseases were all

---

Abbreviations: ARDS, acute respiratory distress syndrome; COVID-19, coronavirus disease 2019; ECMO, extracorporeal membrane oxygenation; LV, left ventricular; LVEF, left ventricular ejection fraction; LGE, late gadolinium enhancement; MRI, magnetic resonance imaging; PEEP, positive end-expiratory pressure; RV, right ventricular; RVLS, right ventricular longitudinal strain.

TABLE 1 | Studies of CMR imaging assessments in patients with COVID-19 and cardiac injury.

Study, publish date	Study type	Location	Study period	Patients	Image type	Mean age & gender	Main test items	Main findings
Huang et al., May 4, 2020 (14)	Retrospective study	Tongji Hospital, Tongji Medical College, Wuhan, China	Since March, 2020	26 hospitalized patients, recovered from COVID-19 with cardiac symptoms, no previous cardiac disease or COPD	CMR	32–45 26% male	◇ Conventional sequences (cine, T2WI, LGE) ◇ Quantitative mapping sequences (T1, T2, T1/T2, ECV mapping) ◇ Oedema ratio ◇ Cardiac function	◇ 15 (58%) T2 signal ↑ and/or positive LGE ◇ 14 (54%) myocardial oedema ◇ Global native T1, T2, ECV values ↑ in COVID-19 patients with positive cardiac MRI findings ◇ RVEF, CO, CI, SV, SV/BSA ↓ in COVID-19 patients with positive cardiac MRI findings ◇ No significant differences of LV function among controls and patients
Puntmann et al., July 27, 2020 (15)	Prospective observational cohort study	University Hospital Frankfurt COVID-19 Registry, Germany	April to June, 2020	100, recovered from COVID-19 including mostly home-based recovery and hospitalized patients, 13% prior CAD, 21% prior COPD or asthma	CMR	45–53 53% male	◇ LVEF ◇ LVEDV index ◇ LV mass index ◇ RVEF ◇ Native T1 and T2 ◇ LGE ◇ Pericardial effusion	◇ LVEF ↓ ◇ RVEF ↓ ◇ 78% abnormal CMR: 73% native T1 ↑, 60% native T2 ↑, 32% myocardial LGE, 22% pericardial LGE ◇ LV volume and mass ↑ ◇ High-sensitivity troponin T was significantly correlated with native T1, native T2 and LV mass ◇ Native T1 and T2 were the best measures to detect COVID-19-related myocardial pathology
Rajpal et al., Sep 11, 2020 (16)	Prospective study	Ohio State, USA	June 2020 to August 2020	26 competitive college athletes, recovered from COVID-19 without hospitalization, no previous cardiac disease or COPD	CMR	19.5 ± 1.5 57.7% male	◇ LGE ◇ LVEF and RVEF ◇ T1 and T2 mapping ◇ LVEDV and RVEDV	◇ 4 athletes had CMR findings consistent with myocarditis ◇ 12 (46%) had LGE, of whom 8 (30.8%) had LGE without concomitant T2 elevation ◇ Mean (SD) T2 in those with suspected myocarditis was 59 ms compared with 51 ms in those without myocarditis. ◇ CMR may provide an excellent riskstratification assessment for myocarditis in athletes who have recovered from COVID-19.

BSA, body surface area; CI, cardiac index; CMR, cardiovascular magnetic resonance; CO, cardiac output; COVID-19, coronavirus disease 2019; ECV, extracellular volume; LV, left ventricular; LVEDV, left ventricular end-diastolic volume; LVEF, left ventricular ejection fraction; LGE, late gadolinium enhancement; RVEF, right ventricular ejection fraction; SV, stroke volume; T2WI, T2-weighted imaging.

TABLE 2 | Studies of echocardiography assessments in patients with COVID-19 and cardiac injury.

Study, publish date	Study type	Location	Study period	Patients	Image type	Mean age & gender	Main test items	Main findings
Argulian et al., May 7, 2020 (17)	Retrospective study	Mount Sinai Morningside Hospital, New York, USA	March 26, 2020 to April 22, 2020	105 hospitalized patients, 31 of whom were intubated and mechanically ventilated during examination	TTE	66 ± 14.6 64% male	◇ RV and LV sizes and function	◇ 32 (31%) RV dilatation ◇ Renal dysfunction is more common in patients with RVD than those without ◇ No differences in LV size and function ◇ 21 (20%) patients died: 13 (41%) deaths were observed in patients with RV dilatation and 8 (11%) in patients without RV dilatation ◇ RV enlargement was significantly associated with mortality
Li et al., April 24, 2020 (7)	Retrospective study	The west branch of Union Hospital, Tongji Medical College, Wuhan, China	February 12, 2020 to March 15, 2020	120 hospitalized patients (Survivors 102 and non-survivors 18), 9.2% prior CVD, 5% prior COPD	TTE, examed in 3–10 days	61 ± 14 58% male	◇ RVFAC ◇ TAPSE ◇ Tricuspid tissue Doppler annular velocities (S') ◇ RVLS ◇ LV volume and function	◇ Male, ARDS, RVLS, RVFAC and TAPSE were significant univariate predictors of higher risk for mortality ◇ RVLS was found to predict higher mortality more accurately ◇ The best cut-off value of RVLS for prediction of outcome was −23%
Szekely et al., May 29, 2020 (5)	Prospective study	Tel Aviv Medical Center, Israel	March 21, 2020 to April 16, 2020	100 hospitalized patients, 16% prior IHD	TTE, examed within 24 h	66.1 ± 17.3 63% male	◇ LV systolic and diastolic function ◇ Valve hemodynamics ◇ RV assessment (TAPSE, RV-S', RVFAC, Tei index, pulmonary acceleration time) ◇ Lung ultrasound	◇ 32% normal echocardiography ◇ 39% RV dilatation with or without dysfunction ◇ 16% LV diastolic dysfunction ◇ 10% LV systolic dysfunction ◇ Patients with elevated troponin (20%) or worse clinical condition had worse RV function
Mahmoud-Elsayed et al., May 24, 2020 (6)	Retrospective study	Queen Elizabeth Hospital Birmingham, United Kingdom	March 22, 2020 to April 17, 2020	74 hospitalized patients, referred for TTE with ≥ 1 clinical indication(s), 9% prior CAD	TTE, examed in 3–10 days	59 ± 13 78% male	◇ Chamber sizes and function ◇ Valvular disease ◇ Pulmonary hypertension	◇ 41% RV dilatation ◇ 27% RVD ◇ 89% LV function was hyper-dynamic or normal ◇ RV impairment was associated with increased D-dimer and CRP levels
Jain et al., June 9, 2020 (18)	Retrospective study	Columbia University Irving Medical Center and New York-Presbyterian Allen Hospital, New York, USA	March 1, 2020 to April 3, 2020	72 hospitalized patients, referred for TTE when having clinical indications, 18.1% prior CAD	TTE, median time was 3 days	50.8–70.3 72.2% male	◇ LV Function ◇ Segmental LV Wall Motion ◇ RV size and systolic function	◇ 34.7% LVEF ≤ 50% ◇ 40.3% RV systolic function ↓ ◇ RV systolic dysfunction was more common than LV systolic dysfunction ◇ patients with elevated hs-cTnT and elevated NT-proBNP were more likely to exhibit reduced LV function
Dweck et al., June 2, 2020 (19)	Prospective international survey	69 countries	April 3 to 20, 2020	1,216, of whom 813 had confirmed COVID-19, and 298 had a high probability when scanning, 26% prior cardiac disease	TTE	52–71 70% male	◇ Ventricular sizes and function	◇ 55% abnormal echocardiogram ◇ 39% LV abnormalities ◇ 33% RV abnormalities ◇ 3% new myocardial infarction ◇ 3% myocarditis ◇ 2% takotsubo cardiomyopathy 15% severe cardiac disease (severe ventricular dysfunction or tamponade)
Rath et al., May 28, 2020 (20)	Prospective study	University Hospital of Tübingen, Germany	February to March, 2020	123 hospitalized patients (Non-survivors 16 and survivors 107), 22.8% prior CAD	TTE, examed in 24h	68 ± 15 70% male	◇ LVEF ◇ RV function (TAPSE, RV-FAC) ◇ Aortic stenosis/regurgitation ◇ Mitral regurgitation ◇ Tricuspid regurgitation	◇ Mean LV function 57% ◇ 48.9% RV dilatation ◇ 30.6% tricuspid regurgitation > 1 ◇ RV-FAC ↓ in non-survivors ◇ Visually estimated impaired RV function ↑ in non-survivors ◇ Impaired LV and RV function, and tricuspid regurgitation > grade 1 were significantly associated with higher mortality

(Continued)

TABLE 2 | Continued

Reference	Study design	Location	Dates	Population	Imaging	Age / Sex	Parameters	Findings
Pagnesi et al., July 1, 2020 (21)	Single-center, observational, cross-sectional study	San Raffaele Scientific Institute in Milan, Italy	March 24, 2020 to April 29, 2020	200 non-ICU inpatients, 7.5% prior CAD, 8.5% prior MI	TTE	55–74 65.5 male	◇ RVEDD ◇ RV length ◇ TAPSE ◇ S'TDI ◇ SPAP	◇ 12% PH, 14.5% RVD ◇ PH (and not RVD) was associated with signs of more severe COVID-19 and with worse in-hospital clinical outcome
D' Andrea et al., June 17, 2020 (22)	Prospective study	4 centers in Italy: "Umberto I Hospital, Monaldi Hospital, M. Scarlato COVID Hospital, Cardarelli Hospital	February 20, 2020 to April 20, 2020	115, 26 of whom suffering cardiac injury	TTE	20–88 60% male	◇ Tricuspid regurgitation ◇ RV tract diameter ◇ Tricuspid Peak E/A ratio ◇ TRV ◇ PASP ◇ MPAP ◇ TAPSE	◇ RV function and pulmonary pressures as independent predictors of COVID pneumonia mortality ◇ Patients with PH and RVD had more frequently a history of prior cardiac comorbidities ◇ Only patients with PH showed signs of more severe SARS- CoV-2 infection
Vasudev et al., July 26, 2020 (23)	Retrospective study	Three hospitals in Northern New Jersey, USA	March 15, 2020 to April 15, 2020	45 hospitalized patients, 20% prior ACS	TTE, during hospitalization	61.4 ± 12.2 51% male	◇ Ventricular size and function ◇ SPAP ◇ Pressure and volume overload	◇ 31.1% LVEF ↓ ◇ 11.1% RVEF ↓ ◇ 13.3% RV dilatation ◇ 22.2% PH ◇ Echocardiography is essential for assessment of COVID-19
Baycan et al., August 8, 2020 (24)	Prospective, single-center study	Goztepe Training and Research Hospital, Istanbul, Turkey	April 15, 2020 to April 30, 2020	100 hospitalized patients, all of whom having normal LVEF (≥50%)	TTE, examined on the first day	55.6 ± 14.4 50% male	◇ LV-GLS ◇ RV-FAC ◇ RV-LS ◇ TAPSE ◇ SPAP	◇ LV-GLS and RV-LS were lower in the severe group compared to the non-severe group ◇ LV-GLS and RV-LS are independent predictors of in-hospital mortality in patients with COVID-19 ◇ RVD is important in determining circulation and respiratory management strategies
Krishnamoorthy et al., August 4, 2020 (25)	Single-center study	The Zena & Michael A Wiener Cardiovascular Institute, New York, USA	–	12, 5 of whom required intubation and/or died, 16.7% prior CAD	TTE	29–60 41.7% male	◇ LVGLS ◇ RVGS ◇ RVFWS ◇ RVSP	◇ 41.7% RVD ◇ 58.3% LVD ◇ RVGS and RVFWS were significantly decreased in the patients who had poor outcomes compared with those who did not ◇ LVGLS was decreased regardless of outcome
Van den Heuvel et al., July 8, 2020 (26)	Single center, cross-sectional study	Radboud University Medical Center, Nijmegen, The Netherlands	April 1, 2020 to May 12, 2020	51 hospitalized patients (ICU 19 and non-ICU 32), 22% prior Cardiac history	TTE	51–68 80% male	◇ LV and RV dimensions ◇ LV function (LVEF, GLS) ◇ RV function (TAPSE, RV S') ◇ Atrial dimensions	◇ 27% LVD ◇ 10% RVD ◇ No relation between elevated Troponin T or NT-proBNP and ventricular dysfunction ◇ Ventricular dysfunction by means of L VEF, GLS, TAPSE and RV S' were not significantly different between ICU and non-ICU patients
Zeng et al., July 28, 2020 (27)	Single-center retrospective study	Shenzhen Third People's Hospital, China	January 11, 2020 to April 1, 2020	416 (ICU 35 and non-ICU 381), 3% prior CAD	TTE, only for severe patients (ICU 31 and non-ICU 26)	33–68 47.6% male	◇ LV and RV sizes ◇ LV and RV function ◇ PASP ◇ Ventricular wall thickness	◇ Ventricular wall thickening ◇ LVEF ↓ in 5 (16%) ICU patients ◇ PASP ↑ in 9 (29%) ICU patients ◇ RV dilatation and RVD in 3 (10%) ICU patients

ARDS, acute respiratory distress syndrome; CAD, coronary atherosclerotic heart disease; COVID-19, coronavirus disease 2019; CVD, cardiovascular disease; ICU, intensive care unit; IHD, ischemic heart disease; LV, left ventricular; LVD, left ventricular dysfunction; LVEF, left ventricular ejection fraction; LVGLS, left ventricular global longitudinal strain; MPAP, mean pulmonary artery pressure; PASP, pulmonary artery systolic pressure; PH, pulmonary hypertension; RV, right ventricular; RVD, right ventricular dysfunction; RVEDD, right ventricular end-diastolic diameter; RVEF, right ventricular ejection fraction; RVFAC, right ventricular fractional area change; RVFWS, right ventricular free wall strain; RVGS, right ventricular global strain; RVLS, right ventricular longitudinal strain; RV S', right ventricular systolic excursion velocity; RVSP, right ventricular systolic pressure; SPAP, systolic pulmonary artery pressure; S' TDI, tissue Doppler imaging S wave; TAPSE, tricuspid annular plane systolic excursion; TRV, tricuspid regurgitation velocity; TTE, transthoracic echocardiography.

recovered and isolated for 14 days, and myocardial edema was found in 54% of patients (14). In Puntmann's study, mostly non-hospitalized patients recovered from COVID-19, 60% of them found myocardial inflammation (16). While COVID-19 patients had cardiac injury, regardless of preexisting disease, severity and overall course of COVID-19 manifestations, time since initial diagnosis, or presence of cardiac symptoms (16). Decreased RV functional parameters, including the RV ejection fraction, cardiac output, the cardiac index, and stroke volume, were found in patients with positive cardiac MRI findings compared with healthy controls ($P < 0.05$). These findings suggest that sustained cardiac involvement, including oedema, fibrosis, and impaired RV contractile function, may remain in patients who recover from COVID-19. Similarly, Puntmann et al. showed that the RV ejection fraction was decreased in patients with COVID-19 compared with healthy controls (15). They also found a reduction in the LV ejection fraction in the recovered COVID-19 cohort. However, Huang et al. showed that LV function was hyperdynamic or normal in the same subgroup (14). The outcomes were inconsistent between these two studies. Regardless of the discrepancy, Puntmann et al. considered that native T1 and T2 were the best indicators with the ability to detect COVID-19-related myocardial pathology (15). Further investigation on the long-term cardiovascular consequences of COVID-19 is required (16).

Echocardiographic Findings

Echocardiography is commonly used for assessing cardiac damage. This technique is easier to perform than cardiac MRI. Conventional echocardiographic evaluation includes cardiac structural assessment, myocardial systolic and diastolic function, and valvular hemodynamics. According to the American Society of Echocardiography, RV dysfunction is present when the following parameters used to quantify RV function are less than low values in the normal range: pulsed Doppler systolic myocardial velocity < 9.5 cm/s, tricuspid annular plane systolic excursion < 17 mm, RV ejection fraction < 45%, and RV fractional area change < 35% (32, 33). RV dilatation is usually observed early in the pressure-overloaded right ventricle. Typically, in the RV-focused view, a basal diameter > 41 mm and an intermediate horizontal diameter > 35 mm indicate RV dilatation (32).

Most inpatients with COVID-19 have RV dilatation or dysfunction. However, LV dysfunction is less common. In a study of 74 patients with COVID-19, 27% presented with RV dysfunction, but LV function was hyperdynamic or normal in 89% (6). Szekely et al. (5) showed that RV dysfunction was more common in patients with elevated troponin levels and a poor clinical grade, whereas the total number of patients with an impaired LV function was relatively smaller. Notably, in several other studies, LV dysfunction was not rare in patients with COVID-19 (18, 23, 25). This discrepancy among studies may be due to differences in the study populations, but RV damage is still universally found by echocardiography in patients with COVID-19. We summarized the results of recent cardiac imaging studies (**Table 2**). Among patients with COVID-19-related myocardial injury, the proportion of RV

dilatation ranged from 13.3 to 48.9% (5, 6, 17, 20, 23). RV dilatation associated with elevated D-dimer levels and C-reactive protein levels was more common in patients with COVID-19 (6, 17, 18, 20). There was no significant difference in the incidence of major comorbidities (hypertension, diabetes and known coronary artery disease), laboratory markers of inflammation (white blood cell count, C-reactive protein) or myocardial injury (troponin) in patients with right ventricular dilatation (17).

Conventional echocardiographic parameters are not sensitive to early RV systolic dysfunction, and therefore, cannot be used for early diagnosis (34). Two-dimensional speckle tracking echocardiography can more accurately evaluate myocardial function and detect subclinical cardiac functional impairment earlier than conventional echocardiography (35, 36), which can measure LV global longitudinal strain (LVGLS), RV longitudinal strain (RVLS), RV free wall strain (RVFWS), and RV global strain (RVGS). In a retrospective study, RVLS was found to predict mortality in patients with COVID-19 more accurately. Therefore, there is potential value of RVLS for risk stratification in COVID-19. The optimal cut-off values for prediction of outcome were calculated to be −23% for RVLS, 43.5% for RV fractional area change, and 23 mm for tricuspid annular systolic displacement (7). Baycan et al. (24) and Krishnamoorthy et al. (25) also evaluated the prognostic value of strain indices. RVGS and RVFWS were significantly reduced in patients with poor clinical outcomes. RVLS is an independent predictor of in-hospital mortality in patients with COVID, while the predictive value of LVGLS for mortality varies in different studies. However, speckle-tracking echocardiography is demanding on image quality. The structure of the chest wall in different patients has a large effect on imaging, and critically ill patients are unable to cooperate in adjusting positions, both of which affect the results.

RV Dysfunction and Prognosis in COVID-19

Cardiac imaging findings have shown that RV damage is common in patients with COVID-19. Concomitant RV damage usually indicates a poor prognosis and affects the clinical outcome of patients. In a study of 120 COVID-19 cases, non-survivors showed elevated pulmonary artery systolic pressure, dilated right heart chambers, and diminished RV function compared with survivors (7). In another study where 28 patients died of COVID-19, 14 had a RV abnormality, but only 2 had LV impairment (6). Indeed, these outcomes all indicate a strong relation between RV dysfunction and poor prognosis. One multivariate analysis revealed that RV enlargement was the only factor significantly associated with mortality (17). Patients with COVID-19 and RV dysfunction often have more severe symptoms (19). Argulian et al. found that renal dysfunction was more common in patients with RV dilatation than those without (17). Therefore, RV dysfunction often predicts the presence of some severe complications, and they may partly account for the high mortality in this population. Additionally, Pagnesi et al. (21) showed that pulmonary hypertension, instead of RV dysfunction, was associated with worse in-hospital clinical outcomes in patients with COVID-19. However, because their study population was non-intensive care unit patients without mechanical ventilation, this may have eliminated the association between COVID-19 and RV involvement.

Although CMR imaging is the gold standard for assessing RV function (30), the high infectivity of COVID-19 and the inability of patients to hold their breath for a long time limit its application. Patients without pre-existing cardiovascular diseases are more likely to have normal echocardiography than those with pre-existing cardiovascular diseases (21). RV dysfunction is more common than LV dysfunction in COVID-19 (23). Patients with RV dysfunction had a higher rate of cardiac comorbidities compared with patients without RV dysfunction (37). The main reasons for performing echocardiography in the previous study were suspected heart failure and elevated cardiac biomarker concentrations (5, 21, 23). Independent predictors of RV abnormalities are suspected RV failure and moderate or severe COVID-19 symptoms (21). To minimize the risk of the spread of infection, at least echocardiography should be performed in patients with suspected heart failure, more cardiac comorbidities, elevated cardiac biomarkers, and severe COVID-19 symptoms. Abnormal transthoracic echocardiography ultimately affects decision-making of clinicians in 16–33.3% of patients (18, 19). It also showed that clinical management was altered in 24.2% of patients because of acute cardiovascular events observed with transthoracic echocardiography (18).

Male was an independent predictor of prognosis (7), while age, weight, and ethnicity were not significantly different in COVID-19 patients with cardiac injury. Patients with a history of established cardiovascular disease or elevated cardiac biomarkers have an increased susceptibility to infection and an increased risk of severe disease progression and death (4, 37, 38). These patients are more likely to have RV dysfunction and pulmonary hypertension, which are independent risk factors for poor prognosis (21, 22). The proportions of echocardiographic abnormalities and serious heart disease are similar after excluding patients with pre-existing heart disease (heart failure, valvular disease, or ischemic heart disease), suggesting that cardiac abnormalities are associated with COVID-19 infection in this population (19).

AETIOLOGY OF COVID-19 WITH RV FUNCTIONAL CHANGES MAY INVOLVE MULTIPLE FACETS

The Right Ventricle Is More Susceptible to Lung Injury Than the Left Ventricle

The transverse section of the right ventricle is crescent-shaped compared with the thick wall of the left ventricle, and the relative surface area of the right ventricle is higher and the volume is lower. The thin RV free wall has greater compliance than the left ventricle. These anatomical features allow acute dilatation of the right ventricle when there is a sharp increase in afterload. RV systolic function is sensitive to increased pressure, and a slight rise in pulmonary circulation resistance causes RV overload and impaired systolic function. The primary

target organ of severe acute respiratory syndrome coronavirus-2 is the lungs. The right ventricle is vulnerable to a slight increase in pulmonary vascular resistance (39), making it more vulnerable to injury than the left ventricle. As the right ventricle continues to expand, RV geometry changes, and the tricuspid annulus dilates insufficiently, resulting in tricuspid regurgitation. Tricuspid regurgitation leads to further RV dilatation and volume overload, which shifts the interventricular septum to the left and affects LV filling and contraction. RV pressure overload increases wall tension, increases myocardial oxygen consumption, and decreases RV oxygen supply during systole. This further leads to myocardial ischaemia and reduces RV contractility. RV dilatation may precede development of acute cor pulmonale (40).

Acute Respiratory Distress Syndrome and RV Dysfunction

COVID-19 mainly affects the respiratory system and the incidence of acute respiratory distress syndrome (ARDS) reported in COVID-19 ranges from 19.6 to 31% (37, 38, 41). ARDS is a severe form of COVID-19, which leads to a dramatic increase in RV afterload and delayed contraction owing to its own pathological effects and mechanical ventilation with a high positive end-expiratory pressure (PEEP). This then reverses the end-systolic transseptal pressure gradient. The incidence of RV dysfunction in ARDS has been reported to be 22–50% (33). There is no robust evidence to verify a definitive causal relationship between RV dysfunction and mortality in ARDS. However, RV dysfunction is undoubtedly associated with increased mortality and poorer prognosis in patients with COVID-19-related ARDS (42). In the setting of ARDS, numerous factors can destroy the pulmonary circulation, including mechanical compression by interstitial oedema, microvascular thrombosis, hypoxic or mediator-induced pulmonary vasoconstriction, and pulmonary vascular muscular remodeling. These factors raise pulmonary arterial pressure and further rapidly increase RV afterload. Pulmonary vascular resistance abates RV ejection and LV pulmonary venous return, while RV dilatation results in LV compression by a septal shift because of an inextensible pericardium. Both of these mechanisms account for the decrease in LV ejection and RV coronary blood flow. Therefore, ARDS-derived pulmonary circulation injury in COVID-19 has a deleterious effect on RV dysfunction (43, 44).

RV dilatation secondary to mechanical ventilation during hospitalization for ARDS requires attention. In the ARDS population, a lung protective ventilation strategy is recommended and mainly refers to PEEP. High PEEP levels cause overinflation of the normal alveoli and compression of intra-alveolar vessels, which lead to high pulmonary vascular resistance and increased RV afterload (43). Therefore, RV dysfunction can be a haemodynamically significant and deleterious consequence of COVID-19-related mechanical ventilation. Notably, Sud et al. showed that there was no meaningful correlation between PEEP and RV dilation on echocardiography in their COVID-19 infection cohort (17). However, they did not deny the possible contribution on RV dilatation from mechanical ventilation.

Pulmonary Embolism and RV Dysfunction

Owing to risk factors, such as virus-induced endothelial injury, vascular inflammation, and hospitalization-related prolonged immobilization, most patients with COVID-19 stay in a hypercoagulable state, and they are vulnerable to venous thrombosis. Poissy et al. studied 107 patients with COVID-19 who were admitted to the intensive care unit (45). They reported a high incidence of pulmonary embolism (20.4%), which was significantly higher than the contemporaneous average level in patients with influenza and in in-hospital patients. An autopsy of patients with COVID-19 showed a high incidence of deep venous thrombosis (58%) and death-causing pulmonary embolism (33%) (46). When thrombus enters pulmonary vessels, it produces mechanical obstruction and stimulates endothelial cells and platelets to release vasoactive mediators (e.g., thromboxane A2, serotonin). This triggers obstruction-related vasoconstriction and increases RV afterload and pulmonary arterial pressure in patients. Oxygen demand from the right ventricle increases, while embolism-associated hypoxemia and hypotension decrease myocardial oxygen supply. This imbalance finally leads to RV dysfunction (47).

Myocardial Injury and a Cytokine Storm

Myocardial injury was recognized early in patients with COVID-19 in China, and it also partly accounts for RV dysfunction. Myocarditis can occur before pulmonary symptoms of shock (48). The possible mechanisms for myocardial injury are as follows. Angiotensin-converting enzyme 2 (ACE2) is highly expressed not only in the lungs, but also in the cardiovascular system, thus possibly mediating viral entry into cardiomyocytes to cause direct damage. Cardiac elevation of troponin-I levels is accompanied by an increase in other inflammatory markers, such as lactate dehydrogenase, ferritin, tumor necrosis factor-α (TNF-α), interleukin-6 (IL-6) and interleukin-8 (IL-8). This could represent a cytokine storm syndrome or secondary haemophagocytic lymphohistiocytosis, which may result in cardiac involvement (49). After viral invasion into the body, T cells become activated, and they produce and release amounts of antiviral cytokines. Because of an imbalanced response among subtypes of T helper cells, a cytokine storm release is induced, which attributes to hyperactivation of monocytes/macrophages. This then leads to tissue damage to multiple organs and causes complications, such as ARDS and cardiac insufficiency.

In ARDS, increased levels of cytokines, such as IL-6, IL-8, TNF-α, can be tested. In particular, IL-6 is an important marker. A previous study reported that elevated circulating IL-6 levels were associated with increased mortality in COVID-19 (50). Targeted therapy against the IL-6 receptor with tocilizumab can be effective in severe COVID-19 cases. A cytokine storm is essentially a protective response to limit spread of the virus, but its exact mechanism of myocardial injury remains unclear. However, cardiomyocyte and endothelial cell death triggered by inflammatory cytokines, such as TNF-α, has been well-documented (51). Ventricular dilatation with a reduction in the ejection fraction may be an adaptive response to myocardial dysfunction. Myocardial depression results from the direct or indirect action of one or more cardioinhibitory substances.

Besides, TNF-α and IL-1, which act as potent inducible nitric oxide synthase inducers, are associated with inhibition of cardiomyocyte function. For one thing, nitric oxide interferes with calcium metabolism in cardiomyocytes, which in turn impairs contractile function. For another, peroxynitrite generated by interaction of nitric oxide with superoxide ions is directly toxic to cardiomyocytes (52). Additionally, Hypoxemia caused by COVID-19 can also induce intracellular calcium overload, leading to apoptosis of cardiomyocytes (53). So, an inflammatory storm, as well as autoimmune activation, can induce extensive vascular and myocardial inflammation, while predisposing to diffuse thrombosis (54).

In summary, the mechanism of myocardial injury varies at different stages of COVID-19. Isolated RV dysfunction can be found in the presence of severe ARDS or pulmonary embolism (55), while diffuse myocardial damage caused by viral toxicity and the host immune response also partly weaken RV function (**Figure 1**). Because of ACE2 expression in the endothelium, virus-induced endothelial shedding and microvascular damage may lead to thrombosis and myocardial infarction (55). ACE2-mediated direct injury may be a major mechanism in the early stages of COVID-19. With aggravation of COVID-19, pulmonary and cardiac injury caused by hypoxia is gradually aggravated. Inflammatory reactions and autoimmune damage leading to exacerbation of disease play a major role in the later stages of COVID-19.

TREATMENT OF RV DYSFUNCTION WITH COVID-19

Medical Treatment

Medical treatment of RV functional impairment includes reducing volume load, enhancing RV contractility, and reducing pulmonary arterial pressure. Diuretics can reduce intravascular volume. The RV Starling curve is flat, and improvement in RV function can only be observed with a large negative fluid balance. Normally, the RV filling pressure needs to be maintained at a slightly increased level at ∼8–12 mmHg. The volume status can be further adjusted on this basis to achieve optimal RV function and cardiac output (56). RV pressure monitoring is also important when circulating hypovolemia results in decreased blood pressure and the requirement for appropriate fluid replacement. Central venous pressure and mixed venous oxygen saturation help determine RV filling and oxygen supply. Echocardiography also helps determine the volume status. RV dilatation with restriction of LV filling indicate excessive preload.

Levosimendan is a novel calcium sensitizer that stabilizes the spatial configuration of myocardial fibrin and increases myocardial contractility. This calcium sensitizer has the advantages of no effect on diastolic function or arrhythmia, and does not increase myocardial oxygen consumption. Levosimendan improves RV myocardial contractility and reduces RV afterload. Morelli et al. showed that levosimendan was an effective treatment option for ARDS with acute right heart dilatation, and it was believed to dilate the pulmonary circulation and improve RV contractility (57).

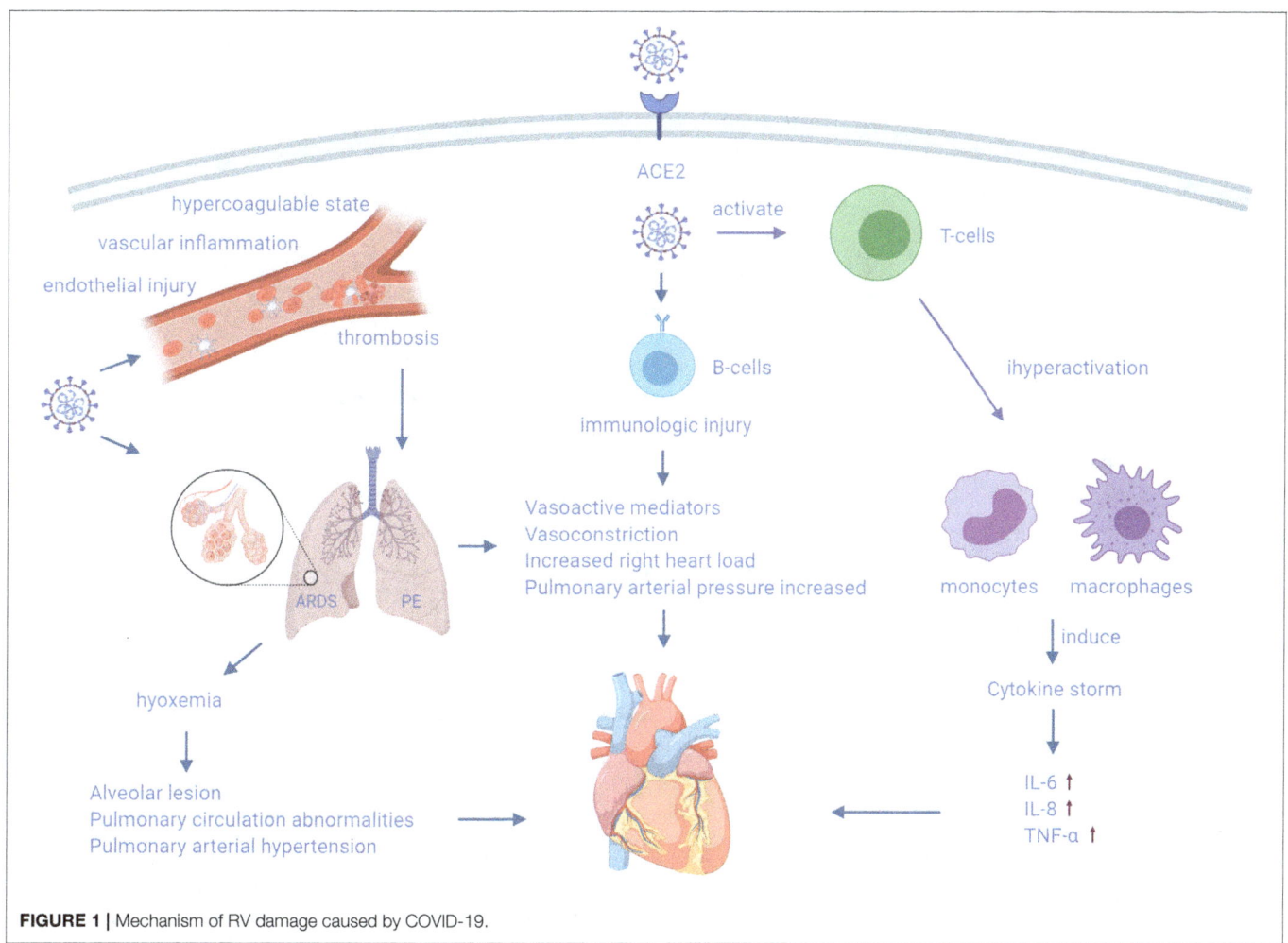

FIGURE 1 | Mechanism of RV damage caused by COVID-19.

Norepinephrine might improve RV function by restoring RV perfusion pressure as suggested in an experimental model of massive pulmonary embolism (58). Intravenous epoprostenol can improve symptoms, hemodynamics, and the survival rate, and enhance RV systolic function (59). Bosentan is a specific endothelin receptor antagonist, which reduces mean pulmonary arterial pressure and increases the cardiac index. Inhaled nitric oxide can selectively dilate pulmonary vessels, improve the ventilation-blood flow ratio, significantly reduce pulmonary vascular resistance, and increase cardiac output, while it has a slight effect on systemic vascular resistance. In patients with pulmonary heart disease caused by ARDS, inhaled nitric oxide reduces pulmonary arterial pressure and pulmonary inflammatory responses (60). In patients with pulmonary embolism and ARDS, prostacyclin is as effective as inhaled nitric oxide in reducing pulmonary arterial pressure, improving gas exchange and oxygenation, increasing cardiac output, and improving RV function (61, 62).

To alleviate inflammation and fibrosis, corticosteroids are considered as potential therapeutic agents for ARDS, which reduce morbidity and mortality, but remain controversial.

High-dose corticosteroid therapy can accelerate improvement of ARDS, reduce mortality, and shorten the duration of invasive mechanical ventilation (63). However, the World Health Organization recommends that systemic corticosteroids should not be routinely used in patients with COVID-19 or COVID-19-associated ARDS (64).

Severe COVID-19 is often associated with thrombosis, and disseminated intravascular coagulation may be present in the majority of fatal cases (65). Prolonged immobilization and hormonal therapy increases the risk of venous thromboembolism. Patients with right heart enlargement are also prone to cardiac thrombosis. Coagulopathy due to COVID-19 may be associated with bacterially-induced infectious coagulopathy. Overproduction of inflammatory cytokines, vascular endothelial injury, and increased levels of damage-associated molecular patterns contribute to thrombosis. Patients who meet the sepsis-induced coagulopathy score criteria or have significantly elevated D-dimer levels may benefit from anticoagulant therapy by mainly using low-molecular-weight heparin (66). Among 449 patients with severe COVID-19, 99 received heparin (mainly low-molecular-weight heparin)

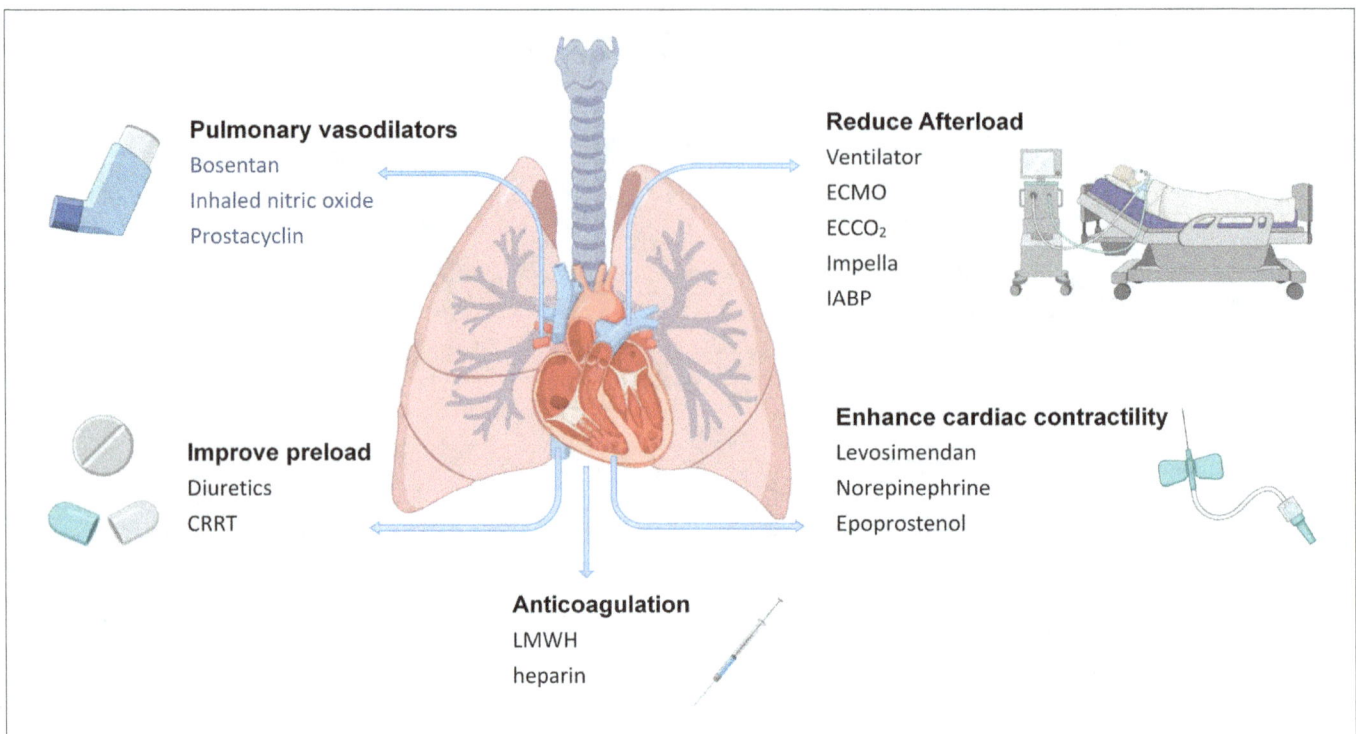

Pulmonary vasodilators
Bosentan
Inhaled nitric oxide
Prostacyclin

Reduce Afterload
Ventilator
ECMO
ECCO$_2$
Impella
IABP

Improve preload
Diuretics
CRRT

Enhance cardiac contractility
Levosimendan
Norepinephrine
Epoprostenol

Anticoagulation
LMWH
heparin

FIGURE 2 | Treatment of RV dysfunction with COVID-19. ECCO$_2$, extracorporeal carbon dioxide removal devices; IABP, intra-aortic balloon pump; LMWH, low molecular weight heparin.

for 7 days or longer, and 28-day mortality was significantly lower in patients with sepsis-induced coagulopathy scores ≥ 4 or D-dimer levels > six times the upper limit of normal using heparin than in non-users (P = 0.029, P = 0.017). Lin et al. (67) also recommended the use of low-molecular-weight heparin in patients with D-dimer values > four times the upper limit of normal. Thrombotic coagulopathy is common in severe patients with COVID-19, and D-dimer is more useful than other coagulation markers for prediction of this disease. However, bleeding complications are relatively uncommon in COVID-19. Therefore, anticoagulant therapy is necessary.

Device-Assisted Therapy

Mechanical ventilation, sedation, and analgesia may lead to increased afterload, increased transpulmonary pressure, and decreased cardiac output. Therefore, mechanical ventilation indications need to be strictly followed. For critically ill patients requiring mechanical ventilation, appropriate mechanical ventilation measures should be implemented to avoid hypoxemia, hypercapnia, a low or high lung volume, and high PEEP. Protective ventilation strategies should also be used when necessary. The principle of mechanical ventilation in patients with right heart failure is to limit plateau pressure and offer PEEP, avoiding hypercapnia, hypoxemia, and pulmonary vasoconstriction. Respiratory settings are adjusted according to the tolerance of the right ventricle, as assessed by ultrasound, to coordinate the balance between recruitment

and hyperventilation resulting from ventilation according to RV function (68). PEEP can dilate the alveoli, compress extra-alveolar capillaries, and cause an increase in pulmonary vascular resistance. This increases afterload and RV volume, resulting in RV dilatation, which in turn affects LV filling. Appropriate PEEP is important for treatment.

When optimized ventilation measures still do not improve hypoxemia in mechanically ventilated patients, extracorporeal membrane oxygenation (ECMO) can be considered. ECMO is used as a rescue therapy for COVID-19 with refractory hypoxemia in accordance with provisional guidelines established by the World Health Organization (69) in 2020. However, because of a lack of relevant trials on the use of ECMO in patients with COVID-19, there is insufficient evidence that these patients can benefit from ECMO. For acute RV failure caused by severe ARDS, extracorporeal carbon dioxide removal devices can be considered for super-protective lung ventilation (tidal volume: 4 mL/kg) (70). Additionally, increased work of breathing, pulmonary oedema, and endogenous PEEP caused by weaning increase RV afterload. Worsening of RV function is an important cause of weaning failure in mechanically ventilated patients. When RV function is impaired in combination with severely impaired LV function, adjunctive therapy with Impella device or intra-aortic balloon counterpulsation can be used. Continuous renal replacement therapy may be considered when volume overload and drug therapy are not effective. COVID-19-related myocardial injury treatments are summarized in **Figure 2**.

FUTURE DIRECTIONS AND CONCLUSIONS

RV dysfunction usually indicates a poor prognosis in the wide array of cardiopulmonary diseases. Assessment of RV function is essential for managing ARDS, acute pulmonary embolism, and pulmonary hypertension. RV dilatation is common in patients with COVID-19. A full understanding of COVID-19-related RV dysfunction is conducive for early identification and precise treatment, and to help improve the prognosis of severe cases and reduce mortality. Early recognition of RV dysfunction allows appropriate treatment to be provided as soon as possible. How to identify RV dysfunction early is important for stratification of disease risk and prognostic evaluation. Echocardiography, cardiac MRI, right heart catheterization, and other examinations are helpful for early identification of RV dysfunction. At the same time, monitoring of biological indicators related to RV function, such as troponins and brain natriuretic peptide, should not be ignored for the suggestive role in RV function. It is recommended to assess RV function as soon as possible, for COVID-19 patients with suspected cardiac injury, elevated cardiac biomarkers, severe respiratory symptoms. RV function is often monitored to optimize haemodynamic and respiratory parameter settings.

Timely medical treatment should be delivered. And device assistance should be implemented if necessary. RV damage reflects an association between myocardial injury and COVID-19. In future medical care, clinicians need to further focus on the morbidity of RV dysfunction in patients with COVID-19. Using cardiac imaging to detect RV dysfunction will provide early information concerning the severity of COVID-19 infection. Performing an appropriate strategy of the right ventricle will be helpful to reduce mortality and improve prognosis in this persistent epidemic.

AUTHOR CONTRIBUTIONS

WL contributed conception and constructing the overall structure and contents. YL wrote the draft and sections of the manuscript. All authors contributed to manuscript revision, read, and approved the submitted version.

ACKNOWLEDGMENTS

We thank Ellen Knapp, PhD, from Liwen Bianji, Edanz Group China (www.liwenbianji.cn/ac), for editing the English text of a draft of this manuscript.

REFERENCES

1. Medicine JHUa. *COVID-19 Dashboard by the Center for Systems Science and Engineering (CSSE) at Johns Hopkins.* (2020). Available online at: https://coronavirus.jhu.edu/map.html (accessed December 6, 2020).

2. Chen C, Chen C, Yan JT, Zhou N, Zhao JP, Wang DW. Analysis of myocardial injury in patients with COVID-19 and association between concomitant cardiovascular diseases and severity of COVID-19. *Zhonghua Xin Xue Guan Bing Za Zhi.* (2020) 48:567–71. doi: 10.3760/cma.j.cn112148-20200225-00123

3. Guo T, Fan Y, Chen M, Wu X, Zhang L, He T, et al. Cardiovascular implications of fatal outcomes of patients with coronavirus disease 2019 (COVID-19). *JAMA Cardiol.* (2020) 5:811–8. doi: 10.1001/jamacardio.2020.1017

4. Shi S, Qin M, Shen B, Cai Y, Liu T, Yang F, et al. Association of cardiac injury with mortality in hospitalized patients with COVID-19 in Wuhan, China. *JAMA Cardiol.* (2020) 5:802–10. doi: 10.1001/jamacardio.2020.0950

5. Szekely Y, Lichter Y, Taieb P, Banai A, Hochstadt A, Merdler I, et al. Spectrum of cardiac manifestations in COVID-19: a systematic echocardiographic study. *Circulation.* (2020) 142:342–53. doi: 10.1161/CIRCULATIONAHA.120.047971

6. Mahmoud-Elsayed HM, Moody WE, Bradlow WM, Khan-Kheil AM, Senior J, Hudsmith LE, et al. Echocardiographic findings in patients with COVID-19 pneumonia. *Can J Cardiol.* (2020) 36:1203–7. doi: 10.1016/j.cjca.2020.05.030

7. Li Y, Li H, Zhu S, Xie Y, Wang B, He L, et al. Prognostic value of right ventricular longitudinal strain in patients with COVID-19. *JACC: Cardiovasc Imaging.* (2020) 13:2287–99. doi: 10.1016/j.jcmg.2020.04.014

8. Matsuura H, Ichida F, Saji T, Ogawa S, Waki K, Kaneko M, et al. Clinical features of acute and fulminant myocarditis in children-2nd nationwide survey by japanese society of pediatric cardiology and cardiac surgery. *Circ J.* (2016) 80:2362–8. doi: 10.1253/circj.CJ-16-0234

9. Ito T, Akamatsu K, Ukimura A, Fujisaka T, Ozeki M, Kanzaki Y, et al. The Prevalence and findings of subclinical influenza-associated cardiac abnormalities among Japanese patients. *Intern Med.* (2018) 57:1819–26. doi: 10.2169/internalmedicine.0316-17

10. Bavishi C, Bonow RO, Trivedi V, Abbott JD, Messerli FH, Bhatt DL. Acute myocardial injury in patients hospitalized with COVID-19 infection: a review. *Prog Cardiovasc Dis.* (2020) 6:682–9. doi: 10.1016/j.pcad.2020.05.013

11. Bonow RO, Fonarow GC, O'Gara PT, Yancy CW. Association of coronavirus disease 2019 (COVID-19) with myocardial injury and mortality. *JAMA Cardiol.* (2020) 5:751–3. doi: 10.1001/jamacardio.2020.1105

12. Chinese Clinical Guidance for COVID-19 Pneumonia Diagnosis and Treatment (7th edition). Published by China National Health Commission on March 4, 2020. Available online at: http://kjfy.meeting.so/msite/news/show/cn/3337.html (accessed March 16, 2020).

13. Deng Q, Hu B, Zhang Y, Wang H, Zhou X, Hu W, et al. Suspected myocardial injury in patients with COVID-19: evidence from front-line clinical observation in Wuhan, China. *Int J Cardiol.* (2020) 311:116–21. doi: 10.1016/j.ijcard.2020.03.087

14. Huang L, Zhao P, Tang D, Zhu T, Han R, Zhan C, et al. Cardiac involvement in patients recovered from COVID-2019 identified using magnetic resonance imaging. *JACC Cardiovasc Imaging.* (2020). doi: 10.1016/j.jcmg.2020.05.004

15. Puntmann VO, Carerj ML, Wieters I, Fahim M, Arendt C, Hoffmann J, et al. Outcomes of cardiovascular magnetic resonance imaging in patients recently recovered from coronavirus disease 2019 (COVID-19). *JAMA Cardiol.* (2020) 5:1265–73. doi: 10.1001/jamacardio.2020.3557

16. Rajpal S, Tong MS, Borchers J, Zareba KM, Obarski TP, Simonetti OP, et al. Cardiovascular magnetic resonance findings in competitive athletes recovering from COVID-19 infection. *JAMA Cardiol.* (2020) 13:e204916. doi: 10.1001/jamacardio.2020.4916

17. Argulian E, Sud K, Vogel B, Bohra C, Garg VP, Talebi S, et al. Right ventricular dilation in hospitalized patients with COVID-19 infection. *JACC Cardiovasc Imaging.* (2020) 13:2459–61. doi: 10.1016/j.jcmg.2020.05.010

18. Jain SS, Liu Q, Raikhelkar J, Fried J, Elias P, Poterucha TJ, et al. Indications and findings on transthoracic echocardiography in COVID-19. *J Am Soc Echocardiogr.* (2020) 33:1278–84. doi: 10.1016/j.echo.2020.06.009

19. Dweck MR, Bularga A, Hahn RT, Bing R, Lee KK, Chapman AR, et al. Global evaluation of echocardiography in patients with COVID-19. *Eur Heart J Cardiovasc Imaging.* (2020) 2:949–58. doi: 10.1093/ehjci/jeaa178

20. Rath D, Petersen-Uribe A, Avdiu A, Witzel K, Jaeger P, Zdanyte M, et al. Impaired cardiac function is associated with mortality in patients with acute COVID-19 infection. *Res Rep Clin Cardiol.* (2020) 109:1491–9. doi: 10.1007/s00392-020-01683-0

21. Pagnesi M, Baldetti L, Beneduce A, Calvo F, Gramegna M, Pazzanese V, et al. Pulmonary hypertension and right ventricular involvement in hospitalised patients with COVID-19. *Heart.* (2020) 106:1324–31. doi: 10.1136/heartjnl-2020-317355

22. D'Andrea A, Scarafile R, Riegler L, Liccardo B, Crescibene F, Cocchia R, et al. Right ventricular function and pulmonary pressures as independent predictors of survival in patients with COVID-19 pneumonia. *JACC: Cardiovasc Imaging.* (2020) 13:2467–8. doi: 10.1016/j.jcmg.2020.06.004

23. Vasudev R, Guragai N, Habib H, Hosein K, Virk H, Goldfarb I, et al. The utility of bedside echocardiography in critically ill COVID-19 patients: early observational findings from three Northern New Jersey hospitals. *Echocardiography.* (2020) 37:1362–5. doi: 10.1111/echo.14825

24. Baycan OF, Barman HA, Atici A, Tatlisu A, Bolen F, Ergen P, et al. Evaluation of biventricular function in patients with COVID-19 using speckle tracking echocardiography. *Int J Cardiovas Imag.* (2020) 15:1–10. doi: 10.1007/s10554-020-01968-5

25. Krishnamoorthy P, Croft LB, Ro R, Anastasius M, Zhao W, Giustino G, et al. Biventricular strain by speckle tracking echocardiography in COVID-19: findings and possible prognostic implications. *Future Cardiol.* (2020). doi: 10.2217/fca-2020-0100

26. van den Heuvel FMA, Vos JL, Koop Y, van Dijk APJ, Duijnhouwer AL, de Mast Q, et al. Cardiac function in relation to myocardial injury in hospitalised patients with COVID-19. *Neth Heart J.* (2020) 28:410–7. doi: 10.1007/s12471-020-01458-2

27. Zeng JH, Wu WB, Qu JX, Wang Y, Dong CF, Luo YF, et al. Cardiac manifestations of COVID-19 in Shenzhen, China. *Infection.* (2020) 48:861–70. doi: 10.1007/s15010-020-01473-w

28. Ferreira VM, Schulz-Menger J, Holmvang G, Kramer CM, Carbone I, Sechtem U, et al. Cardiovascular magnetic resonance in non-ischemic myocardial inflammation: expert recommendations. *J Am Coll Cardiol.* (2018) 72:3158–76. doi: 10.1016/j.jacc.2018.09.072

29. Kammerlander AA, Marzluf BA, Zotter-Tufaro C, Aschauer S, Duca F, Bachmann A, et al. T1 mapping by cmr imaging: from histological validation to clinical implication. *JACC Cardiovasc Imaging.* (2016) 9:14–23. doi: 10.1016/j.jcmg.2015.11.002

30. Friedrich MG, Sechtem U, Schulz-Menger J, Holmvang G, Alakija P, Cooper LT, et al. Cardiovascular magnetic resonance in myocarditis: a JACC white paper. *J Am Coll Cardiol.* (2009) 53:1475–87. doi: 10.1016/j.jacc.2009.02.007

31. Puntmann VO, Valbuena S, Hinojar R, Petersen SE, Greenwood JP, Kramer CM, et al. Society for Cardiovascular Magnetic Resonance (SCMR) expert consensus for CMR imaging endpoints in clinical research: part I—analytical validation and clinical qualification. *J Cardiovasc Magn Reson.* (2018) 20:67. doi: 10.1186/s12968-018-0484-5

32. Lang RM, Badano LP, Mor-Avi V, Afilalo J, Armstrong A, Ernande L, et al. Recommendations for cardiac chamber quantification by echocardiography in adults: an update from the American Society of Echocardiography and the European Association of Cardiovascular Imaging. *J Am Soc Echocardiogr.* (2015) 28:1–39.e14. doi: 10.1016/j.echo.2014.10.003

33. Zochios V, Parhar K, Tunnicliffe W, Roscoe A, Gao F. The Right Ventricle in ARDS. *Chest.* (2017) 152:181–93. doi: 10.1016/j.chest.2017.02.019

34. Carluccio E, Biagioli P, Alunni G, Murrone A, Zuchi C, Coiro S, et al. Prognostic value of right ventricular dysfunction in heart failure with reduced ejection fraction: superiority of longitudinal strain over tricuspid annular plane systolic excursion. *Circ Cardiovasc Imaging.* (2018) 11:e006894. doi: 10.1161/CIRCIMAGING.117.006894

35. Li Y, Xie M, Wang X, Lu Q, Zhang L, Ren P. Impaired right and left ventricular function in asymptomatic children with repaired tetralogy of Fallot by two-dimensional speckle tracking echocardiography study. *Echocardiography.* (2015) 32:135–43. doi: 10.1111/echo.12581

36. Park SJ, Park JH, Lee HS, Kim MS, Park YK, Park Y, et al. Impaired RV global longitudinal strain is associated with poor long-term clinical outcomes in patients with acute inferior STEMI. *Jacc-Cardiovasc Imag.* (2015) 8:161–9. doi: 10.1016/j.jcmg.2014.10.011

37. Huang C, Wang Y, Li X, Ren L, Zhao J, Hu Y, et al. Clinical features of patients infected with 2019 novel coronavirus in Wuhan, China. *Lancet.* (2020) 395:497–506. doi: 10.1016/S0140-6736(20)30183-5

38. Zhou F, Yu T, Du R, Fan G, Liu Y, Liu Z, et al. Clinical course and risk factors for mortality of adult inpatients with COVID-19 in Wuhan, China: a retrospective cohort study. *Lancet.* (2020) 395:1054–62. doi: 10.1016/S0140-6736(20)30566-3

39. Repesse X, Charron C, Vieillard-Baron A. Right ventricular failure in acute lung injury and acute respiratory distress syndrome. *Minerva Anestesiol.* (2012) 78:941–8.

40. Boissier F, Katsahian S, Razazi K, Thille AW, Roche-Campo F, Leon R, et al. Prevalence and prognosis of cor pulmonale during protective ventilation for acute respiratory distress syndrome. *Intensive Care Med.* (2013) 39:1725–33. doi: 10.1007/s00134-013-2941-9

41. Wang D, Hu B, Hu C, Zhu F, Liu X, Zhang J, et al. Clinical characteristics of 138 hospitalized patients with 2019 novel coronavirus-infected pneumonia in Wuhan, China. *JAMA.* (2020) 323:1061–9. doi: 10.1001/jama.2020.1585

42. Li X, Ma X. Acute respiratory failure in COVID-19: is it "typical" ARDS? *Crit Care.* (2020) 24:198. doi: 10.1186/s13054-020-02911-9

43. Nobre C, Thomas B. Right ventricle in ARDS. *Chest.* (2017) 152:215–6. doi: 10.1016/j.chest.2017.04.163

44. Repesse X, Charron C, Vieillard-Baron A. Acute respiratory distress syndrome: the heart side of the moon. *Curr Opin Crit Care.* (2016) 22:38–44. doi: 10.1097/MCC.0000000000000267

45. Poissy J, Goutay J, Caplan M, Parmentier E, Duburcq T, Lassalle F, et al. Pulmonary embolism in patients with COVID-19: awareness of an increased prevalence. *Circulation.* (2020) 142:184–6. doi: 10.1161/CIRCULATIONAHA.120.047430

46. Wichmann D, Sperhake JP, Lutgehetmann M, Steurer S, Edler C, Heinemann A, et al. Autopsy findings and venous thromboembolism in patients With COVID-19: a prospective cohort study. *Ann Intern Med.* (2020) 173:268–77. doi: 10.7326/L20-1206

47. Huisman MV, Barco S, Cannegieter SC, Le Gal G, Konstantinides SV, Reitsma PH, et al. Pulmonary embolism. *Nat Rev Dis Primers.* (2018) 4:18028. doi: 10.1038/nrdp.2018.28

48. Inciardi RM, Lupi L, Zaccone G, Italia L, Raffo M, Tomasoni D, et al. Cardiac involvement in a patient with coronavirus disease 2019 (COVID-19). *JAMA Cardiol.* (2020) 5:819–24. doi: 10.1001/jamacardio.2020.1096

49. Khan IH, Zahra SA, Zaim S, Harky A. At the heart of COVID-19. *J Cardiac Surg.* (2020) 35:1287–94. doi: 10.1111/jocs.14596

50. Ruan QR, Yang K, Wang WX, Jiang LY, Song JX. Clinical predictors of mortality due to COVID-19 based on an analysis of data of 150 patients from Wuhan, China. *Intensive Care Medicine.* (2020) 46:846–8. doi: 10.1007/s00134-020-05991-x

51. Zhu H, Rhee JW, Cheng P, Waliany S, Chang A, Witteles RM, et al. Cardiovascular complications in patients with COVID-19: consequences of viral toxicities and host immune response. *Curr Cardiol Rep.* (2020) 22:32. doi: 10.1007/s11886-020-01302-4

52. Nduka OO, Parrillo JE. The pathophysiology of septic shock. *Crit Care Clin.* (2009) 25:677–702. doi: 10.1016/j.ccc.2009.08.002

53. Clerkin KJ, Fried JA, Raikhelkar J, Sayer G, Griffin JM, Masoumi A, et al. COVID-19 and cardiovascular disease. *Circulation.* (2020) 141:1648–55. doi: 10.1161/CIRCULATIONAHA.120.046941

54. Zheng YY, Ma YT, Zhang JY, Xie X. COVID-19 and the cardiovascular system. *Nat Rev Cardiol.* (2020) 17:259–60. doi: 10.1038/s41569-020-0360-5

55. Boukhris M, Hillani A, Moroni F, Annabi MS, Addad F, Ribeiro MH, et al. Cardiovascular implications of the COVID-19 pandemic: a global perspective. *Can J Cardiol.* (2020) 36:1068–80. doi: 10.1016/j.cjca.2020.05.018

56. Ventetuolo CE, Klinger JR. Management of acute right ventricular failure in the intensive care unit. *Ann Am Thorac Soc.* (2014) 11:811–22. d doi: 10.1513/AnnalsATS.201312-446FR

57. Morelli A, Teboul JL, Maggiore SM, Vieillard-Baron A, Rocco M, Conti G, et al. Effects of levosimendan on right ventricular afterload in patients with acute respiratory distress syndrome: a pilot study. *Crit Care Med.* (2006) 34:2287–93. doi: 10.1097/01.CCM.0000230244.17174.4F

58. Hirsch LJ, Rooney MW, Wat SS, Kleinmann B, Mathru M. Norepinephrine and phenylephrine effects on right ventricular function in experimental canine pulmonary embolism. *Chest.* (1991) 100:796–801. doi: 10.1378/chest.100.3.796

59. Kisch-Wedel H, Kemming G, Meisner F, Flondor M, Kuebler WM, Bruhn S, et al. The prostaglandins epoprostenol and iloprost increase

left ventricular contractility *in vivo*. *Intensive Care Med*. (2003) 29:1574–83. doi: 10.1007/s00134-003-1891-z

60. Hunt JL, Bronicki RA, Anas N. Role of inhaled nitric oxide in the management of severe acute respiratory distress syndrome. *Front Pediatr*. (2016) 4:74. doi: 10.3389/fped.2016.00074

61. Searcy RJ, Morales JR, Ferreira JA, Johnson DW. The role of inhaled prostacyclin in treating acute respiratory distress syndrome. *Ther Adv Respir Dis*. (2015) 9:302–12. doi: 10.1177/1753465815599345

62. Lang IM, Gaine SP. Recent advances in targeting the prostacyclin pathway in pulmonary arterial hypertension. *Eur Respir Rev*. (2015) 24:630–41. doi: 10.1183/16000617.0067-2015

63. Meduri GU, Siemieniuk RAC, Ness RA, Seyler SJ. Prolonged low-dose methylprednisolone treatment is highly effective in reducing duration of mechanical ventilation and mortality in patients with ARDS. *J Intensive Care Med*. (2018) 6:53. doi: 10.1186/s40560-018-0321-9

64. Organization WH. *Infection Prevention and Control During Health Care When Novel Coronavirus (ncov) Infection is Suspected*. (2020). Available online at: https://www.who.int/publications/i/item/10665-331495 (accessed March 19, 2020).

65. Tang N, Li D, Wang X, Sun Z. Abnormal coagulation parameters are associated with poor prognosis in patients with novel coronavirus pneumonia. *J Thromb Haemost*. (2020) 18:844–7. doi: 10.1111/jth.14768

66. Tang N, Bai H, Chen X, Gong JL, Li DJ, Sun ZY. Anticoagulant treatment is associated with decreased mortality in severe coronavirus disease 2019 patients with coagulopathy. *J Thromb Haemost*. (2020) 18:1094–9. doi: 10.1111/jth.14817

67. Lin L, Lu LF, Cao W, Li TS. Hypothesis for potential pathogenesis of SARS-CoV-2 infection-a review of immune changes in patients with viral pneumonia. *Emerg Microbes Infec*. (2020) 9:727–32. doi: 10.1080/22221751.2020.1746199

68. Repesse X, Charron C, Vieillard-Baron A. Acute cor pulmonale in ARDS: rationale for protecting the right ventricle. *Chest*. (2015) 14:259–65. doi: 10.1378/chest.14-0877

69. Organization WH. *Clinical Management of Severe Acute Respiratory Infection When Novel Coronavirus (nCoV) Infection Is Suspected: Interim Guidance*. (2020). Available online at: https://www.who.int/publications/i/item/10665-332299 (accessed January 12, 2020).

70. Tiruvoipati R, Botha JA, Pilcher D, Bailey M. Carbon dioxide clearance in critical care. *Anaesth Intensive Care*. (2013) 41:157–62. doi: 10.1177/0310057X1304100129

2

Hypertension and COVID-19: Ongoing Controversies

Marijana Tadic [1*], Sahrai Saeed [2], Guido Grassi [3], Stefano Taddei [4], Giuseppe Mancia [5] and Cesare Cuspidi [3,6]

[1] Department of Cardiology, University Hospital "Dr. Dragisa Misovic - Dedinje", Belgrade, Serbia, [2] Department of Heart Disease, Haukeland University Hospital, Bergen, Norway, [3] Department of Cardiology, University of Milan-Bicocca, Milan, Italy, [4] Department of Clinical and Experimental Medicine, University of Pisa, Pisa, Italy, [5] University of Milano-Bicocca, Milano and Policlinico di Monza, Monza, Italy, [6] Department of Cardiology, Istituto Auxologico Italiano, Scientific Institute for Research, Hospitalization and Healthcare, Milan, Italy

*Correspondence:
Marijana Tadic
marijana_tadic@hotmail.com

Coronavirus disease 2019 (COVID-19) has become a worldwide pandemic responsible for millions of deaths around the world. Hypertension has been identified as one of the most common comorbidities and risk factors for severity and adverse outcome in these patients. Recent investigations have raised the question whether hypertension represents a predictor of outcome in COVID-19 patients independently of other common comorbidities such as diabetes, obesity, other cardiovascular diseases, chronic kidney, liver, and pulmonary diseases. However, the impact of chronic and newly diagnosed hypertension in COVID-19 patients has been insufficiently investigated. The same is true for the relationship between blood pressure levels and outcomes in COVID-19 patients. It seems that the long discussion about the impact of angiotensin-converting enzyme inhibitors (ACEI) and blockers of angiotensin I receptors (ARB) on severity and outcome in COVID-19 is approaching an end because the large number of original studies and meta-analyses discarded the initial findings about higher prevalence of ACEI/ARB use in patients with unfavorable outcomes. Nevertheless, there are many controversies in the relationship between hypertension and COVID-19. The aim of this review article is to provide a clinical overview of the currently available evidence regarding the predictive value of hypertension, the effect of blood pressure levels, the impact of previously known and newly diagnosed hypertension, and the effect of antihypertensive therapy on the severity and outcomes in COVID-19 patients.

Keywords: hypertension, COVID - 19, blood pressure, antihypertensive therapy, comorbidities

INTRODUCTION

Coronavirus disease 2019 (COVID-19), induced by Severe Acute Respiratory Syndrome Coronavirus 2 (SARS-CoV-2), has become a worldwide pandemic that is responsible for millions of deaths around the world. Hypertension, diabetes, and cardiovascular diseases were soon identified as common comorbidities in COVID-19 patients (1, 2). The following studies revealed that hypertension is an important risk factor for adverse outcomes in COVID-19 patients (3, 4). Initial studies reported hypertension as an independent predictor of hospitalization, an advanced stage of pneumonia, admission to the intensive care unit (ICU), and mortality in these patients (3–5). Later investigations raised the question whether hypertension would be a predictor of outcome in COVID-19 patients independently of diabetes, obesity, and other cardiovascular diseases (6, 7). Furthermore, the majority of studies did not make any distinction between patients with chronic and new-onset of hypertension in COVID-19 patients, which could significantly impact final results. The relationship between blood pressure level and susceptibility to SARS-CoV-2 or outcome in COVID-19 patients has been insufficiently investigated, and potential blood pressure target value in these patients is still unknown.

There was a long discussion regarding the impact of antihypertensive therapy in COVID-19 patients and particularly of angiotensin-converting enzyme inhibitors (ACEI) and blockers of angiotensin I receptors (ARB). After initial reports that showed higher prevalence of use of these medications in COVID-19 patients with cardiac injury and more severe course of disease (8, 9), numerous original studies and meta-analysis reported no relationship with severity or mortality in COVID-19 patients (10, 11) or even benefit of taking renin-angiotensin-aldosterone inhibitors in COVID-19 patients (12, 13).

The aim of this review article is to provide an overview of the current evidence on controversies regarding hypertension in COVID-19 patients: predictive value of hypertension, effect of blood pressure (BP) level and control, influence of new-onset hypertension and impact of antihypertensive therapy.

IS HYPERTENSION AN INDEPENDENT PREDICTOR OF OUTCOME IN COVID-19 PATIENTS?

Initial studies were focused on prevalence of different comorbidities, including the impact of various risk factors on susceptibility, severity and mortality of COVID-19 (3–5). Later investigations revealed association between hypertension and more advanced stages of disease and mortality (14, 15). However, majority of them did not include diabetes and obesity in multivariable analysis.

A recent study demonstrated that hypertension alone was not an independent predictor of outcome, but only in combination with diabetes or some other risk factor (6). One should also notice that some researches did not show any impact of neither hypertension nor diabetes on outcome in COVID-19 patients (16), whereas other investigations reported that both hypertension and diabetes with or without obesity were independently associated with adverse outcome (3).

Bauer et al. suggested that hypertension was independent predictor of severe form of COVID-19 only in patients younger than 65 years, but not in the whole study population (17). On the other hand, diabetes and congestive heart failure were independent predictors both in patients younger than 65 years and in all participants. Barrera et al. included 15,794 participants and reported that hypertension and diabetes separately were significant predictors of ICU and mortality, but not with severe COVID-19 (18). Interestingly, concomitant presence of hypertension and diabetes was not predictor of severe COVID-19 (18).

An investigation that included almost 4,000 critically ill COVID-19 patients that were hospitalized in ICU showed that hypertension, diabetes, cardiovascular diseases,

hypercholesterolemia, chronic kidney disease, and other comorbidities were predictors of mortality in these patients (19). However, among these comorbidities only diabetes and hypercholesterolemia were independent predictors (19). A study that involved only hypertensive patients reported that diabetes was not an independent prognostic factor, whereas age and chronic kidney disease were independent predictors. The same study demonstrated that hypertension, diabetes and obesity were independent predictors of severe COVID-19 in both sexes and obesity was stronger predictor in patients younger than 50 years, whereas the interaction between hypertension and diabetes with age was not noticed (20). However, the authors did not perform adjustment for all comorbidities like in the first mentioned from the same cohort of patients.

Furthermore, the National Cohort Study in England investigated 19,256 COVID-19–related ICU admissions and revealed that patients with type 2 diabetes were at increased risk of mortality independently of hypertension, chronic respiratory disease, chronic heart disease, chronic renal disease, chronic liver disease and other potential risk factors (21). Nevertheless, the recent investigation showed no association between hypertension and mortality or acute respiratory distress syndrome (ARDS) in COVID-19 patients (6). The authors reported that hypertension only together with diabetes was independent predictor of mortality and ARDS in COVID-19 patients (6). Moreover, diabetes alone was also independently related with adverse outcomes in these patients. On the other hand, Gupta et al. revealed that only body mass index ≥ 40 kg/m^2 and coronary artery disease were independent predictors of 28-day mortality in COVID-19 patients (16). Hypertension, diabetes, heart failure and chronic pulmonary obstructive disease were not independently associated with lethal outcome in these patients. **Table 1** summarizes findings from described studies.

There are several major limitations of mentioned studies: retrospective nature, confounding factors that were not measured, lack of information regarding duration of hypertension, diabetes and other comorbidities, as well as missing or incomplete data about antihypertensive and anti-diabetic therapy.

THE INFLUENCE OF BLOOD PRESSURE CONTROL IN COVID-19

Data regarding the impact of BP level on susceptibility, severity or outcome of COVID-19 patients are scarce. Majority of studies and particularly those published at the beginning of pandemic were based on anamnestic data and therefore were not fully reliable. Recently published studies investigated the impact of BP control on outcome in COVID-19 patients and provided more detailed insight (22, 23).

Ran et al. investigated 803 hypertensive patients with COVID-19 and found that average systolic BP was independent predictor of only heart failure development in these COVID-19 patients (22). After adjustment for confounding factors (systolic and diastolic BP on admission, age, sex, smoking, alcohol consumption, and comorbidities (cancer, diabetes, coronary

TABLE 1 | Hypertension as independent predictor of outcome in COVID-19.

Reference	Sample size	Age	Women (%)	Hypertension (%)	Other important findings
Sun et al. (6)	3,400	61 (50–68)	1,751 (51)	1,782 (52)	Hypertension only together with diabetes was independent predictor of mortality and ARDS.
Bauer et al. (17)	1,449	54.7 ± 22.5	920 (63)	525 (36)	Hypertension was independent predictor of severe form of COVID-19 only in patients younger than 65 years, but not in the whole study population.
Barrera et al. (18)	15,794	–	–	–	Hypertension and diabetes separately were significant predictors of ICU and mortality, but not with severe COVID-19.
Grasselli et al. (19)	3,988	63 (56–69)	800 (20)	1,643 (41)	Diabetes and hypercholesterolemia, but not hypertension, were independent predictors of mortality in COVID-19 patients hospitalized in ICU.
Dennis et al. (21)	19,256	66	7,683 (40)	5,657 (29)	Patients with type 2 diabetes were at increased risk of mortality independently of hypertension, chronic respiratory disease, chronic heart disease, chronic renal disease, chronic liver disease and other potential risk factors.
Gupta et al. (16)	2,215	60.5 ± 14.5	779 (35)	1,322 (60)	Body mass index $\geq$ 40 kg/m^2 and coronary artery disease, but not hypertension and diabetes, were independent predictors of 28-day mortality in COVID-19 patients.

ARDS, acute respiratory distress syndrome; ICU, intensive care unit.

heart disease, cerebrovascular disease, COPD, chronic liver disease, and chronic kidney disease), the remaining significant predictors for heart failure were average systolic BP and pulse pressure, and an increase in systolic BP variability was also marginally associated with an increased hazard of heart failure. Increased BP variability was significantly associated with higher risks of mortality and ICU admission, respectively. The authors showed that the risks of COVID-induced heart failure development significantly increased in patients with high systolic BP, but this trend was less evident for diastolic BP (22). This finding implies that high BP is an important predictor of adverse outcome and suggests that systolic BP should be the primary target of BP control in COVID-19 patients. However, high BP variability was related with high risks of mortality and ICU admissions, underlying the importance of maintenance of stable in-hospital BP in these patients. Increased BP variability could reflect increased arterial stiffness and endothelial dysfunction that are associated with cardiovascular events (24, 25). Additional explanation could be a sudden BP decline because of progressive deterioration of underlying conditions.

Chen et al. reported gradual increase in lethal outcome, septic shock, ARDS, respiratory failure, mechanical ventilation and ICU admission from normotensive patients with COVID-19, throughout patients with grade I hypertension, to those with grade II and III hypertension (23). Even though trend existed for all outcomes, one must admit that the significant difference was not noticed between normotensive patients and participants with grade I hypertension, as well as between grade II and III hypertension. Interestingly, the length of disease and symptoms gradually increased with grade of hypertension. In multivariable analysis hypertension grade $\geq$2 was independently associated with adverse events. However, diabetes was not included in multivariable analysis despite its significant proportion among COVID-19 patients in total study population and particularly in hypertensive participants (23).

Determination of the relationship between BP and COVID-19 outcome is not an easy task due to its high variability and dependency on comorbidities. Furthermore, both studies investigated hospitalized patients, which means that BP was measured after admission and not after symptoms onset and therefore COVID-19 could already influence BP.

CHRONIC VS. NEW-ONSET HYPERTENSION IN COVID-19

One of the main challenges in assessment of the relationship between hypertension and COVID-19 is the absence of data regarding the ratio of patients with hypertension before hospital admission. Namely, patients with chronic hypertension have significant endothelial dysfunction, which is crucial in the pathogenesis of cardiovascular complications in COVID-19 (25). Chronically hypertensive patients often have target organ damage that increases susceptibility for SARS-CoV-2 and elevates the risk of unfavorable outcomes in COVID-19 patients.

Data regarding the impact of known and newly diagnosed hypertension in COVID-19 patients are very limited. Ran et al. found that poor BP control was independently associated with adverse outcomes in COVID-19 patients with chronic hypertension (22). Chen et al. reported that stage I chronic hypertension was present in only 37% of hospitalized COVID-19 patients, whereas the prevalence of chronic hypertension stages II and III was significantly higher (61 and 70%, respectively) (23). This shows that newly diagnosed hypertension was present in a significant portion of COVID-19 patients. The investigators demonstrated that unfavorable outcomes (mortality, septic shock, respiratory failure, ARDS, ICU admission) gradually increased with BP elevation (23). However, the authors did not make separate analyses for patients with known and newly diagnosed hypertension.

Xiong et al. showed that almost 40% of patients with known hypertension did not receive any antihypertensive medication (26). Nevertheless, the occurrence of adverse events did not differ between patients who were previously treated with anti-hypertensive medications and those who did not receive therapy despite hypertension. A significant limitation is the small number of hypertensive patients in this study ($n = 71$), which is not enough to make a conclusion (26). One should also keep in mind that the majority of studies regarding COVID-19 have come from China, where traditional medicines are frequently used instead of formal medications, including antihypertensive drugs.

Data regarding the relationship between known and newly diagnosed diabetes among COVID-19 patients potentially might be used as the model for the association between chronic and newly diagnosed hypertension with outcome in these patients. It is already well-established that diabetes is associated with elevated risk of adverse outcomes in COVID-19 patients. Nevertheless, one should notice that COVID-19 could induce diabetes with its metabolic complications and insulin therapy requirement. Li et al. found that newly diagnosed diabetes was associated with higher mortality than known diabetes in hospitalized COVID-19 patients (27). Similar results were reported from the Italian group (28). Higher glucose levels at admission were related to COVID-19 severity, with a stronger association among patients without as compared to those with known diabetes.

It is evident that this topic deserves further investigation because whether newly diagnosed hypertension potentially has a more negative effect than chronic hypertension should be explained, in the same way as the comparison of newly diagnosed diabetes with known diabetes. This would have significant clinical and particularly therapeutic implications in COVID-19 patients.

ANTIHYPERTENSIVE THERAPY IN COVID-19

SARS-CoV-2 enters human host cells upon binding to angiotensin-converting enzyme 2 (ACE2)—a molecule functioning both as the main trans-membrane receptor for the virus and a component of the renin-angiotensin system —the key BP regulating cascade. Because renin-angiotensin-system inhibitors increase ACE2 levels, the potential negative effect of ACEI or ARB has been largely discussed since the beginning of COVID-19 pandemic. This hypothesis was supported by initial findings that these medications were more frequently used in COVID-19 patients with cardiac injury or in those with severe form of disease (8, 9). Nevertheless, later reports failed to show any negative relationship between adverse outcome and use of ACEI and ARB in COVID-19 patients (10–13).

A large study from the United Kingdom that included 16,866 patients with COVID-19 events and 70,137 matched controls showed that ACEIs and ARBs were associated with lower risk of COVID-19 diagnosis (28). In fully adjusted analyses, calcium channel blockers and thiazide diuretics were also associated with lower risk of COVID-19. Interestingly, beta-blockers were initially associated with increased risk, but this relationship

disappeared in a multivariable-adjusted model (28). In adjusted analyses, patients treated with ACEIs or ARBs had similar mortality to patients treated with beta-blockers, calcium channel antagonists, and other antihypertensive medications or patients receiving no antihypertensive therapy (28).

A study that analyzed 880 COVID-19 patients from Germany and the Netherlands reported that use of ACEI/ARB and diuretics was not related to worse outcomes; instead, use of beta-blockers was associated with better outcomes, and use of calcium channel blockers with poorer outcomes (29). The model was adjusted only for age, sex, and diabetes and therefore not fully conclusive, if we consider the fact that many other confounding factors (comorbidities in the first place) were not included (29). There is a hypothesis that some beta-blockers, such as carvedilol, unlike ACEI and ARB, decrease the expression of ACE2 and suppress the properties of interleukin-6, which potentially could help in treatment of COVID-19 patients (30). However, this still remains in the domain of hypothesis.

Gao et al. reported no difference in mortality, time from onset of symptoms to discharge, COVID-19 severity, and percentage of ventilation between the cohort of patients who were treated with ACEI/ARB and those treated with beta-blockers, calcium channel blockers, and diuretics (31). Unfortunately, the authors did not investigate the influence of each antihypertensive class separately. Other Chinese study reported no association between any antihypertensive class (ACEI/ARB, beta-blockers, calcium channel blockers, and diuretics) and the composite endpoint, which was defined as admission to an ICU, need for mechanical ventilation, or a fatal outcome (26).

A Massachusetts community-based observational study showed that no antihypertensive medications were related to increased risk of severe COVID-19 (17). The authors investigated each of five antihypertensive classes separately. Similar results were reported in a large meta-analysis that included 2,100,587 participants (32). The investigators observed no association between prior usage of antihypertensive medications, including ACEIs/ARBs, calcium channel blockers, beta-blockers, or diuretics, and the risk or severity of COVID-19. Interestingly, when the analysis included only hypertensive patients, prior usage of ACEIs/ARBs was related to lower severity and mortality of COVID-19.

The large Italian population-based study that matched 6,272 COVID-19 patients and 30,759 subjects according to sex, age, and municipality of residence, showed that therapy with ACEIs and ARBs was more prevalent in COVID-19 patients than among their counterparts because of higher prevalence of CV disease in COVID-19 patients (33). Nevertheless, there was no association between use of ACEIs or ARBs and the risk of COVID-19.

Considering the confusion about the use of ACEI/ARBs in COVID-19 patients with hypertension that appeared at the beginning of the pandemic, hypertension societies around the globe were forced to publish statements that should encourage the maintenance of ongoing antihypertensive therapy and the following of current guidelines (34), which include the use of ACEI/ARB and the avoidance of replacing or switching ACEI/ARB to another antihypertensive medication (35–37).

Large recently published studies and meta-analysis have significantly reduced initial uncertainties regarding the use of ACEI and ARB in treatment of COVID-19 patients. Available data indicate that all antihypertensive classes are safe in this group of patients. However, prospective studies with a large number of patients with accurate data regarding antihypertensive therapy before and during COVID-19 would be very much appreciated.

DIFFERENCES AMONG COUNTRIES

Data regarding incidence and mortality of COVID-19 significantly changed during pandemic and particularly between different countries. Sorci et al. used data on the temporal trajectory of the case fatality rate provided by the European Center for Disease Prevention and Control, as well as country-specific data (38). The authors reported that temporal trajectories of case fatality rate vary significantly among countries. The main factors associated with temporal changes were comorbidities, demographic, economic, and political parameters. Countries with the highest prevalence of cardiovascular, cancer, and chronic respiratory diseases showed the highest levels of COVID-19 CFR (37). However, these are still preliminary data because information from all countries is updated on a daily basis and final conclusions will be published once the pandemic is over.

FUTURE DIRECTIONS

Many questions regarding the effects of hypertension, BP level, BP control, and antihypertensive therapy have been raised since the beginning of COVID-19 pandemic. A large number of studies have been published over a very short time period, which unfortunately does not guarantee their quality. Many questions remained without adequate answers. This is particularly true for the influence of BP levels and control on outcomes for COVID-19 patients. There is still not enough evidence about the effects of known and newly diagnosed hypertension on the severity and outcomes of COVID-19 for patients. A large number of studies considered the association of different antihypertensive classes of medications with the outcomes in these patients, but almost all of them are retrospective investigations or meta-analyses. It is evident that well-conducted research with a significant number of hypertensive patients is necessary to resolve current controversies in the relationship between hypertension and COVID-19.

AUTHOR CONTRIBUTIONS

MT: writing the article. SS: searching the literature and review. ST, GG, and GM: detailed review with constructive remarks that substantially changed the article. CC: conceptualization of the article and constructive review. All authors contributed to the article and approved the submitted version.

REFERENCES

1. Guan WJ, Ni ZY, Hu Y, Liang WH, Ou CQ, He JX, et al. Clinical characteristics of coronavirus disease 2019 in China. *N Engl J Med.* (2020) 382:1708–20. doi: 10.1056/NEJMoa2002032
2. Wu C, Chen X, Cai Y, Xia J, Zhou X, Xu S, et al. Risk factors associated with acute respiratory distress syndrome and death in patients with coronavirus disease 2019. Pneumonia in Wuhan, China. *JAMA Intern Med.* (2020) 180:934–43. doi: 10.1001/jamainternmed.2020.0994
3. Giannouchos TV, Sussman RA, Mier JM, Poulas K, Farsalinos K. Characteristics and risk factors for COVID-19 diagnosis and adverse outcomes in Mexico: an analysis of 89,756 laboratory-confirmed COVID-19 cases. *Eur Respir J.* (2020) 30:2002144. doi: 10.1183/13993003.02144-2020
4. Wang Z, Deng H, Ou C, Liang J, Wang Y, Jiang M, et al. Clinical symptoms, comorbidities and complications in severe and non-severe patients with COVID-19: A systematic review and meta-analysis without cases duplication. *Medicine.* (2020) 99:e23327. doi: 10.1097/MD.0000000000023327
5. de Almeida-Pititto B, Dualib PM, Zajdenverg L, Dantas JR, de Souza FD, Rodacki M, et al. Severity and mortality of COVID 19 in patients with diabetes, hypertension and cardiovascular disease: a meta-analysis. *Diabetol Metab Syndr.* (2020) 12:75. doi: 10.1186/s13098-020-00586-4
6. Sun Y, Guan X, Jia L, Xing N, Cheng L, Liu B, et al. Independent and combined effects of hypertension and diabetes on clinical outcomes in patients with COVID-19: a retrospective cohort study of Huoshen mountain hospital and Guanggu Fangcang Shelter Hospital. *J Clin Hypertens.* (2020). doi: 10.1111/jch.14146. [Epub ahead of print].
7. Mehraeen E, Karimi A, Barzegary A, Vahedi F, Afsahi AM, Dadras O, et al. Predictors of mortality in patients with COVID-19-a systematic review. *Eur J Integr Med.* (2020) 40:101226. doi: 10.1016/j.eujim.2020.101226
8. Guo T, Fan Y, Chen M, Wu X, Zhang L, He T, et al. Cardiovascular implications of fatal outcomes of patients with coronavirus disease 2019 (COVID-19). *JAMA Cardiol.* (2020) 5:811–8. doi: 10.1001/jamacardio.2020.1017
9. Feng Y, Ling Y, Bai T, Xie Y, Huang J, Li J, et al. COVID-19 with different severities: a multicenter study of clinical features. *Am J Respir Crit Care Med.* (2020) 201:1380–8. doi: 10.1164/rccm.202002-0445OC
10. Zhang G, Wu Y, Xu R, Du X. Effects of renin-angiotensin-aldosterone system (RAAS) inhibitors on disease severity and mortality in patients with COVID-19: a meta-analysis. *J Med Virol.* (2020). doi: 10.1002/jmv.26695. [Epub ahead of print].
11. Savarese G, Benson L, Sundström J, Lund LH. Association between renin-angiotensin-aldosterone system inhibitor use and COVID-19 hospitalization and death: A 1,4 million patient nation-wide registry analysis. *Eur J Heart Fail.* (2020). doi: 10.1002/ejhf.2060. [Epub ahead of print].
12. Ssentongo AE, Ssentongo P, Heilbrunn ES, Lekoubou A, Du P, Liao D, et al. Renin-angiotensin-aldosterone system inhibitors and the risk of mortality in patients with hypertension hospitalised for COVID-19: systematic review and meta-analysis. *Open Heart.* (2020) 7:e001353. doi: 10.1136/openhrt-2020-001353
13. Wang Y, Chen B, Li Y, Zhang L, Wang Y, Yang S, et al. The use of renin-angiotensin-aldosterone system (RAAS) inhibitors is associated with a lower risk of mortality in hypertensive COVID-19 patients: a systematic review and meta-analysis. *J Med Virol.* (2020). doi: 10.1002/jmv.26625. [Epub ahead of print].
14. Rodilla E, Saura A, Jiménez I, Mendizábal A, Pineda-Cantero A, Lorenzo-Hernández E, et al. Association of hypertension with all-cause mortality among hospitalized patients with COVID-19. *J Clin Med.* (2020) 9:3136. doi: 10.3390/jcm9103136
15. Zhang J, Wu J, Sun X, Xue H, Shao J, Cai W, et al. Association of hypertension with the severity and fatality of SARS-CoV-2 infection: a meta-analysis. *Epidemiol Infect.* (2020) 148:e106. doi: 10.1017/S095026882000117X
16. Gupta S, Hayek SS, Wang W, Chan L, Mathews KS, Melamed ML, et al. Factors associated with death in critically ill patients with coronavirus disease 2019 in the US. *JAMA Intern Med.* (2020) 180:1–12. doi: 10.1001/jamainternmed.2020.3596

17. Bauer AZ, Gore R, Sama SR, Rosiello R, Garber L, Sundaresan D, et al. Hypertension, medications, and risk of severe COVID-19: a Massachusetts community-based observational study. *J Clin Hypertens.* (2020). doi: 10.1111/jch.14101. [Epub ahead of print].

18. Barrera FJ, Shekhar S, Wurth R, Moreno-Pena PJ, Ponce OJ, Hajdenberg M, et al. Prevalence of diabetes and hypertension and their associated risks for poor outcomes in Covid-19 patients. *J Endocr Soc.* (2020) 4:bvaa102. doi: 10.1210/jendso/bvaa102

19. Grasselli G, Greco M, Zanella A, Albano G, Antonelli M, Bellani G, et al. Risk factors associated with mortality among patients with COVID-19 in intensive care units in Lombardy, Italy. *JAMA Intern Med.* (2020) 180:1345–55. doi: 10.1001/jamainternmed.2020.3539

20. Denova-Gutiérrez E, Lopez-Gatell H, Alomia-Zegarra JL, López-Ridaura R, Zaragoza-Jimenez CA, Dyer-Leal DD, et al. The association of obesity, type 2 diabetes, and hypertension with severe coronavirus disease 2019 on Admission among Mexican patients. *Obesity.* (2020) 28:1826–32. doi: 10.1002/oby.22946

21. Dennis JM, Mateen BA, Sonabend R, Thomas NJ, Patel KA, Hattersley AT, et al. Type 2 diabetes and COVID-19-related mortality in the critical care setting: a national cohort study in England, march-july (2020). *Diabetes Care.* (2020) 23:dc201444. doi: 10.2337/figshare.13034210

22. Ran J, Song Y, Zhuang Z, Han L, Zhao S, Cao P, et al. Blood pressure control and adverse outcomes of COVID-19 infection in patients with concomitant hypertension in Wuhan, China. *Hypertens Res.* (2020) 43:1267–76. doi: 10.1038/s41440-020-00541-w

23. Chen R, Yang J, Gao X, Ding X, Yang Y, Shen Y, et al. Influence of blood pressure control and application of renin-angiotensin-aldosterone system inhibitors on the outcomes in COVID-19 patients with hypertension. *J Clin Hypertens.* (2020). doi: 10.1111/jch.14038. [Epub ahead of print].

24. Vlachopoulos C, Aznaouridis K, Stefanadis C. Prediction of cardiovascular events and all-cause mortality with arterial stiffness: a systematic review and meta-analysis. *J Am Coll Cardiol.* (2010) 55:1318–27. doi: 10.1016/j.jacc.2009.10.061

25. Nägele MP, Haubner B, Tanner FC, Ruschitzka F, Flammer AJ. Endothelial dysfunction in COVID-19: Current findings and therapeutic implications. *Atherosclerosis.* (2020) 314:58–62. doi: 10.1016/j.atherosclerosis.2020.10.014

26. Xiong TY, Huang FY, Liu Q, Peng Y, Xu YN, Wei JF, et al. Hypertension is a risk factor for adverse outcomes in patients with coronavirus disease 2019: a cohort study. *Ann Med.* (2020) 52:361–66. doi: 10.1080/07853890.2020.1802059

27. Li H, Tian S, Chen T, Cui Z, Shi N, Zhong X, et al. Newly diagnosed diabetes is associated with a higher risk of mortality than known diabetes in hospitalized patients with COVID-19. *Diabetes Obes Metab.* (2020). doi: 10.1111/dom.14099. [Epub ahead of print].

28. Fadini GP, Morieri ML, Boscari F, Fioretto P, Maran A, Busetto L, et al. Newly-diagnosed diabetes and admission hyperglycemia predict COVID-19 severity by aggravating respiratory deterioration. *Diabetes Res Clin Pract.* (2020) 168:108374. doi: 10.1016/j.diabres.2020.108374

29. Rezel-Potts E, Douiri A, Chowienczyk PJ, Gulliford MC. Antihypertensive medications and COVID-19 diagnosis and mortality: population based case-control analysis in the United Kingdom. *medRxiv [Preprint].* (2020). doi: 10.1101/2020.09.25.20201731

30. Pinto-Sietsma SJ, Flossdorf M, Buchholz VR, Offerhaus J, Bleijendaal H, Beudel M, et al. Antihypertensive drugs in COVID-19 infection. *Eur Heart J Cardiovasc Pharmacother.* (2020) 6:415–6. doi: 10.1093/ehjcvp/pvaa058

31. Gao C, Cai Y, Zhang K, Zhou L, Zhang Y, Zhang X, et al. Association of hypertension and antihypertensive treatment with COVID-19 mortality: a retrospective observational study. *Eur Heart J.* (2020) 41:2058–66. doi: 10.1093/eurheartj/ehaa433

32. Ren L, Yu S, Xu W, Overton JL, Chiamvimonvat N, Thai PN. Lack of association of antihypertensive drugs with the risk and severity of COVID-19: a meta-analysis. *J Cardiol.* (2020). doi: 10.1016/j.jjcc.2020.10.015. [Epub ahead of print].

33. Mancia G, Rea F, Ludergnani M, Apolone G, Corrao G. Renin-angiotensin-aldosterone system blockers and the risk of Covid-19. *N Engl J Med.* (2020) 382:2431–40. doi: 10.1056/NEJMoa2006923

34. Williams B, Mancia G, Spiering W, Agabiti Rosei E, Azizi M, Burnier M, et al. 2018 ESC/ESH guidelines for the management of arterial hypertension. The task force for the management of arterial hypertension of the European society of cardiology and the European society of hypertension: the task force for the management of arterial hypertension of the European society of cardiology and the European society of hypertension. *J Hypertens.* (2018) 36:2284–309. doi: 10.1097/HJH.0000000000001961

35. Iaccarino G, Borghi C, Cicero AFG, Ferri C, Minuz P, Muiesan ML, et al. Renin-angiotensin system inhibition in cardiovascular patients at the time of COVID19: much ado for nothing? A statement of activity from the directors of the board and the scientific directors of the Italian society of hypertension. *High Blood Press Cardiovasc Prev.* (2020) 27:105–8. doi: 10.1007/s40292-020-00380-3

36. De Simone G. *Position Statement of the ESC Council on Hypertension on ACE-Inhibitors and Angiotensin Receptor Blockers.*

37. *BSH & BCS Joint Statement on ACEi or ARB in Relation to COVID-19.* Available online at: https://www.britishcardiovascularsociety.org/news/ACEi-or-ARB-and-COVID-19

38. Sorci G, Faivre B, Morand S. Explaining among-country variation in COVID-19 case fatality rate. *Sci Rep.* (2020) 10:18909. doi: 10.1038/s41598-020-75848-2

3

Post-ST-Segment Elevation Myocardial Infarction Follow-Up Care during the COVID-19 Pandemic and the Possible Benefit of Telemedicine

Audrey A. Y. Zhang [1†], Nicholas W. S. Chew [1*†], Cheng Han Ng [2], Kailun Phua [3], Yin Nwe Aye [1], Aaron Mai [2], Gwyneth Kong [2], Kalyar Saw [1], Raymond C. C. Wong [1,2], William K. F. Kong [1,2], Kian-Keong Poh [1,2], Koo-Hui Chan [1,2], Adrian Fatt-Hoe Low [1,2], Chi-Hang Lee [1,2], Mark Yan-Yee Chan [1,2], Ping Chai [1,2], James Yip [1,2], Tiong-Cheng Yeo [1,2], Huay-Cheem Tan [1,2] and Poay-Huan Loh [1,2]

[1] Department of Cardiology, National University Heart Centre, National University Health System, Singapore, Singapore,
[2] Yong Loo Lin School of Medicine, National University of Singapore, Singapore, Singapore, [3] Department of Medicine, National University Hospital, Singapore

*Correspondence:
Nicholas W. S. Chew
nicholas_ws_chew@nuhs.edu.sg

†These authors have contributed equally to this work

Background: Infectious control measures during the COVID-19 pandemic have led to the propensity toward telemedicine. This study examined the impact of telemedicine during the pandemic on the long-term outcomes of ST-segment elevation myocardial infarction (STEMI) patients.

Methods: This study included 288 patients admitted 1 year before the pandemic (October 2018–December 2018) and during the pandemic (January 2020–March 2020) eras, and survived their index STEMI admission. The follow-up period was 1 year. One-year primary safety endpoint was all-cause mortality. Secondary safety endpoints were cardiac readmissions for unplanned revascularisation, non-fatal myocardial infarction, heart failure, arrythmia, unstable angina. Major adverse cardiovascular events (MACE) was defined as the composite outcome of each individual safety endpoint.

Results: Despite unfavorable in-hospital outcomes among patients admitted during the pandemic compared to pre-pandemic era, both groups had similar 1-year all-cause mortality (11.2 vs. 8.5%, respectively, $p = 0.454$) but higher cardiac-related (14.1 vs. 5.1%, $p < 0.001$) and heart failure readmissions in the pandemic vs. pre-pandemic groups (7.1 vs. 1.7%, $p = 0.037$). Follow-up was more frequently conducted via teleconsultations (1.2 vs. 0.2 per patient/year, $p = 0.001$), with reduction in physical consultations (2.1 vs. 2.6 per patient/year, $p = 0.043$), during the pandemic vs. pre-pandemic era. Majority achieved guideline-directed medical therapy (GDMT) during pandemic vs. pre-pandemic era (75.9 vs. 61.6%, $p = 0.010$). Multivariable Cox regression demonstrated achieving medication target doses (HR 0.387, 95% CI 0.164–0.915, $p = 0.031$) and GDMT (HR 0.271, 95% CI 0.134–0.548, $p < 0.001$) were independent predictors of lower 1-year MACE after adjustment.

Conclusion: The pandemic has led to the wider application of teleconsultation, with increased adherence to GDMT, enhanced medication target dosing. Achieving GDMT was associated with favorable long-term prognosis.

Keywords: COVID-19, telemedicine, telehealth, ST-segment elevation myocardial infarction, pandemic

INTRODUCTION

The coronavirus-2019 (COVID-19) pandemic has demanded the rapid adaptation of healthcare operations in implementing measures to reduce the infectious rate but to also maintain the standard of patient care. Patients with cardiovascular disease are at increased risk of contracting the COVID-19 infection with a poorer outcome (1). The universally adopted strategy of social distancing as a measure to "flatten the curve" have resulted in a decrease in traditional physical consultations and the wider adaptation of teleconsultations. Teleconsultations, or telemedicine in general, offers virtual clinic consultations and monitoring which has gained traction as appropriate viable alternative for safe and efficient medical care. Its role has gained attention given the benefits of removing the risk of hospital exposure for these vulnerable patients during the pandemic. As the application of telemedicine expands, it becomes increasingly important to understand its impact on patient care and clinical outcomes.

During the pandemic, there has been a substantial reduction in patients presenting with ST-segment elevation myocardial infarction (STEMI) requiring primary percutaneous coronary intervention (PPCI) compared to the pre-pandemic era (2). Despite the decrease in PPCI case volume, the opposite effect of worse overall in-hospital STEMI performance metrics and short-term clinical outcomes were observed during the pandemic (3, 4). At present, little is known about the follow-up care of these STEMI patients during the pandemic and the potential role of telemedicine in the management of such patients following hospital discharge. This study is the first to examine the trend in teleconsultations for post-STEMI patients during the pandemic, and its association with optimal medical therapy, target medication doses, cardiovascular risk factor control and long-term clinical outcomes.

METHODS

Setting and Design

This is a retrospective single-center study of patients with STEMI who presented to a major PCI-capable hospital in Singapore, and survived the index STEMI admission. Consecutive patients were enrolled into two study groups according to the date of their index admission: (1) Pre-pandemic, from 1 October 2018 to 31 December 2018, and (2) pandemic, from 1 January 2020 to 31 March 2020. Those who did not survive the index admission were excluded from the study. There were no patients who were admitted during both study periods. The follow-up was 1 year following the index STEMI admission. For at least 1 year post-STEMI, the cardiologists of the center visit would traditionally follow up with these patients closely whilst on dual-antiplatelet therapy. It was highly unlikely for these patients to be followed up by other cardiologists outside of the center visit, although these patients might be followed up by doctors from other sub-specialties based on their comorbidities. The time period for the pre-pandemic group was carefully chosen to allow a control with the closest temporal proximity to the COVID-19 pandemic period, without its 1-year post-STEMI follow-up being affected by the pandemic.

During the pandemic, particularly when the Disease Outbreak Response was heightened to its second highest level on 7 February 2020, the standard post-STEMI care after hospital discharge had to be rapidly revamped with increased adaptation of telemedicine. This involved virtual consultations that were conducted via a secure audio-visual telecommunication system between the patients and healthcare providers. Patients were encouraged to subscribe to the hospital telemedicine service and were either provided with or used their own equipment to measure blood pressure, pulse rate and body weight. Patients were also offered remote vital signs monitoring conducted daily for 1 month post-STEMI. Prescriptions were optimized based on the virtual assessment and delivered to the patient's homes. The main goal of teleconsultation during the COVID-19 pandemic was not to provide superior care to the standard face-to-face consultations, but to provide these patients with "health maintenance strategy" individualized to their needs and risk factor control targets (5, 6). The teleconsultation integrated virtual consultations, symptomology assessment, evaluation of home monitoring vitals such as blood pressure, patient education, drug tolerance and adherence, quality of life, and anticoagulation tolerance (7). Physical face-to-face consultations were still conducted, albeit less frequently, during the pandemic and these consultations involved serum testing for cardiovascular risk factor control. Serum measurements of glycated A1c (HbA1c), low-density lipoprotein (LDL) cholesterol, creatinine, estimated glomerular filtration rates (eGFR) and international normalized ratio (INR) (as appropriate) were taken during the physical consultations. Hence, these study periods were carefully chosen to compare the effectiveness of telemedicine on post-STEMI care during the pandemic, vs. the standard post-STEMI care during the pre-pandemic era. Patients with recurrent STEMI presentations during subsequent study periods were excluded to avoid duplication. During the pandemic, the hospital was actively involved in the care for COVID-19 patients.

None of the patients in the study were diagnosed with COVID-19. In our institution, the COVID-19 patients would be co-managed by the pandemic and the Cardiology inpatient teams. Once the COVID-19 patients have been de-isolated with negative COVID-19 polymerase chain reaction tests, they will be transferred under the Cardiology team's care. All patients, regardless of the COVID-19 status, will be reviewed outpatient in the Cardiology clinics. The COVID-19 status of the patients do not have any implications on their post-STEMI management.

Data Collection

Data on demographic and clinical characteristics were retrospectively collected from the hospital STEMI registry. This included past medical history, cardiovascular risk factors, presentation type, presentation route, complications during index admission, and medications on discharge. Angiographic data were also collected from the electronic medical records. Follow-up outpatient data on the number of outpatient consultations (including physical consultations, teleconsultations and cardiac rehabilitation), remote vital signs monitoring uptake, reported symptoms in clinic, and post-discharge medications were obtained. Serial measurements of Hba1c, LDL, and systolic blood pressure during the follow-up period were collected.

Guideline-directed medical therapy for STEMI was defined as being on dual antiplatelet therapy (aspirin and P2Y12 inhibitor), statin, β-blocker, with the option of angiotensin-converting enzyme inhibitor or angiotensin receptor blocker (ACEI/ARB) if the post-STEMI left ventricular ejection fraction (LVEF) was ≤40% or the patient had diabetes mellitus (8, 9), unless these medications were clinically contraindicated in the individual. Patients who were on oral anticoagulation had to complete a month of triple antithrombotic therapy followed by concomitant oral anticoagulation and single antiplatelet, to be considered as being on guideline-directed medical therapy. β-blocker and angiotensin-converting enzyme inhibitors (ACEI) or angiotensin II receptor blocker (ARB) doses were recorded on discharge and at follow-up clinic. Achieving target dose intensity of β-blocker and ACEI/ARB was based on the type and dose of the medication in accordance to a standardized algorithm as defined by our previous study (10). Guideline-directed medical therapy at follow-up was recorded in any of the outpatient clinic visits during the first year post-STEMI. The presence of guideline-directed medical therapy during the outpatient follow-up was used for the multivariable analyses. Our institution adopted the protocol for dual antiplatelet therapy in accordance to the European Society of Cardiology (11) and American College of Cardiology/American Heart Association (12) guidelines in administering a potent $P2Y_{12}$ inhibitor (prasugrel or ticagrelor), or clopidogrel if these are unavailable or contraindicated, and is usually prescribed before percutaneous coronary intervention is performed. Dual antiplatelet therapy was maintained over 12 months unless contraindicated.

Study Outcomes

All study outcomes were measured during the 1-year follow-up from the discharge date of the index admission. The primary safety endpoint was all-cause mortality. Secondary safety endpoints were cardiac readmissions for unplanned revascularisation, non-fatal MI, heart failure, arrhythmia, unstable angina, and major adverse cardiovascular events (MACE). MACE was defined as the composite outcome of each individual safety endpoints.

Secondary efficacy outcomes measured were (1) prescription of guideline-directed medical therapy, (2) achieving target dose intensities of β-blocker and ACEI/ARB (10), and (3) cardiovascular risk factor control (systolic blood pressure, LDL, and HbA1c).

Statistical Analyses

Categorical variables were described as percentages and continuous variables as mean with standard deviation (SD). Continuous variables were assessed with one-way analysis of variance (ANOVA). Categorical variables were evaluated with Pearson's chi-square test (or Fisher's Exact Test where appropriate). The multivariable Cox regression model was constructed to evaluate the association of telemedicine and 1-year MACE, as well as telemedicine and all-cause mortality, which included variables such as achieving medication target doses, guideline-directed medical therapy, remote vital signs monitoring, age, diabetes mellitus, chronic kidney disease, LVEF, smoking status, admission in the pandemic era, and presented with out-of-hospital cardiac arrest and/or cardiogenic shock. These co-variates were carefully chosen as they are traditional prognostic factors in STEMI patients.

Furthermore, *post-hoc* logistic regression was performed to evaluate the association of telemedicine and achieving guideline-directed medical therapy or medication target doses, which included co-variates such as age, smoking status, admission in the pandemic era, out-of-hospital cardiac arrest and cardiogenic shock, LVEF, gender, ethnicity, and presence of symptoms post-discharge. A p-value of < 0.05 was considered statistically significant. All statistical analyses were performed using IBM SPSS Statistics for Windows, Version 25.0. Armonk, NY. This study was conducted in accordance to the revised Declaration of Helsinki and approved by the institutional and local ethics committee (NHG DSRB No. 2013/00442). As the study involved retrospective analysis of clinically acquired data, the institutional review board waived the need for written patient consent.

RESULTS

Baseline Characteristics

Table 1 displays the baseline characteristics of the study population. A total of 320 patients with STEMI who underwent primary PCI were reviewed retrospectively from the local STEMI registry. A total of 17 patients were lost to follow-up, with 6 patients from the pre-pandemic era and 11 from the pandemic era. All patients included in the analysis completed 1-year of follow-up. There were 15 inpatient deaths, 9 and 6 of whom were from the pandemic and pre-pandemic eras, respectively. After excluding inpatient deaths in the index hospitalization, 288 patients who survived their index admission were recruited in the study analysis. There were 170 (59.0%) STEMI patients in the pandemic group, and 118 (41.0%) in the pre-pandemic group. Baseline demographic characteristics and past medical history were similar between both groups. There were more evolved MI

TABLE 1 | Baseline characteristics of study participants with ST-segment elevation myocardial infarction during index admission according to pre-pandemic or pandemic era.

	Total (*n* = 288)	Pandemic (*n* = 170)	Pre-pandemic (*n* = 118)	*P*-value
Demographic				
Age, years	59 (13)	59 (13)	58 (12)	0.626
Sex, female	46 (16.0)	29 (17.1)	17 (14.4)	0.546
Ethnicity				0.448
Chinese	142 (49.3)	88 (51.8)	54 (45.8)	
Malay	58 (20.1)	29 (17.1)	29 (24.6)	
Indian	66 (22.9)	39 (22.9)	27 (22.9)	
Other	22 (7.6)	14 (8.2)	8 (6.8)	
Medical history				
Smoking status				0.952
Non-smoker	130 (45.1)	78 (45.9)	52 (44.1)	
Active smoker	124 (43.1)	72 (42.4)	52 (44.1)	
Ex-smoker	34 (11.8)	20 (11.8)	14 (11.9)	
Hypertension	169 (58.7)	98 (57.6)	71 (60.2)	0.669
Diabetes	113 (39.2)	70 (41.2)	43 (36.4)	0.418
Hyperlipidaemia	179 (62.2)	100 (58.8)	79 (66.9)	0.162
Previous myocardial infarction	38 (13.2)	20 (11.8)	18 (15.3)	0.389
Previous PCI	45 (15.6)	21 (12.4)	24 (20.3)	0.066
Previous CABG	5 (1.7)	1 (0.6)	4 (3.4)	0.073
Stroke	14 (4.9)	8 (4.7)	6 (5.1)	0.883
Chronic kidney disease	23 (8.0)	15 (8.8)	8 (6.8)	0.529
Atrial fibrillation	8 (2.8)	4 (2.4)	4 (3.4)	0.598
Previous heart failure	9 (3.1)	6 (3.5)	3 (2.5)	0.636
Family history of premature CAD	37 (12.8)	28 (16.5)	9 (7.6)	**0.027**
Index admission				
Presentation type				**<0.001**
STEMI	248 (86.1)	136 (80.0)	112 (94.9)	
Evolved MI	23 (8.0)	23 (13.5)	0	
Out-of-hospital cardiac arrest	17 (5.9)	11 (6.5)	6 (5.1)	
Presentation route				0.156
Direct visit	199 (69.1)	112 (65.9)	87 (73.7)	
Interhospital transfers	89 (30.9)	58 (34.1)	31 (26.3)	
Complications				
Heart failure (Killip class 3)	34 (11.8)	26 (15.3)	8 (6.8)	**0.028**
Sepsis	23 (8.0)	18 (10.7)	5 (4.2)	**0.049**
New onset atrial fibrillation	16 (5.6)	14 (8.2)	2 (1.7)	**0.017**
Major bleed	27 (9.4)	18 (10.6)	9 (7.6)	0.397
Cardiogenic shock	21 (7.3)	13 (7.6)	8 (6.8)	0.781
Stroke	3 (1.0)	3 (1.8)	0	0.147
Acute kidney injury	53 (18.4)	27 (15.9)	26 (22.0)	0.185
Inotrope requirement	34 (11.8)	22 (12.9)	12 (10.2)	0.473
Requiring intubation	36 (12.5)	25 (14.7)	11 (9.3)	0.174
Requiring CABG	7 (2.5)	5 (3.2)	2 (1.7)	0.442
Length of stay, days	6 (7)	6 (8)	5 (5)	0.226
LVEF on discharge, %	46 (12)	44 (13)	49 (10)	**0.002**
Angiographic characteristics				
Radial access	210 (73.0)	128 (75.3)	82 (70.1)	0.451
Multivessel disease	140 (48.6)	85 (50.0)	55 (46.6)	0.571
Number of stents				0.616
0	36 (19.3)	30 (19.7)	6 (17.1)	

(Continued)

TABLE 1 | Continued

	Total (*n* = 288)	Pandemic (*n* = 170)	Pre-pandemic (*n* = 118)	*P*-value
1	120 (64.2)	95 (62.5)	25 (71.4)	
2	26 (13.9)	22 (14.5)	4 (11.4)	
3	5 (2.7)	5 (3.3)	0	
Door-to-balloon time, minutes	88 (145)	96 (172)	80 (103)	0.390
Discharge medications Aspirin	269 (93.4)	160 (94.1)	109 (92.4)	0.557
P2Y12 inhibitor	281 (97.6)	170 (100)	111 (94.1)	**0.001**
Oral anticoagulation	13 (4.5)	8 (4.7)	5 (4.2)	0.851
Betablocker	231 (82.5)	136 (84.0)	95 (80.5)	0.454
ACEI/ARB	191 (68.2)	113 (69.8)	78 (66.1)	0.517
Statin	269 (93.7)	157 (92.9)	112 (94.9)	0.488
Guideline-directed medical therapy	220 (76.4)	131 (77.1)	83 (75.4)	0.748

Categorical data presented as n (%). Continuous data presented as mean values (standard deviation).
ACEI, angiotensin converting enzyme inhibitor; ARB, angiotensin receptor blocker; CABG, coronary artery bypass graft; CAD, Coronary artery disease; LVEF, left ventricular ejection fraction; MI, myocardial infarction; PCI, percutaneous coronary intervention; STEMI, ST segment elevation myocardial infarction.
Statistically significant P values are highlighted in bold.

TABLE 2 | Characteristics of study participants with ST-segment elevation myocardial infarction during 1-year follow-up based on pre-pandemic or pandemic era.

	Total (*n* = 288)	Pandemic (*n* = 170)	Pre-pandemic (*n* = 118)	*P*-value
Outpatient consultations				
Total consultations	3.6 (3.1)	4.1 (3.5)	2.7 (2.2)	**<0.001**
Physical consultations	2.4 (1.7)	2.1 (1.6)	2.6 (1.7)	**0.043**
Teleconsultations	0.8 (1.7)	1.2 (1.9)	0.2 (1.1)	**0.001**
Cardiac rehabilitation	0.17 (0.74)	0.1 (0.7)	0.3 (0.7)	**<0.001**
Remote vital signs monitoring	97 (33.7)	59 (34.7)	38 (32.2)	0.659
Reported symptoms				
Typical chest pain	3 (1.2)	1 (0.7)	2 (1.9)	0.386
Atypical chest pain	22 (8.7)	12 (8.2)	10 (9.3)	0.741
Dyspnoea	21 (8.3)	10 (6.8)	11 (10.3)	0.320
Palpitations	3 (1.2)	3 (2.0)	0	0.137
Orthopnoea/PND/lower limb oedema	30 (11.8)	20 (13.6)	10 (9.3)	0.299
Post-discharge medications				
Aspirin	269 (93.4)	160 (94.1)	109 (92.4)	0.557
P2Y12 inhibitor	251 (87.8)	154 (90.6)	97 (83.6)	0.077
Oral anticoagulation	22 (7.6)	12 (7.1)	10 (8.5)	0.656
Beta-blocker	220 (76.9)	136 (80.0)	84 (72.4)	0.135
ACEI/ARB	202 (70.6)	126 (74.1)	76 (65.6)	0.117
Statin	263 (92.0)	158 (92.9)	105 (90.5)	0.459

Categorical data presented as n (%). Continuous data presented as mean values (standard deviation).
ACEI, angiotensin converting enzyme inhibitor; ARB, angiotensin receptor blocker; PND, paroxysmal nocturnal dyspnea.
Total consultations include physical and teleconsultations.
Statistically significant P values are highlighted in bold.

(13.5% vs. none, $p < 0.001$) and out-of-hospital cardiac arrest (6.5 vs. 5.1%, $p < 0.001$) in the pandemic group compared to the pre-pandemic group. Those who were admitted during the pandemic had higher incidence of unfavorable inpatient clinical progress compared to those admitted during the pre-pandemic era, such as Killip class 3 heart failure (15.3 vs. 6.8%, $p = 0.028$), sepsis (10.7 vs. 4.2%, $p = 0.049$), new onset atrial fibrillation (8.2 vs. 1.7%, $p = 0.017$) and lower LVEF (44 vs. 49%, $p = 0.002$). Importantly, there was no difference in discharge medications between the pandemic and pre-pandemic groups, apart from P2Y12 inhibitor use (100 vs. 94.1%, $p = 0.001$, respectively). Of the 7 patients discharged without P2Y12 inhibitor, only 1 was on concomitant oral anticoagulation with aspirin. The prescription of guideline-directed medical therapy on discharge between both groups was similar ($p = 0.748$).

Telemedicine, Guideline-Directed Medical Therapy, Target Drug Dose Intensity, and Cardiovascular Risk Factor Control

The characteristics of study participants during follow-up are described in **Table 2**. The average number of physical consultations per patient over a 1-year period during the pandemic was lower than that in the pre-pandemic era (2.1 vs. 2.6 visits per patient per year, respectively, $p = 0.043$). Conversely, there was higher average number of teleconsultations per patient during the pandemic compared to the pre-pandemic era over the 1-year follow-up (1.2 vs. 0.2 teleconsultations per patient per year, respectively, $p = 0.001$). Cardiac rehabilitation visits were fewer during the pandemic compared to pre-pandemic era (mean of 0.1 vs. 0.3 per patient per year, respectively, $p < 0.001$).

During follow-up, all first visit post-myocardial infarction clinic consultations were physical consultations. The mean duration from discharge to first physical consultation was longer during the pandemic compared to pre-pandemic era (50 ± 39 vs. 39 ± 31 days, respectively, $p = 0.005$), with also longer mean duration between the first physical consultation to second physical consultation during the pandemic compared to pre-pandemic era (128 ± 84 vs. 98 ± 67 days, respectively,

$p = 0.008$). There was no statistical difference in the uptake of remote vital signs monitoring between both study groups.

The pandemic era observed a significantly greater proportion of patients being on guideline-directed medical therapy (75.9%) compared to the pre-pandemic era (61.6%, $p = 0.010$) on follow-up. There was a trend towards achieving medication target doses in both β-blocker (19.4 vs. 15.3%, respectively, $p = 0.363$) and ACEI/ARB (9.5 vs. 5.9%, respectively, $p = 0.278$) during the pandemic compared to the pre-pandemic era.

We observed some differences in cardiovascular risk factor control and laboratory measurements from admission to outpatient surveillance between the pandemic and pre-pandemic periods. Firstly, LDL during index admission was similar in both pandemic and pre-pandemic groups (3.09 vs. 3.14 mmol/L, respectively, $p = 0.588$). Throughout the 1-year follow-up, similar improvement in LDL was achieved in the pandemic and pre-pandemic groups on the first clinic visit (1.81 vs. 1.52 mmol/L, respectively, $p = 0.124$), second visit (1.73 vs. 1.69 mmol/L, respectively, $p = 0.788$) and third visit (1.95 vs. 1.24 mmol/L, respectively, $p = 0.179$). Secondly, the percentage of patients with Hba1c ≥7% was similar between the pandemic and pre-pandemic eras during admission (30.7 vs. 29.0%, respectively, $p = 0.536$) and first clinic visit (29.4 vs. 32.6%,

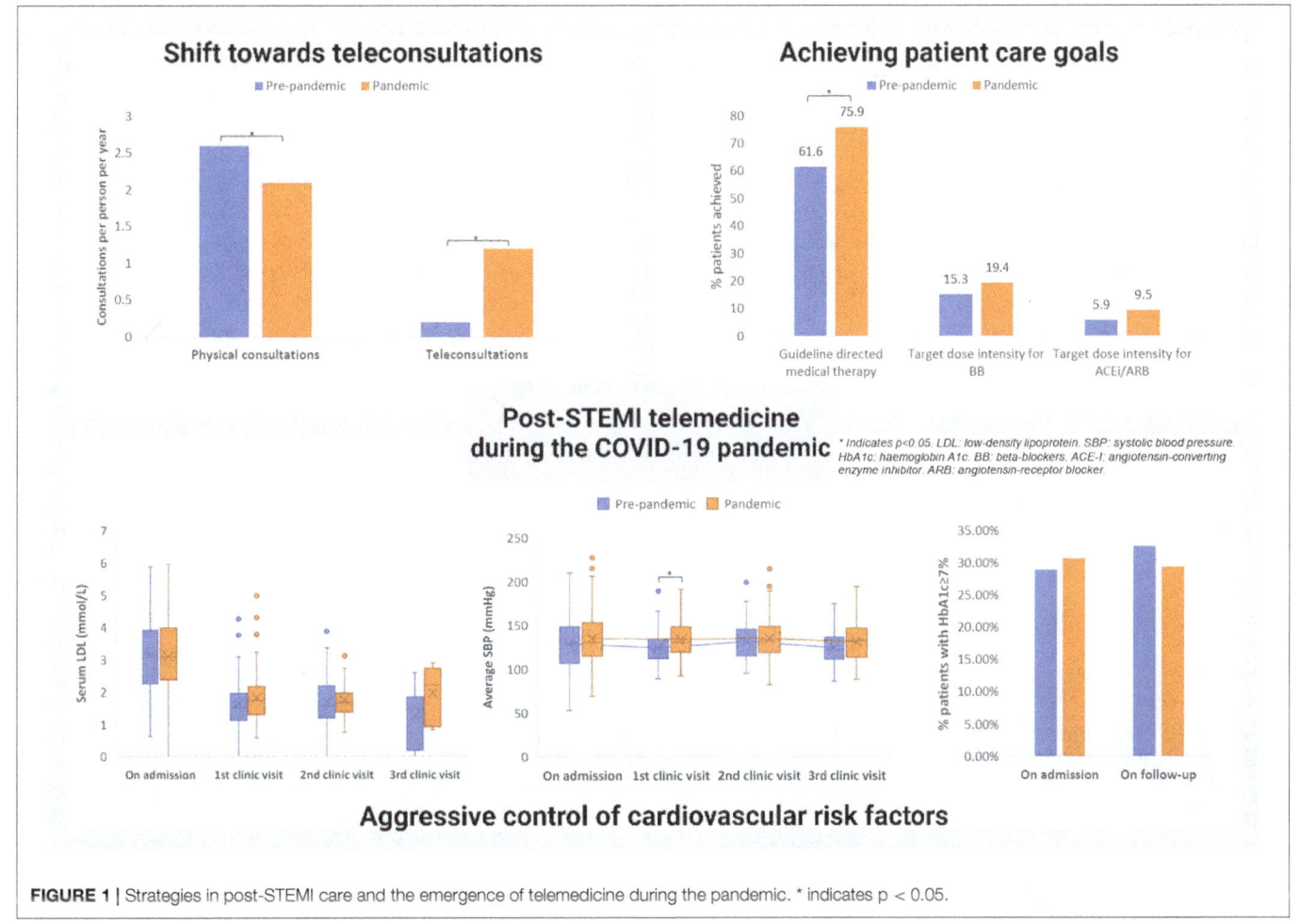

FIGURE 1 | Strategies in post-STEMI care and the emergence of telemedicine during the pandemic. * indicates p < 0.05.

respectively, $p = 0.734$). Thirdly, the average systolic blood pressure measured on discharge (134 vs. 128 mmHg, $p = 0.09$) and first clinic visit (133 vs. 123 mmHg, $p < 0.001$) was higher during the pandemic vs. the pre-pandemic eras; however such difference was no longer observed subsequently during the second (132 vs. 131 mmHg, $p = 0.235$) and third visit (130 vs. 123 mmHg, $p = 0.174$). These findings are summarized in **Figure 1**.

Study Safety End-Point

The 1-year all-cause mortality rates were similar between both groups ($p = 0.454$). However, there was an overall increased cardiac readmissions in the pandemic vs. the pre-pandemic era (14.1 vs. 5.1%, $p < 0.001$). There were increased heart failure readmissions in the pandemic (7.1%) compared to pre-pandemic era (1.7%, $p = 0.037$). No differences in unplanned revascularisation ($p = 0.787$), non-fatal MI ($p = 0.336$), arrhythmia ($p = 0.239$), unstable angina ($p = 0.701$) and MACE ($p = 0.112$) were observed between the two groups (**Table 3**).

On the multivariable Cox regression analysis, there was no significant association between teleconsultation and 1-year MACE [adjusted hazards ratio [aHR] 1.938, 95% confidence interval [CI] 0.896–4.190, $p = 0.093$]. Patients who achieved medication target doses (aHR 0.387, 95% CI 0.164–0.915, $p = 0.031$) and guideline-directed medical therapy (aHR 0.271, 95% CI 0.134–0.548, $p < 0.001$) were significantly associated with decreased rates of MACE after adjusting for important confounders (**Table 4**). There was also no significant association between teleconsultation and 1-year all-cause mortality (aHR 0.867, 95% CI 0.203–3.706, $p = 0.847$) after adjusting for important confounders (**Supplementary Material 1**)

In addition, the association between telemedicine and guideline-directed medical therapy or medication target doses was explored. *Post-hoc* multivariable logistic regression demonstrated that having teleconsultations was significantly associated with achieving guideline-directed medical

therapy [odds ratio [OR] 3.472, 95% CI 1.537–7.843, $p = 0.003$] but not achieving medication target doses (OR 1.272, 95% CI 0.636–2.542, $p = 0.496$), after adjusting for important confounders.

DISCUSSION

The conventional post-STEMI care has been drastically affected by the COVID-19 pandemic, and healthcare institutions have been required to adapt quickly to the stringent infectious control measures without compromising STEMI care. To our knowledge, this study is the first to systematically examine real-world data of the impact of COVID-19 pandemic on the standard of follow-up care and outcomes of STEMI patients over the ensuing year following hospital discharge. Our study has revealed several important findings. Firstly, despite exclusion of those who died while inpatient, patients admitted with STEMI during the pandemic had worse in-hospital outcomes such as increased rates of sepsis, new onset atrial fibrillation, heart failure and reduced left ventricular ejection fraction, compared to the pre-pandemic counterparts. Yet, during the 1-year follow-up, both these groups of patients had similar rates of all-cause mortality, but there were more frequent overall cardiac readmissions and heart failure readmission among those admitted during the pandemic era. This was in conjunction with the wider adaptation of teleconsultations, albeit a reduction of physical consultations, during the pandemic. Secondly, there were significantly more patients achieving guideline-directed medical therapy during the pandemic compared to the pre-pandemic era. Thirdly, there was also a trend toward increased rate of achieving medication target doses of β-blocker and ACEI/ARB therapy during the pandemic vs. the pre-pandemic era. Despite this, patients in the pandemic era had substantially higher mean LDL levels

---

TABLE 3 | Safety and efficacy end-points of the study population during 1-year follow-up post-index ST-segment elevation myocardial infarction admission.

	Total (*n* = 288)	Pandemic (*n* = 170)	Pre-pandemic (*n* = 118)	*P*-value
Safety end-point				
All-cause mortality	29 (10.1)	19 (11.2)	10 (8.5)	0.454
Cardiac readmission				
Unplanned revascularisation	3 (1.0)	2 (1.2)	1 (0.8)	0.787
Non-fatal MI	5 (1.7)	4 (2.4)	1 (0.8)	0.336
Heart failure	14 (4.9)	12 (7.1)	2 (1.7)	**0.037**
Arrythmia	2 (0.7)	2 (1.2)	0	0.239
Unstable angina	6 (2.1)	4 (2.4)	2 (1.7)	0.701
Major adverse cardiac events	59 (20.4)	43 (25.2)	16 (13.6)	0.112
Efficacy end-point				
Guideline-directed medical therapy	202 (70.2)	129 (75.9)	72 (61.6)	**0.010**
Achieving target dose intensity				
ACEI/ARB	23 (8.0)	16 (9.5)	7 (5.9)	0.278
Beta-blocker	51 (17.7)	33 (19.4)	18 (15.3)	0.363

Categorical data presented as n (%).
ACEI, angiotensin converting enzyme inhibitor; ARB, angiotensin receptor blocker; MI, myocardial infarction.
Statistically significant P values are highlighted in bold.

TABLE 4 | Cox regression for 1-year MACE in patients who survived index admission of STEMI.

Variables	Adjusted hazards ratio (95% confidence ratio)	p-value
Teleconsultation	1.938 (0.896–4.190)	0.093
Achieving medication target doses	0.387 (0.164–0.915)	**0.031**
Post-discharge guideline-directed medical therapy	0.271 (0.134–0.548)	**<0.001**
Remote vital signs monitoring	0.512 (0.216–1.213)	0.128
Age	1.024 (1.000–1.050)	0.055
Diabetes mellitus	1.369 (0.706–2.655)	0.353
Chronic kidney disease	3.057 (1.291–7.238)	**0.011**
Left ventricular ejection fraction	0.944 (0.921–0.969)	**<0.001**
Smoker/Ex-smoker	0.609 (0.297–1.246)	0.174
Out-of-hospital cardiac arrest/cardiogenic shock	0.842 (0.348–2.037)	0.702
Admission in pandemic era	1.905 (0.827–4.390)	0.130

Statistically significant P values are highlighted in bold.

on follow-up, albeit statistically non-significant, than those in the pre-pandemic era. Fourthly, for patients who survived the index STEMI admission, achieving medication target doses and guideline-directed medical therapy during the follow-up were independently associated with a lower 1-year MACE. Even though teleconsultation was not an independent predictor of MACE, our findings highlight that teleconsultation had a significant association with achieving guideline-directed medical therapy during follow-up.

As demonstrated by a recent meta-analysis on the global impact of the COVID-19 pandemic on STEMI care (3), short-term STEMI outcomes have been shown to be unfavorable with delayed symptom onset-to-door time, door-to-balloon time, lower LVEF on discharge, suboptimal reperfusion following PCI, increased duration of intensive care unit stay and increased in-hospital mortality during the pandemic era compared to the pre-pandemic era. Similarly, our study has shown worse STEMI metrics during the index admission even after excluding those who did not survive. There were higher overall cardiac related readmissions, particularly heart failure readmissions, in the pandemic compared to pre-pandemic eras. The study sample size, however, might be too small to detect small significant differences in readmission rates in the other subgroups. Despite this, our findings revealed similar 1-year follow-up mortality between both groups. Moreover, achieving medication target doses and guideline-directed medical therapy during follow-up are independent predictors of reducing the risk of MACE. Whether teleconsultation affects the overall outcome of patients with STEMI remains to be investigated. However, it allows for safer and regular follow-up during the pandemic, with drug optimisation for patients in the early post-STEMI period. Importantly, as demonstrated by the present study that patients admitting during the pandemic had worse clinical outcomes during the index admission, this could have increased the demand for closer outpatient surveillance with increased teleconsultations particularly for patients with worse severity of cardiac disease. This might be reflected by the large standard deviation of the average number of teleconsultations in this study. Telemedicine indeed offers a synergistic avenue, in conjunction with physical consultations, in enhancing more frequent

surveillance which is particularly important during the pandemic whilst maintaining the stringent infection control measures. Beyond the pandemic, teleconsultation has been shown to be cost-effective particularly for patients with myocardial infarction, as this important window of follow-up helps ameliorate adverse post-STEMI remodeling, and reduces the potential for the detrimental consequences of chronic heart failure (13).

Our recent published data displayed an increase in STEMI cases during the pandemic compared to the pre-pandemic era, which was partly due to the our regional STEMI network strategy in centralizing primary PCI service at our hospital, taking advantage of the geographical proximity of healthcare hospitals within the West of Singapore allowing timely inter-hospital transfers (14). Our previous study (4) also demonstrated that no significant door-to-balloon delay in inter-hospital transfers between the pandemic and pre-pandemic periods. This allowed the other hospitals to divert resources in providing care for the COVID-19 cases. Moreover, patients admitted during the pandemic had higher incidence of heart failure, sepsis, atrial fibrillation and lower LVEF, compared to those in the pre-pandemic period, which might play a role on the follow-up requirements during the pandemic.

Although telemedicine is a viable alternative, it is not a complete replacement for physical face-to-face consultations. In our study, there was increased overall cardiac related and heart failure readmissions during the pandemic compared to the pre-pandemic era. This could partly be due to the increased in-hospital complications during the pandemic era, such as increased prevalence of Killip class 3 heart failure at presentation and lower LVEF, compared to the pre-pandemic era. However, one might speculate that this observation suggests the limitation of teleconsultation follow-up when it comes to patients at risk of heart failure especially during the early stage following STEMI since it is limited by the absence of face-to-face clinical examination of fluid status and the lack of traditional parameter measurements in clinics such as body weight (15, 16). Nevertheless, the increasing evidence for telemedicine in heart failure management appears promising with several reviews demonstrating significant reduction in heart failure-related hospital admission compared to the conventional care

(17–21). Various trials including Telemedical Interventional Monitoring in Heart Failure (TIM-HF I and TIM-HF II) have shown improved patient education, medication adherence rates, lower mortality, overall hospital admissions and heart failure admissions, with improved quality of life for patients and reduced healthcare costs with the use of telemedicine (22, 23). Hence, patients might require closer monitoring during early stage following STEMI especially those with unfavorable risk factors such as lower LVEF (10).

Teleconsultations allow rapid titration of guideline-directed medical therapy and the increased likelihood of achieving medication target doses. Despite the restrictions during the pandemic, patients were more likely to be on guideline-directed medical therapy with similar medication target dose intensities, compared to their pre-pandemic counterparts. Our study echoes previous landmark trials such that patients achieving guideline-directed medical therapy and target doses have significantly lower rate of MACE (24, 25), especially in the setting of reduced LVEF. Several reviews demonstrated significant benefits in telemedicine for HbA1c (26, 27) and LDL reductions (28, 29), although the evidence for telemedical interventions on lowering blood pressure and body mass index remains mixed (30–32). However, our study highlights the concerns regarding aggressive cardiovascular risk factor control during the pandemic. Even though we demonstrated non-significant differences between pandemic and pre-pandemic groups in terms of LDL control over the 1-year follow-up period, the absolute differences between the serial LDL levels are clinically significant. Clinicians need to be aware of the potentiality of inadequate cardiovascular risk factor control particularly in the pandemic when lifestyle and diet might be changed during the lockdown. Teleconsultation remains the cornerstone of post-STEMI care during the pandemic with timely consultations, prompt initiation and titration of optimal medical therapy, whilst ensuring social distancing and reducing the patient's exposure to the hospital. As it will take time for the telemedicine program to adapt and evolve with the dynamic demands of the pandemic, it is a possibility that there might be variations in follow-up efficacy and efficiency within each of the study groups. However, given the small study sample size, the correlation of monthly variations with clinical outcomes is likely to be underpowered to draw any conclusions. Nevertheless, these are invaluable lessons that we should take beyond the pandemic in reducing waiting and traveling time, and clinic delays, whilst maintaining the standard of post-STEMI care (33–35). The institution is constantly evolving its telemedicine programmes in conjunction with regular physical consultations, and also integrating allied health care practitioner-led remote intensive management in addition to the cardiologist-led standard care (10).

Further studies are needed to evaluate patient's perspective and potential hurdles of telemedicine. Potential hurdles to implementation of telemedicine include patient-related factors associated with older age, low health literacy, cognitive dysfunction, privacy and security concerns (6, 36, 37). In the face of constant evolution of modalities to deliver digital healthcare, the European Society of Cardiology recommends the development of specific training programs for patients, caregivers and medical staff to assist them in understanding the capabilities and limitations of telemedicine (36).

CLINICAL IMPLICATIONS

With enhanced pandemic control measures, there is a pressing need to reduce physical consultations. Telemedicine plays an important role during the pandemic to bridge this gap in providing adequate follow-up to ensure optimisation of medical therapy post-STEMI and maintaining intensive cardiovascular risk factor control (21). It has, at least in part, contributed to the comparable 1-year post-STEMI outcomes between the pandemic and pre-pandemic eras among our patients, despite the adverse in-hospital STEMI metrics observed during the pandemic. These lessons from the pandemic serve a vital and broader role for the future with the emergence of telemedicine in post-STEMI care.

LIMITATIONS

Although this study is the first to examine the feasibility, efficacy, and safety of telemedicine in post-STEMI care during the pandemic, our study has several limitations that merit consideration. Firstly, this is a single-center retrospective observational study with a small sample size, and hence it is not possible to infer causality between telemedicine and the observed clinical outcomes. Nevertheless, our study offers real-world data based on consecutive patients enrolled in our STEMI database, and it reflects the actual follow-up processes that transitioned from physical consultations to teleconsultations during the pandemic. Secondly, the care provided to our control group (pre-pandemic group) might not be representative of care standard that was in line with the current recommendations. Nevertheless, it was chosen as it was the most recent period possible during which the 1-year follow-up care was not affected by the pandemic. Thirdly, teleconsultation was not standardized across all attending physicians and follow-up intervals varied among the patients given the nature of the study and resource constraints during the pandemic. Fourthly, the general attitudes to health and the stresses faced by patients and healthcare providers may also differ during pre-pandemic and pandemic era. For example, the pandemic might motivate the adoption of healthier lifestyle and healthier choices; on the other hand, the social distancing and compulsory home isolation may compel a more sedentary lifestyle (38). New challenges for healthcare providers during the pandemic include the need to comply to social distancing while ensuring the rapport with patients and quality of care are not compromised, and also identifying patients at higher risk of complications in a remote setting (39). However, this study was not designed to evaluate these additional factors which might have an impact on clinical outcomes and cardiovascular risk factor control.

However, our study findings represent actual clinical practice based on the physician's clinical judgment and discretion. Moreover, telemedicine consists of both virtual telehealth clinics and the utility of digital healthcare technologies. However, our study was not designed to evaluate the deliverance of digital healthcare. Overall, the results of the study need to be interpreted with caution, as the study observations might be related to the complex interplay between the COVID-19 pandemic, telemedicine and other non-measurable factors. This retrospective cohort provides, for the first time, real-world data of the dynamic change in hospital follow-up processes in STEMI follow-up with drastic decrease in physical consultations due to social distancing policies and the rapid emergence of telemedicine. With the inherent limitations of a real-world cohort study in this ever-changing landscape during a pandemic, the preliminary findings shed light on the invaluable lessons of teleconsultation adaptation, but controlling for external influences of the pandemic is evidently not possible. Furthermore, we were not able to evaluate if the number of total consultations correlated with improvement in outcomes as the number of consultations was determined by both the routine follow-up as well as the patient's individual need for closer surveillance.

CONCLUSION

Despite the unfavorable in-hospital STEMI metrics of patients admitted during the pandemic, their 1-year mortality rate was similar to those admitted during the pre-pandemic era.

The pandemic led to wider adaptation of teleconsultation which might partly contribute to increased use of guideline-directed medical therapy and meeting medication target dosing. Guideline-directed medical therapy was associated with better outcomes regardless of telemedicine or the pandemic. Telemedicine, at its core, should not be considered a replacement of the traditional face-to-face doctor-patient interactions, but a synergistic extension of post-STEMI care. The invaluable lessons of telemedicine during the pandemic should be extended for future post-STEMI care.

IRB INFORMATION

This study was approved by the local institution review board (NHG DSRB No. 2013/00442).

AUTHOR CONTRIBUTIONS

All authors listed have made a substantial, direct and intellectual contribution to the work, and approved it for publication.

REFERENCES

1. Ganatra S, Hammond SP, Nohria A. The novel coronavirus disease (COVID-19) threat for patients with cardiovascular disease and cancer. *JACC CardioOncol.* (2020) 2:350–55. doi: 10.1016/j.jaccao.2020.03.001
2. De Luca G, Verdoia M, Cercek M, Jenson LO, Vavlukis M, Calmac L, et al. Impact of COVID-19 pandemic on mechanical reperfusion for patients with STEMI. *J Am Coll Cardiol.* (2020) 76:2321–30. doi: 10.1016/j.jacc.2020.09.546
3. Chew NW, Ow ZGW, Teo VXY, Heng RRY, Ng CH, Lee CH, et al. The global impact of the COVID-19 pandemic on STEMI care: a systematic review and meta-analysis. *Can J Cardiol.* (2021) 37:1450–9. doi: 10.1016/j.cjca.2021.04.003
4. Chew NW, Sia CH, Wee HL, Loh JDB, Rastogi S, Kojodjojo P, et al. Impact of the COVID-19 pandemic on door-to-balloon time for primary percutaneous coronary intervention - results from the Singapore Western STEMI Network. *Circ J.* (2021) 85:139–49. doi: 10.1253/circj.CJ-20-0800
5. Cleland JGF, Clark RA, Pellicori P, Inglis SC. Caring for people with heart failure and many other medical problems through and beyond the COVID-19 pandemic: the advantages of universal access to home telemonitoring. *Eur J Heart Fail.* (2020) 22:995–8. doi: 10.1002/ejhf.1864
6. Tersalvi G, Winterton D, Cioffi GM, Ghidini S, Roberto M, Biasco L, et al. Telemedicine in heart failure during COVID-19: a step into the future. *Front Cardiovasc Med.* (2020) 7:612818. doi: 10.3389/fcvm.2020.612818
7. Nan J, Jia R, Meng S, Jin Y, Chen W, Hu H. The impact of the COVID-19 pandemic and the importance of telemedicine in managing acute st segment elevation myocardial infarction patients: preliminary experience and literature review. *J Med Syst.* (2021) 45:9. doi: 10.1007/s10916-020-01703-6
8. O'Gara PT, Kushner FG, Ascheim DD, Casey DE Jr, Chung MK, de Lemos JA, et al. 2013 ACCF/AHA guideline for the management of ST-elevation myocardial infarction: a report of the American College of Cardiology Foundation/American Heart Association Task Force on Practice Guidelines. *Circulation.* (2013) 127:e362–425. doi: 10.1161/CIR.0b013e3182742c84
9. Ibanez B, James S, Agewall S, Antunes MJ, Bucciarelli-Ducci C, Bueno H, et al. 2017 ESC Guidelines for the management of acute myocardial infarction in patients presenting with ST-segment elevation: the Task Force for the management of acute myocardial infarction in patients presenting with ST-segment elevation of the European Society of Cardiology (ESC). *Eur Heart J.* (2018) 39:119–77. doi: 10.1093/eurheartj/ehx393
10. Chan MY, Koh KWL, Poh SC, Marchesseau S, Singh D, Han Y, et al. Remote postdischarge treatment of patients with acute myocardial infarction by allied health care practitioners vs standard care: the IMMACULATE randomized clinical trial. *JAMA Cardiol.* (2020) 6:830–5. doi: 10.1001/jamacardio.2020.6721
11. Valgimigli M, Bueno H, Byrne RA, Collet JP, Costa F, Jeppsson A, et al. 2017 ESC focused update on dual antiplatelet therapy in coronary artery disease developed in collaboration with EACTS: the Task Force for dual antiplatelet therapy in coronary artery disease of the European Society of Cardiology (ESC) and of the European Association for Cardio-Thoracic Surgery (EACTS). *Eur Heart J.* (2018) 39:213–60. doi: 10.1093/eurheartj/ehx419
12. Levine GN, Bates ER, Bittl JA, Brindis RG, Fihn SD, Fleisher LA, et al. 2016 ACC/AHA guideline focused update on duration of dual antiplatelet therapy in patients with coronary artery disease. *Circulation.* (2016) 134:e123–55. doi: 10.1161/CIR.0000000000000404
13. Roth GA, Johnson C, Abajobir A, Abd-Allah F, Abera SF, Abyu G, et al. Global, regional, and national burden of cardiovascular diseases for 10 causes, 1990 to 2015. *J Am Coll Cardiol.* (2017) 70:1–25. doi: 10.1016/j.jacc.2017.04.052
14. Phua K, Chew NWS, Sim V, Zhang AA, Rastogi S, Kojodjojo P, et al. One-year outcomes of patients with ST-segment elevation myocardial infarction during the COVID-19 pandemic. *J Thromb Thrombolysis.* (2021) 1–11 doi: 10.1007/s11239-021-02557-6
15. Tse G, Chan C, Gong M, Meng L, Zhang J, Su XL, et al. Telemonitoring and hemodynamic monitoring to reduce hospitalization rates in heart

failure: a systematic review and meta-analysis of randomized controlled trials and real-world studies. *J Geriatr Cardiol.* (2018) 15:298–309. doi: 10.11909/j.issn.1671-5411.2018.04.008

16. Emani S. Remote monitoring to reduce heart failure readmissions. *Curr Heart Fail Rep.* (2017) 14:40–7. doi: 10.1007/s11897-017-0315-2

17. Conway A, Inglis SC, Clark RA. Effective technologies for noninvasive remote monitoring in heart failure. *Telemed J E Health.* (2014) 20:531–8. doi: 10.1089/tmj.2013.0267

18. Kotb A, Cameron C, Hsieh S, Wells G. Comparative effectiveness of different forms of telemedicine for individuals with heart failure (HF): a systematic review and network meta-analysis. *PLoS ONE.* (2015) 10:e0118681. doi: 10.1371/journal.pone.0118681

19. Piotrowicz E. The management of patients with chronic heart failure: the growing role of e-Health. *Expert Rev Med Devices.* (2017) 14:271–277. doi: 10.1080/17434440.2017.1314181

20. Yun JE, Park JE, Park HY, Lee HY, Park DA. Comparative effectiveness of telemonitoring versus usual care for heart failure: a systematic review and meta-analysis. *J Card Fail.* (2018) 24:19–28. doi: 10.1016/j.cardfail.2017.09.006

21. Carbo A, Gupta M, Tamariz L, Palacio A, Levis S, Nemeth Z, et al. Mobile technologies for managing heart failure: a systematic review and meta-analysis. *Telemed J E Health.* (2018). doi: 10.1089/tmj.2017.0269

22. Koehler F, Winkler S, Schieber M, Sechtem U, Stangl K, Böhm M, et al. Telemedical Interventional Monitoring in Heart Failure (TIM-HF), a randomized, controlled intervention trial investigating the impact of telemedicine on mortality in ambulatory patients with heart failure: study design. *Eur J Heart Fail.* (2010) 12:1354–62. doi: 10.1093/eurjhf/hfq199

23. Koehler F, Koehler K, Prescher S, Sechtem U, Stangl K, Böhm M, et al. Mortality and morbidity 1 year after stopping a remote patient management intervention: extended follow-up results from the telemedical interventional management in patients with heart failure II (TIM-HF2) randomised trial. *Lancet Digit Health.* (2020) 2:e16–24. doi: 10.1016/S2589-7500(19)30195-5

24. Dargie HJ. Effect of carvedilol on outcome after myocardial infarction in patients with left-ventricular dysfunction: the CAPRICORN randomised trial. *Lancet.* (2001) 357:1385–90. doi: 10.1016/S0140-6736(00)04560-8

25. Effect of ramipril on mortality and morbidity of survivors of acute myocardial infarction with clinical evidence of heart failure. The Acute Infarction Ramipril Efficacy (AIRE) Study Investigators. *Lancet.* (1993) 342:821–8.

26. Eberle C, Stichling S. Clinical improvements by telemedicine interventions managing type 1 and type 2 diabetes: systematic meta-review. *J Med Internet Res.* (2021) 23:e23244. doi: 10.2196/23244

27. Eberle C, Stichling S. Effect of Telemetric interventions on glycated hemoglobin A1c and management of type 2 diabetes mellitus: systematic meta-review. *J Med Internet Res.* (2021) 23:e23252. doi: 10.2196/23252

28. Akbari M, Lankarani KB, Naghibzadeh-Tahami A, Tabrizi R, Honarvar B, Kolahdooz F, et al. The effects of mobile health interventions on lipid profiles among patients with metabolic syndrome and related disorders: a systematic review and meta-analysis of randomized controlled trials. *Diabetes Metab Syndr.* (2019) 13:1949–55. doi: 10.1016/j.dsx.2019.04.011

29. Lau D, McAlister FA. Implications of the COVID-19 pandemic for cardiovascular disease and risk-factor management. *Can J Cardiol.* (2021) 37:722–32. doi: 10.1016/j.cjca.2020.11.001

30. Parati G, Pellegrini D, Torlasco C. How digital health can be applied for preventing and managing hypertension. *Curr Hypertens Rep.* (2019) 21:40. doi: 10.1007/s11906-019-0940-0

31. Timpel P, Oswald S, Schwarz PEH, Harst L. Mapping the evidence on the effectiveness of telemedicine interventions in diabetes, dyslipidemia, and hypertension: an umbrella review of systematic reviews and meta-analyses. *J Med Internet Res.* (2020) 22:e16791. doi: 10.2196/16791

32. Huang JW, Lin YY, Wu NY. The effectiveness of telemedicine on body mass index: a systematic review and meta-analysis. *J Telemed Telecare.* (2019) 25:389–401. doi: 10.1177/1357633X18775564

33. Kronenfeld JP, Penedo FJ. Novel Coronavirus (COVID-19): telemedicine and remote care delivery in a time of medical crisis, implementation, and challenges. *Transl Behav Med.* (2021) 11:659–63. doi: 10.1093/tbm/ibaa105

34. Orlando JF, Beard M, Kumar S. Systematic review of patient and caregivers' satisfaction with telehealth videoconferencing as a mode of service delivery in managing patients' health. *PLoS ONE.* (2019) 14:e0221848. doi: 10.1371/journal.pone.0221848

35. Knox L, Rahman RJ, Beedie C. Quality of life in patients receiving telemedicine enhanced chronic heart failure disease management: a meta-analysis. *J Telemed Telecare.* (2017) 23:639–49. doi: 10.1177/1357633X16660418

36. Frederix I, Caiani EG, Dendale P, Anker S, Bax J, Böhm A, et al. ESC e-cardiology working group position paper: overcoming challenges in digital health implementation in cardiovascular medicine. *Eur J Prev Cardiol.* (2019) 26:1166–77. doi: 10.1177/2047487319832394

37. Walker RC, Tong A, Howard K, Palmer SC. Patient expectations and experiences of remote monitoring for chronic diseases: Systematic review and thematic synthesis of qualitative studies. *Int J Med Inform.* (2019) 124:78–85. doi: 10.1016/j.ijmedinf.2019.01.013

38. Esther T. Van der Werf, Martine Busch, Meik C. Jong, Hoenders HJR. Lifestyle changes during the first wave of the COVID-19 pandemic: a cross-sectional survey in the Netherlands. *BMC Public Health.* (2021) 21:1226. doi: 10.1186/s12889-021-11264-z

39. Verhoeven V, Tsakitzidis G, Philips H, Royen PV. Impact of the COVID-19 pandemic on the core functions of primary care: will the cure be worse than the disease? A qualitative interview study in Flemish GPs. *BMJ Open.* (2020) 10:e039674. doi: 10.1136/bmjopen-2020-039674

4

Impact of Angiotensin-Converting Enzyme Inhibitors and Angiotensin Receptor Blockers on the Inflammatory Response and Viral Clearance in COVID-19 Patients

Linna Huang [1,2,3†], Ziying Chen [1,2,3,4†], Lan Ni [5], Lei Chen [6], Changzhi Zhou [7], Chang Gao [8], Xiaojing Wu [1,2,3], Lin Hua [9], Xu Huang [1,2,3], Xiaoyang Cui [1,2,3], Ye Tian [1,2,3], Zeyu Zhang [1,2,3] and Qingyuan Zhan [1,2,3*]

[1] Center for Respiratory Diseases, China-Japan Friendship Hospital, Beijing, China, [2] Department of Pulmonary and Critical Care Medicine, China-Japan Friendship Hospital, Beijing, China, [3] National Clinical Research Center for Respiratory Diseases, Beijing, China, [4] Peking University Health Science Center, Beijing, China, [5] Department of Pulmonary and Critical Care Medicine, Zhongnan Hospital of Wuhan University, Wuhan, China, [6] Department of Pulmonary and Critical Care Medicine, Tongji Hospital, Tongji Medical College, Huazhong University of Science and Technology, Wuhan, China, [7] Department of Pulmonary and Critical Care Medicine, The Central Hospital of Wuhan, Wuhan, China, [8] Department of Critical Care Medicine, The First Affiliated Hospital of Soochow University, Suzhou, China, [9] School of Biomedical Engineering, Capital Medical University, Beijing, China

*Correspondence:
Qingyuan Zhan
drzhanqy@163.com

† These authors have contributed equally to this work

Objectives: To evaluate the impact of angiotensin-converting enzyme inhibitors (ACEIs) or angiotensin receptor blockers (ARBs) on the inflammatory response and viral clearance in coronavirus disease 2019 (COVID-19) patients.

Methods: We included 229 patients with confirmed COVID-19 in a multicenter, retrospective cohort study. Propensity score matching at a ratio of 1:3 was introduced to eliminate potential confounders. Patients were assigned to the ACEI/ARB group ($n = 38$) or control group ($n = 114$) according to whether they were current users of medication.

Results: Compared to the control group, patients in the ACEI/ARB group had lower levels of plasma IL-1β [(6.20 ± 0.38) vs. (9.30 ± 0.31) pg/ml, $P = 0.020$], IL-6 [(31.86 ± 4.07) vs. (48.47 ± 3.11) pg/ml, $P = 0.041$], IL-8 [(34.66 ± 1.90) vs. (47.93 ± 1.21) pg/ml, $P = 0.027$], and TNF-α [(6.11 ± 0.88) vs. (12.73 ± 0.26) pg/ml, $P < 0.01$]. Current users of ACEIs/ARBs seemed to have a higher rate of vasoconstrictive agents (20 vs. 6%, $P < 0.01$) than the control group. Decreased lymphocyte counts [(0.76 ± 0.31) vs. $(1.01 \pm 0.45)*10^9$/L, $P = 0.027$] and elevated plasma levels of IL-10 [(9.91 ± 0.42) vs. (5.26 ± 0.21) pg/ml, $P = 0.012$] were also important discoveries in the ACEI/ARB group. Patients in the ACEI/ARB group had a prolonged duration of viral shedding [(24 ± 5) vs. (18 ± 5) days, $P = 0.034$] and increased length of hospitalization [(24 ± 11) vs. (15 ± 7) days, $P < 0.01$]. These trends were similar in patients with hypertension.

Conclusions: Our findings did not provide evidence for a significant association between ACEI/ARB treatment and COVID-19 mortality. ACEIs/ARBs might decrease proinflammatory cytokines, but antiviral treatment should be enforced, and hemodynamics should be monitored closely. Since the limited influence on the ACEI/ARB treatment, they should not be withdrawn if there was no formal contraindication.

Keywords: ACE inhibitor, ARB, inflammatory response, viral clearance, COVID-19

INTRODUCTION

Up to March 31, 2020, the total number of patients with coronavirus disease 2019 has risen sharply to nearly 700,000 globally, with a mortality rate of nearly 5%. Meanwhile, this epidemic seems to be spreading at an exponential rate and has become an urgent public health emergency of international concern.

Several large retrospective studies have revealed that pre-existing cardiovascular disease and diabetes were the most frequent comorbidities of coronavirus disease 2019 (COVID-19) patients (1–3); these patients even had a higher risk of mortality (4, 5) than those with underlying respiratory disease. Angiotensin-converting enzyme inhibitors (ACEIs) and angiotensin receptor blockers (ARBs) are widely prescribed for these patients. ACEIs/ARBs have an impact on the renin-angiotensin system (RAS) and are postulated to attenuate pulmonary and systemic inflammatory responses, reducing the severity and mortality of viral pneumonia-related acute respiratory distress syndrome (6–8), ultimately by angiotensin-converting enzyme 2 (ACE2) upregulation through the ACE2-Ang-(1-7)-Mas axis (9).

The molecular biology of severe acute respiratory syndrome coronavirus 2 (SARS-CoV-2) is well-established, as it appears to bind to its target cells through ACE2, which is expressed by epithelial cells of the lung, to enable it to infect host cells (10, 11). The expression of ACE2 is substantially increased in patients who are treated with ACE inhibitors and ARBs (12), which promotes SARS-CoV-2 entry into the body, increasing the risk of developing COVID-19 (13, 14).

The controversial pathogenesis as well as the mixed results of several clinical studies (15, 16) of pneumonia with other pathogens made it difficult for physicians to determine whether the use of ACE inhibitors or ARBs should be terminated in patients with COVID-19.

To date, the actual impact of ACE inhibitor and ARB prescriptions on COVID-19 patients has not been assessed in current studies. Therefore, we aimed to evaluate the clinical manifestations and outcomes, especially inflammatory responses and viral clearance, by a multicenter, retrospective cohort study.

MATERIALS AND METHODS

Study Design and Population

We retrospectively included patients with microbiologically confirmed cases of COVID-19 according to the World Health Organization (WHO) (17) and official Chinese guidelines (18) in a multicenter retrospective cohort study performed at three tertiary hospitals in Wuhan, Hubei Province, China (Tongji Hospital, Tongji Medical College, Huazhong University of Science and Technology; Zhongnan Hospital of Wuhan University; and the Central Hospital of Wuhan) from February 15, 2020 to March 25, 2020. Patients included in our study were all assessed for eligibility on the basis of positive SARS-CoV-2 nucleic acid testing results by reverse transcription-polymerase chain reaction (RT-PCR) with nasopharyngeal swab samples. However, it was not possible to determine whether the patients had pneumonia, as not all were available for CT scans.

Exclusion Criteria

(1) Patients younger than 18 years old.

(2) Patients still hospitalized at the end of the study.

All patients were treated according to the standard protocols for antiviral, antibiotic, glucocorticoid, and Chinese medicine treatments.

The ethics committee of China-Japan Friendship Hospital approved this study (2020-21-K16). Written informed consent was waived due to the rapid emergence of this infectious disease.

Group Division

We divided the patients into two groups. The ACEI/ARB group included patients who were current users of ACE inhibitors or ARB medication, while non-current users were included as the control group. Patients in the ACEI/ARB group were further divided into subgroups of a continued medication group and a terminated medication group according to the application of ACE inhibitors or ARBs during hospitalization.

Data Collection and Analysis

We collected data on the following parameters from the hospital electronic medical record systems, nursing records, laboratory examination systems, and radiological examinations and obtained standardized data collection forms: demographic characteristics, comorbidities, medication history within 1 month, symptoms at admission, laboratory finding changes from day 1 to day 14, radiological manifestations, treatment during hospitalization and outcome data that contained the rate of in-hospital death and progression, the duration of viral shedding, the length of hospital stay and the time from onset to death or discharge. The primary outcome was mortality at discharge, while the secondary outcomes we observed included the duration of hospital stay, the duration of viral shedding and the differences in inflammatory cytokines.

Patients with cardiovascular disease and diabetes are often taking a combination of medications with statins (19) and oral hypoglycemic agents, especially thiazolidinediones, which have been reported to have an impact on the level of ACE2 by several studies (14, 20). To further control for potential confounders, data on the use of statins, thiazolidinediones and other antihypertensive agents (α receptor blocking agents, β receptor blocking agents, calcium channel blockers and diuretics) prior to admission in each group were calculated within 90 days (6).

Two researchers also independently reviewed the data collection forms to double check the data collected. Any missing or uncertain records of the epidemiological, medication and symptom data were collected and clarified through direct communication with patients and their families.

We compared the two groups in terms of the above aspects to identify the differences between current users and non-users prior to admission. Then, among the current users of ACEIs/ARBs, an analysis was conducted by comparing the dynamic changes in indicators involved in immune status and inflammatory reactions, as well as the outcomes between patients who continued and terminated medication during hospitalization. As hypertension itself could activate the RAS, patients with hypertension were excluded to avoid potential confounders. A comparison of the immune status, inflammatory reactions and outcomes between the ACEI/ARB and control groups in patients without hypertension was conducted.

Cytokine and Chemokine Measurement

To evaluate the impact of coronavirus and additional ACE inhibitors or ARBs on the production of cytokines or chemokines in the acute phase of the illness, plasma cytokines and chemokines [interleukin 1β (IL-1β), IL-2R, IL-6, IL-8, IL-10, and tumor necrosis factor α (TNF-α)] were measured using chemiluminescent immunoassays (CLIAs) (CFDA approved) by Siemens IMMULITE 1000 for patients according to the manufacturer's instructions.

Definitions

Medications classified as ACE inhibitors were benazepril, perindopril and fosinopril, while the ARBs of the included patients were candesartan, irbesartan, valsartan, olmesartan, telmisartan, and losartan.

Patients were considered a current user of medication if they had a supply of medication to last until the date of hospitalization assuming an 80% compliance rate (6, 21). The patients who did not meet the definition were regarded as non-current users. ACE inhibitors or ARBs were considered to be continued if they were given more than 50% of the days during hospitalization (8); otherwise, they were considered to be terminated.

In-hospital progression was defined as a decline in PaO_2/FiO_2 of more than 100 mmHg or the need for invasive positive pressure ventilation (IPPV) and/or extracorporeal membrane oxygenation (ECMO) during hospitalization.

The duration of viral shedding was defined as the duration of the SARS-CoV-2 RNA test result becoming negative from positive. All patients were routinely reexamined for SARS-CoV-2 nucleic acid testing every 5 days to assess whether it had turned negative.

Shock was defined according to the interim guidance of the WHO for novel coronavirus (22). Acute kidney injury (AKI) was identified and classified on the basis of the highest serum creatinine level or urine output criteria according to the Kidney Disease Improving Global Outcomes Classification (KDIGO) (22, 23). Respiratory failure, coagulation and liver failure were defined as a Sequential Organ Failure Assessment (SOFA) score greater than or equal to two points.

Statistical Analysis

Descriptive statistics included proportions for categorical variables and the mean (standard deviation) or median (interquartile range) for continuous variables. Data were unadjusted unless specifically stated otherwise.

Processing of Missing Data

When the missing rate of vital variables involved in our study was <15%, we used SAS predictive mean matching imputation to replace missing values within each variable, while the variables were abandoned when the missing rate reached 20%.

Processing of the Unbalanced Sample Size: Propensity Score Matching

The propensity score matching (PSM) method was applied at a ratio of 1:3 between the ACEI/ARB group and the control group. The Sequential Organ Failure Assessment (SOFA) score, Charlson's comorbidity index (CCI), and body mass index (BMI) were matched variables in PSM to derive the cohort. The overall balance test was conducted to confirm that the baseline data of the two groups matched successfully.

Proportions were compared using χ^2 or Fisher's exact tests, and continuous variables were compared using the t-test or Wilcoxon rank sum test, as appropriate. Statistical significance was defined as a two-tailed P-value of ≤ 0.05. SAS software, version 9.4 (SAS Institute Inc.) was used for all analyses.

RESULTS

From February 15, 2020 to March 25, 2020, a total of 229 patients with confirmed cases of COVID-19 were admitted; 51 patients were current users of ACEIs/ARBs, while the other 178 patients were non-current users of the medication. The PSM method was applied at a ratio of 1:3 between the ACEI/ARB group ($n = 38$) and the control group ($n = 114$). The SOFA score and CCI were matched variables in PSM to derive the cohort. Thirteen cases in the ACEI/ARB group and 64 cases in the control group were not matched successfully. The overall balance test was with no significant difference between the two groups ($P = 0.872$). Among the patients with ACEI/ARB medication, 18 continued medication during hospitalization, while the other 20 terminated medication (**Figure 1**). The mean age was 57 ± 12 years, male patients accounted for 52% ($n = 79$), the SOFA score was 1.5 (1–2.3) points, and the CCI was 1 (1–2) prior to admission.

Comparisons of Baseline Prior Hospitalization Between the ACEI/ARB and Control Groups

The ACEI/ARB group included more patients with hypertension (67 vs. 22%, $P < 0.01$) than the control group. The demographic characteristics, other comorbidities, severity of the condition and possible medication histories might have influenced the ACE2 level but did not differ significantly between the two groups. No significant difference was found between the two groups in

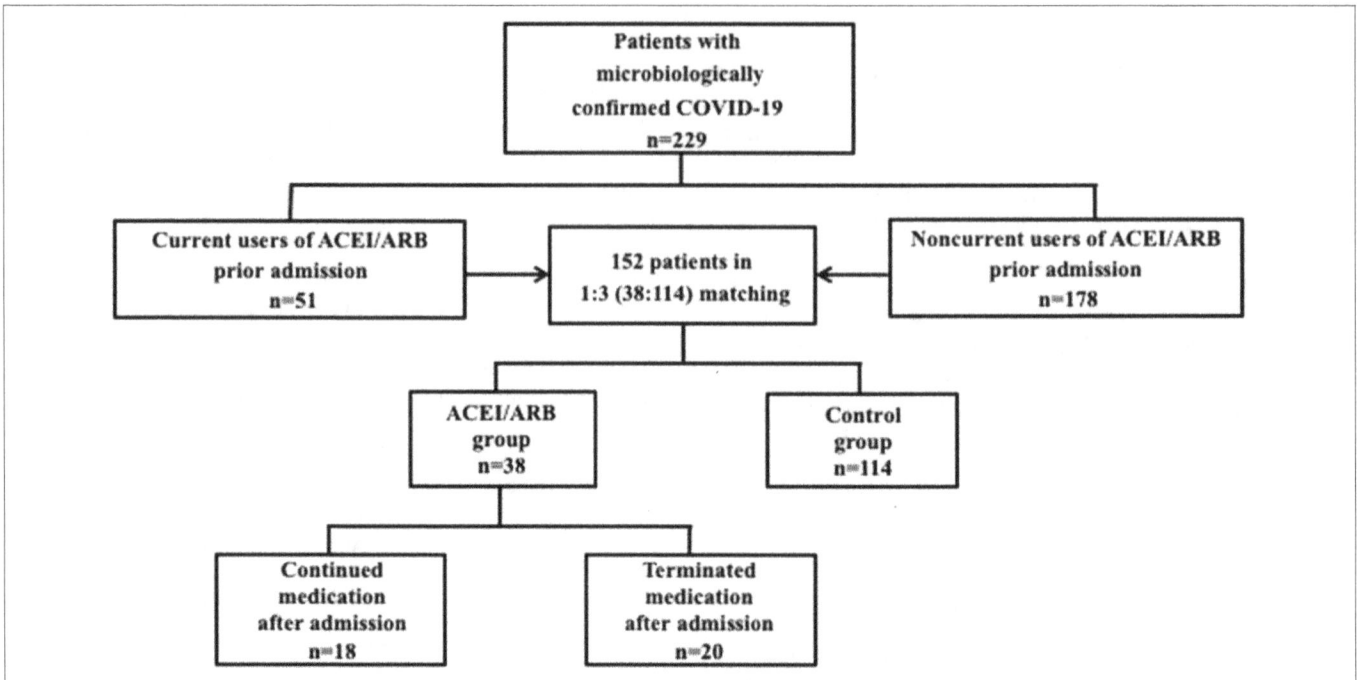

FIGURE 1 | Flowchart. A flowchart illustrated the enrollment of patients in our study. From February 15, 2020 to March 25, 2020, a total of 229 patients with confirmed cases of COVID-19 were admitted; 51 patients were current users of ACEIs/ARBs, while the other 178 patients were non-current users of the medication. The PSM method was applied at a ratio of 1:3 between the ACEI/ARB group (*n* = 38) and the control group (*n* = 114). The SOFA score and CCI were matched variables in PSM to derive the cohort. Among the patients with ACEI/ARB medication, 18 continued medication during hospitalization, while the other 20 terminated medication.

time from onset to hospitalization and to COVID-19 diagnosis (**Table 1**).

Comparisons of Clinical Symptoms, Laboratory Examinations, and Radiological Manifestations on Admission Between the ACEI/ARB and Control Groups

The symptoms, including fever, cough, hemoptysis, dyspnea, fatigue/myalgia and diarrhea, as well as vital signs, with the exception of systolic blood pressure, were not significantly different between the ACEI/ARB group and the control group. Although systolic blood pressure was lower in the study group (116 ± 14 vs. 124 ± 13 mmHg, $P = 0.031$), it was within the normal range. For laboratory examinations, patients with ACE inhibitor or ARB medication had lower lymphocyte counts [(0.76 ± 0.31) vs. (1.01 ± 0.45) $*10^9$/L, $P = 0.027$] than the control group (**Table 2**).

The first measurements of the inflammatory factors, including IL-1β, IL-2R, IL-6, IL-8, IL-10, and TNFα, were taken within 3 days of admission; while the most (97%, 147/152) were within 24 h. The time from COVID-19 diagnose to measurements was (3 ± 2) days. Besides, as the missing rate reached 12–15%, SAS predictive mean matching imputation was applied to replace missing values in each group. The missing rates of IL-2R, serum ferritin, erythrocyte sedimentation rate (ESR) and C-reactive protein (CRP) were as high as 25–35%; therefore, they were abandoned in the statistical analysis. Patients in the

ACEI/ARB group had slightly lower levels of proinflammatory cytokines, including IL-1β [(6.20 ± 0.38) vs. (9.30 ± 0.31) pg/ml, $P = 0.020$], IL-6 [(31.86 ± 4.07) vs. (48.47 ± 3.11) pg/ml, $P = 0.041$], IL-8 [(34.66 ± 1.90) vs. (47.93 ± 1.21) pg/ml, $P = 0.027$], and TNF-α [(6.11 ± 0.88) vs. (12.73 ± 0.26) pg/ml, $P < 0.01$], and higher levels of the anti-inflammatory cytokine IL-10 [(9.91 ± 0.42) vs. (5.26 ± 0.21) pg/ml, $P = 0.012$] than the control group (**Table 2**).

Comparison of Organ Function, Treatment and Outcomes During Hospitalization Between the ACEI/ARB and Control Groups

Current users of ACEIs/ARBs seemed to have a higher rate of vasoconstrictive agent application (18 vs. 7%, $P < 0.01$) than the control group; however, the percentages of respiratory failure, shock, AKI, coagulation failure, and liver failure were not different between the two groups. In addition, the necessities for invasive IPPV and ECMO were not decreased in the ACEI/ARB group (**Table 3**).

The duration of viral shedding [(24 ± 5) vs. (18 ± 5) days, $P = 0.034$], length of hospital stay [(24 ± 11) vs. (15 ± 7) days, $P < 0.01$], and time from onset to death or discharge [(32 ± 10) vs. (25 ± 7) days, $P < 0.01$] were longer in the ACEI/ARB group than in the control group, while no difference was found in the rate of in-hospital progression or death (**Table 3**).

TABLE 1 | Baseline variables in the two groups prior to admission.

	All ($n = 152$)	ACEI/ARB group ($n = 38$)	Control group ($n = 114$)	P
Age, years, mean ± SD	57 ± 12	57 ± 11	58 ± 18	0.671
Gender (men), number (%)	79 (52%)	19 (51%)	60 (53%)	0.533
Body mass index, kg/m², mean ± SD	21.0 ± 6.9	21.1 ± 6.4	21.0 ± 7.0	0.838
Comorbidities, number (%)				
Hypertension	55 (36%)	30 (67%)	25 (22%)	<0.001[b]
Diabetes	37 (24%)	10 (27%)	27 (24%)	0.217
Coronary heart disease	17 (11%)	6 (16%)	11 (10%)	0.071
Chronic heart failure	6 (4%)	2 (5%)	4 (4%)	0.622
Underlying lung disease	18 (12%)	7 (18%)	11 (10%)	0.094
Chronic kidney disease	2 (1%)	1 (3%)	1 (1%)	0.512
Chronic liver dysfunction	3 (2%)	0 (0%)	3 (3%)	0.425
Malignancy	3 (2%)	0 (0%)	3 (3%)	0.186
History of smoking, number (%)	23 (15%)	8 (21%)	15 (13%)	0.081
Other medication history within 90 days, number (%)				
Corticosteroids	0 (0%)	0 (0%)	0 (0%)	1
Immunosuppressants	0 (0%)	0 (0%)	0 (0%)	1
Statins	21 (14%)	6 (16%)	15 (13%)	0.214
Thiazolidinediones	1 (1%)	0 (0%)	1 (1%)	0.996
α receptor blocking agent	4 (3%)	1 (3%)	3 (3%)	0.820
β receptor blocking agent	19 (13%)	5 (13%)	14 (12%)	0.731
CCB	19 (13%)	5 (13%)	14 (12%)	0.731
Diuretics	16 (11%)	4 (11%)	12 (11%)	1
SOFA Score, points (IQR)	1.5 (1–2.3)	1.5 (1–2.5)	1.5 (1–2)	0.879
CCI, points (IQR)	1 (1–2)	1 (1–2)	1 (1–2)	1
Treatment before hospital, number (%)				
Methylprednisolone	10 (7%)	3 (8%)	7 (6%)	0.091
Antibiotic therapy	92 (61%)	22 (58%)	70 (61%)	0.429
Antiviral therapy	102 (67%)	22 (57%)	80 (70%)	0.239
Time from onset to hospital admission, days, mean ± SD	10 ± 6	11 ± 3	10 ± 6	0.296
Time from onset to diagnosis, days, mean ± SD	7 ± 5	7 ± 5	7 ± 2	0.8

[b]$P < 0.01$; CCB, calcium channel blocker; SOFA, Sequential Organ Failure Assessment; CCI, Charlson's Comorbidity Index (18).

Subgroup Analyses: Comparison Between Patients Who Continued and Terminated Medication During Hospitalization

Among the patients in the ACEI/ARB group, 18 continued medication during hospitalization, while the other 20 terminated medication for several reasons. The baseline variables were with no significant difference between the two groups (**Supplementary Table 1**). The dynamic changes in lymphocytes and inflammatory factors at the first, seventh, and fourteenth days after hospitalization as well as the outcomes were compared between the two groups. The missing rates of IL-2R and IL-8 at seven days and 14 days after admission were extremely high and were not included in the analysis. Patients with continued use of ACEIs/ARBs had consistently lower levels of lymphocytes, IL-1β, IL-6, and TNF-α but maintained higher levels of IL-10 on the seventh and fourteenth days than patients who terminated medication during hospitalization. However, the patients who terminated the medication had a trend of elevated lymphocyte counts [day 1, day 7, day 14: (0.82 ± 0.47) vs. (1.41 ± 0.74) vs. (1.69 ± 0.45)*10⁹/L, $P = 0.029$] and IL-1β [day 1, day 7, day 14: (6.03 ± 3.19) vs. (10.78 ± 6.88) vs. (13.75 ± 5.26) pg/ml,

$P < 0.01$] from the first day to the fourteenth day (**Figure 2, Supplementary Table 2**).

The duration of viral shedding [(27 ± 4) vs. (21 ± 5) days, $P = 0.032$], length of hospital stay [(26 ± 10) vs. (20 ± 3) days, $P = 0.044$], and time from onset to death or discharge [(34 ± 9) vs. (29 ± 10) days, $P = 0.019$] were longer in the continued medication group than in the terminated medication group. The rates of in-hospital progression and death were not significantly different between the two groups (**Table 4**).

Subgroup Analyses: A Comparison of the Immune Status, Inflammatory Reactions and Outcomes Between the ACEI/ARB and Control Groups in Patients With Hypertension

Among 55 patients with hypertension, 30 patients were divided into the study group (ACEI/ARB group), and the other 25 patients were in the control group.

Compared with the control group, the patients in the study group had lower levels of IL-1β [(6.33 ± 0.56) vs. (8.27 ± 0.14)

TABLE 2 | Clinical, laboratory findings, and radiological manifestations in the two groups on admission.

	All (*n* = 152)	ACEI/ARB group (*n* = 38)	Control group (*n* = 114)	*P*
Initial symptoms, number (%)				
Fever (≥37.3°C)	140 (92%)	35 (92%)	105 (92%)	0.981
Cough	109 (72%)	27 (70%)	82 (72%)	0.866
Productive cough	60 (39%)	16 (42%)	44 (39%)	0.605
Hemoptysis	3 (2%)	1 (3%)	2 (2%)	0.263
Dyspnea	78 (51%)	20 (53%)	58 (51%)	0.432
Fatigue or myalgia	67 (44%)	16 (43%)	51 (45%)	0.619
Diarrhea	46 (30%)	12 (31%)	34 (30%)	0.764
Initial signs, mean ± SD				
Highest temperature, °C	38.4 ± 0.7	38.5 ± 1.1	38.3 ± 0.4	0.461
Respiratory rate, breaths/min	23 ± 3	22 ± 3	23 ± 3	0.709
Heart rate, beats/min	96 ± 11	97 ± 8	96 ± 14	0.338
Systolic blood pressure, mmHg	123 ± 10	116 ± 14	124 ± 13	0.031[a]
SpO$_2$, %	94 ± 4	93 ± 3	94 ± 4	0.741
FiO$_2$, %	40 ± 18	42 ± 15	40 ± 17	0.302
Laboratory examination, mean ± SD				
Blood routine				
WBC, *10^9/L	5.94 ± 3.00	6.27 ± 3.21	5.80 ± 2.97	0.085
Neutrophil count, *10^9/L	4.40 ± 2.99	5.21 ± 3.29	4.39 ± 3.01	0.097
Lymphocytes, *10^9/L	0.89 ± 0.40	0.76 ± 0.31	1.01 ± 0.45	0.027[a]
Biochemical examination				
ALT, U/L	43 ± 4	42 ± 4	43 ± 4	0.747
AST, U/L	40 ± 5	44 ± 4	40 ± 5	0.841
TBIL, mmol/L	11.3 ± 5.2	11.0 ± 5.9	11.4 ± 5.0	0.660
Scr, μmol/L	79.2 ± 2.7	77.5 ± 2.2	80.1 ± 3.6	0.915
LDH, U/L	295 ± 89	301 ± 77	294 ± 91	0.617
TnT, pg/ml	11 ± 1	12 ± 1	11 ± 1	0.770
NT-proBNP, pg/ml	401 ± 55	411 ± 55	397 ± 51	0.528
Inflammatory factors				
IL-1β, pg/ml	8.02 ± 0.33	6.20 ± 0.38	9.30 ± 0.31	0.020[a]
IL-2R, U/ml	796.02 ± 27.40	724.25 ± 52.30	807.23 ± 26.21	0.246
IL-6, pg/ml	47.11 ± 3.26	31.86 ± 4.07	48.47 ± 3.11	0.041[a]
IL-8, pg/ml	46.03 ± 1.85	34.66 ± 1.90	47.93 ± 1.21	0.027[a]
IL-10, pg/ml	6.37 ± 0.37	9.91 ± 0.42	5.26 ± 0.21	0.012[b]
TNF-α, pg/ml	11.21 ± 0.44	6.11 ± 0.88	12.73 ± 0.26	<0.001[b]
PCT, ng/ml	0.27 ± 0.07	0.26 ± 0.03	0.29 ± 0.08	0.619
Coagulation function				
PT, s	14 ± 3	14 ± 1	14 ± 1	0.995
APTT, s	42 ± 5	44 ± 3	42 ± 5	0.881
D-Dimer, μg/ml	2.19 ± 0.44	2.33 ± 0.47	2.12 ± 0.46	0.448
Chest CT manifestations, number (%)				
Bilateral lesion	82 (54%)	19 (49%)	63 (55%)	0.374
GGO	89 (59%)	19 (49%)	70 (61%)	0.310
Consolidation	36 (24%)	11 (29%)	25 (22%)	0.229

[a]*P* < 0.05; [b]*P* < 0.01; *SpO$_2$, saturation of peripheral oxygen; FiO$_2$, fraction of inspiration; ALT, alanine aminotransferase; AST, aspartate aminotransferase; TBIL, total bilirubin; Scr, creatinine; LDH, lactate dehydrogenase; TnT, troponin T; NT-proBNP, N-terminal pro-brain natriuretic peptide; IL-1β, interleukin-1β; IL-2R, interleukin-2R; IL-6, interleukin-6; IL-8, interleukin-8; IL-10, interleukin-10; TNF-α, tumor necrosis factor-α; PCT, procalcitonin; PT, prothrombin time; APTT, activated partial thromboplastin time; GGO, ground-glass opacity.*

pg/ml, *P* = 0.026], IL-6 [(40.16 ± 12.59) vs. (52.33 ± 14.09) pg/ml, *P* = 0.030], and IL-8 [(31.60 ± 2.97) vs. (42.83 ± 3.27) pg/ml, *P* = 0.030] on admission. Regarding clinical outcomes, the duration of viral shedding [(26 ± 6) vs. (19 ± 4) days, *P* = 0.029] and time from onset to death or discharge [(30 ± 10) vs. (24 ± 8) days, *P* = 0.031] were longer in the study group than in the

TABLE 3 | Organ function, treatments and outcomes in the two groups during hospitalization.

	All (n = 152)	ACEI/ARB group (n = 38)	Control group (n = 114)	P
Organ failure*, number (%)				
Respiratory failure	25 (16%)	8 (20%)	17 (15%)	0.092
Shock	13 (9%)	4 (11%)	8 (7%)	0.060
AKI	15 (10%)	4 (11%)	11 (10%)	0.829
Coagulation failure	3 (2%)	1 (3%)	2 (2%)	0.664
Liver failure	15 (10%)	4 (11%)	11 (10%)	0.796
Treatment, number (%)				
Antibiotics	105 (69%)	24 (64%)	81 (71%)	0.461
Antiviral treatment	145 (95%)	36 (92%)	109 (96%)	0.334
Glucocorticoids	49 (32%)	11 (30%)	38 (33%)	0.612
Intravenous immunoglobin	36 (24%)	9 (23%)	27 (24%)	0.552
Standard oxygen therapy	132 (87%)	35 (92%)	97 (85%)	0.080
HFNO	28 (18%)	7 (18%)	21 (18%)	0.927
NPPV	18 (12%)	5 (12%)	13 (11%)	0.327
IPPV	17 (11%)	4 (11%)	13 (11%)	0.629
ECMO	4 (3%)	1 (3%)	3 (3%)	0.994
Vasoconstrictive agents	15 (10%)	7 (18%)	8 (7%)	<0.01[b]
Outcome				
In-hospital progression[#], number (%)	28 (18%)	6 (16%)	22 (19%)	0.326
In-hospital death, number (%)	15 (10%)	4 (10%)	11 (10%)	0.983
Hospital length of stay, days, mean ± SD	17 ± 8	24 ± 11	15 ± 7	<0.01[b]
Duration of viral shedding, days, mean ± SD	19 ± 3	24 ± 5	18 ± 5	0.034[a]
Time from onset to death or discharge, days, mean ± SD	27 ± 9	32 ± 10	25 ± 7	<0.01[b]

[a]$P < 0.05$; [b]$P < 0.01$; *Shock was defined according to the interim guidance of the WHO for novel coronavirus (22, 23). AKI was identified and classified on the basis of the highest serum creatinine level or urine output criteria according to kidney disease, improving global outcome classification (23, 24). Respiratory failure, coagulation and liver failure were defined as a SOFA score greater than or equal to two points. [#]Defined as a decline in $PaO_2/FiO_2 > 100$ mmHg or the need for IPPV and/or ECMO during hospitalization. AKI, acute kidney injury; HFNO, high flow nasal oxygenation; NPPV, noninvasive positive pressure ventilation; IPPV, invasive positive pressure ventilation; ECMO, extracorporeal membrane oxygenation.

control group; however, no difference was detected in the rate of in-hospital progression and death between the two groups.

DISCUSSION

To our knowledge, this is the first study to thoroughly evaluate the inflammatory responses and viral clearance of COVID-19 patients treated with ACEIs/ARBs by a multicenter, retrospective cohort control study and to allow dynamic observation of inflammatory responses by continuous monitoring from the first to the fourteenth day after admission.

The major findings of our study were that ACEIs/ARBs inhibited the proinflammatory response but promoted the anti-inflammatory response and persistently decreased lymphocytes, thus extending the duration of viral shedding and the length of hospital stay. Antiviral treatments should be enforced in those patients. In addition, since current users of ACEIs/ARBs seem to have a higher necessity of vasoconstrictive agents, hemodynamics should be monitored closely during medication use. The message to the physician was that the influence on the ACEI/ARB treatment was limited, and they should not be withdrawn if there was no formal contraindication.

Inflammation is mediated by proinflammatory cytokines and anti-inflammatory cytokines. Inappropriate elevated expression of proinflammatory cytokines can result in sepsis, tissue destruction, or death (21, 24). Our study revealed that the plasma levels of IL-1β, IL-6, IL-8, and TNF-α in patients taking ACEI/ARBs were lower than those in patients not without medication; in addition, persistently lower levels of proinflammatory factors were maintained in patients who continued medication during hospitalization, which was consistent with the previous experimental results by Gullestad et al. (25) with the conclusion that high-dose enalapril was associated with a significant decrease in IL-6 activity in patients with severe chronic heart failure. The specific organ and systemic inflammatory responses were postulated to attenuate through a reduction in the level of cytokines, which might be explained by the attenuating effects of ACE inhibitors through the deactivation of the ACE-AngII-AT1 axis but the stimulation of the ACE2-Ang-(1-7)-Mas axis in a feedback mechanism (9, 26, 27) as a negative regulator with attenuated cytokines and thus protecting the patients from organ injury. Consequently, some authors (28, 29) have speculated that the use of ACEIs/ARBs might actually be a potentially beneficial intervention in those with COVID-19.

Apart from organ protection by attenuating the inflammatory response, basic investigation has shown that bradykinin and substance P produced by ACE inhibitors sensitize the sensory

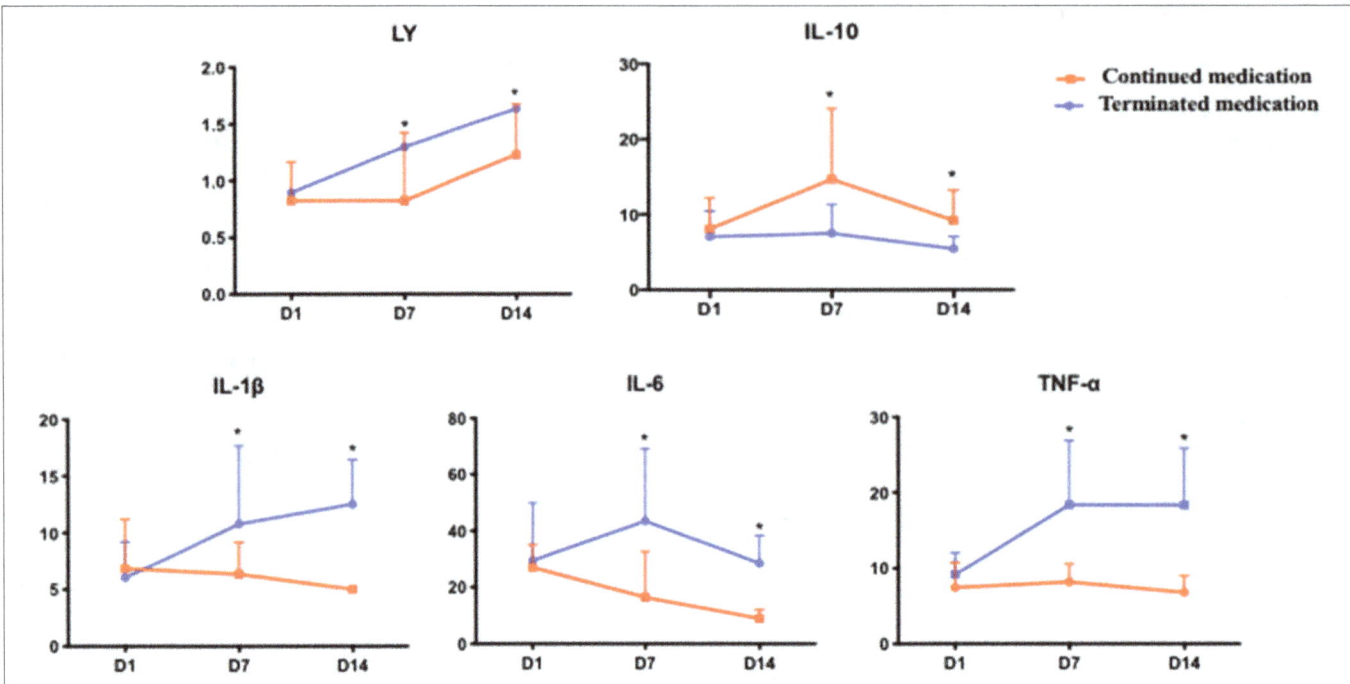

FIGURE 2 | The dynamic changes in the lymphocyte counts and inflammatory factors between patients who continued and those who terminated ACEIs/ARBs during hospitalization. Patients with continued use of ACEIs/ARBs had consistently lower levels of lymphocytes, IL-1β, IL-6, and TNF-α but maintained higher levels of IL-10 on the seventh and fourteenth days than patients who terminated medication during hospitalization. However, the patients who terminated the medication had a trend of elevated lymphocyte counts and IL-1β from the first day to the fourteenth day. *$p < 0.01$.

TABLE 4 | Outcomes in patients who continued and those who terminated ACEIs/ARBs during hospitalization.

Outcomes	Continued ACEIs/ARBs (n = 18)	Terminated ACEIs/ARBs (n = 20)	P
In-hospital progression[#]	3 (17%)	3 (15%)	0.611
In-hospital death	2 (11%)	2 (10%)	0.709
Duration of viral shedding, days	27 ± 4	20 ± 5	0.032[a]
Hospital length of stay, days	26 ± 10	20 ± 3	0.044[a]
Time from onset to death or discharge, days	34 ± 9	29 ± 10	0.019[a]

[a]$P < 0.05$; [#]Defined as a decline in $PaO_2/FiO_2 > 100$ mmHg or the need for IPPV and/or ECMO during hospitalization.

nerves of the airways and enhance the cough reflex (30, 31), which plays a protective role against pathogens. These two mechanics made it possible to improve the outcome in patients with pneumonia. Mortensen et al. (6) found a significant decrease in mortality, the length of hospital stay, and mechanical ventilation in patients taking ACE/ARBs who were hospitalized with pneumonia compared to a matched cohort. A meta-analysis (32) that included 19 studies noted that patients taking ACE inhibitors were associated with a significant approximately one-third reduction in the risk of pneumonia compared with controls. In addition, a recent study (8) by Christopher Henry also observed lower rates of death and intubation with continued use of ACE inhibitors than with terminated use (OR = 0.25; 95% CI, 0.09–0.64) throughout the hospital stay in cases of viral pneumonia not due to coronavirus. Unfortunately, our study did not find decreased mortality in patients with current use of ACEI/ARBs, even though we analyzed patients with continued medication during hospitalization and combined with hypertension to avoid potential confounding factors. The most likely explanation was that our study included a small number of patients, while most of their patients had mild cases as determined by SOFA scores and without excessive inflammatory reactions, which was the target for ACE inhibitors or ARBs.

What noteworthy was that ACEI/ARBs increased the necessity of vasoconstrictive agents. It could be explained by the nature of the antihypertensive agents and came as a revelation to us that the hemodynamics should be monitored closely during medication.

Our research also revealed that ACE inhibitors or ARBs led to prolonged viral shedding and extended the length of hospitalization. SARS-CoV-2 appears to bind to its target cells through angiotensin-converting enzyme 2 (ACE2). ACE inhibitors or ARBs upregulate ACE2 receptor expression in humans (33) by blocking the classic ACE pathway; thus, it is theoretically possible that the pre-existing use of these drugs might predispose a person to infection with a greater viral load of SARS-CoV-2 (13). This hypothesis was supported by the evidence of Ferrario that there was a 4.7-fold increase in cardiac ACE2 mRNA by an ACE inhibitor (34). Decreased lymphocyte counts and elevated plasma levels of IL-10 were also important discoveries in patients with ACEI/ARBs. Moreover, the lymphocyte counts in patients with continued use of medication during hospitalization recovered slowly, as observed by successive monitoring on the first to fourteenth days. The immune status was weakened by lymphocytopenia and elevated anti-inflammatory cytokines in patients taking ACEI/ARBs, which might be another reason for the slow viral clearance. As the important criterion for discharge was the negative conversion of the SARS-CoV-2, prolonged viral shedding led to an extended length of hospitalization. This might be the defect of the ACEI/ARBs and might explain the mixed results and controversy about their prescription in COVID-19 patients. For this reason, antiviral therapy in patients taking ACEI/ARBs should be reinforced, and their viral load should be monitored closely.

An autopsy report revealed that mononuclear inflammatory infiltration dominated by lymphocytes was observed in the lungs, but no virus inclusion bodies were found (35). We could then propose a hypothesis that cytokines released by inflammatory storms secondary to viral infection might be more important in the death of critically ill patients with COVID-19 than the viral infection itself in a certain period. From this perspective, it is possible that ACEI/ARBs might improve the outcome in critically ill patients with excessive inflammatory responses or severe multiple organ failure; when the inflammatory storm gradually diminishes, the focus of therapy should be on clearance of the virus and the enhancement of the immune system. Prospective cohort and randomized controlled trials are needed to confirm this hypothesis and examine potential mechanisms of action.

Our study was limited by the small number of patients included and by not strictly excluding confounding factors. We especially noticed that the number of patients with hypertension was much higher in the ACEI/ARB group, which might be an important confounding factor. However, by subgroup analyze in patients with hypertension, we found similar results. The prospective randomized controlled studies designed by increasing the sample size and strictly excluding potential confounders to explore the impact of ACE/ARBs on inflammatory responses, viral clearance and the mortality in COVID-19 patients should be encouraged in the future.

AUTHOR CONTRIBUTIONS

All authors made substantial contributions to the conception and design of the study or to the data acquisition, analysis, or interpretation, reviewed and approved the final manuscript, and significantly contributed to this study. QZ took full responsibility for the integrity of the submission and publication and was involved in the study design. LHuang and ZC involved in data collection, had full access to all of the data in the study, took responsibility for the integrity of the data and were responsible for data verification, as well as the drafting of the manuscript. LHua took the responsibility for statistical analysis and the accuracy of the data analysis. Others involved in data collection, had full access to all of the data in the study, and took responsibility for the integrity of the data.

REFERENCES

1. Yang X, Yu Y, Xu J, Shu H, Xia J, Liu H, et al. Clinical course and outcomes of critically ill patients with SARS-CoV-2 pneumonia in Wuhan, China: a single-centered, retrospective, observational study. *Lancet Respir Med.* (2020) 8:e26. doi: 10.1016/S2213-2600(20)30079-5

2. Guan WJ, Ni ZY, Hu Y, Liang WH, Ou CQ, He JX, et al. Clinical characteristics of Covid-19 in China. *N Engl J Med.* (2020) 382:1859–62. doi: 10.1056/NEJMc2005203

3. Zhang JJ, Dong X, Cao YY, Yuan YD, Yang YB, Yan YQ, et al. Clinical characteristics of 140 patients infected with SARS-CoV-2 in Wuhan, China. *Allergy.* (2020) 75:1730–41. doi: 10.1111/all.14238

4. Wu C, Chen X, Cai Y, Xia J, Zhou X, Xu S, et al. Risk factors associated with acute respiratory distress syndrome and death in patients with coronavirus disease 2019 pneumonia in Wuhan, China. *JAMA Intern Med.* (2020) 180:934–43. doi: 10.1001/jamainternmed.2020.0994

5. Zhou F, Yu T, Du R, Fan G, Liu Y, Liu Z, et al. Clinical course and risk factors for mortality of adult inpatients with COVID-19 in Wuhan, China: a retrospective cohort study. *Lancet.* (2020) 395:1054–62. doi: 10.1016/S0140-6736(20)30566-3

6. Mortensen EM, Pugh MJ, Copeland LA, Restrepo MI, Cornell JE, Anzueto A, et al. Impact of statins and angiotensin-converting enzyme inhibitors on mortality of subjects hospitalised with pneumonia. *The Eur Respir J.* (2008) 31:611–7. doi: 10.1183/09031936.00162006

7. Wu A, Good C, Downs JR, Fine MJ, Pugh MJ, Anzueto A, et al. The association of cardioprotective medications with pneumonia-related outcomes. *PLoS ONE.* (2014) 9:e85797. doi: 10.1371/journal.pone.0085797

8. Henry C, Zaizafoun M, Stock E, Ghamande S, Arroliga AC, White HD. Impact of angiotensin-converting enzyme inhibitors and statins on viral pneumonia. *Proceedings.* (2018) 31:419–23. doi: 10.1080/08998280.2018.1499293

9. Tan WSD, Liao W, Zhou S, Mei D, Wong WF. Targeting the renin-angiotensin system as novel therapeutic strategy for pulmonary diseases. *Curr Opin Pharmacol.* (2018) 40:9–17. doi: 10.1016/j.coph.2017.12.002

10. Walls AC, Park YJ, Tortorici MA, Wall A, McGuire AT, Veesler D. Structure, function, and antigenicity of the SARS-CoV-2 spike glycoprotein. *Cell.* (2020) 181:281–92.e6. doi: 10.1016/j.cell.2020.02.058

11. Hoffmann M, Kleine-Weber H, Schroeder S, Kruger N, Herrler T, Erichsen S, et al. SARS-CoV-2 cell entry depends on ACE2 and TMPRSS2 and is blocked by a clinically proven protease inhibitor. *Cell.* (2020) 181:271–80.e8. doi: 10.1016/j.cell.2020.02.052

12. Li XC, Zhang J, Zhuo JL. The vasoprotective axes of the renin-angiotensin system: physiological relevance and therapeutic implications in cardiovascular, hypertensive and kidney diseases. *Pharmacological Res.* (2017) 125(Pt A):21–38. doi: 10.1016/j.phrs.2017.06.005

13. Thomson G. COVID-19: social distancing, ACE2 receptors, protease inhibitors and beyond? *Int J Clin Pract.* (2020) 74:e13503. doi: 10.1111/ijcp.13503

14. Fang L, Karakiulakis G, Roth M. Are patients with hypertension and diabetes mellitus at increased risk for COVID-19 infection? *Lancet Respir Med.* (2020) 8:e21. doi: 10.1016/S2213-2600(20)30116-8

15. Okaishi K, Morimoto S, Fukuo K, Niinobu T, Hata S, Onishi T, et al. Reduction of risk of pneumonia associated with use of angiotensin I converting enzyme inhibitors in elderly inpatients. *Am J Hypertens.* (1999) 12(8 Pt 1):778–83. doi: 10.1016/S0895-7061(99)00035-7

16. Van de Garde EM, Souverein PC, van den Bosch JM, Deneer VH, Leufkens HG. Angiotensin-converting enzyme inhibitor use and pneumonia risk in a general population. *Eur Respir J.* (2006) 27:1217–22. doi: 10.1183/09031936.06.00110005

17. World Health Organization. *Clinical Management of Severe Acute Respiratory Infection When Novel Coronavirus (nCoV) Infection is Suspected: Interim Guidance.* (2020). Available online at: https://www.who.int/publications-detail/clinical-management-of-severe-acute-respiratory-infection-when-novel-coronavirus-(ncov)-infection-is-suspected

18. National Health Commission of the People's Republic of China. *Chinese Management Guideline for COVID-19 (Version 7.0).* (2020). Available online at: http://211.136.65.146/cache/www.nhc.gov.cn/yzygj/s7653p/202003/46c9294a7dfe4cef80dc7f5912eb1989/files/ce3e6945832a438eaae415350a8ce964.pdf?ich_args2=65-11155015043898_f32a0b9f969d8670abb9ee3d42d8e898_10001002_9c896c2ad2caf0d59239518939a83798_0ad7c3e0d3161a7f69a04f61b3ce861b.

19. Chopra V, Rogers MA, Buist M, Govindan S, Lindenauer PK, Saint S, et al. Is statin use associated with reduced mortality after pneumonia? A systematic review and meta-analysis. *Am J Med.* (2012) 125:1111–23. doi: 10.1016/j.amjmed.2012.04.011

20. Wan Y, Shang J, Graham R, Baric RS, Li F. Receptor recognition by the novel coronavirus from Wuhan: an analysis based on decade-long structural studies of SARS coronavirus. *J Virol.* (2020) 94:e00127-20. doi: 10.1128/JVI.00127-20

21. Mortensen EM, Nakashima B, Cornell J, Copeland LA, Pugh MJ, Anzueto A, et al. Population-based study of statins, angiotensin II receptor blockers, and angiotensin-converting enzyme inhibitors on pneumonia-related outcomes. *Clin Infect Dis.* (2012) 55:1466–73. doi: 10.1093/cid/cis733

22. Huang C, Wang Y, Li X, Ren L, Zhao J, Hu Y, et al. Clinical features of patients infected with 2019 novel coronavirus in Wuhan, China. *Lancet.* (2020) 395:497–506. doi: 10.1016/S0140-6736(20)30183-5

23. Kidney Disease: Improving Global Outcomes (KDIGO) Acute Kidney Injury Work Group. *KDIGO Clinical Practice Guideline for Acute Kidney Injury.* (2012). Available online at: https://kdigo.org/wp-content/uploads/2016/10/KDIGO-2012-AKI-Guideline-English.pdf (accessed January 23, 2020).

24. Nathan C. Points of control in inflammation. *Nature.* (2002) 420:846–52. doi: 10.1038/nature01320

25. Gullestad L, Aukrust P, Ueland T, Espevik T, Yee G, Vagelos R, et al. Effect of high- versus low-dose angiotensin converting enzyme inhibition on cytokine levels in chronic heart failure. *J Am Coll Cardiol.* (1999) 34:2061–7. doi: 10.1016/S0735-1097(99)00495-7

26. Duprez DA. Role of the renin-angiotensin-aldosterone system in vascular remodeling and inflammation: a clinical review. *J Hypertension.* (2006) 24:983–91. doi: 10.1097/01.hjh.0000226182.60321.69

27. Marchesi C, Paradis P, Schiffrin EL. Role of the renin-angiotensin system in vascular inflammation. *Trends Pharmacol Sci.* (2008) 29:367–74. doi: 10.1016/j.tips.2008.05.003

28. Liu Y, Yang Y, Zhang C, Huang F, Wang F, Yuan J, et al. Clinical and biochemical indexes from 2019-nCoV infected patients linked to viral loads and lung injury. *Sci China Life Sci.* (2020) 63:364–74. doi: 10.1007/s11427-020-1643-8

29. Sun M, Yang JM, Sun YP, Su GH. Inhibitors of RAS might be a good choice for the therapy of COVID-19 pneumonia. *Zhonghua Jie He He Hu Xi Za Zhi.* (2020) 43:219–22. doi: 10.3760/cma.j.issn.1001-0939.2020.03.016

30. Fox AJ, Lalloo UG, Belvisi MG, Bernareggi M, Chung KF, Barnes PJ. Bradykinin-evoked sensitization of airway sensory nerves: a mechanism for ACE-inhibitor cough. *Nat Med.* (1996) 2:814–7. doi: 10.1038/nm0796-814

31. Tomaki M, Ichinose M, Miura M, Hirayama Y, Kageyama N, Yamauchi H, et al. Angiotensin converting enzyme (ACE) inhibitor-induced cough and substance P. *Thorax.* (1996) 51:199–201. doi: 10.1136/thx.51.2.199

32. Caldeira D, Alarcao J, Vaz-Carneiro A, Costa J. Risk of pneumonia associated with use of angiotensin converting enzyme inhibitors and angiotensin receptor blockers: systematic review and meta-analysis. *BMJ.* (2012) 345:e4260. doi: 10.1136/bmj.e4260

33. Vuille-dit-Bille RN, Camargo SM, Emmenegger L, Sasse T, Kummer E, Jando J, et al. Human intestine luminal ACE2 and amino acid transporter expression increased by ACE-inhibitors. *Amino Acids.* (2015) 47:693–705. doi: 10.1007/s00726-014-1889-6

34. Turgeon RD, Kolber MR, Loewen P, Ellis U, McCormack JP. Higher versus lower doses of ACE inhibitors, angiotensin-2 receptor blockers and beta-blockers in heart failure with reduced ejection fraction: systematic review and meta-analysis. *PLoS ONE.* (2019) 14:e0212907. doi: 10.1371/journal.pone.0212907

35. Wang H-j, Du S-h, Yue X, Chen C-x. Review and prospect of pathological features of corona virus disease. *Fa Yi Xue Za Zhi.* (2020) 36:16–20. doi: 10.12116/j.issn.1004-5619.2020.01.004

5

Frequent Constriction-Like Echocardiographic Findings in Elite Athletes Following Mild COVID-19: A Propensity Score-Matched Analysis

Bálint Károly Lakatos [1]*, Márton Tokodi [1], Alexandra Fábián [1], Zsuzsanna Ladányi [1], Hajnalka Vágó [1,2], Liliána Szabó [1], Nóra Sydó [1,2], Emese Csulak [1], Orsolya Kiss [1,2], Máté Babity [1], Anna Réka Kiss [1], Zsófia Gregor [1], Andrea Szűcs [1], Béla Merkely [1,2†] and Attila Kovács [1†]

[1] Heart and Vascular Center, Semmelweis University, Budapest, Hungary, [2] Department of Sports Medicine, Semmelweis University, Budapest, Hungary

*Correspondence:
Bálint Károly Lakatos
lakatos.balint@
med.semmelweis-univ.hu

† These authors have contributed equally to this work

Background: The cardiovascular effects of SARS-CoV-2 in elite athletes are still a matter of debate. Accordingly, we sought to perform a comprehensive echocardiographic characterization of post-COVID athletes by comparing them to a non-COVID athlete cohort.

Methods: 107 elite athletes with COVID-19 were prospectively enrolled (P-CA; 23 ± 6 years, 23% female) 107 healthy athletes were selected as a control group using propensity score matching (N-CA). All athletes underwent 2D and 3D echocardiography. Left (LV) and right ventricular (RV) end-diastolic volumes (EDVi) and ejection fractions (EF) were quantified. To characterize LV longitudinal deformation, 2D global longitudinal strain (GLS) and the ratio of free wall vs. septal longitudinal strain (FWLS/SLS) were also measured. To describe septal flattening (SF—frequently seen in P-CA), LV eccentricity index (EI) was calculated.

Results: P-CA and N-CA athletes had comparable LV and RVEDVi (P-CA vs. N-CA; 77 ± 12 vs. 78 ± 13mL/m2; 79 ± 16 vs. 80 ± 14mL/m2). P-CA had significantly higher LVEF (58 ± 4 vs. 56 ± 4%, $p < 0.001$), while LVGLS values did not differ between P-CA and N-CA (−19.0 ± 1.9 vs. −18.8 ± 2.2%). EI was significantly higher in P-CA (1.13 ± 0.16 vs. 1.01 ± 0.05, $p < 0.001$), which was attributable to a distinct subgroup of P-CA with a prominent SF ($n = 35$, 33%), further provoked by inspiration. In this subgroup, the EI was markedly higher compared to the rest of the P-CA (1.29 ± 0.15 vs. 1.04 ± 0.08, $p < 0.001$), LVEDVi was also significantly higher (80 ± 14 vs. 75 ± 11 mL/m2, $p < 0.001$), while RVEDVi did not differ (82 ± 16 vs. 78 ± 15mL/m2). Moreover, the FWLS/SLS ratio was significantly lower in the SF subgroup (91.7 ± 8.6 vs. 97.3 ± 8.2, $p < 0.01$). P-CA with SF experienced symptoms less frequently (1.4 ± 1.3 vs. 2.1 ± 1.5 symptom during the infection, $p = 0.01$).

Conclusions: Elite athletes following COVID-19 showed distinct morphological and functional cardiac changes compared to a propensity score-matched control athlete group. These results are mainly driven by a subgroup, which presented with some echocardiographic features characteristic of constrictive pericarditis.

Keywords: athlete's heart, COVID-19, speckle-tracking analysis, 3D echocardiography, constrictive pericaditis

INTRODUCTION

The COVID-19 pandemic represents an unprecedented challenge to the healthcare systems worldwide with still increasing patient numbers. While the infection was initially thought to be affecting mainly the respiratory tract, current evidence suggests that the cardiovascular consequences of COVID-19 are not negligible (1). SARS-CoV-2-related myocardial injury is frequently reported as a worrisome manifestation, whereas prior cardiovascular disorders are strong negative prognostic factors for the course of the infection (2, 3).

Fortunately, COVID-19 is often asymptomatic or associated with only mild symptoms, especially in the young (4). Still, the potential cardiac effects of an uncomplicated SARS-CoV-2 infection need to be further explored.

Elite athletes are a distinguished group of young individuals as a relatively high proportion of them underwent (or will undergo) the infection. This is attributable to their high-risk profile: a young community with frequent social interactions; the majority of sport disciplines include direct physical contact; and wearing a mask during training sessions or competitions is rarely a realistic expectation (5). While the vast majority of young athletes experience an uncomplicated disease course, it is important to emphasize that high-intensity training and related cardiac adaptation may even exaggerate the adverse effects of COVID-19, as it does for other cardiac or non-cardiac disorders (6). Initial reports demonstrated that a considerable proportion of athletes may have detectable myocardial damage; however, the lack of proper control groups limited the generalizability of these results (7–10). Recent studies also proposed the possibility of pericardial involvement (10, 11). Nevertheless, all of the aforementioned studies utilized cardiac magnetic resonance (cMR), an imaging modality that can hardly be incorporated into the routine return to play examination protocol. As a potential alternative, the clinical value of state-of-the-art echocardiographic techniques, such as 3D echocardiography and speckle-tracking echocardiography (STE) should be also tested.

Accordingly, we sought to perform a comprehensive echocardiographic characterization of post-COVID athletes and compare them to a propensity score (PS)-matched healthy athlete cohort.

MATERIALS AND METHODS

Patient Characteristics

We consecutively enrolled elite athletes undergoing "return to play" examinations between September and December 2020 at our Center's Sports Cardiology Department (study protocol approved by the National Public Health Center; no: ETT TUKEB IV/10282-1/2020/EKU). The study protocol complies with the Declaration of Helsinki, and participants gave written informed consent to every procedure. SARS-CoV-2 infection was diagnosed by real-time polymerase chain reaction (rt-PCR) or by serum immunoglobulin G (IgG) antibody titer measurement. All athletes were officially released from quarantine defined by having two negative rt-PCR assays of nasopharyngeal swab specimens following the infection and/or

passing the appropriate quarantine period (10 or 14 days depending on the time of enrollment). All of the athletes completed a questionnaire regarding the nature and duration of their SARS-CoV-2 infection, based on the recommendation of the National Institute of Health (12). Detailed medical history and training regimen were obtained along with the routine physical examination and 12-lead electrocardiogram. Body surface area (BSA) was calculated using the Mosteller formula (13). Subjects with previously documented uncommon echocardiographic and/or electrocardiographic features or with suboptimal echocardiographic image quality for further analysis ($n = 5$) and athletes who suspended regular training in the preceding 6 months before their SARS-CoV-2 infection ($n = 2$) were excluded.

To enable the appropriate pairwise comparison of COVID vs. non-COVID athletes, PS-matching was performed with the optimal pair matching algorithm (14). Our institutional database comprising 425 elite athletes served as the pool for the matching. First, propensity scores were calculated based on age, BSA, and weekly training hours. Then, each COVID athlete was paired with one non-COVID athlete from our institutional database, targeting the collective optimization of the overall criterion (i.e., minimizing the mean of the within-pair difference in propensity score). Matching was applied in males and females separately to ensure that each COVID athlete is paired with a non-COVID athlete of the same sex. PS-matching was performed in R (version 3.6.3, R Foundation for Statistical Computing, Vienna, Austria) using the MatchIt package (version 3.0.2).

Conventional Echocardiography

Echocardiographic loops were recorded using a Vivid E95 ultrasound system equipped with a 4Vc-D phased-array transducer (GE Vingmed Ultrasound, Horten, Norway). Cardiac chambers were quantified according to current guidelines (15). Left ventricular (LV) wall thicknesses and diameters were measured in the parasternal long-axis view at the level of mitral valve coaptation. Relative wall thickness (RWT) was calculated as 2*posterior wall thickness/LV end-diastolic internal diameter. LV diastolic eccentricity index was measured from parasternal short-axis view at the level of the papillary muscles, defined as the ratio of the distances between the anterior-to-posterior wall and the septal-to-lateral wall in end-diastole. Left- and right atrial volumes were measured using the Simpson method and were indexed to BSA. LV diastolic inflow by pulsed-wave Doppler at the level of the mitral valve coaptation was obtained to determine early (E) and late diastolic (A) peak velocities, their ratio, and E-wave deceleration time. Pulsed-wave tissue Doppler imaging (TDI) was used to measure systolic (s'), early (e'), and late diastolic (a') velocities at the mitral lateral and medial annuli. The ratio of E-wave velocity to averaged e' velocities of the mitral medial and lateral annuli was calculated, serving as an estimate of LV filling pressures. Tricuspid annular plane systolic excursion (TAPSE) was measured by M-mode as the peak longitudinal excursion of the tricuspid annulus on an apical four-chamber view. Inferior vena cava (IVC) diameters estimated right atrial pressure (RAP), pulmonary arterial systolic pressure (PASP), diastolic pressure (PADP), mean pressure (PAMP), and also pulmonary vascular resistance (PVR) were quantified according to the current echocardiographic recommendations (16). The presence of a visually detectable septal flattening or pericardial effusion was evaluated during postprocessing by a single expert operator (B.L.) blinded to the study groups.

Speckle-Tracking Analysis

ECG-gated, LV-focused apical long axis, four- and two-chamber view loops targeting a frame rate over 50 FPS were obtained for further analysis. STE was performed by a single expert operator (B.L.) blinded to the study groups using dedicated semi-automatic software (EchoPAC v204 AFI, GE). The software automatically detects the myocardial region of interest (ROI) of the given acquisition and tracks its motion throughout the cardiac cycle. If necessary, the ROI was adjusted manually in order to provide adequate tracking. Segments with poor tracking quality (driven by the software's recommendation) were excluded from the analysis; however, subjects with three or more excluded segments were not included in the study (none). The software automatically calculates global longitudinal strain (GLS) and segmental longitudinal strain (LS) values as well. By averaging the segmental data of the free wall (FW—average LS of inferior, posterior, lateral, and anterior segments) and septal (S—average LS of infero- and anteroseptal segments) regions, we have quantified FWLS and SLS, respectively.

3D Echocardiography

LV- and RV-focused ECG-gated full volume 3D datasets were obtained from apical four-chamber view using multi-beat reconstruction from 4 cardiac cycles. Offline analyses of these datasets focused on the LV and RV were performed by the same expert, blinded operator using conventionally available software packages (4D LV Analysis 3 and RV-Function 2, TomTec Imaging Systems GmbH, Unterschleissheim, Germany). The algorithm automatically generates LV and RV endocardial contours, which were manually corrected on multiple short- and long-axis planes throughout the entire cardiac cycle. We determined the LV and RV end-diastolic volume index (EDVi), end-systolic volume index (ESVi), and stroke volume index (SVi) normalized to BSA. To quantify global ventricular function, LV and RV ejection fractions (EF) were also calculated.

Statistical Analysis

All values are expressed as mean ± standard deviation, or median and interquartile range (IQR). The distribution of the variables was assessed by the Shapiro-Wilk normality test. An unpaired two-sided Student's t-test, in case of normal distribution, or a Mann-Whitney U test, in case of non-normal distribution, was performed to compare the continuous variables of the study groups. Fisher's exact test was used to compare the incidence of symptoms between groups. A $p < 0.05$ was used as the criterion for statistical significance.

Intra- and interobserver variability of the most relevant parameters were also assessed. The operator of the first measurements (B.L.) and a second expert reader (A.F.), both blinded to the study groups, repeated the measurements in a randomly chosen subset of 5–5 athletes from each group. Lin's concordance correlation coefficient and coefficient of variation were calculated.

RESULTS

One hundred and seven post-COVID athletes (handball $n = 37$, ice hockey $n = 26$, water polo $n = 26$, basketball $n = 12$, speedskating $n = 2$, other $n = 4$) were included in the current analysis. Athletes were asymptomatic at the time of examination with the exception of the loss of taste and/or smell in a handful of cases ($n = 12$), as these symptoms frequently exceed the period of active infection (17). A total of 59 subjects (55%) were completely asymptomatic throughout the disease course. The symptom burden of the study group is summarized in **Supplementary Table 1**. The athletes were symptomatic for a median of 4 [IQR: 1–7] days and presented for the return to play examinations 22 [IQR: 17–25] days following the first rt-PCR or IgG positivity.

The mean age of the post-COVID athletes was 23 ± 6 years. There were no differences in age, BSA and training hours between the post-COVID and the PS-matched non-COVID athletes, indicating successful matching. Systolic and diastolic blood pressures also did not differ between post-COVID and non-COVID athletes, while heart rate was significantly lower in the post-COVID group (**Table 1**).

Basic echocardiographic parameters of the left and right heart are shown in **Table 2**. LV wall thicknesses and RWT were significantly lower in the post-COVID group. Transmitral E/A ratio was higher in the post-COVID group, along with a longer deceleration time. TDI-derived mitral lateral and medial velocities were significantly higher in the post-COVID group resulting in a lower E/e' ratio; however, e' lateral/e' medial ratio was significantly lower. 2D RV, left and right atrial dimensions did not differ between the study groups. Maximal IVC diameter and right atrial pressure were significantly lower in the post-COVID group, whereas other estimated pulmonary artery pressures were comparable between post-COVID athletes and PS-matched non-COVID athletes. TAPSE/PASP ratio was also similar (**Table 2**).

3D echocardiographic and 2D LV STE parameters are summarized in **Table 3**. 3D LV and RV EDVi were comparable between groups, whereas 3D LV ESVi was significantly lower in post-COVID athletes, resulting in elevated LV EF. 2D GLS, SLS, and FWLS were comparable between the post-COVID and non-COVID groups; however, a lower FWLS/SLS ratio was detected in the post-COVID athletes.

Interestingly, LV diastolic eccentricity index was significantly higher in the post-COVID subjects (1.13 ± 0.16 vs. 1.01 ± 0.05, $p < 0.001$). This finding was mainly driven by a subgroup ($n = 35/107$; 33%) of post-COVID athletes, in which an early-diastolic septal flattening (SF) was present consistently throughout the entire echocardiographic examination on multiple views, showing an inspiratory enhancement (**Figure 1**, **Supplementary Video 1**). This phenomenon was not detected in

TABLE 1 | Baseline characteristics of the post-COVID and the non-COVID athlete groups.

	Post-COVID athletes ($n = 107$)	Non-COVID athletes ($n = 107$)	p-value
Age (years)	22.9 ± 6.1	22.7 ± 7.0	0.82
Female (n [%])	25 (23%)	25 (23%)	1
Height (cm)	182.9 ± 10.0	181.8 ± 12.0	0.45
Weight (kg)	80.2 ± 15.3	80.6 ± 17.0	0.87
BSA (m²)	2.0 ± 0.2	2.0 ± 0.3	0.93
SBP (mmHg)	130.3 ± 15.1	134.0 ± 15.8	0.09
DBP (mmHg)	79.4 ± 11.3	77.4 ± 9.2	0.16
HR (1/min)	62.9 ± 10.6	66.6 ± 13.3	**<0.05**
Training per week (hours)	13.1 ± 6.0	14.5 ± 6.4	0.08

BSA, body surface area; SBP, systolic blood pressure; DBP, diastolic blood pressure. HR, heart rate. Bold values indicate a p < 0.05.

TABLE 2 | Conventional echocardiographic left- and right heart parameters in the post-COVID and the non-COVID athlete groups.

	Post-COVID athletes ($n = 107$)	Non-COVID athletes ($n = 107$)	p-value
LVIDd (mm)	51.8 ± 4.4	51.4 ± 5.4	0.56
IVSd (mm)	9.4 ± 1.8	10.4 ± 1.8	**<0.01**
PWd (mm)	8.4 ± 1.3	9.0 ± 1.3	**<0.01**
RWT (%)	0.33 ± 0.05	0.35 ± 0.05	**<0.001**
LAVi (mL/m²)	26.4 ± 6.5	27.9 ± 8.6	0.16
Transmitral E wave (cm/s)	81.7 ± 16.0	82.3 ± 20.6	0.79
Transmitral A wave (cm/s)	50.2 ± 12.3	57.4 ± 15.5	**<0.001**
E/A	1.68 ± 0.40	1.49 ± 0.43	**<0.001**
DT (ms)	192.7 ± 40.8	176.6 ± 39.3	**<0.01**
E/e' average	4.64 ± 0.88	5.55 ± 1.50	**<0.001**
Mitral lateral s' (cm/s)	12.8 ± 2.5	12.1 ± 2.3	**<0.05**
Mitral lateral e' (cm/s)	19.7 ± 3.2	17.7 ± 3.2	**<0.001**
Mitral lateral a' (cm/s)	8.3 ± 2.0	7.6 ± 1.8	**<0.01**
Mitral medial s' (cm/s)	10.3 ± 1.5	9.6 ± 1.4	**<0.01**
Mitral medial e' (cm/s)	15.6 ± 2.7	13.0 ± 2.6	**<0.001**
Mitral medial a' (cm/s)	8.4 ± 1.4	7.5 ± 1.8	**<0.001**
e' lateral/e' septal	1.29 ± 0.21	1.40 ± 0.27	**<0.001**
LV diastolic eccentricity index	1.13 ± 0.16	1.01 ± 0.05	**<0.001**
RV basal diameter (mm)	34.3 ± 4.2	33.7 ± 4.3	0.27
TAPSE (mm)	24.7 ± 3.9	23.6 ± 4.2	0.05
RAVi (mL/m²)	28.0 ± 6.6	28.1 ± 8.1	0.89
PASP (mmHg)	20.7 ± 4.3	20.4 ± 5.2	0.61
PADP (mmHg)	6.9 ± 2.3	7.0 ± 2.8	0.76
PAMP (mmHg)	13.4 ± 4.2	12.3 ± 3.7	0.19
IVC max (mm)	13.2 ± 3.0	16.0 ± 4.1	**<0.001**
IVC min (mm)	11.3 ± 6.0	9.3 ± 6.7	0.39
RAP (mmHg)	3.5 ± 1.8	4.2 ± 2.3	**<0.05**
RVOT VTI (cm)	20.0 ± 3.5	18.8 ± 3.4	**<0.05**
PVR (Wood units)	1.24 ± 0.21	1.21 ± 0.26	0.51
TAPSE/PASP	1.23 ± 0.30	1.24 ± 0.42	0.86
Prevalence of mild pericardial effusion (n [%])	41 (38%)	10 (9%)	**<0.001**

LVIDd, left ventricular end-diastolic diameter; IVSd, interventricular septal thickness; PWd, posterior wall thickness; RWT, relative wall thickness; LAVi, left atrial volume index; DT: deceleration time; LV eccentricity index, left ventricular eccentricity index; RV basal diamater, right ventricular basal diameter; TAPSE, tricuspid annular plane systolic excursion; RAVi, right atrial volume index; PASP, pulmonary arterial systolic pressure; PADP, pulmonary arterial diastolic pressure; PAMP, pulmonary arterial mean pressure; IVC, inferior vena cava; RAP, right atrial pressure; RVOT VTI, right ventricular outflow tract velocity-time integral; PVR, pulmonary vascular resistance. Bold values indicate a p < 0.05.

TABLE 3 | Comparison of 3D and speckle-tracking echocardiographic data between the post-COVID and the non-COVID athlete groups.

	Post-COVID athletes (*n* = 107)	Non-COVID athletes (*n* = 107)	*p*-value
3D LVEDVi (mL/m^2)	76.7 ± 12.2	78.3 ± 13.3	0.39
3D LVESVi (mL/m^2)	32.4 ± 6.3	34.7 ± 7.4	**0.01**
3D LVSVi (mL/m^2)	44.4 ± 7.5	43.5 ± 7.3	0.4
3D LVEF (%)	57.9 ± 4.3	55.8 ± 4.2	**<0.001**
3D RVEDVi (mL/m^2)	78.9 ± 15.5	79.6 ± 14.2	0.72
3D RVESVi (mL/m^2)	35.4 ± 8.4	36.6 ± 8.6	0.32
3D RVSVi (mL/m^2)	43.5 ± 8.5	43.1 ± 7.1	0.72
3D RVEF (%)	55.3 ± 4.5	54.3 ± 4.7	0.14
2D LVGLS (%)	−19.0 ± 1.9	−18.8 ± 2.2	0.51
2D FWLS (%)	−18.6 ± 2.1	−18.6 ± 2.2	0.97
2D SLS (%)	−19.6 ± 2.1	−19.0 ± 2.4	0.06
2D FWLS/SLS (%)	95.5 ± 8.7	98.3 ± 6.8	**<0.01**

LVEDVi, left ventricular end-diastolic index; LVESVi, left ventricular end-systolic volume index; LVSVi, left ventricular stroke volume index; LVEF, left ventricular ejection fraction; RVEDVi, right ventricular end-diastolic volume index; RVESVi, right ventricular end-systolic volume index; RVSVi, right ventricular stroke volume index; RVEF, right ventricular ejection fraction; LVGLS, left ventricular global longitudinal strain; FWLS, free wall longitudinal strain; SLS, septal longitudinal strain; FWLS/SLS, free wall to septal longitudinal strain ratio. Bold values indicate a p < 0.05.

any athletes of the PS-matched non-COVID group. Therefore, we have also assessed the differences between the athletes with and without SF within the post-COVID group.

Post-COVID athletes with SF were younger; however, they did not differ in other anthropometric or basic hemodynamic measures and in average weekly training hours (**Supplementary Table 2**).

The presence of detectable (trivial) pericardial effusion was more frequent in the SF subgroup of post-COVID athletes compared to the corresponding subset of PS-matched non-COVID athletes (41% vs. 12%, $p < 0.01$). Post-COVID athletes with SF and without SF did not differ in terms of the number of symptomatic days (3 [IQR: 0–7.0] days vs. 5 [IQR: 2.5–8.0] days, $p = 0.09$), the time between the onset of symptoms and the examination (24 [IQR: 17.5–37.5] days vs. 23 [IQR: 18.0–29.0] days, $p = 0.65$), or the time elapsed between the first positive PCR or IgG and the examination (22.5 [IQR: 17.0–25.0] days vs. 21 [IQR: 17.0–25.0] days, $p = 0.70$). The incidence of fever (34 vs. 29%, $p = 0.66$), coughing (9 vs. 7%, $p = 0.71$), headache (29 vs. 44%, $p = 0.15$), and loss of smell and/or taste (47 vs. 52%, $p = 0.54$) were also comparable between the athlete groups. Interestingly, chest pain (0 vs. 15%, $p = 0.01$) and fatigue (17 vs. 34%, $p = 0.04$) were reported more frequently in post-COVID athletes without SF (**Figure 2**). When the symptom burden was summed as a "composite symptom score", athletes with SF generally had fewer symptoms (1.4 ± 1.3 vs. 2.1 ± 1.5 symptom during the infection, $p = 0.01$, **Figure 2**).

Regarding basic echocardiographic measures, post-COVID athletes with SF showed significantly higher E/A ratio, while RAP and PADP were also found to be significantly higher compared to post-COVID athletes without SF (**Supplementary Table 2**). LV diastolic eccentricity index was markedly higher in post-COVID athletes with SF, while it was comparable between post-COVID athletes without SF and their matched non-COVID athletes (1.04 ± 0.08 vs. 1.00 ± 0.04, $p = 0.14$). Regarding

3D echocardiographic measures, post-COVID athletes with SF had significantly higher LV EDVi and LV ESVi compared to post-COVID athletes without SF, while RV morphological measures along with LV and RV EF were similar (**Table 4**). 2D LV GLS did not differ between the post-COVID athlete subgroups; however, the FWLS/SLS ratio was significantly lower in athletes with SF compared to those without (**Figure 3**). During the last phase of the enrollment and already having our awareness at SF and related STE-based alterations, we have referred athletes presented with SF to cMR examination ($n = 5$). Notably, no myopericardial involvement was detected by cMR in these cases. Detailed case reports are presented in **Supplementary Table 3**.

Intra- and interobserver variability of the key echocardiographic parameters showed good intra- and interreader agreements (**Supplementary Table 4**).

DISCUSSION

Our study is the first to investigate a relatively high number of European elite athletes who underwent mild COVID-19, while also comparing them to a PS-matched healthy athlete group using a comprehensive echocardiographic approach. We have shown that post-COVID athletes show distinct changes in cardiac morphology and function compared to matched non-COVID athletes. Of note, the vast majority of these alterations was attributable to a subpopulation of athletes in whom an inspiration-enhanced early diastolic SF could be detected. In these athletes, the E/A ratio of mitral inflow, the 3D echocardiography-derived LV volumes were significantly higher, along with a significantly lower FWLS/SLS ratio.

The earliest reports from China already mentioned the high prevalence of elevated cardiac necroenzymes and the commonly deteriorated LV functional measures in COVID-19 patients (18). With the worldwide expansion of the pandemic, several other studies demonstrated the high frequency of cardiac

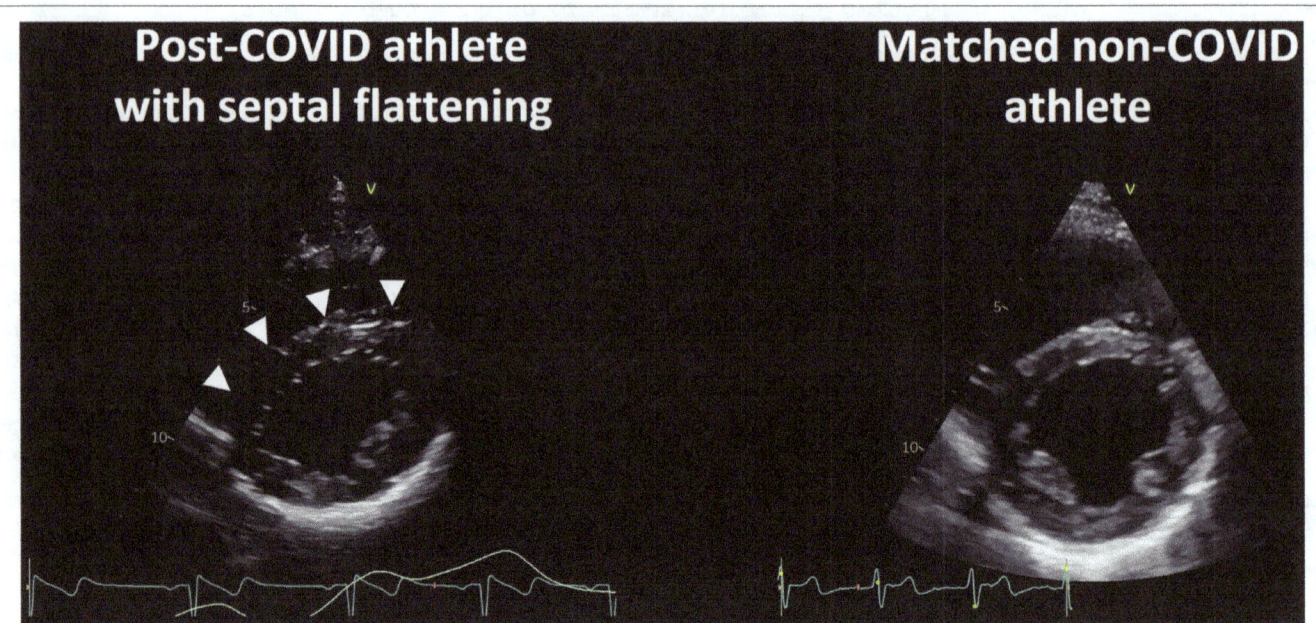

FIGURE 1 | Representative case of the post-COVID septal flattening (SF) in athletes. Parasternal short-axis views at the level of the papillary muscles at mid-diastole in a young athlete underwent asymptomatic SARS-CoV-2 infection and his matched control. In the post-COVID athlete, a prominent SF can be seen with early diastolic dominance and inspiratory enhancement (left, SF shown by arrows), compared to the propensity score-matched control (right).

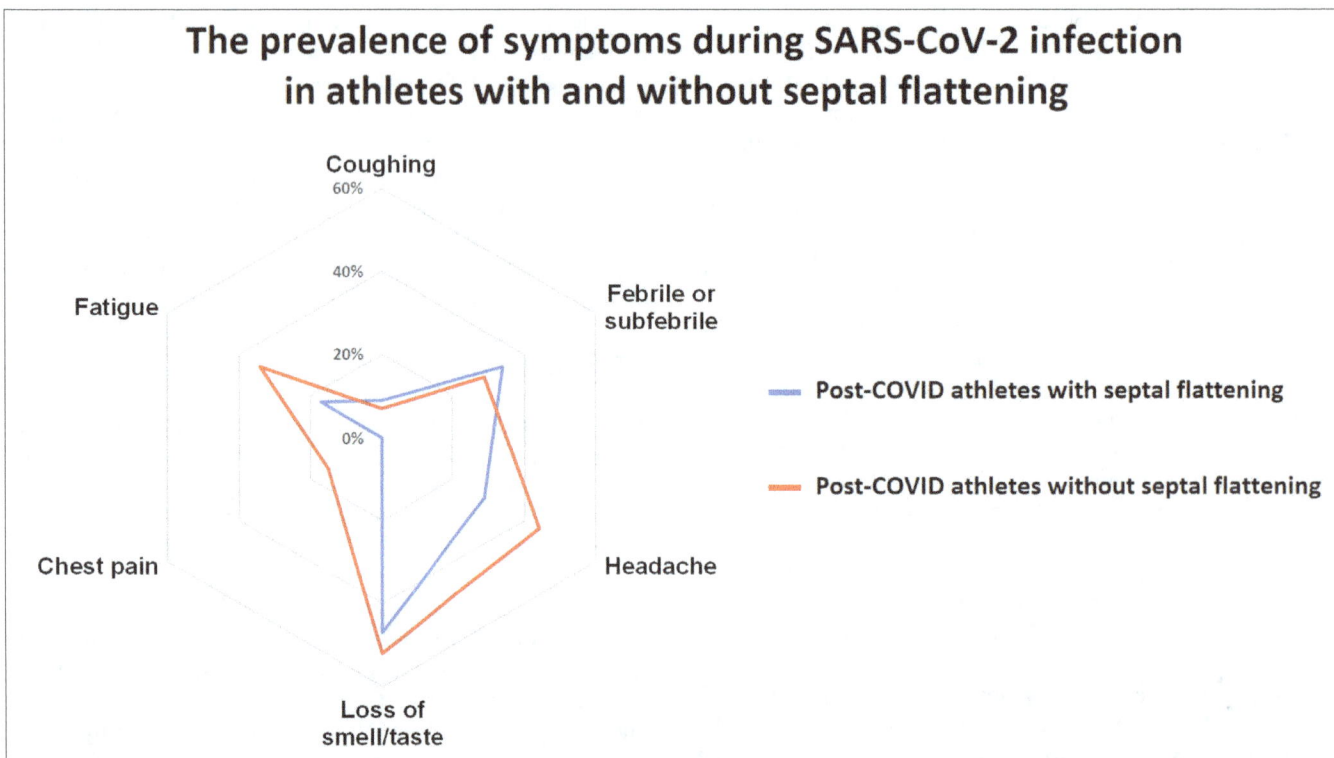

FIGURE 2 | Radar chart comparisons of the most relevant symptoms in post-COVID athletes with our without septal flattening (SF). Athletes with SF (blue line) and without SF (red line) did not differ in the incidence of fever or subfebrility, coughing, headache or the lost of smell and/or taste. On the other hand, chest pain and fatigue were significantly more frequent in athletes without SF. In general, athletes with SF were less symptomatic, as shown by the smaller area of the radar chart compared to athletes without SF (see details in text).

TABLE 4 | Echocardiographic comparison of post-COVID athletes with vs. without septal flattening.

	Post-COVID athletes with SF (*n* = 35)	Post-COVID athletes without SF (*n* = 72)	*p*-value
LV diastolic eccentricity index	1.29 ± 0.15	1.04 ± 0.08	**<0.001**
3D LVEDVi (mL/m²)	80.1 ± 14.4	74.9 ± 10.7	**<0.05**
3D LVESVi (mL/m²)	34.5 ± 8.0	31.3 ± 5.1	**<0.05**
3D LVSVi (mL/m²)	46.2 ± 8.2	43.5 ± 7.1	0.09
3D LVEF (%)	57.5 ± 4.6	58.1 ± 4.1	0.52
3D RVEDVi (mL/m²)	82.1 ± 15.9	77.7 ± 15.3	0.3
3D RVESVi (mL/m²)	36.5 ± 9.8	35.9 ± 7.6	0.37
3D RVSVi (mL/m²)	44.7 ± 7.8	42.9 ± 8.8	0.31
3D RVEF (%)	55.6 ± 5.5	55.2 ± 4.0	0.68
2D LVGLS (%)	−18.9 ± 1.9	−19.0 ± 2.0	0.70
2D FWLS (%)	−18.3 ± 2.0	−18.8 ± 2.1	0.20
2D SLS (%)	−20.0 ± 2.3	−19.4 ± 2.0	0.16
2D FWLS/SLS (%)	91.7 ± 8.6	97.3 ± 8.2	**<0.001**

SF, septal flattening; LVEDVi, left ventricular end-diastolic index; LVESVi, left ventricular end-systolic volume index; LVSVi, left ventricular stroke volume index; LVEF, left ventricular ejection fraction; RVEDVi, right ventricular end-diastolic volume index; RVESVi, right ventricular end-systolic volume index; RVSVi, right ventricular stroke volume index; RVEF, right ventricular ejection fraction; LVGLS, left ventricular global longitudinal strain; FWLS, free wall longitudinal strain; SLS, septal longitudinal strain; FWLS/SLS, free wall to septal longitudinal strain ratio. Bold values indicate a p < 0.05.

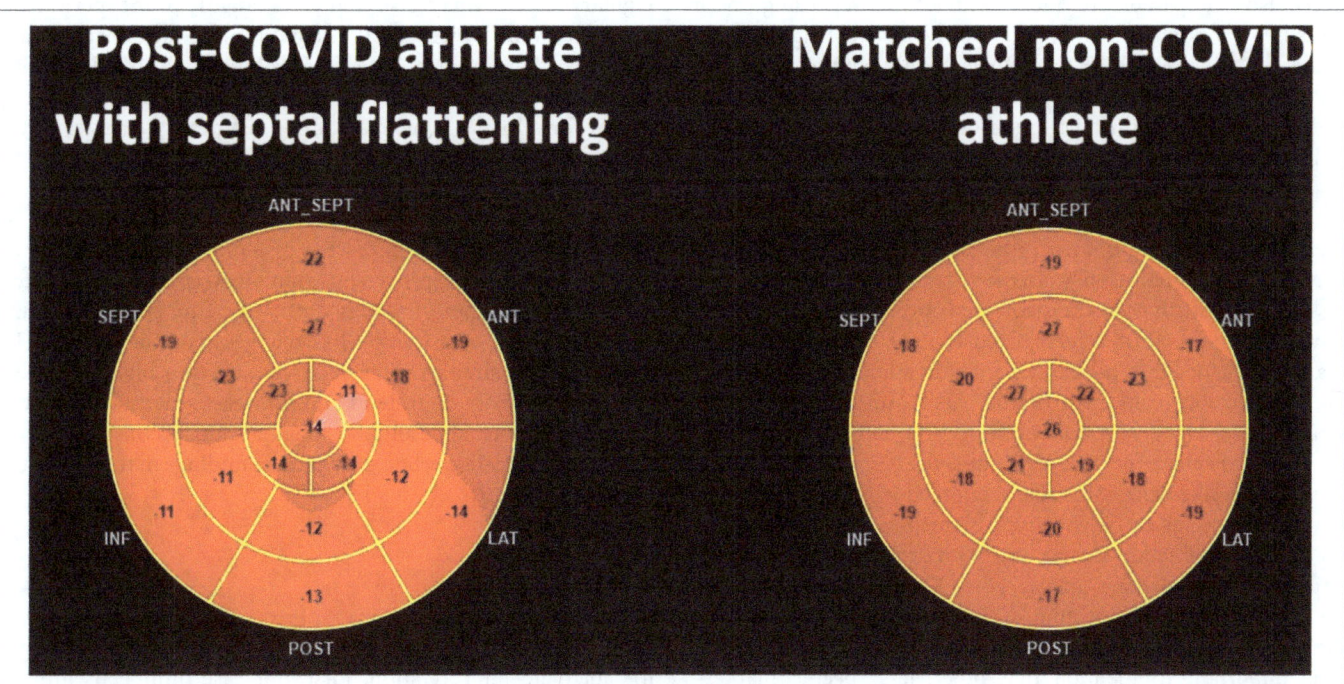

FIGURE 3 | The "Hot Septum Sign" in a post-COVID athlete with septal flattening. While left ventricular global longitudinal strain is preserved, a relative decrease in the free wall segments can be noted (left), suggestive of a characteristic feature of pericardial constriction. In the matched control, segmental strain values of the septum and free wall do not markedly differ (right).

damage; however, the investigations were mainly focused on the severe/critical cases (19). Nowadays, evidence is growing that mild or even asymptomatic disease courses do not exclude myocardial involvement of COVID-19 (20). Special considerations are needed in the case of elite athletes following SARS-CoV-2 infection, even though these young, exceptionally healthy individuals usually undergo COVID-19 with no or very mild symptoms. Robust evidence suggests that even minor cardiac alterations can be exaggerated by high-intensity exercise,

and this can worsen the course of various diseases (6). Therefore, the detailed characterization of the athlete's heart following COVID-19 is a relevant clinical demand.

In our post-COVID population, LV wall thicknesses and RWT were significantly lower compared to the matched control athletes. These findings may correspond to the effects of short-term detraining: LV wall thicknesses are known to decrease even after a few weeks of suspended athletic activity along with unaltered ventricular volumes (21, 22). Regarding functional measures, LV EF was found to be significantly higher in the post-COVID group, with unaltered LV GLS. While data are conflicting regarding the resting LV systolic function of the athlete's heart, low-normal values are commonly reported; therefore, an increase in LV EF following detraining may be expected (23).

In a subpopulation of our post-COVID elite athletes, an early diastolic SF was detected with inspiratory enhancement, commonly resulting in marked LV eccentricity (**Figure 1**, **Supplementary Video 1**). This phenomenon may be attributable to a handful of causes. Previous studies examining sedentary COVID-19 patients and also elite athletes reported alterations of the myocardium with a septal predominance (such as decreased septal LS, or increased native T1 values and/or late gadolinium enhancement of the septum) suggestive of SARS-CoV-2-related myocarditis (7, 11). Nevertheless, in viral myocarditis, segmental or global wall motion abnormalities would be expected rather than a bouncing septal motion with preserved deformation.

COVID-19 is also known to affect the pulmonary vasculature (24). However, in our post-COVID cohort, Doppler-based estimated pulmonary pressures did not markedly differ from matched control athletes, and post-COVID athletes with SF were also comparable to those without SF regarding these measures. Of note, estimated RAP and PADP were significantly higher in athletes with SF, nevertheless, only with a borderline statistical significance. Moreover, a COVID-related imbalance between intrapericardial and intrathoracic pressures should also be considered.

The aforementioned study of Brito et al. reported a surprisingly high prevalence of pericardial involvement in their study enrolling student athletes (11). While acute viral pericarditis does not usually alter myocardial function, previous results suggest that a transient pericardial constriction-like physiology may occur, which could explain the SF (25). As a marker of a possible pericardial inflammation, the prevalence of a detectable (although trivial) pericardial effusion was significantly higher in our post-COVID athletes compared to their matched non-COVID athletes. Furthermore, this constriction-like behavior is also reinforced by the phenomenon that the SF seems to be enhanced by inspiration and becomes the most prominent during early diastole (**Figure 1**) (26). Regarding STE-markers, in our post-COVID athletes with SF, the characteristic "hot septum" sign can be seen as shown by the STE-derived FWLS/SLS ratio (**Figure 3**) (27, 28). Of note, it is important to mention that other, less specific markers of constrictive physiology, such as increased E/A ratio and PADP, can also be measured in this subpopulation. In line with the cMR findings of the post-COVID population of Brito and colleagues, LV volumes were significantly higher in the post-COVID group with SF (11). This may be attributable to the partially similar methodology of cMR and a "multi-beat" 3D echocardiographic acquisition: during expiratory breathhold, the enhanced ventricular interdependence of the constrictive physiology may result in increased LV volumes (26).

Interestingly, SF was more common in athletes with generally fewer symptoms. This corresponds to previous large-scale cMR data demonstrating that all athletes with confirmed inflammatory heart disease were only minimally symptomatic (9). Moreover, in another study, pericardial enhancement was significantly more common in asymptomatic athletes (11). In a large retrospective cardiac surgery registry, post-surgery constrictive pericarditis patients were characterized by more commonly detected postoperative pericardial effusion and a higher LVEF (29). These results may indicate that the main driver of disease progression is the interplay of ongoing serous membrane inflammation and more pronounced friction of the pericardial sac by a hyperdynamic LV. Theoretically, athletes with fewer symptoms are likely to continue training during the infection, potentially creating a similar pathophysiological scenario.

However, it is important to mention that in those cases where cMR was also performed, no signs of pericardial inflammation or constriction were detected. Considering that the main body of data about the reverse remodeling after abrupted training is derived from small sample studies of the early 90's, it is plausible that a temporary change in the pericardial constraint is a benign phenomenon of athletic detraining (HIV). Hemodynamic overload is proved to induce not only myocardial, but pericardial remodeling as well (HIV). Therefore, it is suspected that intense regular exercise may also induce changes of the pericardial structure. While myocardial deconditioning is known to take place over the course of a few weeks of abrupted training regime, the altered characteristics of the pericardium may persist for a longer time, resulting in temporary changes of the pericardial constraint.

The current Sports Cardiology and Exercise Guideline of the European Society of Cardiology recommends at least 30 days of suspended training in the case of pericarditis, however, in the absence of a proven inflammatory process the clinical implications of these findings are hard to judge (HIV).In the case of persistent constriction-like changes in the SF post-COVID group, an impaired peak exercise capacity has high possibility (HIV)., Follow-up of athletes and further research are urged to explain the appearance and the potential clinical consequences of the constriction-like echocardiographic findings in the context of the athlete's heart.

LIMITATIONS

Our study carries limitations that have to be acknowledged for adequate interpretation. First, our case number is limited. Nevertheless, the number of subjects is considered to be relatively high as compared to current COVID-19-related data in athletes. The population has a male predominance; therefore, the study was not powered to examine the role of gender differences. In the post-COVID athlete group, echocardiographic loops prior to the SARS-CoV-2 infection were not available. Therefore, PS-matching was used to provide a matched control athlete group. The observed changes were often subtle and only statistically significant. The most common causes of SF are pulmonary hypertension and constrictive pericarditis, and the gold-standard evaluation method for both these diseases is still right (and left-) heart catheterization (26). For obvious ethical reasons, such invasive procedures were not performed in the mainly asymptomatic/paucisymptomatic post-COVID athlete group. However, various echocardiographic pressure estimates and other functional parameters were quantified, which may also adequately assess the characteristic features of such diseases. Nevertheless, certain indirect markers of pericardial constriction, such as mitral and/or tricuspid inflow variation, hepatic vein flow and M-mode assessment of the septal motion were not obtained. Computed tomography was not included in this study; therefore, possible pulmonary involvement of the post-COVID athletes was not evaluated. cMR examinations were only performed in a handful of athletes; therefore, the gold-standard measurements of cardiac volumes are not available, and cMR markers of myopericardial inflammation were not assessed in the majority of the subjects. The cMR acquisitions were obtained during breath holding, therefore, free breathing loops confirming the septal flattening were not available. Respirometry was not part of our routine echocardiographic image acquisition protocol (used only in a few cases in the post-COVID group); therefore, the inspiratory enhancement of the SF was not tested consistently. Assessment of the long-term consequences and clinical importance of these findings requires further work and follow-up.

CONCLUSIONS

Our results suggest that even mild SARS-CoV-2 infection may significantly affect cardiac morphology and function in elite athletes. The observed alterations are mainly attributable to a subgroup of athletes, in whom some features of pericardial constriction could be detected, such as pericardial effusion, early diastolic SF with inspiratory enhancement, and STE-derived "hot

septum" sign. Interestingly, these athletes seemed to experience fewer symptoms during the course of the infection. Considering that current guidelines usually propose a more thorough return to play examinations in symptomatic athletes only, our data is especially alarming, as many of our athletes presented with SF would not have been eligible for a detailed assessment (30). The pathophysiological background and clinical relevance of these findings are unclear and require further research. Nevertheless, our data support the use of a comprehensive echocardiographic protocol applying advanced techniques in the return to play examination of elite athletes.

AUTHOR CONTRIBUTIONS

BL, MT, AF, MB, and AK contributed to the conception of the study design. BL, HV, LS, NS, EC, OK, MB, AK, ZG, and AS performed the measurents. BL, MT, AF, ZL, LS, and EC managed the database. BL and MT perfomed the statistical analysis. BL, MB and AK wrote the draft of the manuscript. MT, AF, HV, LS, NS, EC, OK, AS, and MB reviewed it. BL, MT, and MB prepared the figures. All authors contributed to the article and approved the submitted version.

SUPPLEMENTARY MATERIAL

Supplementary Video 1 | Post-COVID athlete with septal flattening (SF). An early diastolic dominance of the SF can be seen with inspiratory enhancement (as shown on the parallel ECG and respirometry tracing).

REFERENCES

1. Guzik TJ, Mohiddin SA, Dimarco A, Patel V, Savvatis K, Marelli-Berg FM, et al. COVID-19 and the cardiovascular system: implications for risk assessment, diagnosis, and treatment options. *Cardiovasc Res.* (2020) 116:1666–87. doi: 10.1093/cvr/cvaa106

2. Peng Y, Meng K, He M, Zhu R, Guan H, Ke Z, et al. Clinical characteristics and prognosis of 244 cardiovascular patients suffering from coronavirus disease in Wuhan, China. *J Am Heart Assoc.* (2020) 9:e016796. doi: 10.1161/JAHA.120.016796

3. Bae S, Kim SR, Kim MN, Shim WJ, Park SM. Impact of cardiovascular disease and risk factors on fatal outcomes in patients with COVID-19 according to age: a systematic review and meta-analysis. *Heart.* (2021) 107:373–80. doi: 10.1136/heartjnl-2020-317901

4. Barek MA, Aziz MA, Islam MS. Impact of age, sex, comorbidities and clinical symptoms on the severity of COVID-19 cases: a meta-analysis with 55 studies and 10014 cases. *Heliyon.* (2020) 6:e05684. doi: 10.1016/j.heliyon.2020.e05684

5. Watson A, Haraldsdottir K, Biese K, Goodavish L, Stevens B, McGuine T. The association of COVID-19 incidence with sport and face mask use in United States high school athletes. *medRxiv.* (2001) 2019.21250116. doi: 10.4085/1062-6050-281-21

6. Guasch E, Mont L. Diagnosis, pathophysiology, and management of exercise-induced arrhythmias. *Nat Rev Cardiol.* (2017) 14:88–101. doi: 10.1038/nrcardio.2016.173

7. Rajpal S, Tong MS, Borchers J, Zareba KM, Obarski TP, Simonetti OP, et al. Cardiovascular magnetic resonance findings in competitive athletes recovering from COVID-19 infection. *JAMA Cardiol.* (2020). doi: 10.1001/jamacardio.2020.4916

8. Vago H, Szabo L, Dohy Z, Merkely B. Cardiac magnetic resonance findings in patients recovered from COVID-19: initial experiences in elite athletes. *JACC Cardiovasc Imaging.* (2020) 14:1279–81. doi: 10.1016/j.jcmg.2020.11.014

9. Martinez MW, Tucker AM, Bloom OJ, Green G, Difiori JP, Solomon G, et al. Prevalence of inflammatory heart disease among professional athletes with prior COVID-19 infection who received systematic return-to-play cardiac screening. JAMA Cardiol. (2021) 6:745–52. doi: 10.1001/jamacardio.2021.0565

10. Moulson N, Petek BJ, Drezner JA, Harmon KG, Kliethermes SA, Patel MR, et al. SARS-CoV-2 cardiac involvement in young competitive athletes. *Circulation.* (2021) 144:256–66. doi: 10.1161/CIRCULATIONAHA.121.054824

11. Brito D, Meester S, Yanamala N, Patel HB, Balcik BJ, Casaclang-Verzosa G, et al. High prevalence of pericardial involvement in college student athletes recovering from COVID-19. *JACC Cardiovasc Imaging.* (2020) 14:541–55. doi: 10.1016/j.jcmg.2020.10.023

12. NIH. *Coronavirus Disease 2019 (COVID-19). Treatment Guidelines* (2019:130). Avaliable online at: https://covid19treatmentguidelines.nih.gov/ (accessed May 12, 2021).

13. Mosteller RD. Simplified calculation of body-surface area. *N Engl J Med.* (1987) 317:1098. doi: 10.1056/NEJM198710223171717

14. Gu XS, Rosenbaum PR. Comparison of multivariate matching methods: structures, distances, and algorithms. *J Comput Graph Stat.* (1993) 2:405–20. doi: 10.1080/10618600.1993.10474623

15. Lang RM, Badano LP, Mor-Avi V, Afilalo J, Armstrong A, Ernande L, et al. Recommendations for cardiac chamber quantification by echocardiography in adults: an update from the American society of echocardiography and the European association of cardiovascular imaging. *J Am Soc Echocardiogr.* (2015) 28:1–39. doi: 10.1016/j.echo.2014.10.003

16. Rudski LG, Lai WW, Afilalo J, Hua L, Handschumacher MD, Chandrasekaran K, et al. Guidelines for the echocardiographic assessment of the right heart in adults: a report from the American society of echocardiography endorsed by the European association of echocardiography, a registered branch of the European society of cardiology, and the canadian society of echocardiography. *J Am Soc Echocardiogr.* (2010) 23:685–713. doi: 10.1016/j.echo.2010.05.010

17. Boscolo-Rizzo P, Borsetto D, Fabbris C, Spinato G, Frezza D, Menegaldo A, et al. Evolution of altered sense of smell or taste in patients with mildly symptomatic COVID-19. *JAMA Otolaryngol Head Neck Surg.* (2020) 146:729–32. doi: 10.1001/jamaoto.2020.1379

18. Shi S, Qin M, Shen B, Cai Y, Liu T, Yang F, et al. Association of cardiac injury with mortality in hospitalized patients with COVID-19 in Wuhan, China. *JAMA Cardiol.* (2020) 5:802–10. doi: 10.1001/jamacardio.2020.0950

19. Parohan M, Yaghoubi S, Seraji A. Cardiac injury is associated with severe outcome and death in patients with coronavirus disease 2019 (COVID-19) infection: a systematic review and meta-analysis of observational studies. *Eur Heart J Acute Cardiovasc Care.* (2020) 9:665–77. doi: 10.1177/2048872620937165

20. Puntmann VO, Carerj ML, Wieters I, Fahim M, Arendt C, Hoffmann J, et al. Outcomes of cardiovascular magnetic resonance imaging in patients recently recovered from coronavirus disease 2019 (COVID-19). *JAMA Cardiol.* (2020) 5:1265–73. doi: 10.1001/jamacardio.2020.3557

21. Maron BJ, Pelliccia A, Spataro A, Granata M. Reduction in left ventricular wall thickness after deconditioning in highly trained olympic athletes. *Br Heart J.* (1993) 69:125–8. doi: 10.1136/hrt.69.2.125

22. Olah A, Kovacs A, Lux A, Tokodi M, Braun S, Lakatos BK, et al. Characterization of the dynamic changes in left ventricular morphology and function induced by exercise training and detraining. *Int J Cardiol.* (2019) 277:178–85. doi: 10.1016/j.ijcard.2018.10.092

23. Lakatos BK, Molnár AÁ, Kiss O, Sydó N, Tokodi M, Solymossi B, et al. Relationship between cardiac remodeling and exercise capacity in elite athletes: incremental value of left atrial morphology and function assessed by three-dimensional echocardiography. *J Am Soc Echocardiogr.* (2020) 33:101–9. doi: 10.1016/j.echo.2019.07.017

24. Ackermann M, Verleden SE, Kuehnel M, Haverich A, Welte T, Laenger F, et al. Pulmonary vascular endothelialitis, thrombosis, and angiogenesis in Covid-19. *N Engl J Med.* (2020) 383:120–8. doi: 10.1056/NEJMoa2015432

25. Sato K, Ayache A, Kumar A, Cremer PC, Griffin B, Popovic ZB, et al. Improvement in left ventricular mechanics following medical treatment of constrictive pericarditis. Heart. (2021) 107:828–35. doi: 10.1136/heartjnl-2020-317304

26. Syed FF, Schaff HV, Oh JK. Constrictive pericarditis–a curable diastolic heart failure. *Nat Rev Cardiol.* (2014) 11:530–44. doi: 10.1038/nrcardio.2014.100

27. Kusunose K, Dahiya A, Popovic ZB, Motoki H, Alraies MC, Zurick AO, et al. Biventricular mechanics in constrictive pericarditis comparison with restrictive cardiomyopathy and impact of pericardiectomy. *Circ Cardiovasc Imaging.* (2013) 6:399–406. doi: 10.1161/CIRCIMAGING.112.000078

28. Argulian EDH. "Hot septum" sign of constrictive pericarditis. *JACC Case Reports.* (2020) 2:186–90. doi: 10.1016/j.jaccas.2019.12.024

29. Matsuyama K, Matsumoto M, Sugita T, Nishizawa J, Yoshioka T, Tokuda Y, et al. Clinical characteristics of patients with constrictive pericarditis after coronary bypass surgery. *Jpn Circ J.* (2001) 65:480–2. doi: 10.1253/jcj.65.480

30. Wilson MG, Hull JH, Rogers J, Pollock N, Dodd M, Haines J, et al. Cardiorespiratory considerations for return-to-play in elite athletes after COVID-19 infection: a practical guide for sport and exercise medicine physicians. *Br J Sports Med.* (2020) 54:1157–61. doi: 10.1136/bjsports-2020-102710

6

In silico Drug Screening Approach using L1000-Based Connectivity Map and its Application to COVID-19

Takaharu Asano[1], Sarvesh Chelvanambi[1], Julius L. Decano[1], Mary C. Whelan[1], Elena Aikawa[1,2,3] and Masanori Aikawa[1,2,3,4*]

[1] Center for Interdisciplinary Cardiovascular Sciences, Cardiovascular Division, Department of Medicine, Brigham and Women's Hospital and Harvard Medical School, Boston, MA, United States, [2] Center for Excellence in Vascular Biology, Cardiovascular Division, Department of Medicine, Brigham and Women's Hospital and Harvard Medical School, Boston, MA, United States, [3] Department of Human Pathology, I.M. Sechenov First Moscow State Medical University of the Ministry of Health, Moscow, Russia, [4] Channing Division of Network Medicine, Department of Medicine, Brigham and Women's Hospital and Harvard Medical School, Boston, MA, United States

*Correspondence:
Masanori Aikawa
maikawa@bwh.harvard.edu

Conventional drug screening methods search for a limited number of small molecules that directly interact with the target protein. This process can be slow, cumbersome and has driven the need for developing new drug screening approaches to counter rapidly emerging diseases such as COVID-19. We propose a pipeline for drug repurposing combining *in silico* drug candidate identification followed by *in vitro* characterization of these candidates. We first identified a gene target of interest, the entry receptor for the SARS-CoV-2 virus, angiotensin converting enzyme 2 (ACE2). Next, we employed a gene expression profile database, L1000-based Connectivity Map to query gene expression patterns in lung epithelial cells, which act as the primary site of SARS-CoV-2 infection. Using gene expression profiles from 5 different lung epithelial cell lines, we computationally identified 17 small molecules that were predicted to decrease ACE2 expression. We further performed a streamlined validation in the normal human epithelial cell line BEAS-2B to demonstrate that these compounds can indeed decrease ACE2 surface expression and to profile cell health and viability upon drug treatment. This proposed pipeline combining *in silico* drug compound identification and *in vitro* expression and viability characterization in relevant cell types can aid in the repurposing of FDA-approved drugs to combat rapidly emerging diseases.

Keywords: L1000, connectivity map (CMap), ACE2, COVID-19, drug repurposing, lung epithelial cell

INTRODUCTION

Coronavirus disease 2019 (COVID-19), which is caused by the infection of severe acute respiratory syndrome coronavirus 2 (SARS-CoV-2), broke out in December 2019. The World Health Organization designated COVID-19 as a global pandemic in March of 2020. Since then, multiple variants have emerged, spread globally, and continue to hit the health, life, and economy of people worldwide even with the advent of various vaccines designed to provide immunity against the virus. Intensive research efforts have revealed that morbidity, severity, and mortality from COVID-19 are strongly associated with various cardiovascular comorbidities (1). Since COVID-19 infection of lung epithelium could directly signal toward an increased risk for cardiovascular diseases (2), reducing productive infection of these cells becomes an important strategy to not only counter acute infection but prevent progression to cardiovascular diseases. Acute infections of viruses such as influenza virus (3), HIV (4), and SARS-CoV-2 (5) have been shown to have a direct impact on cardiovascular health and act as the initial insult that increases the incidence of cardiovascular disease in these patients. However, due to the massive number of patients globally infected by the virus, increase in cardiovascular disease prevalence due to infection with SARS-CoV-2 virus could severely burden the cardiovascular healthcare system in the future. Therefore, repurposing FDA approved drugs to contain SARS-CoV-2 infection can be an effective strategy to limit the risk of developing cardiovascular diseases in these patients.

The first step of SARS-CoV-2 invasion into human host cells is implemented by the SARS-CoV-2 spike protein binding to a host cell receptor, angiotensin-converting enzyme 2 (ACE2) (6). Inhibiting the spike protein and ACE2 interaction is, therefore, one of the promising drug targets for combating COVID-19 (7). Most current studies aim to inhibit the interaction by drugs that binds to the spike protein or ACE2 protein (7, 8).

In case drug targets are known, target-based drug discovery, in which a specific drug target that associates a target disease is identified and then hit compounds that interact with the target are searched for, is a proven strategy to generate new drugs (9). Conventional drug screening methods used in this strategy such as high-throughput screening (HTS), however, search for a limited number of small molecules that directly interact with the target protein. Moreover, this process can be slow, cumbersome and has driven the need for developing new drug screening approaches to counter rapidly emerging diseases like COVID-19.

The Connectivity Map (CMap) is a database of gene expression profiles induced by exposing a variety of cell types to various perturbagens including small molecules and has been expanded to have over one million gene expression profiles using over 20,000 small molecules through the introduction of L1000 assay technology (10, 11). L1000-based CMap has been widely used for rapid drug repurposing and the core idea is to identify small molecules that induce a gene expression profile canceling or mimicking the differential gene expression caused by diseases (12, 13). This approach is a kind of phenotypic screening, which is a counter approach to the target-based drug discovery and identifies small molecules that provide nice phenotypes (e.g., gene expression) to cells or animals first and then investigates the mechanism. Phenotypic screening has attracted attention recently because it was shown to be the most successful approach for first-in-class drugs (9, 14). As described above, although the conventional L1000-based CMap approach is an attractive way to find drugs that the conventional methods could overlook, it hardly has been applied to target-based drug discovery because this approach requires decreased and/or increased gene set, not a single target gene.

In this study, we propose a pipeline for drug repurposing that applies the L1000-based CMap to a single gene target, ACE2 which is the entry receptor for the SARS-CoV-2 virus. Using gene expression profiles from 5 different lung epithelial cell lines which act as the primary site of SARS-CoV-2 infection, we computationally identify small molecules that were predicted to decrease ACE2 expression. We further perform a streamlined validation in the normal human epithelial cell line BEAS-2B to identify the potential of these compounds to decrease ACE2 surface expression as well as profile cell health and viability upon drug treatment. This proposed pipeline combining *in silico* drug compound identification and *in vitro* expression and viability characterization in relevant cell types can aid in the repurposing of FDA-approved drugs to combat rapidly emerging diseases.

MATERIALS AND METHODS

L1000-Based CMap Dataset

Level 5 gene expression profiles of L1000-based CMap were downloaded from GSE92742 and GSE70138. This dataset has the gene expression profiles in a total of 591,697 conditions consisting of various combinations of perturbagens, cell types, doses, and time points. The profile values mean mRNA expression levels compared to control (the background of the plate). Each gene expression profile comprises 12,328 genes, 978 of which are measured directly (called landmark genes). Of the remaining genes, 9,196 are well-inferred genes the expression levels of which correlate to the actual measured levels with p-values ≤ 0.05, and the other 2,154 less-well inferred genes. ACE2 is in the well-inferred genes.

Cell Culture and Reagents

BEAS-2B normal human epithelial cell line was purchased from ATCC (Catalog number: CRL-9609) and cultured according to vendor instructions using BEGM kit from LONZA (Catalog number: CC-3170). Cells were cultured on 96-well black μ-plate from ibidi (Catalog Number: 89626) for imaging studies. Tanespimycin (abcam ab141433), Acetylcysteine (Cayman, 20261), Amifostine (Cayman 14398), Bortezomib (Ayman 10008822), FK-866 (Cayman 13287), Gemcitabine (Cayman 11690), Idarubicin (Cayman 14176), NVP-AUY922 (Cayman 10012698), NVP-BEZ235 (Cayman 10565), PIK-75 (Cayman 10009210), SN-38 (Cayman 15362), Tretinoin (Cayman 11017), YM-155 (Cayman 11490), Ingenol (Cayman 14031), Sulforaphane (LKT S8044), CD-437 (Sigma C5865), and Parbendazole (Sigma 1498706) were dissolved in DMSO. 1000x concentration working solution was used for downstream experimentation.

Immuno-Fluorescent Staining With High Content Imaging (HCI) for Quantifying ACE2 Expression

BEAS-2B cells were treated overnight with indicated drugs at indicated doses. Cells were then washed twice with PBS and fixed in 4% Paraformaldehyde for 15 min at room temperature. Cells were then stained with primary anti-human ACE2 antibody (Abcam ab239924) or isotype control for 1 h at 4°C with gentle shaking. Cells were then washed thrice with PBS and stained using AF555 labeled secondary antibody. Hoescht 33342 was used as nuclear counterstain.

Sixteen images were captured per well using 20x objective of an Image Express Pico (Molecular Devices) and analyzed using 2 color cell scoring system. Isotype control stained well was used to identify threshold for detecting ACE2 positivity in cells.

Cell Viability Measurement

BEAS-2B cells were plated in 96 well plates at 70% confluency and treated for 48 h with each drug at indicated doses. Cell mitochondrial activity was profiled using CyQuant MTT Cell Viability Assay (Thermo Fisher, Catalog Number V13154) following manufacturer instructions. The absorbance at 590 nm was quantified using Spectramax i3 (Molecular Devices). Cytotoxicity was quantified using CyQuant LDH Cytotoxicity Assay (Thermo Fisher Catalog Number C20301) following manufacturer instructions. Briefly, 50 μl of media supernatant from each well was used to quantify cell toxicity and was normalized to cells lysed with 10x cell lysis buffer as 100% cell death. Absorbance was measured at 490 nm and 680 nm with the 680 nm absorbance used to determine background plate absorbance. Mitochondrial Super Oxide production was quantified using MitoSOX™ Red Mitochondrial Superoxide Indicator (Thermo Fisher Catalog Number M36008) using manufacturer instructions. Hoescht 33342 was used as a nuclear counterstain. Sixteen images were captured per well using 20x objective of the Image Express Pico and analyzed using 2 color cell scoring system to determine average Mitochondrial Superoxide Intensity per cell.

FACS Staining

BEAS-2B cells were treated with indicated doses of drugs overnight and cells detached using accutase. Cells were resuspended in Stain Buffer with FBS (BD Biosciences) and stained with Fixed Viability Stain (FVS-780 BD Biosciences) followed by staining with ACE2-AF647 antibody (Biolegend). Cells stained with isotype AF647 antibody (BD Biosciences) were used to draw gates for ACE2 positivity. Cells were acquired on Cytek Aurora and data analyzed using Flowjo 10.8.

Statistical Methods

ACE2 expression and cell viability data were analyzed using a Python library, SciPy. FACS data was analyzed using Graphpad Prism 9.0. Student's t-test with Welch's correction was used to compare the effect of each treatment to control (vehicle) treated samples. Comparisons between the effects of each candidates were not performed.

RESULTS

Preprocessing for Drug Screening

The following filters were applied to the L1000-based CMap dataset to identify small molecules that are effective to COVID-19 therapy before searching for small molecules that decrease ACE2 expression (**Figure 1**).

Perturbagen Selection

A perturbagen is a reagent used to treat cells and measure the resulting biological response includes CRISPR/Cas9 constructs, short hairpin RNA (shRNA), open reading frames (ORFs), biological agents, small molecules, and so forth. The goal of this study was to identify small molecules suitable for

rapid drug repurposing. Drug Repurposing Hub is a curated and annotated collection of FDA-approved drugs, clinical trial drugs, and pre-clinical tool compounds with a companion information resource, and the mechanisms of action of 6,232 drugs are explicitly stated in it (drug information version: 3/24/2020) (15). L1000-based CMap dataset contains 20,547 small molecules, and 2,760 small molecules out of them overlap with these 6,232 drugs. We therefore extracted the gene expression profiles in conditions treated with these 2,760 small molecules, resulting 160,003 profiles induced by exposing 82 cell types to 2,760 small molecules with up to 177.6 μM for 3, 6, 24, or 48 h.

Dose Selection

Each small molecule was measured at various dosages within the database. To compare these dosages and to increase ease of handling, doses from a similar range were converted to a single value as indicated in **Supplementary Table 1**. Among available dosages, 0.0001–100 μM, the most used dosage was 10 μM and the profiles using over 1 μM dosage dominate 68.5% of the total. These dosages over 1 μM were eliminated due to concerns about cytotoxicity and the need to identify drugs that would work at low doses and minimal side-effects to reduce gene expression of ACE2.

Time-Point Selection

Drugs for COVID-19 need to work within hours to reduce ACE2 expression since that would be the ideal window for drug intervention of a patient testing positive for SARS-CoV-2. The available time-points were 3, 6, and 24 h after the dose selection. We removed the timepoints over 24 h to identify fast-acting drug candidates. This step provided 5,411 profiles induced by exposing 67 cell types to 300 small molecules with 0.0003–0.3162 μM for 3 or 6 h.

Cell Type Selection

After the time-point selection, 67 cell types derived from 14 organs such as large intestine, lung, breast, etc. were available. Each cell type shows a different gene expression profile even though the same small molecule is applied. It is advisable to use the gene expression profiles in a specific cell type of interest. However, human lung epithelial cells such as BEAS-2B that are suitable for model host cells in COVID-19 study are not included in L1000-based CMap. We thus selected 5 cell types (A549, CORL23, H1299, NCIH596, and SKLU1) derived from lung in the dataset. Of note, all five cell types were from lung epithelial cell lines derived from various tumors. The gene expression profiles in conditions using these 5 cell types were extracted, resulting 588 profiles induced by exposing 5 cell types to 80 small molecules with 0.0003–0.3162 μM for 6 h.

The 588 profiles came from 485 unique conditions. Finally, the gene expression levels were averaged over the same conditions, resulting the preprocessed dataset that has 485 profiles induced by exposing 5 cell types to 80 small molecules with 0.0003–0.3162 μM for 6 h.

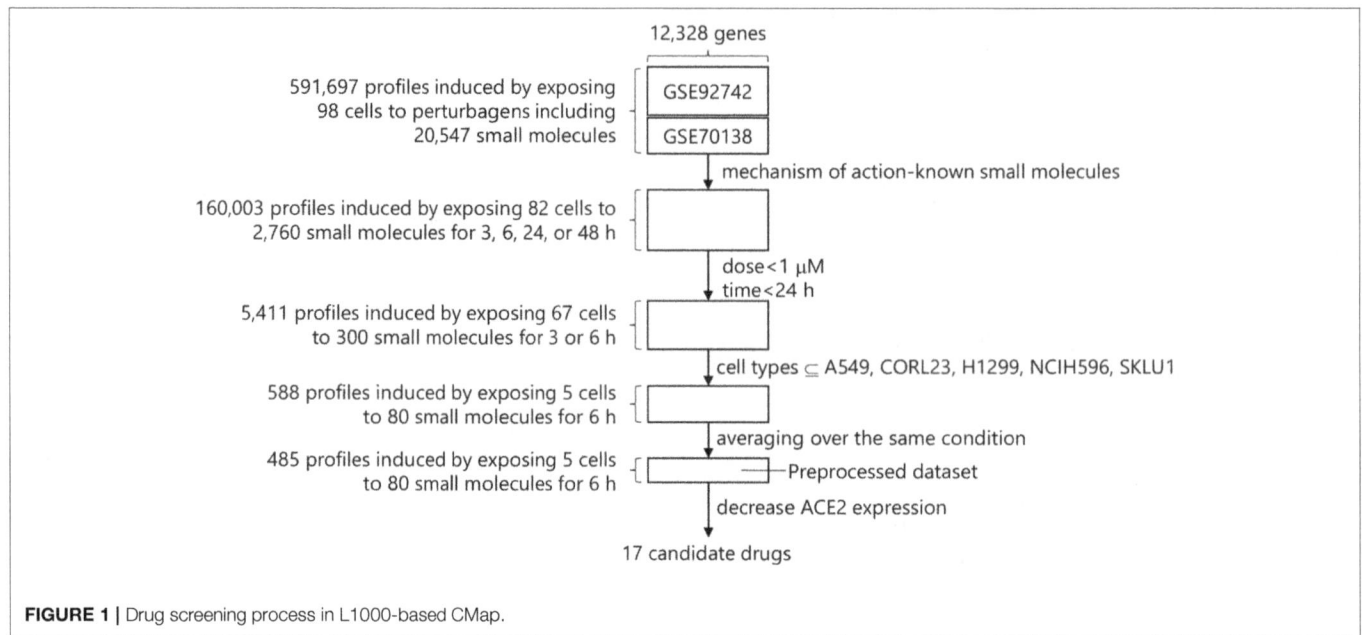

FIGURE 1 | Drug screening process in L1000-based CMap.

Identification of Small Molecules That Decrease ACE2 Expression

We focused on the expression levels of ACE2 and extracted the combinations of the small molecules and their dosages that decrease ACE2 expression (i.e., show the negative ACE2 expression levels) in each cell type. As for A549, since 214 combinations were identified, the top 10 combinations with the lower ACE2 expression levels were selected. In the other 4 cell types, 4, 4, 6, and 5 combinations were identified in CORL23, H1299, NCIH596, and SKLU1, respectively. Out of these 29, 19 combinations were unique. We removed 0.0032 μM veliparib which was commercially unavailable and 0.01 μM idarubicin, while keeping the larger dose, 0.1 μM idarubicin. As a result, 17 small molecules and their optimal dosages in 6 h were obtained as the drug repurposing candidates. The ACE2 expression levels in each cell type treated with these 17 small molecules with their optimal dosages are shown in **Table 1**.

NVP-AUY922 and tanespimycin are heat shock protein (HSP) inhibitors. NVP-BEZ235 and PIK-75 are PI3K inhibitors. CD-437 and tretinoin are retinoid receptor agonists. SN-38 and idarubicin are topoisomerase inhibitors. The other 9 small molecules have different mechanisms of action. The candidates cover a wide variety of mechanisms of action. On the other hand, most small molecules have been developed for cancer drugs except for acetylcysteine, ingenol, and sulforaphane.

For 9 among 17 small molecules, ACE2 expression levels were available in all 5 cell types (**Table 1**). The ACE2 expression levels were quite different in each cell even though the same small molecules are applied with the same doses, suggesting the other 8 small molecules whose ACE2 levels were available only in A549 also have different ACE2 expression levels depending on the cell types. On the other hand, these small molecules show negative ACE2 expression levels in at least 1 cell type, suggesting that these

small molecules have a potential to decrease ACE2 expression in human lung epithelial cells.

For 13 among 17 small molecules, ACE2 expression levels at 6 dose points in A549 were available in the preprocessed dataset. The dose-response of ACE2 expression levels in each small molecule are shown in **Figure 2**. The top 6 small molecules with lower ACE2 levels in A549 in **Table 1** (acetylcysteine, CD-437, NVP-BEZ235, amifostine, ingenol, and NVP-AUY922) decreased ACE2 expression almost dose-dependently within the ranges up to their optimal doses. These small molecules are expected to decrease ACE2 expression in A549, human adenocarcinoma alveolar basal epithelial cells.

In-vitro Pipeline for Evaluation of Predicted Drug Repurposing Candidates That Reduce ACE2 Expression in Human Lung Epithelial Cells

Evaluation of Cytotoxicity Profile of Drug Repurposing Candidates in Normal Human Immortalized Bronchial Epithelial Cells

The first *in vitro* step in our drug repurposing validation pipeline was to evaluate the effect of the various predicted small molecules in impacting cellular health and viability. As listed in **Table 1**, these compounds have a wide range of mechanisms of action. Stringent characterization of the effect of a treating relevant cell type with these compounds was therefore performed.

The five lung epithelial cell lines utilized in the L1000 were tumor-derived lung epithelial cell lines. Evaluating the effectiveness of these predicted drug repurposing candidates in reducing ACE2 expression in COVID-19 infected patients, however, required analysis in a non-tumor lung epithelial cell

TABLE 1 | The identified 17 small molecules, their optimal doses, mechanisms of action, and ACE2 expression levels in each cell type.

Drug name (uM)	Mechanism of action	Cell type				
		A549	CORL23	H1299	NCIH596	SKLU1
Acetylcysteine (0.01)	Mucolytic agent	−2.29				
CD-437 (0.1)	Retinoid receptor agonist	−1.74				
NVP-BEZ235 (0.0316)	mTOR inhibitor, PI3K inhibitor	−1.47				
Amifostine (0.3162)	Reducing agent	−1.47				
Ingenol (0.01)	PKC activator	−1.45		No data		
NVP-AUY922 (0.1)	HSP inhibitor	−1.41				
Tretinoin (0.3162)	Retinoid receptor agonist, retinoid receptor ligand	−1.40				
Sulforaphane (0.001)	Anticancer agent, aryl hydrocarbon receptor antagonist	−1.32				
Bortezomib (0.0316)	NFkB pathway inhibitor, proteasome inhibitor	−0.54	0.13	0.13	−0.80	−0.96
Parbendazole (0.3162)	Tubulin polymerization inhibitor	−0.53	0.01	0.80	−0.80	−0.09
Idarubicin (0.1)	Topoisomerase inhibitor	−0.47	0.70	−1.44	0.00	0.46
Tanespimycin (0.3162)	HSP inhibitor	−0.23	0.00	0.09	0.39	0.07
SN-38 (0.3162)	Topoisomerase inhibitor	−0.19	−0.37	−0.55	−0.38	0.20
FK-866 (0.1)	Niacinamide phosphoribosyltransferase inhibitor	0.06	−0.79	0.41	−0.50	0.10
Gemcitabine (0.1)	Ribonucleotide reductase inhibitor	0.09	0.63	0.94	0.50	−1.28
YM-155 (0.3162)	Survivin inhibitor	0.36	0.00	−0.82	−0.57	−0.17
PIK-75 (0.1)	DNA protein kinase inhibitor, PI3K inhibitor	2.32	0.45	−1.04	0.54	−0.37

The small molecules are sorted based on the ACE2 expression levels in A549. The numbers in brackets beside drug names are their optimal dosages (μM). Gray area means no data in the preprocessed dataset.

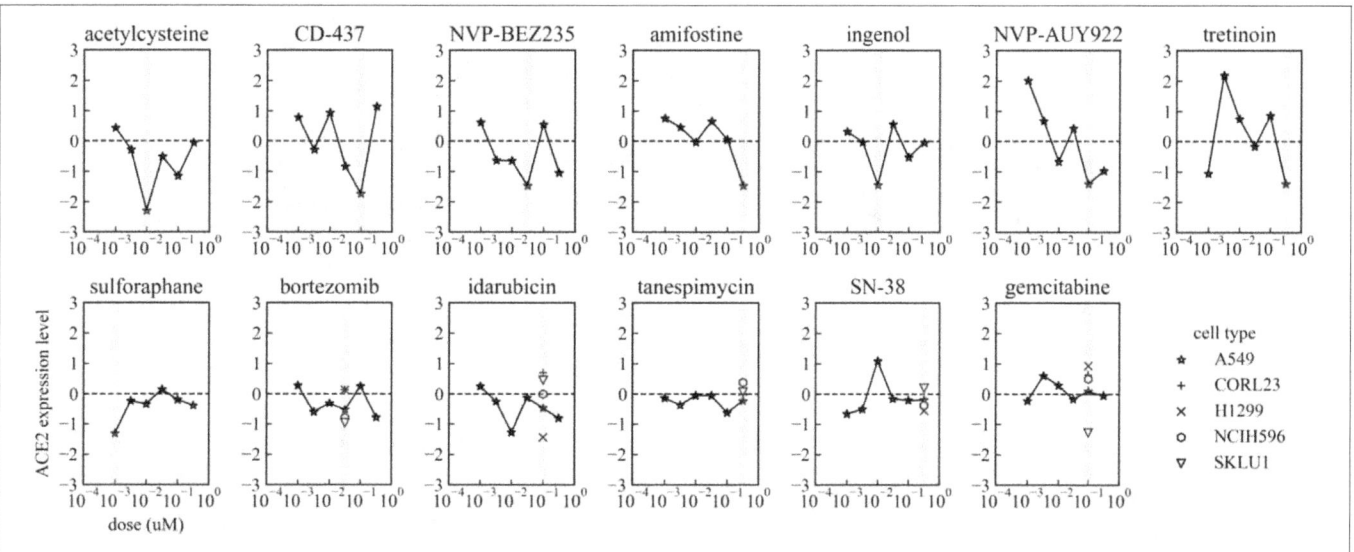

FIGURE 2 | Dose-response of ACE2 expression levels in each small molecule in A549. Gray vertical bars mean the optimal dosages in each small molecule indicated in **Table 1**. ACE2 expression levels in CORL23, H1299, NCIH596, and SKLU1 are also shown in Bortezomib, Idarubicin, Tanespimycin, SN-38, and Gemcitabine.

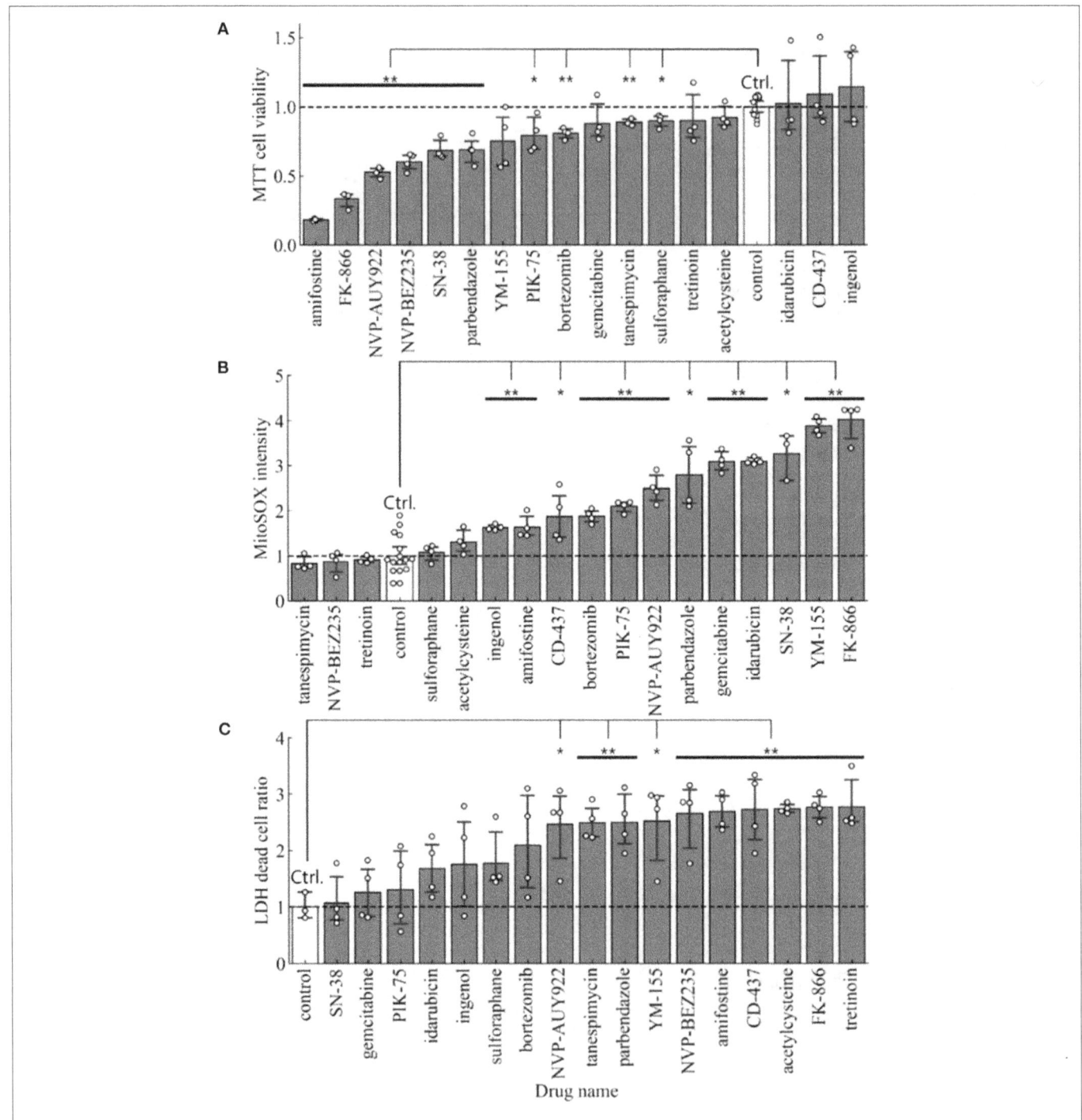

FIGURE 3 | Cell toxicity assay in BEAS-2B treated with each of 17 small molecules and the control. **(A)** Cell viability measured by MTT assay ($n = 4$ in samples and $n = 12$ in control), **(B)** Mitochondrial Super Oxide production measured by MitoSOX assay ($n = 4$ in samples and $n = 16$ in control), and **(C)** Cytotoxicity measured by LDH assay ($n = 4$). Error bars mean 95% confidence interval. *$p < 0.05$, **$p < 0.01$.

setting. BEAS-2B is a normal human immortalized bronchial epithelial cell line, which has been extensively used to study cellular and molecular mechanisms involved in lung. This study therefore used BEAS-2B as a host cell model that could be infected by SARS-CoV-2.

For cell toxicity studies, the BEAS-2B cells were treated with indicated amounts of each drug repurposing candidate, and cell health was evaluated using multiple orthogonal measures. MTT assay measured the amount viable cells in each well by quantifying the amount of MTT converted to formazan crystals.

The average absorbance in cells receiving vehicle were used to normalize the effect of each drug repurposing candidate. Therefore, a ratio <1.0 indicates treatments which exerted a negative effect on cell viability when compared to control cells. In this analysis, all compounds other than CD-437, Idarubicin and Ingenol had a ratio <1.0 (**Figure 3A**). Comparison of cell viability using Student's t-test ($p < 0.05$) showed that 10 out of 17 drug repurposing candidates had a statistically significant lower viability as indicated by MTT assay.

To further characterize whether mitochondrial stress was present upon treatment with these drug re-purposing candidates, we evaluated mitochondrial specific superoxide species production using MitoSOX. We used an HCI strategy to quantify the intensity of mitochondrial superoxide species and compared the average intensity of mitochondrial superoxide per cell in each treatment. A ratio >1.0, therefore, indicated higher levels of mitochondrial reactive oxygen species production upon treatment with the respective drug-repurposing candidates as described in **Figure 3B**. NVP-BEZ235, Tanespimycin and Tretinoin were the three compounds with ratio <1.0. All other compounds had elevated mitochondrial superoxide species when compared to control treatment. Comparison of MitoSOX intensity using Student's t-test ($p < 0.05$) showed that 12 out of 17 drug repurposing candidates had a statistically significant increase in mitochondrial stress as indicated by MitoSOX staining.

Finally, we used a third method to characterize the effect of these drug repurposing candidates in cell cytotoxicity using Lactate Dehydrogenase (LDH) assay. This assay measures the amount of LDH released out into the supernatant from dead cells with leaky plasma membrane. All readouts were normalized to wells where 100% of cells were lysed using a cell lysis buffer. Compared to this number, the average percentage of dead cells in each well was calculated. Again, percent cell death was normalized to control wells receiving vehicle treatment (**Figure 3C**). Therefore, a ratio >1.0 indicates elevated levels of cytotoxicity. All drug repurposing candidates showcased a ratio >1.0 indicated increased cell death upon treatment. Comparison of cell death using Student's t-test ($p < 0.05$) showed that 10 out of 17 drug repurposing candidates had a statistically significant increased cell death as indicated by LDH cytotoxicity assay.

Consensus Ranking of Cytotoxicity in Normal Human Lung Epithelial Cell Lines

To compile the three formats used to evaluate cytotoxicity in BEAS-2B cells treated with our drug repurposing candidates, we built a consensus ranking table comprising of MTT, MitoSOX and LDH cytotoxicity assays. **Table 2** depicts the consensus ranking based on these three assays and ranks small molecules based on low cytotoxicity across all three formats. In this consensus ranking analysis, the following seven candidates, Ingenol, Sulforaphane, Tanespimycin, Idarubicin, CD-437, PIK-75, and Gemcitabine showed a consistently low cytotoxic profile at indicated doses in BEAS-2B lung epithelial cells. This identification of small molecules with favorable safety profile in target cell type is required for our drug repurposing pipeline in order to find suitable candidates for treatment where low

TABLE 2 | Consensus ranking comprising of MTT, MitoSOX, and LDH cytotoxicity assay.

Drug name	Cyto toxicity ranking			
	MTT	**MitoSOX**	**LDH**	**Ave.**
Control	4	4	1	3.0
Ingenol	1	7	6	4.7
Sulforaphane	7	5	7	6.3
Tanespimycin	8	1	10	6.3
Idarubicin	3	15	5	7.7
CD-437	2	9	15	8.7
PIK-75	11	11	4	8.7
Gemcitabine	9	14	3	8.7
Acetylcysteine	5	6	16	9.0
Tretinoin	6	3	18	9.0
Bortezomib	10	10	8	9.3
NVP-BEZ235	15	2	13	10.0
SN-38	14	16	2	10.7
NVP-AUY922	16	12	9	12.3
Parbendazole	13	13	11	12.3
Amifostine	18	8	14	13.3
YM-155	12	17	12	13.7
FK-866	17	18	17	17.3

Each value means ranking of low toxicity (i.e., high number means high toxicity). Drugs are sorted based on the average ranking over 3 assays.

cytotoxic side effects are crucial for applicability of identified small molecules.

Evaluation of ACE2 Surface Expression in Human Lung Epithelial Cells With Predicted Candidates for Drug Repurposing

The next step in our drug repurposing pipeline was to determine the effect of these predicted drug repurposing candidates to reduce surface expression of ACE2. For this study, ACE2 surface expression serves as the most important determinant since we were evaluating the capacity of these small molecules to reduce the prevalence of surface receptors to which the SARS-CoV-2 spike protein can bind to and subsequently infect target cells. We thus used immuno-fluorescent staining to quantify surface expression of human ACE2 expression using HCI followed by a cell scoring system using red staining intensity for ACE2 and cell calling using Hoescht 33342 nuclear counterstain. A representative image for ACE2 staining in BEAS-2B is shown in **Figure 4A**. Thresholds for determining ACE2 expression were established using cells stained with isotype primary antibody followed by secondary antibody staining. Cell calling was performed using nuclear counter stain and establishing appropriate cell diameter to detect all cells within 4 different fields of view. Using these parameters, we observed cells that were high for ACE2 expression and others that expressed ACE2 at low levels (**Figure 4B**). Of note, even when looking with the normal immortalized cell line, we observed heterogeneity in ACE2 expression across cells. Using this categorization strategy, we will

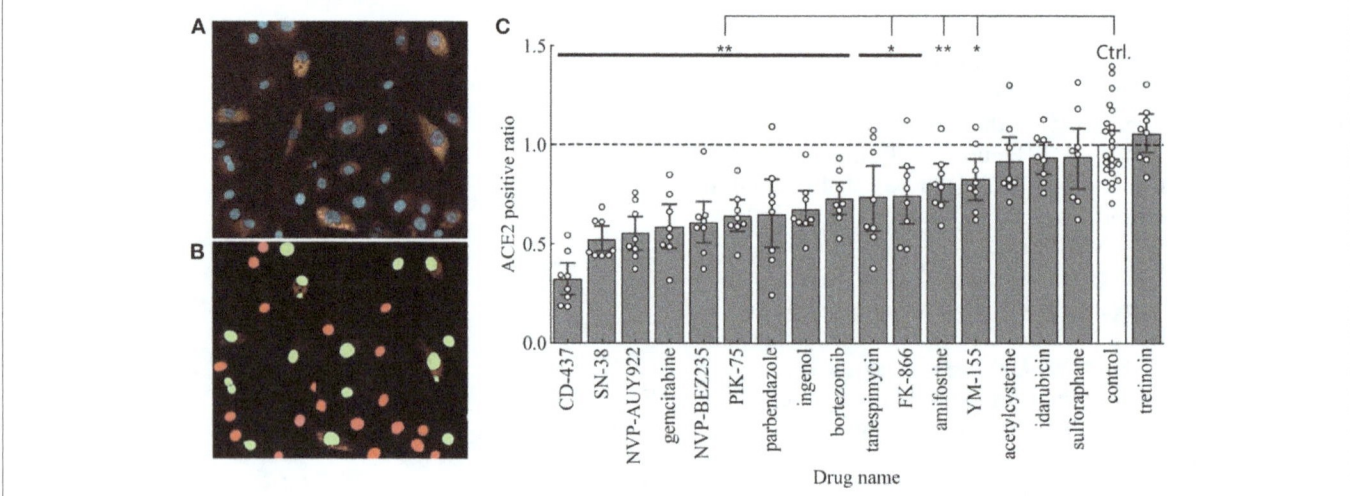

FIGURE 4 | (A) Representative image showing ACE2 staining in BEAS-2B. ACE2-high expressed (ACE2 positive) cells are detected and then ACE2 positive ratio is calculated. **(B)** Representative cell scoring masks indicating ACE2 expressing cells (Green) and ACE2 negative cells (Red). **(C)** ACE2 positive ratios in each drug treatment compared to the control ($n = 8$ in samples and $n = 23$ in control). Error bars mean 95% confidence interval. $*p < 0.05$, $**p < 0.01$.

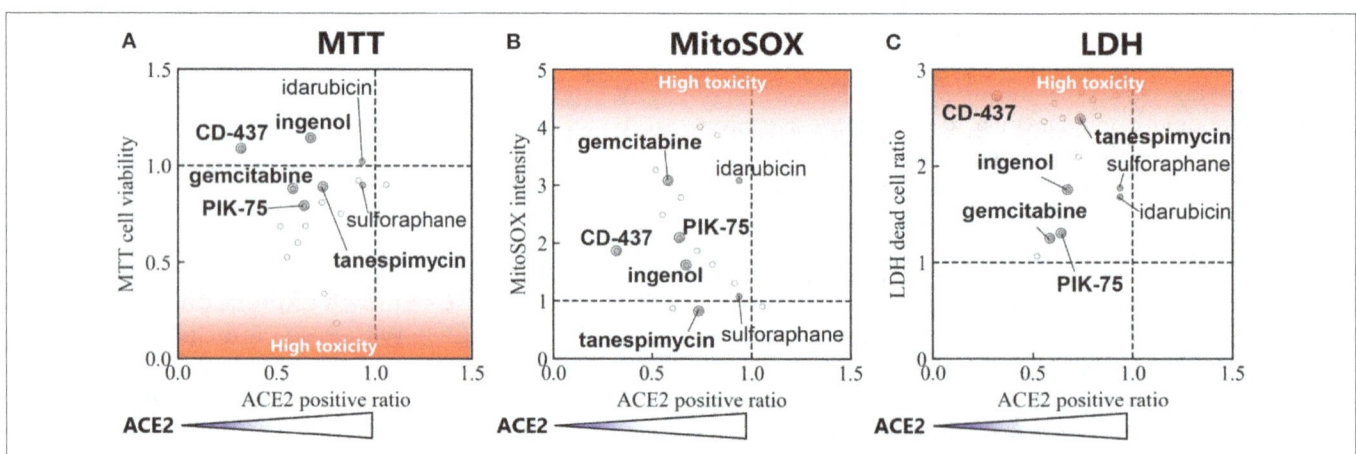

FIGURE 5 | Correlation between ACE2 positive ratio vs. cell toxicity. Correlation between ACE2 positive ratio and **(A)** cell viability measured by MTT assay, **(B)** MitoSOX Assay, and **(C)** LDH assay. The locations of the top 7 small molecules with reduced cytotoxicity in **Table 2** are labeled.

use the nomenclature of ACE2 high- or low-expressed cells to determine the effect of our various treatments in modifying ACE2 expression in a lung epithelial cell population. The number ratios of high-expressed cells in the total cell number were calculated as ACE2 positive ratios in each small molecule treatment and were normalized with the ACE2 positive ratio of the control (no treatment).

The ACE2 positive ratios after our candidate treatments are shown in **Figure 4C**. Using Student's t-test ($p < 0.05$) to compare to control treated BEAS-2B cells, 13 out of 17 treatments showed a statistically significant reduction in surface ACE2 expression. In this regard, the top 3 small molecules with the higher decreasing level of ACE2 positive ratio are CD-437, SN-38, and NVP-AUY922.

Integration of ACE2 Expression and Cell Viability Data to Identify Top Drug Repurposing Candidates

This pipeline follows the L1000 powered identification of small molecule candidates for drug repurposing by evaluating the effect of these compounds in affecting both cell health and surface ACE2 expression. Therefore, correlation analysis was performed in order to narrow down the candidates and identify small molecules that could be used to reduce ACE2 expression without inducing high levels of cell death specifically in our target cell type BEAS-2B (**Figure 5**). Three correlation matrices were constructed to compare the effect of each candidate in affecting cell health as well as the potency with which they reduced ACE2 expression. Using this matrix, Ingenol, CD-437, Tanespimycin, PIK-75, and Gemcitabine were five compounds that consistently

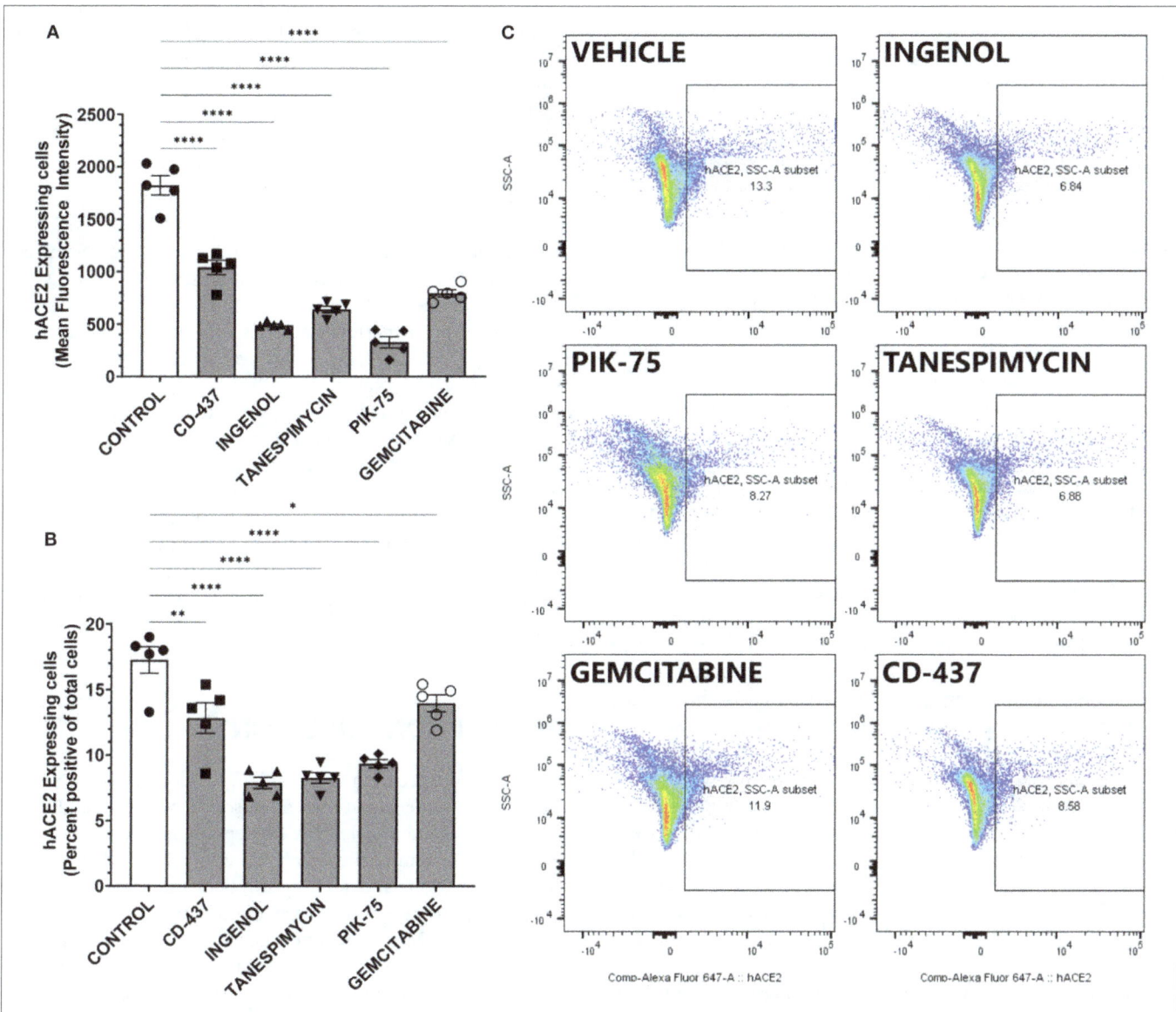

FIGURE 6 | ACE2 expression measure by FACS in BEAS-2B treated with the 5 repurposing candidates. **(A)** mean ACE2 expression ($n = 5$). **(B)** ACE2 positive ratio. Error bar means standard deviation ($n = 5$). *$p < 0.05$, **$p < 0.01$, ****$p < 0.0001$. **(C)** Representative scatter plot showing percent positive ACE2 surface expression in BEAS-2B cells.

showed low cytotoxicity and effective downregulation of surface ACE2 expression. This data suggests that these five candidates identified using our novel drug repurposing pipeline can be evaluated for large scale studies in preventing SARS-CoV-2 infection by targeting ACE2 expression levels.

Validation of Identified Top Candidates Combining Viability and ACE2 Expression

The top five candidates with low toxicity and potent decrease in ACE2 expression were further validated using an orthogonal platform, Fluorescence Assisted Cell Sorting. This platform allows for the quantification of surface ACE2 expression in viable, living cells. Furthermore, quantitative analysis can be performed

in an unbiased fashion in a large number of cells. BEAS-2B cells were treated with indicated doses of drugs and then percent positive cells for surface ACE2 were determined using control cells treated with isotype antibody (**Supplementary Figure 1**). All five candidates produced statistically significant reductions in both the overall amount of surface ACE2 receptors and the mean fluorescent intensity of ACE2 staining in viable BEAS-2B cells (**Figure 6A**). Furthermore, the fraction of cells determined to be positive for ACE2 expression (**Figures 6B,C**) also showed statistically significant reductions with all five compounds identified using our pipeline. Taken together, our data suggest that intervention with these five small molecule compounds can decrease the number of viable cells susceptible to SARS-CoV-2 infection by altering surface ACE2 expression.

DISCUSSION

We identified 17 candidate small molecules that possibly decrease ACE2 expression by processing the L1000-based CMap dataset with focusing on the drug repurposing for COVID-19 (**Table 1** and **Figure 1**). These candidates decreased ACE2 mRNA levels within 6 h in the lung epithelial cell lines in the preprocessed dataset (**Table 1** and **Figure 2**). This suggests that the decrease in ACE2 mRNA levels likely led to reduced ACE2 surface expression in the target cells BEAS-2B derived from the same organ. Indeed, most candidates decreased ACE2 expression on the surface of BEAS-2B (**Figure 4**). These results indicate that our L1000-powered drug screening effectively identifies small molecules that modulate a single drug target. Further investigation, however, is required to address the mechanism of action for ACE2 suppression by these compounds as well as the effects on ACE2 expression in other cell types.

On the other hand, the identified small molecules were mostly drugs that have been developed for cancer treatment, therefore, their cytotoxic effects in BEAS-2B were evaluated using MTT, MitoSOX, and LDH assays. Over half candidates showed significant cytotoxicity or cell viability reduction in each assay (**Figure 3**). To identify small molecules that consistently show a low cytotoxic profile, we built a consensus ranking table (**Table 2**). The top 2 small molecules with the lowest toxicity were Ingenol and Sulforaphane. Ingenol is an FDA-approved drug for keratosis. Sulforaphane is a naturally occurring isothiocyanate found in cruciferous vegetables such as broccoli. These facts support the validity of this table.

Our goal was to obtain the drug repurposing candidates that could be used to reduce surface ACE2 expression without inducing high cell toxicity. Therefore, correlation analysis was performed to narrow down the candidates (**Figure 5**). In this correlation matrix, Ingenol, CD-437, Tanespimycin, PIK-75, and Gemcitabine consistently showed low cytotoxicity and effective downregulation of surface ACE2 expression. These were five compounds, out of the top 7 with low toxicity in **Table 2**, that show significant ACE2 reduction in **Figure 4**. Moreover, additional validation experiments demonstrated that all these five candidates decreased the surface ACE2 expression in living BEAS-2B (**Figure 6**). These results suggest that these five candidates can be evaluated for large scale studies in preventing SARS-CoV-2 infection by targeting ACE2 expression levels.

Our proposed pipeline consists of L1000-powered drug screening and the further narrowing of the drug repurposing candidates based on their cytotoxic effect. As described above, the L1000 screening can be applied to a single target, allowing us to apply this method to target-based drug discovery which is a gold standard strategy. The small molecules identified by this method are different from those by conventional screenings like HTS because our approach focuses on the target gene mRNA level instead of the target protein. In addition, conventional L1000-CMap approaches have no applicability to target-based drug discovery because it requires a gene set rather than a single gene. Furthermore, our pipeline can be adapted to a wide range of cell types including endothelial cells and monocytes. This is of interest since viruses including HIV and SARS-CoV-2 have been shown to specifically induce pulmonary endothelial cell activation (16, 17). Our cell types of interest in the present study were epithelial cells. We thus used the identified compounds in this cell type to perform a series of assays to evaluate cell health and stress. COVID-19, however, affects other cell types. Application of our pipeline to other cell types could include various additional functional assays depending on the cell type of interest, for example, angiogenesis assays in endothelial cells, or measuring pro-inflammatory chemokine secretion in monocytes. Thus, our pipeline provides a novel screening method that is different from both HTS and conventional L1000-CMap approaches, contributing to the repurposing of FDA approved drugs to combat rapidly emerging diseases as well as other diseases like vascular calcification that conventional approaches have yet found the therapeutic options.

AUTHOR CONTRIBUTIONS

TA and SC: conception and design, collection of data, data analysis and interpretation, manuscript writing, and final approval of the manuscript. JD: conception and design and final approval of the manuscript. MW: collection of data, data analysis and interpretation, and final approval of the manuscript. EA: financial support, administrative support, and final approval of the manuscript. MA: conception and design, financial support, administrative support, data interpretation, manuscript editing, and final approval of the manuscript. All authors contributed to the article and approved the submitted version.

ACKNOWLEDGMENTS

The authors thank John Tigges and Brandy Pinckney from Flow Cytometry Core Facility of Beth Israel Deaconess Medical Center (MA, USA) for helping us with setting-up of the flow cytometry analysis.

REFERENCES

1. Brandão SCS, Ramos J, de OX, Dompieri LT, Godoi, E. T. A. M., et al. Is Toll-like receptor 4 involved in the severity of COVID-19 pathology in patients with cardiometabolic comorbidities? *Cytok*

Growth Factor Rev. (2021) 58:102–10. doi: 10.1016/j.cytogfr.2020.09.002

2. Jha PK, Vijay A, Halu A, Uchida S, Aikawa M. Gene expression profiling reveals the shared and distinct transcriptional signatures in human lung epithelial cells infected with SARS-CoV-2, MERS-CoV, or

SARS-CoV: potential implications in cardiovascular complications of COVID-19. *Front Cardiovasc Med.* (2021) 7:1–15. doi: 10.3389/fcvm.202 0.623012

3. Lu H, Chelvanambi S, Poirier C, Saliba J, March KL, Clauss M, et al. EMAPII monoclonal antibody ameliorates influenza A virus-induced lung injury. *Mol Ther.* (2018) 26:2060–9. doi: 10.1016/j.ymthe.2018.05.017

4. Chelvanambi S, Gupta SK, Chen X, Ellis BW, Maier BF, Colbert TM, et al. HIV-Nef protein transfer to endothelial cells requires Rac1 activation and leads to endothelial dysfunction: implications for statin treatment in HIV patients. *Circ Res.* (2019) 125:805–20. doi: 10.1161/CIRCRESAHA.119.315082

5. Nishiga M, Wang DW, Han Y, Lewis DB, Wu JC. COVID-19 and cardiovascular disease: from basic mechanisms to clinical perspectives. *Nat Rev Cardiol.* (2020) 17:543–58. doi: 10.1038/s41569-020-0413-9

6. Rabi FA, Al Zoubi MS, Al-Nasser AD, Kasasbeh GA, Salameh DM. Sars-cov-2 and coronavirus disease 2019: what we know so far. *Pathogens.* (2020) 9:231. doi: 10.3390/pathogens9030231

7. Gil C, Ginex T, Maestro I, Nozal V, Barrado-Gil L, Cuesta-Geijo MÁ, et al. COVID-19: drug targets and potential treatments. *J Med Chem.* (2020) 63:12359–86. doi: 10.1021/acs.jmedchem.0c00606

8. Kifle ZD, Ayele AG, Enyew EF. Drug repurposing approach, potential drugs, and novel drug targets for COVID-19 treatment. *J Environ Public Health.* (2021) 2021:6631721. doi: 10.1155/2021/6631721

9. Swinney DC, Anthony J. How were new medicines discovered? *Nat Rev Drug Discov.* (2011) 10:507–19. doi: 10.1038/nrd3480

10. Lamb J, Crawford ED, Peck D, Modell JW, Blat IC, Wrobel MJ, et al. The Connectivity Map: using gene-expression signatures to connect small molecules, genes, and disease. *Science.* (2006) 313:1929–35. doi: 10.1126/science.1132939

11. Subramanian A, Narayan R, Corsello SM, Peck DD, Natoli TE, Lu X, et al. A next generation connectivity map: L1000 platform and the first 1,000,000 profiles. *Cell.* (2017) 171:1437–52.e17. doi: 10.1016/j.cell.2017. 10.049

12. Duan Q, Reid SP, Clark NR, Wang Z, Fernandez NF, Rouillard AD, et al. L1000CDS2: LINCS L1000 characteristic direction signatures search engine. *Npj Syst Biol Appl.* (2016) 2:1–12. doi: 10.1038/npjsba.2016.15

13. Musa A, Ghoraie LS, Zhang SD, Glazko G, Yli-Harja O, Dehmer M, et al. A review of connectivity map and computational approaches in pharmacogenomics. *Brief Bioinform.* (2018) 19:506–23. doi: 10.1093/bib/bbw112

14. Swinney DC. Phenotypic vs. Target-based drug discovery for first-in-class medicines. *Clin Pharmacol Ther.* (2013) 93:299–301. doi: 10.1038/clpt.2012.236

15. Corsello SM, Bittker JA, Liu Z, Gould J, McCarren P, Hirschman JE, et al. The drug repurposing hub: a next-generation drug library and information resource. *Nat Med.* (2017) 23:405–8. doi: 10.1038/nm.4306

16. Chelvanambi S, Bogatcheva NV, Bednorz M, Agarwal S, Maier B, Alves NJ, et al. HIV-Nef protein persists in the lungs of aviremic patients with HIV and induces endothelial cell death. *Am J Respir Cell Mol Biol.* (2019) 60:357–66. doi: 10.1165/rcmb.2018-0089OC

17. Clauss M, Chelvanambi S, Cook C, Elmergawy R, Dhillon N. Viral bad news sent by evail. *Viruses.* (2021) 13:1–13. doi: 10.3390/v13061168

7

Incidence of Venous Thromboembolism in Hospitalized Coronavirus Disease 2019 Patients

Chi Zhang[1†], Long Shen[2†], Ke-Jia Le[1†], Mang-Mang Pan[1], Ling-Cong Kong[2], Zhi-Chun Gu[1*], Hang Xu[3*], Zhen Zhang[4], Wei-Hong Ge[3] and Hou-Wen Lin[1]

[1] Department of Pharmacy, Renji Hospital, School of Medicine, Shanghai Jiaotong University, Shanghai, China, [2] Department of Cardiology, Renji Hospital, School of Medicine, Shanghai Jiaotong University, Shanghai, China, [3] Department of Pharmacy, Nanjing Drum Tower Hospital, The Affiliated Hospital of Nanjing University Medical School, Nanjing, China, [4] Department of Pharmacy, Roswell Park Comprehensive Cancer Center, Buffalo, NY, United States

*Correspondence:
Zhi-Chun Gu
guzhichun213@163.com
Hang Xu
njglyyxh@126.com

[†] These authors have contributed equally to this work and share first authorship

Background: Emerging evidence shows that coronavirus disease 2019 (COVID-19) is commonly complicated by coagulopathy, and venous thromboembolism (VTE) is considered to be a potential cause of unexplained death. Information on the incidence of VTE in COVID-19 patients, however, remains unclear.

Method: English-language databases (PubMed, Embase, Cochrane), Chinese-language databases (CNKI, VIP, WANFANG), and preprint platforms were searched to identify studies with data of VTE occurrence in hospitalized COVID-19 patients. Pooled incidence and relative risks (RRs) of VTE were estimated by a random-effects model. Variations were examined based on clinical manifestations of VTE (pulmonary embolism-PE and deep vein thrombosis-DVT), disease severity (severe patients and non-severe patients), and rate of pharmacologic thromboprophylaxis (≥ 60 and $<60\%$). Sensitivity analyses were conducted to strengthen the robustness of results. Meta-regression was performed to explore the risk factors associated with VTE in COVID-19 patients.

Results: A total of 17 studies involving 1,913 hospitalized COVID-19 patients were included. The pooled incidence of VTE was 25% (95% CI, 19–31%; I^2, 95.7%), with a significant difference between the incidence of PE (19%; 95% CI, 13–25%; I^2, 93.2%) and DVT (7%; 95% CI, 4–10%; I^2, 88.3%; $P_{interaction} < 0.001$). Higher incidence was observed in severe COVID-19 patients (35%; 95 CI%, 25–44%; I^2, 92.4%) than that in non-severe patients (6%; 95 CI%, 3–10%; I^2, 62.2%; $P_{interaction} < 0.001$). The high rate of pharmacologic thromboprophylaxis in COVID-19 patients ($\geq 60\%$) was associated with a lower incidence of VTE compared with the low pharmacologic thromboprophylaxis rate ($<60\%$) (19 vs. 40%; $P_{interaction} = 0.052$). Severe patients had a 3.76-fold increased risk of VTE compared with non-severe patients (RR, 4.76; 95% CI, 2.66–8.50; I^2, 47.0%). Sensitivity analyses confirmed the robustness of the primacy results.

Conclusions: This meta-analysis revealed that the estimated VTE incidence was 25% in hospitalized COVID-19 patients. Higher incidence of VTE was observed in COVID-19 patients with a severe condition or with a low rate of pharmacologic thromboprophylaxis. Assessment of VTE risk is strongly recommended in COVID-19 patients, and effective measures of thromboprophylaxis should be taken in a timely manner for patients with high risk of VTE.

Keywords: COVID-19, venous thromboembolism, pulmonary embolism, incidence, thromboprophylaxis, anticoagulation

INTRODUCTION

Coronavirus disease 2019 (COVID-19) has spread globally, resulting in an unprecedented health crisis. As of 5 July 2020, there has been 11,125,245 cases of COVID-19 worldwide, of which 528,204 patients have died (1). Remarkably, emerging evidence shows that COVID-19 is commonly complicated by coagulopathy, and venous thromboembolism (VTE) is considered to be a potential cause of unexplained death, especially in severe COVID-19 patients (2, 3). A variety of potential risk factors of VTE exist among COVID-19 patients, including virus infection, respiratory failure, mechanical ventilation, and the use of a central venous catheter (4). The occurrence of VTE in COVID-19 patients, which includes pulmonary embolism (PE) and deep vein thrombosis (DVT), has been reported in several studies (5, 6). Thrombotic complications have been found in 31% of Intensive Care Unit (ICU) patients with COVID-19 in a Dutch teaching hospital (5), while 23% of PE incidence has been reported in a French hospital (7). At present, the incidence of VTE in this viral infection remains uncertain, however, understanding the precise incidence of VTE in COVID-19 patients is critically important for decision making on thromboprophylaxis. Accordingly, the present study summarizes all available evidence for a comprehensive and rigorous systematic review focused on VTE incidence in hospitalized COVID-19 patients, thus providing a panoramic view of this issue.

METHODS

This study was performed according to the standards of the Cochrane Handbook and the Preferred Reporting Items for Systematic Reviews and Meta-Analyses (PRISMA) statement (8). All supporting data is available within the article and the **Supplementary File**.

Data Sources and Searches

The databases of PubMed, Embase, Cochrane Library databases, as well as the Chinese databases of the China National Knowledge Infrastructure (CNKI), China Science and Technology Journal Database (VIP), and the WANFANG databases were electronically searched from inception to 8 May 2020, using search terms related to COVID-19. Full details of the search terms used are presented in **Table S1**. Preprint articles were retrieved from MedRxiv (https://www.medrxiv.

org), BioRxiv (https://www.biorxiv.org), and SSRN (https://www.ssrn.com). The references of identified records were also screened manually to find any further relevant articles.

Study Selection and Outcomes

To be included, studies had to meet the following entry criteria: (1) included SARS-CoV-2 infected and hospitalized adult patients; (2) reported the data of VTE, PE, or DVT confirmed by computed tomography pulmonary angiography (CTPA) and/or ultrasonography. Two authors (CZ and LS) independently reviewed titles and abstracts of all studies, and assessed full texts of retrieved studies, with any discrepancies being resolved *via* consultation with a third author (ZG). The primary outcomes of this study were the incidence of VTE in hospitalized COVID-19 patients and corresponding relative risk in comparison between severe and non-severe patients. COVID-19 disease severity was defined according to the Clinical Management of COVID-19 (Interim guidance 27 May 2020) released by the World Health Organization (WHO). Criteria for severe cases included any of the following: (1) Respiratory rate >30 per min; (2) blood oxygen saturation (SPO2) < 93% at rest; (3) partial pressure of arterial oxygen to fraction of inspired oxygen ratio <300; or (4) more than 50% of lung infiltrates within 24–48 h. Patients needing mechanical respiratory support or presenting with septic shock or multiple organ dysfunction or failure constituted critical cases.

Data Extraction and Quality Assessment

All data from eligible studies were abstracted using *a priori* designed form, which included study characteristics (study name; country and period; population and number), clinical characteristics (mean age; gender ratio; previous VTE; the comorbidities of hypertension, diabetes, and cancer; and pharmacologic thromboprophylaxis rate), and data on VTE (occurrence number and total number of COVID-19 patients). The pharmacologic thromboprophylaxis rate was calculated as follows: the number of COVID-19 patients who received prophylactic anticoagulants (e.g., low molecular weight heparin [LMWH] or unfractionated heparin intravenously [UFH])/ total number of COVID-19 patients in the study. A rate of ≥60% was considered as a high proportion of pharmacologic thromboprophylaxis. The methodological quality of included studies was assessed according to the Newcastle-Ottawa Scale (NOS) (9). The NOS was modified according to our study design with a total of eight scores and the following six dimensions: (1)

representative of the cases; (2) ascertainment of the exposure; (3) ascertainment of the outcome; (4) ascertainment of the outcome for quality control; (5) control for factors of age and gender; and (6) control for factors related to VTE. A study could receive a maximum of one point for the first four dimensions and a maximum of two points for the last two dimensions. Total scores with ≥ 5 points represented a relatively good quality.

Data Synthesis and Statistical Analysis

All statistical analyses were performed using Stata version 13.0 (Statacorp, College Station, Texas, USA). The pooled incidence of VTE in hospitalized COVID-19 patients and associated 95% confidence intervals (95%CI) was calculated using a random-effects model, and relative risks (RRs) of VTE occurrence comparing severe with non-severe patients was also calculated. Heterogeneity among studies was assessed using the Cochran Q-test and I^2 index, with $I^2 > 50\%$ indicating considerable heterogeneity (10). Subgroup analysis was conducted by different manifestations of VTE (PE and DVT), severity of illness (severe patients and non-severe patients), and the pharmacologic thromboprophylaxis rate of patients (<60 and ≥60%). The interaction analysis (P for interaction) was applied to evaluate the risk difference of different subgroups. To strengthen the robustness of the results, leave-1-out sensitivity analyses were performed to explore whether a single study had an excessive influence on VTE incidence. Meta-regression was conducted to explore the potential risks associated with VTE. Funnel plots and Begg's test and Egger's test were carried out to qualitatively and quantitatively evaluate the presence of publication bias when more than 10 studies were available in a single analysis (11).

RESULTS

Study Selection and Study Characteristics

The process of study selection is outlined in **Figure 1**. A total of 4,449 records were identified through database searching, with 181 being from English-language databases, 31 from Chinese-language databases, and 4,237 from preprint platforms. Through reviewing the titles and abstracts, 28 duplicates were removed, and 4,272 records were excluded. The remaining 149 full-text articles were reviewed and 132 articles were excluded for the following reasons: irrelevant articles ($n = 27$), articles not reporting outcome of VTE ($n = 82$), case report or meta-analyses ($n = 16$), and repetition with another database ($n = 7$). Eventually, 17 retrospective studies (1, 5–8, 12–23) involving 1,913 hospitalized COVID-19 patients were included, 13 being from English-language databases, one from a Chinese-language database, and three from preprint platforms. Among them, six studies reported on patients in China, while 11 studies reported on patients in Europe, including the Netherlands, France, and Italy. The sample size of the involved studies varied from 16 to 420 patients. The detailed characteristics of included studies are presented in **Table 1**. Information of VTE and potential risk factors are summarized in **Table S2**. Of 17 studies, nine involved patients who had clinical suspicion of VTE and six included patients who were screened by CT or ultrasound. One study

involved a population with both clinical suspicion and screening and one did not report the related information. Among 17 studies, 10 reported on patients who were prophylactically treated with anticoagulant therapy (**Table S3**), of which, five studies reported the dosage of LMWH (2,850 IU once to 6,000 IU twice). A high pharmacologic thromboprophylaxis rate was reported in seven studies, ranging from 66.7 to 100%.

Study Quality

All included studies satisfied the following risk bias items: representative of the cases; ascertainment of the exposure; ascertainment of the outcome; and ascertainment of the outcome for quality control. In total, 13 studies (82.3%) presented both age and gender ratio of the included patients, while seven studies (41.2%) reported more than three clinical characteristics (two points) and eight studies (47.1%) reported one or two clinical characteristics (one point). Accordingly, all 17 included studies were considered as being of relatively good quality (**Table S4**).

Incidence of VTE

Figure 2 provides the full view of VTE incidence in hospitalized COVID-19 patients. The overall pooled incidence of VTE was 25% (95% CI, 19–31%; I^2, 95.7%) (**Figure S1**). The incidence of PE and DVT was significantly different ($P_{interaction} < 0.001$), with the event rate being 19% (95% CI, 13–25%; I^2, 93.2%; **Figure S2**) and 7% (95% CI, 4–10%; I^2, 88.3%; **Figure S3**), respectively. Considering the disease severity of COVID-19, a higher incidence was observed in severe patients (35%; 95 CI%, 25–44%; I^2, 92.4%; **Figure S4**) than that in non-severe patients (6%; 95 CI%, 3–10%; I^2, 62.2%; **Figure S5**; $P_{interaction} < 0.001$). Because anticoagulation for thromboprophylaxis could decrease the occurrence of VTE, the high pharmacologic thromboprophylaxis rate of above 60% was associated with a lower incidence of VTE (19%; 95 CI%, 10–28%; I^2, 92.8%; **Figure S6**) when compared to the low pharmacologic thromboprophylaxis rate of below 60% (40%; 95 CI%, 20–60%; I^2, 89.7%; **Figure S6**; $P_{interaction} = 0.052$). Sensitivity analysis, by removing a single study at a time, confirmed the robustness of primacy results (**Table S5**).

Comparison of VTE Risk With Severe vs. Non-severe Patients

A total of 99 VTE events were found in 327 severe patients with the event rate of 30.3%. Comparatively, 34 VTE events were observed in 904 non-severe patients with a low event rate of 3.8%. Accordingly, severe patients were at a higher risk of VTE compared to non-severe patients (RR, 4.76; 95% CI, 2.66–8.50; I^2, 47.0%) (**Figure 3**). Leave-1-out sensitivity analysis was consistent with the primacy result (**Table S6**).

Risk Factors Associated With VTE

Meta-regression was conducted to assess the potential risk factors associated with VTE incidence. Seven variables (mean age, gender ratio, previous VTE, the comorbidities of hypertension, diabetes, cancer, and pharmacologic thromboprophylaxis rate)

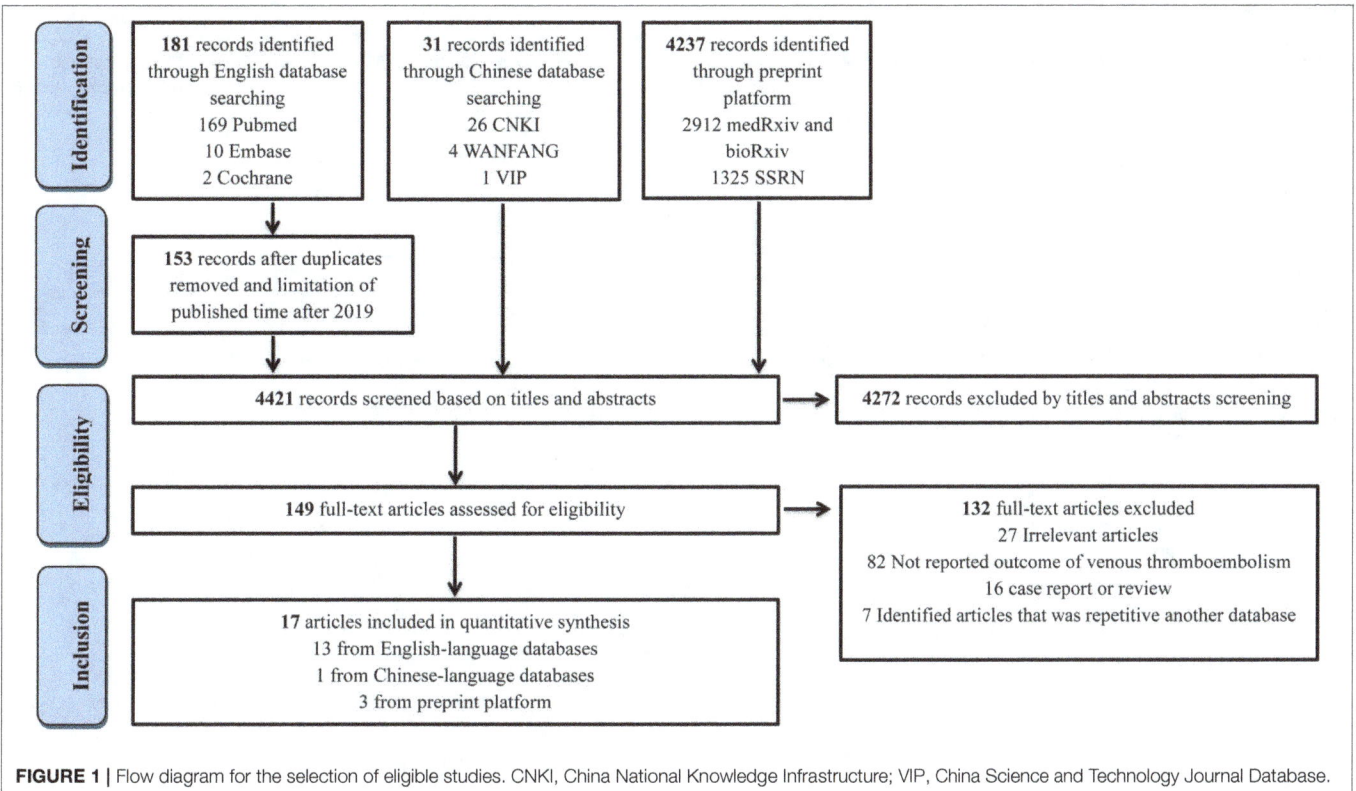

FIGURE 1 | Flow diagram for the selection of eligible studies. CNKI, China National Knowledge Infrastructure; VIP, China Science and Technology Journal Database.

were evaluated, and none of them were detected to be related to the incidence of VTE (**Table S7**).

Publication Bias

The funnel plots for VTE incidence as well as PE and DVT incidence were all asymmetrical on visual inspection. The corresponding P-values for the Egger's test were <0.001, <0.001, and <0.001, and the corresponding P-values for the Begg's test were 0.26, 0.009, and 0.003, respectively (**Figure S7**). Because of limited study numbers in comparison to severe and non-severe patients (seven studies), a funnel plot was not performed.

DISCUSSION

The true incidence of VTE in patients with COVID-19 remains uncertain. This is the first systematic review and meta-analysis to provide a comprehensive overview of VTE occurrence based on 17 retrospective studies involving 1,913 hospitalized COVID-19 patients. The overall VTE incidence was 25%, with the event rate of PE and DVT being 19 and 7%, respectively. Considering disease severity, a higher incidence was observed in severe patients (35%) than in non-severe patients (6%). Moreover, a high pharmacologic thromboprophylaxis rate of above 60% was associated with a lower incidence of VTE (19%) compared to a low pharmacologic thromboprophylaxis rate of below 60% (40%). Severe patients had a 3.76-fold increased risk of VTE compared to non-severe patients. The prevalence of VTE in COVID-19 patients seemed to be high, especially for severe

patients. Therefore, it is important to improve the awareness of thromboprophylaxis for COVID-19 infection.

It was reported that a high proportion of severe and critically ill COVID-19 patients showed major coagulation disorders (24, 25). In our meta-analysis, a higher incidence of VTE was also found in severe patients (35%) than in non-severe patients (6%), with a risk ratio of 4.76. The results were similar to recent preliminary studies on COVID-19, in which the event rate of VTE for ICU patients was 2.18–4.42 folds than that of general ward patients (7, 20). In fact, the prevalence of VTE appeared to be higher in ICU patients than in patients in other disease conditions, with the mean rate of VTE diagnosis being 12.7% (26). The higher risk of VTE in ICU patients mainly resulted from both individual patient related risk factors (e.g., age, history of VTE, cancer) and ICU-specific risk factors (e.g., sedation, immobilization, central venous catheters) (27), therefore, pharmacological VTE prophylaxis is strongly recommended to critically ill patients by clinical guidelines (28). It is speculated that COVID-19 is probably an additional risk factor for VTE in hospitalized patients (29). As for severe or critically ill patients with COVID-19, the release of large amounts of inflammatory mediators and the application of hormones and immunoglobulin might exacerbate the blood hypercoagulability (23, 30). Rapid deterioration in oxygen saturation and increased dead space ventilation could also be factors of VTE events (31). Moreover, severe COVID-19 patients could present with a high fever, dehydration, as well as immobilization (32), which might also lead to VTE (33, 34). Therefore, underestimated prevalence

TABLE 1 | Characteristics of the included studies.

Study	Country/period	Population/number	Mean age (y)	Male (%)	Previous VTE (%)	Hypertension (%)	Diabetes (%)	Cancer (%)	Pharmacologic thromboprophylaxis rate (%)
Beun et al. (12)	Netherlands/NR	ICU/75	60.5	50	NR	NR	NR	NR	NR
Bi et al. (8)	China/2020.1.11–2020.3.10	Mild-moderate and severe-critical/420	NR	47.6	NR	11.7	5.7	0.2	NR
Chen et al. (1)	China/2020.1.1–2020.2.29	Mild-moderate and severe-critical/25	65	60	4	40	20	NR	80
Cui et al. (13)	China/2020.1.20–2020.3.22	ICU/81	59.9	46	NR	25	10	NR	0
Ding et al. (14)	China/2020.1.1–2020.2.3	NR/56	54.6	53.57	NR	NR	NR	NR	NR
Grillet et al. (7)	France/2020.3.15–2020.4.14	Non-ICU and ICU/100	66	70	NR	NR	20	20	NR
Helms et al. (15)	France/2020.3.3–2020.3.31	ICU/150	63	81.3	5.3	NR	NR	NR	66.7
Klok et al. (5)	Netherlands/NR-2020.4.5	ICU/184	64	76	NR	NR	NR	2.7	100
Li et al. (18)	China/2020.1.1–2020.2.13	Suspected PE/24	63	63.6	0	63.6	NR	NR	NR
Llitjos et al. (19)	France/2020.3.19–2020.4.11	ICU/26	68	77	4	85	NR	NR	31
Lodigiani et al. (20)	Italy/2020.2.13–2020.4.10	Non-ICU and ICU/362	66	68	0	47.2	22.7	6.4	Overall: 81.2%; ICU: 100%; Non-ICU: 78.3%
Leonard-Lorant et al. (17)	France/2020.3.1–2020.3.31	Non-ICU and ICU/106	63.3	66	NR	NR	NR	NR	39.6
Middeldorp et al. (21)	Netherlands/NR-2020.4.12	Non-ICU and ICU/198	61	66	5.6	NR	NR	3.5	100
Poissy et al. (6)	France/2020.2.27–2020.3.31	ICU/107	NR	NR	0.93	NR	NR	NR	NR
Ranucci et al. (22)	Italy/2020.3.8-NR	ICU/16	61	93.75	0	NR	NR	NR	100
Tavazzi et al. (16)	Italy/2020.2.21-NR	ICU/54	68	83	NR	NR	NR	NR	100
Xing et al. (23)	China/NR	Moderate and severe-critical/20	NR	60	NR	NR	NR	NR	NR

NR, not reported; ICU, intensive care unit; VTE, venous thromboembolism; PE, pulmonary embolism.

of VTE and inadequate thromboprophylaxis might exist among critically ill COVID-19 patients (35). It was reported that even on standard doses of thromboprophylaxis, the incidence of thrombotic complications was still as high as 31% for ICU patients with COVID-19 infection (5). Accordingly, routinely screening for VTE by CTPA or ultrasound, as well as the use of full-dose anticoagulation, are now recommended for critically ill COVID-19 patients by some experts.

To increase the awareness of thrombotic complications, the assessment of VTE risk should be strongly recommended, for the sake of taking timely and effective preventive measures for patients at high risk of VTE. It is recognized that prevention of VTE is required in all severe or critically ill patients in absence of anticoagulation contraindication (30, 36). For mild or moderate patients with COVID-19, determination of VTE

risk might be exerted using the PADUA risk assessment model for medical patients and the CAPRINI prediction score for surgical patients, as there are currently no new VTE risk assessment models that are specialized for COVID-19 patients (30). Therefore, measures of thromboprophylaxis could be taken without delay in patients with high or moderate risk of VTE. Importantly, dynamic and repeated assessment for thrombotic risk should also be conducted in the course of treatment, including routine coagulation tests, concomitant medications, and invasive procedures, to adjust the antithrombotic regimen in a timely manner. Furthermore, the regular evaluation of bleeding risk should not be neglected in COVID-19 patients, and should be carefully balanced against the risk of thrombosis.

Anticoagulants are definitely the cornerstone for VTE prevention. Therefore, COVID-19 patients with high VTE risk

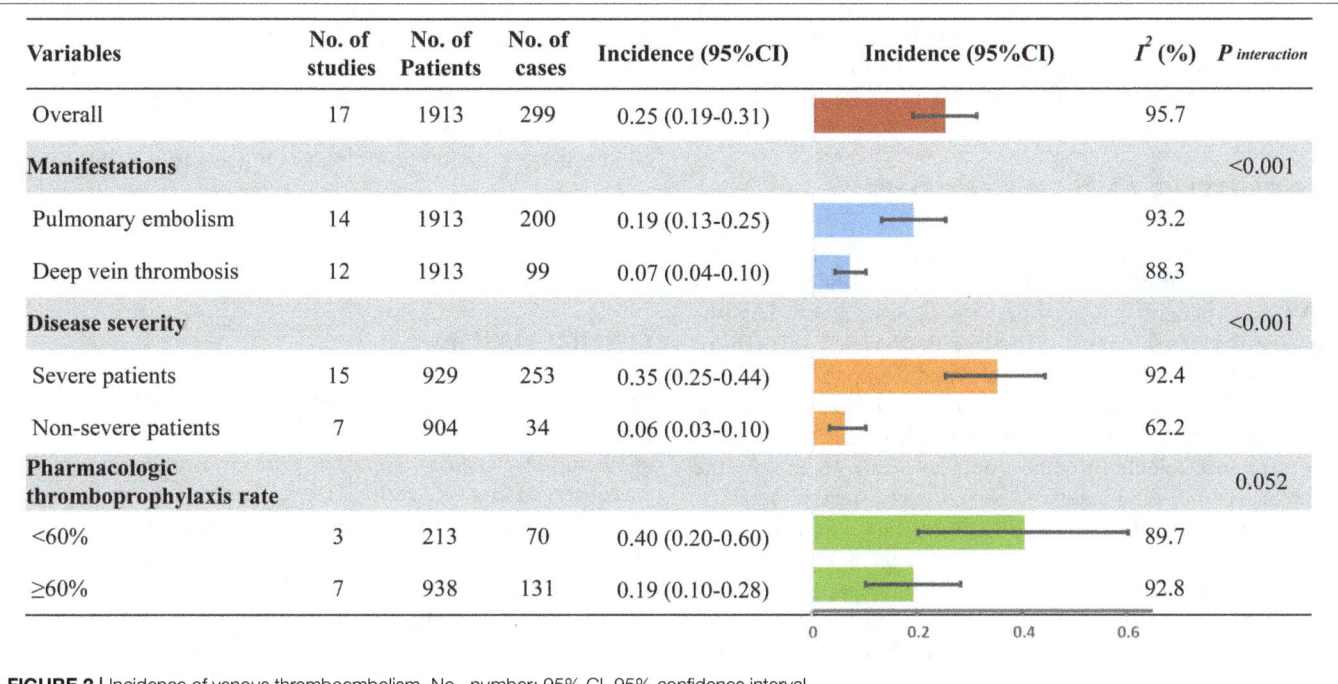

Variables	No. of studies	No. of Patients	No. of cases	Incidence (95%CI)	Incidence (95%CI)	I^2 (%)	$P_{interaction}$
Overall	17	1913	299	0.25 (0.19-0.31)		95.7	
Manifestations							<0.001
Pulmonary embolism	14	1913	200	0.19 (0.13-0.25)		93.2	
Deep vein thrombosis	12	1913	99	0.07 (0.04-0.10)		88.3	
Disease severity							<0.001
Severe patients	15	929	253	0.35 (0.25-0.44)		92.4	
Non-severe patients	7	904	34	0.06 (0.03-0.10)		62.2	
Pharmacologic thromboprophylaxis rate							0.052
<60%	3	213	70	0.40 (0.20-0.60)		89.7	
≥60%	7	938	131	0.19 (0.10-0.28)		92.8	

FIGURE 2 | Incidence of venous thromboembolism. No., number; 95% CI, 95% confidence interval.

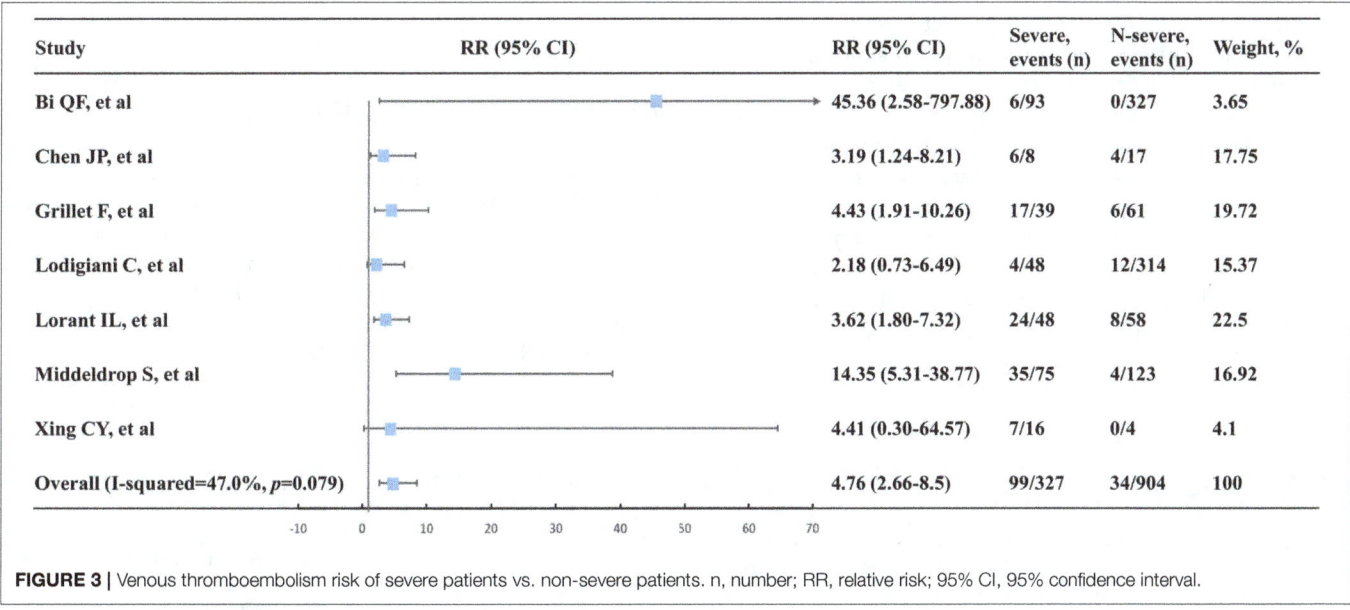

Study	RR (95% CI)	RR (95% CI)	Severe, events (n)	N-severe, events (n)	Weight, %
Bi QF, et al		45.36 (2.58-797.88)	6/93	0/327	3.65
Chen JP, et al		3.19 (1.24-8.21)	6/8	4/17	17.75
Grillet F, et al		4.43 (1.91-10.26)	17/39	6/61	19.72
Lodigiani C, et al		2.18 (0.73-6.49)	4/48	12/314	15.37
Lorant IL, et al		3.62 (1.80-7.32)	24/48	8/58	22.5
Middeldrop S, et al		14.35 (5.31-38.77)	35/75	4/123	16.92
Xing CY, et al		4.41 (0.30-64.57)	7/16	0/4	4.1
Overall (I-squared=47.0%, p=0.079)		4.76 (2.66-8.5)	99/327	34/904	100

FIGURE 3 | Venous thromboembolism risk of severe patients vs. non-severe patients. n, number; RR, relative risk; 95% CI, 95% confidence interval.

should receive pharmacologic thromboprophylaxis, unless there are absolute contraindications (37, 38). As found in this study, the high pharmacologic thromboprophylaxis rate of above 60% was associated with a lower incidence of VTE (19 vs. 40%) compared with the low pharmacologic thromboprophylaxis rate of below 60%. A recent study involving 449 severe COVID-19 patients revealed that LMWH users appeared to be associated with better prognosis compared with non-users (39). Remarkably, prophylactic daily LMWH or twice daily subcutaneous UFH are now recommended for all hospitalized COVID-19 patients by the WHO as well as the International Society on Thrombosis and Haemostasis (ISTH) (23, 37, 40). Nevertheless, prophylactic dose of anticoagulation is supposed to be insufficient to contrast the hypercoagulable state presented by many COVID-19 patients in response to a cytokine storm syndrome (41). A substantial number of patients with standard doses of thromboprophylaxis could still suffer from thrombotic complications, which was also observed in some studies involved in our meta-analysis (5, 16, 20). These findings are strongly suggestive of a higher dose of anticoagulation for patients at high risk of VTE.

Given the relatively high VTE occurrence found in early reports, it might therefore be appropriate to conduct a universal thromboprophylaxis strategy for all hospitalized COVID-19 patients (42), however, more evidence is needed to support these considerations.

STRENGTHS AND LIMITATIONS

This is the first systematic review and meta-analysis that estimates the relatively precise incidence of VTE in hospitalized COVID-19 patients. A comprehensive search of English-language databases, Chinese-language databases, and preprint platforms was conducted, and a revised NOS tool was used to assess the study quality appropriately. Subgroup analyses were conducted by clinical manifestations, disease severity, as well as pharmacologic thromboprophylaxis rate, to explore the differences on VTE incidence. Nevertheless, several intrinsic limitations still remained in this study. First, in this meta-analysis, 17 retrospective studies with three being from preprint platforms were included. Because of the unexpected outbreak of COVID-19, timely information and initial experiences are urgently needed by medical workers to decide on the most optimal therapy for infected patients. Given that journal publications requires peer review and is a time-consuming process, preprints might provide a mechanism for rapidly communicating research, although they are recognized as being less reliable than peer reviewed journal publications. In order to perform a comprehensive meta-analysis, we analyzed as many studies as we could find in this field. Additionally, all studies included were retrospective, which could inevitably introduce heterogeneity to the results. Further studies published in journals as well as high quality studies are therefore needed to obtain more reliable results. Second, given the difficulty of performing CTPA or ultrasonography under strict isolation, it might be difficult to fully illuminate the exact prevalence and nature of VTE in COVID-19. Third, patient-level information about comorbidities and concomitant medication was unavailable to explore the potential risk factors of VTE. Furthermore, whether patients were on thromboprophylaxis or not, as well as different pharmacologic thromboprophylaxis rates, could also contribute to heterogeneity. In addition, the association between the occurrence of VTE and coagulation indicators, such as D-dimers and fibrin degradation products, was not assessed in this study.

CONCLUSION

This meta-analysis revealed that the estimated VTE incidence was 25% in hospitalized COVID-19 patients, with the incidence of PE and DVT being 19 and 7%, respectively. Higher incidence was observed in severe patients (35%) than in non-severe patients (6%). The high pharmacologic thromboprophylaxis rate was associated with a lower incidence of VTE compared with the low pharmacologic thromboprophylaxis rate. Assessment of VTE risk is therefore strongly recommended in COVID-19 patients, and effective measures of thromboprophylaxis should be taken for patients at high risk of VTE in a timely manner.

AUTHOR CONTRIBUTIONS

Z-CG and HX are the guarantors of the entire manuscript. CZ, LS, and K-JL contributed to the study conception and design, critical revision of the manuscript for important intellectual content, and final approval of the version to be published. M-MP, L-CK, ZZ, W-HG, and H-WL contributed to the data acquisition, analysis, and interpretation. All authors contributed to the article and approved the submitted version.

REFERENCES

1. Chen J, Wang X, Zhang S, Liu B, Wu X, Wang Y, et al. Findings of acute pulmonary embolism in COVID-19 patients. *Lancet Infect Dis.* (2020). doi: 10.2139/ssrn.3548771.[Epub ahead of print].
2. Kollias A, Kyriakoulis KG, Dimakakos E, Poulakou G, Stergiou GS, Syrigos K. Thromboembolic risk and anticoagulant therapy in COVID-19 patients: emerging evidence and call for action. *Br J Haematol.* (2020) 189:846–7. doi: 10.1111/bjh.16727
3. Wang T, Chen R, Liu C, Liang W, Guan W, Tang R, et al. Attention should be paid to venous thromboembolism prophylaxis in the management of COVID-19. *Lancet Haematol.* (2020) 7:e362–3. doi: 10.1016/S2352-3026(20)30109-5
4. Violi F, Pastori D, Cangemi R, Pignatelli P, Loffredo L. Hypercoagulation and antithrombotic treatment in coronavirus 2019: a new challenge. *Thromb Haemost.* (2020) 120:949–56. doi: 10.1055/s-0040-17 10317
5. Klok FA, Kruip M, van der Meer NJM, Arbous MS, Gommers D, Kant KM, et al. Incidence of thrombotic complications in critically ill ICU patients with COVID-19. *Thromb Res.* (2020) 191:145–7. doi: 10.1016/j.thromres.2020. 04.013
6. Poissy J, Goutay J, Caplan M, Parmentier E, Duburcq T, Lassalle F, et al. Pulmonary embolism in COVID-19 patients: awareness of an increased prevalence. *Circulation.* (2020) 142:184–6. doi: 10.1161/CIRCULATIONAHA.120.047430
7. Grillet F, Behr J, Calame P, Aubry S. Acute pulmonary embolism associated with COVID-19 pneumonia detected by pulmonary CT Angiography. *Radiology.* (2020). doi: 10.1148/radiol.2020 201544. [Epub ahead of print].
8. Bi Q, Hong C, Meng J, Wu Z, Zhou P, Ye C, et al. Characterization of clinical progression of COVID-19 patients in Shenzhen, China. *MedRxiv.* (2020). doi: 10.1101/2020.04.22.20076190
9. Stang A. Critical evaluation of the Newcastle-Ottawa scale for the assessment of the quality of non-randomized studies in meta-analyses. *Eur J Epidemiol.* (2010) 25:603–5. doi: 10.1007/s10654-010-9491-z
10. Higgins JP, Thompson SG, Deeks JJ, Altman DG. Measuring inconsistency in meta-analyses. *BMJ.* (2003) 327:557–60. doi: 10.1136/bmj.327.7414.557

11. Liberati A, Altman DG, Tetzlaff J, Mulrow C, Gotzsche PC, Ioannidis JP, et al. The PRISMA statement for reporting systematic reviews and meta-analyses of studies that evaluate health care interventions: explanation and elaboration. *J Clin Epidemiol.* (2009) 62:e1–34. doi: 10.1016/j.jclinepi.2009.06.006

12. Beun R, Kusadasi N, Sikma M, Westerink J, Huisman A. Thromboembolic events and apparent heparin resistance in patients infected with SARS-CoV-2. *Int J Lab Hematol.* (2020) 42(Suppl.1):19–20. doi: 10.1111/ijlh.13230

13. Cui S, Chen S, Li X, Liu S, Wang F. Prevalence of venous thromboembolism in patients with severe novel coronavirus pneumonia. *J Thromb Haemost.* (2020) 18:1421–4. doi: 10.1111/jth.14830

14. Ding Y, Huang Z, Zhao S, Li X, Wang X, Xie Y. Clinical and imaging characteristics of corona virus disease 2019 (COVID-19). *Radiol Practice.* (2020) 35:281–5. doi: 10.1016/j.jrid.2020.04.003

15. Helms J, Tacquard C, Severac F, Leonard-Lorant I, Ohana M, Delabranche X, et al. High risk of thrombosis in patients with severe SARS-CoV-2 infection: a multicenter prospective cohort study. *Intensive Care Med.* (2020) 46:1089–98. doi: 10.1007/s00134-020-06062-x

16. Tavazzi G, Civardi L, Caneva L, Mongodi S, Mojoli F. Thrombotic events in SARS-CoV-2 patients: an urgent call for ultrasound screening. *Intensive Care Med.* (2020) 46:1121–3. doi: 10.1007/s00134-020-06040-3

17. Leonard-Lorant I. Acute pulmonary embolism in COVID-19 patients on CT angiography and relationship to D-dimer levels. *Radiology.* (2020). doi: 10.1148/radiol.2020201561. [Epub ahead of print].

18. Li T, Kicska G, Kinahan PE, Zhu C, Oztek MA, Wu W. Clinical and imaging findings in COVID-19 patients complicated by pulmonary embolism. *MedRxiv.* (2020). doi: 10.1101/2020.04.20.20064105

19. Llitjos JF, Leclerc M, Chochois C, Monsallier JM, Ramakers M, Auvray M, et al. High incidence of venous thromboembolic events in anticoagulated severe COVID-19 patients. *J Thromb Haemost.* (2020) 18:1743–6. doi: 10.1111/jth.14869

20. Lodigiani C, Iapichino G, Carenzo L, Cecconi M, Ferrazzi P, Sebastian T, et al. Venous and arterial thromboembolic complications in COVID-19 patients admitted to an academic hospital in Milan, Italy. *Thromb Res.* (2020) 191:9–14. doi: 10.1016/j.thromres.2020.04.024

21. Middeldorp S. Incidence of venous thromboembolism in hospitalized patients with COVID-19. *J Thromb Haemost.* (2020). doi: 10.1111/jth.14888. [Epub ahead of print].

22. Ranucci M, Ballotta A, Di Dedda U, Bayshnikova E, Dei Poli M, Resta M, et al. The procoagulant pattern of patients with COVID-19 acute respiratory distress syndrome. *J Thromb Haemost.* (2020) 18:1747–51. doi: 10.1111/jth.14854

23. Xing C, Li Q, Du H, Kang W, Lian J, Yuan L. Lung ultrasound findings in patients with COVID-19 pneumonia. *Crit Care.* (2020) 24:174. doi: 10.1186/s13054-020-02876-9

24. Chen N, Zhou M, Dong X, Qu J, Gong F, Han Y, et al. Epidemiological and clinical characteristics of 99 cases of 2019 novel coronavirus pneumonia in Wuhan, China: a descriptive study. *Lancet.* (2020) 395:507–13. doi: 10.1016/S0140-6736(20)30211-7

25. Huang C, Wang Y, Li X, Ren L, Zhao J, Hu Y, et al. Clinical features of patients infected with 2019 novel coronavirus in Wuhan, China. *Lancet.* (2020) 395:497–506. doi: 10.1016/S0140-6736(20)30183-5

26. Malato A, Dentali F, Siragusa S, Fabbiano F, Kagoma Y, Boddi M, et al. The impact of deep vein thrombosis in critically ill patients: a meta-analysis of major clinical outcomes. *Blood Transfus.* (2015) 13:559–68. doi: 10.2450/2015.0277-14

27. Minet C, Potton L, Bonadona A, Hamidfar-Roy R, Somohano CA, Lugosi M, et al. Venous thromboembolism in the ICU: main characteristics, diagnosis and thromboprophylaxis. *Crit Care.* (2015) 19:287. doi: 10.1186/s13054-015-1003-9

28. Schunemann HJ, Cushman M, Burnett AE, Kahn SR, Beyer-Westendorf J, Spencer FA, et al. American Society of Hematology 2018 guidelines for management of venous thromboembolism: prophylaxis for hospitalized and non-hospitalized medical patients. *Blood Adv.* (2018) 2:3198–225. doi: 10.1182/bloodadvances.2018022954

29. Zhang L, Feng X, Zhang D, Jiang C, Mei H, Wang J, et al. Deep vein thrombosis in hospitalized patients with coronavirus disease 2019 (COVID-19) in Wuhan, China: prevalence, risk factors, and outcome. *Circulation.* (2020) 142:114–28. doi: 10.1161/CIRCULATIONAHA.120.046702

30. Zhai Z, Li C, Chen Y, Gerotziafas G, Zhang Z, Wan J, et al. Prevention and treatment of venous thromboembolism associated with coronavirus disease 2019 infection: a consensus statement before guidelines. *Thromb Haemost.* (2020) 120:937–48. doi: 10.1055/s-0040-1710019

31. Aryal MR, Gosain R, Donato A, Pathak R, Bhatt VR, Katel A, et al. Venous thromboembolism in COVID-19: towards an ideal approach to thromboprophylaxis, screening, and treatment. *Curr Cardiol Rep.* (2020) 22:52. doi: 10.1007/s11886-020-01327-9

32. Subbarao K, Mahanty S. Respiratory virus infections: understanding COVID-19. *Immunity.* (2020) 52:905–9. doi: 10.1016/j.immuni.2020.05.004

33. Ettema HB, Kollen BJ, Verheyen CC, Buller HR. Prevention of venous thromboembolism in patients with immobilization of the lower extremities: a meta-analysis of randomized controlled trials. *J Thromb Haemost.* (2008) 6:1093–8. doi: 10.1111/j.1538-7836.2008.02984.x

34. Elias S, Hoffman R, Saharov G, Brenner B, Nadir Y. Dehydration as a possible cause of monthly variation in the incidence of venous thromboembolism. *Clin Appl Thromb Hemost.* (2016) 22:569–74. doi: 10.1177/1076029616649435

35. Hippensteel JA, Burnham EL, Jolley SE. Prevalence of venous thromboembolism in critically ill patients with COVID-19. *Br J Haematol.* (2020). doi: 10.1111/bjh.16908. [Epub ahead of print].

36. Song JC, Wang G, Zhang W, Zhang Y, Li WQ, Zhou Z. Chinese expert consensus on diagnosis and treatment of coagulation dysfunction in COVID-19. *Mil Med Res.* (2020) 7:19. doi: 10.1186/s40779-020-00247-7

37. Bikdeli B, Madhavan MV, Jimenez D, Chuich T, Dreyfus I, Driggin E, et al. COVID-19 and thrombotic or thromboembolic disease: implications for prevention, antithrombotic therapy, and follow-up: JACC state-of-the-art review. *J Am Coll Cardiol.* (2020) 75:2950–73. doi: 10.1016/j.jacc.2020.04.031

38. Moores LK, Tritschler T, Brosnahan S, Carrier M, Collen JF, Doerschug K, et al. Prevention, diagnosis and treatment of venous thromboembolism in patients with COVID-19: CHEST guideline and expert panel report. *Chest.* (2020). doi: 10.1016/j.chest.2020.05.559. [Epub ahead of print].

39. Tang N, Bai H, Chen X, Gong J, Li D, Sun Z. Anticoagulant treatment is associated with decreased mortality in severe coronavirus disease 2019 patients with coagulopathy. *J Thromb Haemost.* (2020) 18:1094–9. doi: 10.1111/jth.14817

40. Thachil J, Tang N, Gando S, Falanga A, Cattaneo M, Levi M, et al. ISTH interim guidance on recognition and management of coagulopathy in COVID-19. *J Thromb Haemost.* (2020) 18:1023–6. doi: 10.1111/jth.14810

41. Porfidia A, Pola R. Venous thromboembolism and heparin use in COVID-19 patients: juggling between pragmatic choices, suggestions of medical societies. *J Thromb Thrombolysis.* (2020) 50:68–71. doi: 10.1007/s11239-020-02125-4

42. Spyropoulos AC, Levy JH, Ageno W, Connors JM, Hunt BJ, Iba T, et al. Scientific and standardization committee communication: clinical guidance on the diagnosis, prevention and treatment of venous thromboembolism in hospitalized patients with COVID-19. *J Thromb Haemost.* (2020). doi: 10.1111/jth.14929. [Epub ahead of print].

8

Vascular Inflammation as a Therapeutic Target in COVID-19 "Long Haulers": HIITing the Spot?

Regitse Højgaard Christensen [1,2]* and Ronan M. G. Berg [1,3,4,5]

[1] Centre for Physical Activity Research, Rigshospitalet, University of Copenhagen, Copenhagen, Denmark, [2] Department of Cardiology, Rigshospitalet, University of Copenhagen, Copenhagen, Denmark, [3] Department of Biomedical Sciences, Faculty of Health and Medical Sciences, University of Copenhagen, Copenhagen, Denmark, [4] Department of Clinical Physiology, Nuclear Medicine & Positron Emission Tomography (PET), Rigshospitalet, University of Copenhagen, Copenhagen, Denmark, [5] Neurovascular Research Laboratory, Faculty of Life Sciences and Education, University of South Wales, Newport, United Kingdom

*Correspondence:
Regitse Højgaard Christensen
regitse.hoejgaard.christensen@
regionh.dk

Keywords: COVID-19 complications, high-intensity exercise, cardiovascular disease, systemic inflammation, exercise

BACKGROUND

In the wake of the first wave of the ongoing global pandemic, it has become imminently clear that coronavirus disease 2019 (COVID-19) has brought with it a whole new clinical syndrome: "long COVID" (1, 2). Hence, after recovery from the acute viral infection, a remarkably large proportion of patients, who initially coined themselves "long haulers" in social media-based patient communities for COVID-19 survivors suffer from persistent and often invalidating symptoms, including dyspnoea, chest pain, tachycardia, post-viral brain fog, exercise intolerance, and extreme fatigue to mention a few (3, 4). According to recent studies $\sim$10% of all individuals infected with the causative acute respiratory syndrome-coronavirus-2 (SARS-CoV-2), and as many as nine out of 10 patients that have required hospitalization because of COVID-19 develop long COVID that persists for at least 4 months, according to the currently available data (4). Time will tell whether the symptoms associated with long COVID are transient or ever-lasting phenomena.

Long COVID will expectedly have a huge impact on the morbidity burden and quality of life in many COVID-19 survivors in the future, and when considering the extent of the global pandemic with currently more than 40 million verified cases, it will expectedly have substantial consequences, both in terms of economic cost and health care capacity throughout the world. It is thus widely recognized that there is an impending need for implementing evidence-based patient-tailored safe and effective rehabilitation schemes, but due to the paucity of data on this, the structure and specificity of such schemes remain obscure. While it is widely recognized that some exercise is better than none and more intense exercise is superior to less intense exercise, opinion papers and guidelines published over the past year have consistently refuted high-intensity interval training (HIIT) as an option for rehabilitation after COVID-19 (5–10). On the basis of the known pathophysiology of COVID-19 and the physiological effects of HIIT, we will however argue in favor of the opposite stand, that is, that HIIT should be considered as one of the rehabilitation interventions of choice for alleviating or even reversing the symptoms of long COVID.

COVID-19 IS (ALSO) A VASCULAR DISEASE

Even though COVID-19 is primarily a viral pneumonia, its multiorgan involvement, both in the acute phase and when considering the persistent systems in long COVID, stresses that this is far from the whole story. Over the past months, several studies have highlighted the presence of a substantial vascular component in the pathophysiology of the disease (11–14). Indeed, COVID-19 is associated with severe vascular inflammation, both in the pulmonary and extrapulmonary vasculature, both on the macro- and microvascular level (11). This involves diffuse endothelial damage with pyroptosis and apoptosis as well as a procoagulant change of the vascular endothelium. Consequently, both pulmonary and extrapulmonary thromboembolism are common complications, that may both determine the initial clinical presentation and the long-term consequences of COVID-19 in many patients (15).

The main mechanisms of the universal vascular component of COVID-19 may both involve the mode of entry of the virus into host cells and the immune response to the virus. The causative severe acute respiratory syndrome coronavirus 2 (SARS-CoV-2) invades host endothelial cells through endocytosis which is facilitated by the angiotensin converting enzyme 2 receptor and the transmembrane protease serine 2 which are expressed in practically all organs throughout the body (16).

In terms of the immune response, a type 3 hypersensitivity reaction has been reported to contribute to vascular inflammation in COVID 19, at least in some cases (17). This type of immune reaction takes place when an excess or slight excess of soluble antigens lead to the accumulation of immune complexes, which then precipitate inside the tissues, in particular blood vessels, where they may cause so-called "leukocytoclastic vasculitis," which is a procoagulant condition that affects both the macro- and microvasculature.

Another immune mechanism, which is probably important regardless of whether a type 3 reaction takes place, is the highly proinflammatory cytokine response to SARS-CoV-2, which is prominent both in milder and very severe cases, and which some have designated a "cytokine storm" (18, 19). This involves vast elevations in the classical pro-inflammatory cytokines, TNF-α and IL-1β, which have prominent effects on the endothelium. Hence, TNF-α facilitates the development of a procoagulant endothelium by increasing the expression of endothelial cellular adhesion molecules and genes critical for coagulation, such as tissue factor and decreased thrombomodulin, resulting in a pro-thrombotic state (20, 21). Moreover, TNF-α suppresses endothelial nitric oxide synthase and cyclooxygenase 1, which further compounds endothelial dysfunction (22). Furthermore, IL-1β, which is a downstream cytokine of TNF-α in the initial cytokine cascade triggered by an invading pathogen, is a potent trigger of vascular inflammation, among other things by enhancing monocyte and leukocyte infiltration in the vascular wall. This has most convincingly been demonstrated in studies of infants with non-functional IL-1 receptor antagonist (IL-1ra) function and thus uninhibited IL-1β signal transduction, which leads to severe universal vasculitis (23, 24).

In the following sections we will argue that because the multiorgan involvement of COVID-19 may largely reflect universal vascular inflammation, HIIT is an alluring contender for alleviating and perhaps preventing long COVID.

THE ANTI-INFLAMMATORY EFFECT OF EXERCISE

Physical exercise is a fundamental physiological stressor that is capable of inducing ubiquitous adaptations in nearly all cells, in nearly all tissues and organs (25). This involves the skeletal muscle "secretome" of myokines that are released from contracting skeletal muscle, and which exerts various functions through autocrine, paracrine, and endocrine functions, including marked immunomodulatory effects (**Figure 1**) (26). To this end, the low-grade inflammation, which is a common manifestation of aging has been demonstrated to be reversed by exercise of both moderate to strenuous intensity in randomized controlled trials in the elderly (27). Of note, IL-6 is the first detectable myokine released into the bloodstream during exercise. This is triggered by contraction-induced glycogen depletion in skeletal muscle and its concentration in blood increases exponentially depending on the intensity and duration of exercise (25). Therefore, exercise modalities involving large muscle groups produce the greatest IL-6 response. HIIT regimens or marathons can result in IL-6 increase of 100-fold, although increases of 2–10-fold are more common in exercise regimes of more moderate intensity or duration (28).

Once released, recent studies indicate that IL-6 directly stimulates cardiac exercise adaptations (29) and also affects the vasculature by mobilizing natural killer and dendritic cells to the blood stream (30), which are critically involved in viral clearance. The principal immunomodulatory function of IL-6 released during exercise is however to stimulate the release of IL-10 and IL-1ra by monocytes (31), while also reducing the expression of genes encoding several pro-inflammatory cytokines, including TNF-α and IL-1β. IL-10 also directly inhibits the synthesis of TNF-α (32) while IL-1ra inhibits IL-1β signaling. Additionally, IL-10 negatively interferes with tissue factor expression, thus exerting an anti-coagulant effect in the vasculature (**Figure 1**) (33).

By increasing viral clearance, while also aberrating TNF-α and IL-1β signaling, and alleviating the associated procoagulant state, exercise may thus reduce vascular inflammation in COVID-19.

HIIT: IS IT EFFECTIVE AND/OR SAFE IN COVID-19?

Given that the anti-inflammatory effects of exercise depends critically on the intensity of exercise, intense modalities that involve large muscle groups, such as HIIT protocols, have the potential to produce marked anti-inflammatory effects in target tissues in a time-efficient fashion (28, 34, 35).

HIIT has become increasingly popular in various rehabilitation schemes in patients with lung diseases, mostly because patients with respiratory symptoms are often unable to engage in classical continuous exercise regimens at an intensity sufficient to induce a training adaptation, but during HIIT relatively high intensities are often tolerated (36). Another advantage of HIIT, which is also a benefit in the scientific study of exercise adaptations, is its highly standardized and reproducible nature and that it evokes measurable physiological adaptations much faster than continuous training, i.e., within 2 weeks in healthy volunteers (36). Hence, although an acute HIIT bout elicits apparently similar plasma IL-6 as an iso-energetic continuous exercise bout, the higher intensities and total workloads that may be tolerated during HIIT in

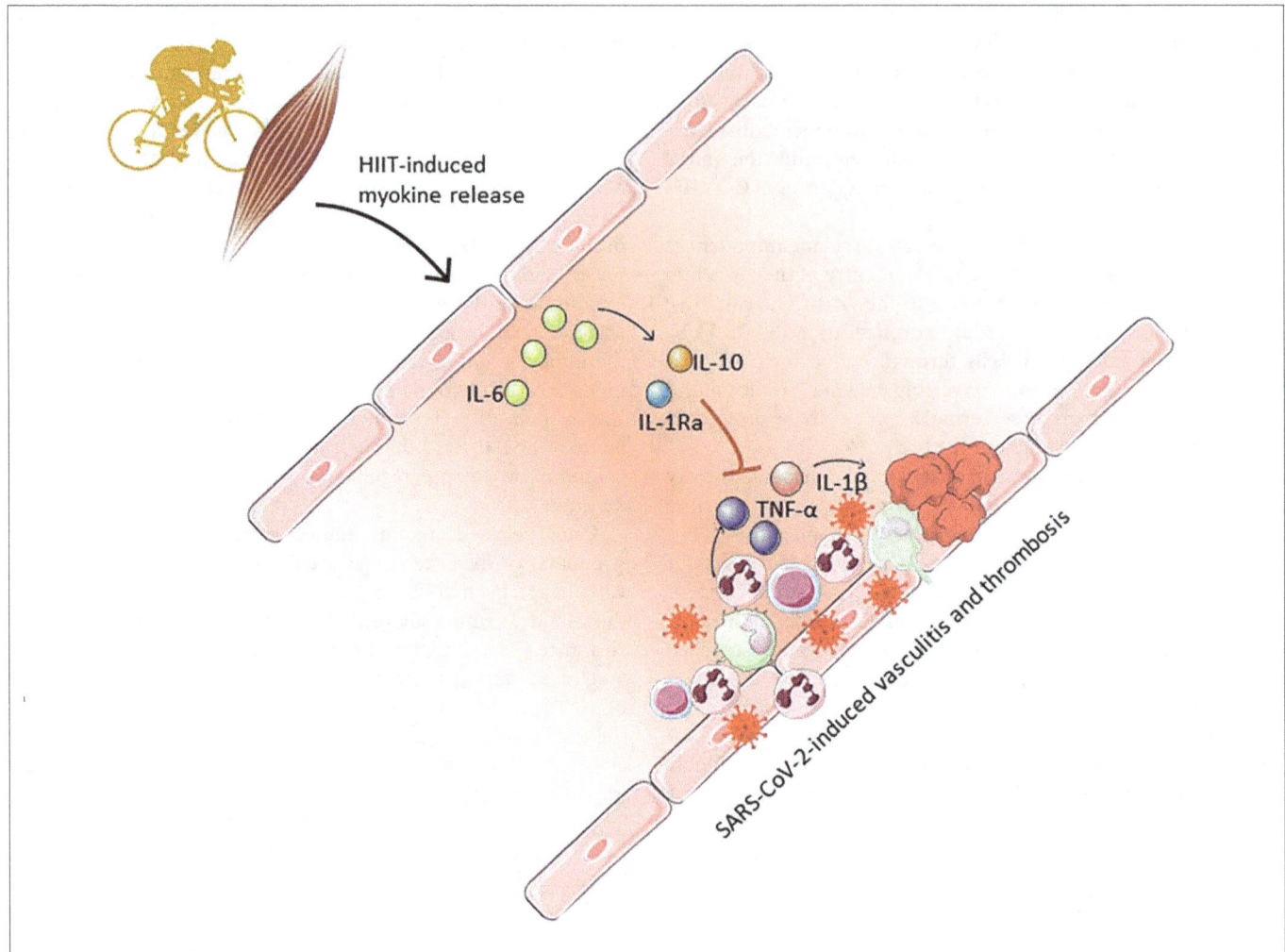

FIGURE 1 | High-intensity interval training (HIIT)-induced myokines (IL-6, IL-10 and IL-1Ra) may counter-act systemic vasculitis through an anti-inflammatory response, namely inhibition of TNFα and IL-1β-mediated activation of pro-coagulant and pro-inflammatory pathways. Clipart provided by Servier Medical Art (60).

various disease states compounds the exercise-induced anti-inflammatory effects (37, 38). Hence, HIIT has been shown to reduce disease-related TNF-α in an animal model of diabetes (39), and furthermore has specific suggested effects related to vascular inflammation, including reduced chemokine chemotaxis and enhanced endothelial repair reported in reviews and meta-analyses conducted on diverse populations of both normal overweight and obese individuals (40–42). This may both reflect the imminent effects of the high-intensity intervals on the IL-6 response as well as on the vasculature *per se*, i.e., due to the pronounced changes in vascular shear stress between intervals (43).

Of all the potential exercise interventions that may be prescribed in COVID-19, HIIT is nonetheless the most controversial. Several aspects of HIIT have been highlighted to disfavor it in this context, including presumed immunosuppressive effects that could increase viral susceptibility and decrease viral clearance (5, 44) and the potential risk of sudden cardiac arrest due to COVID-19-induced residual

cardiovascular pathology (45). Due to the latter, the American College of Sports Medicine (ASCM) and experts endorsed by the section of Sports Cardiology & Exercise of the European Association of Preventive Cardiology (EAPC) have recommend that even athletes accustomed to high exercise intensities should resume to exercise only after a complete cardiovascular evaluation and in a gradual manner following a COVID-19 infection (6–10).

Concerns relating to viral susceptibility and clearance are directly contradicted by the known effects of exercise on immune function, including the effects on NK and dendritic cells described above (30). Accordingly, others have also stressed the potential of HIIT as a means to enhance immune surveillance and regulation while also exerting anti- rather than pro-inflammatory effects in COVID-19 survivors (46, 47).

In terms of the concerns of increasing the risk of adverse cardiovascular outcomes by HIIT in COVID-19 survivors, other reports suggest otherwise (48). Hence, a recent, admittedly small retrospective study of 28 discharged

COVID-19 survivors reported that rehabilitation triggered by HIIT, with endurance training at the maximum tolerated exercise load was both safe and feasible (49). To this end HIIT has successfully been implemented as a rehabilitation strategy in other "high risk" populations, as demonstrated in larger studies on patients at risk or with prevalent ischaemic heart disease, heart failure, chronic obstructive pulmonary disease, cystic fibrosis, and asthma with effects on parameters such as cardiorespiratory fitness (VO_2 peak) and exercise capacity with few reports of severe adverse events, even in patients with left ventricular assist devices (36, 41, 50–59). The rate of cardiovascular complications has been reported of 1 per 23,182 h of high-intensity exercise (51) and later studies have confirmed that HIIT is safe in patients with cardiovascular disease (53). As of now, no studies have thus provided any documentation to indicate that high intensity exercise regimes such as HIIT are not safe in COVID-19 survivors.

CONCLUSION

While the major focus in handling the burgeoning COVID-19 pandemic has hitherto been on reducing the spread of disease and mortality rates, the startlingly high prevalence and severity of long COVID in survivors heralds an aftermath of similar proportions. This may put health care systems throughout the world on the spot in the years to come, and clinical studies that seek to identify and implement effective rehabilitation strategies are thus of utmost importance. We thus believe that the following questions should be addressed by such studies in the very near near future: "When should HIIT be initiated in COVID-19 patients?," "Which specific HIIT protocol should be instigated in COVID-19 patients?" and "What are the effects on HIIT-based rehabilitation on cardio-pulmonary function, symptom burden, and quality of life in patients with long COVID?". HIIT may comprise a valuable component of the rehabilitation intervention in this context, given that its anti-inflammatory effects may target the prominent disease-specific vascular inflammation that is likely a substantial pathogenetic component of the "long haul" of COVID-19.

AUTHOR CONTRIBUTIONS

RC and RB conceived and wrote the initial draft of the manuscript. All authors provided critical input at all stages, and were involved in drafting and editing subsequent versions of the manuscript, read, and approved the final version of the manuscript.

REFERENCES

1. Alwan NA, Attree E, Blair JM, Bogaert D, Bowen MA, Boyle J, et al. From doctors as patients: a manifesto for tackling persisting symptoms of covid-19. *BMJ*. (2020) 370:m3565. doi: 10.1136/bmj.m3565
2. Bos LDJ, Brodie D, Calfee CS. Severe COVID-19 infections—knowledge gained and remaining questions. *JAMA Intern Med*. (2020) 181:9–11. doi: 10.1001/jamainternmed.2020.6047
3. Rubin R. As their numbers grow, COVID-19 "Long Haulers" stump experts. *JAMA*. (2020) 1:23–5. doi: 10.1001/jama.2020.17709
4. Carfi A, Bernabei R, Landi F. Persistent symptoms in patients after acute COVID-19. *JAMA*. (2020) 324:603–5. doi: 10.1001/jama.2020.12603
5. Rahmati-Ahmadabad S. Exercise against SARS-CoV-2 (COVID-19): does workout intensity matter? (A mini review of some indirect evidence related to obesity). *Obes Med*. (2020) 19:100245. doi: 10.1016/j.obmed.2020.100245
6. Bhatia RT, Marwaha S, Malhotra A, Iqbal Z, Hughes C, Börjesson M, et al. Exercise in the severe acute respiratory syndrome Coronavirus-2 (SARS-CoV-2) era: a question and answer session with the experts endorsed by the section of sports cardiology & exercise of the European association of preventive cardiology (EAPC). *Eur J Prev Cardiol*. (2020) 27:1242–51. doi: 10.1177/2047487320930596
7. Verwoert GC, de Vries ST, Bijsterveld N, Willems AR, vd Borgh R, Jongman JK, et al. Return to sports after COVID-19: a position paper from the dutch sports cardiology section of the Netherlands society of cardiology. *Netherlands Hear J*. (2020) 28:391–5. doi: 10.1007/s12471-020-01469-z
8. Dores H, Cardim N. Return to play after COVID-19: a sport cardiologist's view. *Br J Sports Med*. (2020) 54:8–9. doi: 10.1136/bjsports-2020-102482
9. Denay KL, Breslow RG, Turner MN, Nieman DC, Roberts WO, Best TM. ACSM call to action statement: COVID-19 considerations for sports and physical activity. *N Engl J Med*. (2020) 383:120–8. doi: 10.1249/JSR.0000000000000739
10. Kennedy FM, Sharma S. COVID-19, the heart and returning to physical exercise. *Occup Med*. (2020) 70:467–9. doi: 10.1093/occmed/kqaa154
11. Ackermann M, Verleden SE, Kuehnel M, Haverich A, Welte T, Laenger F, et al. Pulmonary vascular endothelialitis, thrombosis, and angiogenesis in Covid-19. *N Engl J Med*. (2020) 383:120–8. doi: 10.1056/NEJMoa2015432
12. Iba T, Connors JM, Levy JH. The coagulopathy, endotheliopathy, and vasculitis of COVID-19. *Inflamm Res*. (2020) 69:1181–9. doi: 10.1007/s00011-020-01401-6
13. Vacchi C, Meschiari M, Milic J, Marietta M, Tonelli R, Alfano G, et al. COVID-19-associated vasculitis and thrombotic complications: from pathological findings to multidisciplinary discussion. *Rheumatology*. (2020) 59:e147–50. doi: 10.1093/rheumatology/keaa581
14. Verdoni L, Mazza A, Gervasoni A, Martelli L, Ruggeri M, Ciuffreda M, et al. An outbreak of severe kawasaki-like disease at the italian epicentre of the SARS-CoV-2 epidemic: an observational cohort study. *Lancet*. (2020) 395:1771–8. doi: 10.1016/S0140-6736(20)31103-X
15. Madjid M, Safavi-Naeini P, Solomon SD, Vardeny O. Potential effects of Coronaviruses on the cardiovascular system: a review. *JAMA Cardiol*. (2020) 10:1–10. doi: 10.1001/jamacardio.2020.1286
16. Libby P. The heart in COVID-19: primary target or secondary bystander? *JACC Basic Transl Sci*. (2020) 5:537–42. doi: 10.1016/j.jacbts.2020.04.001
17. Roncati L, Ligabue G, Fabbiani L, Malagoli C, Gallo G, Lusenti B, et al. Type 3 hypersensitivity in COVID-19 vasculitis. *Clin Immunol*. (2020) 217:108487. doi: 10.1016/j.clim.2020.108487
18. Ronit A, Berg RMG, Bay J, Haugaard AK, Ahlström MG, Burgdorf KS, et al. Compartmental immunophenotyping and cytomorphology in COVID-19 ARDS: a case series. *J Allergy Clin Immunol*. (2020) 147:81–91. doi: 10.1016/j.jaci.2020.09.009
19. Cao X. COVID-19: immunopathology and its implications for therapy. *Nat Rev Immunol*. (2020) 20:269–70. doi: 10.1038/s41577-020-0308-3
20. Tremoli E, Camera M, Toschi V, Colli S. Tissue factor in atherosclerosis. *Atherosclerosis*. (1999) 144:273–83. doi: 10.1016/S0021-9150(99)00063-5
21. Hot A, Lenief V, Miossec P. Combination of IL-17 and TNFα induces a pro-inflammatory, pro-coagulant and pro-thrombotic phenotype in human endothelial cells. *Ann Rheum Dis*. (2012) 71:768–76. doi: 10.1136/annrheumdis-2011-200468

22. Vallance P, Collier J, Bhagat K. Infection, inflammation, and infarction: does acute endothelial dysfunction provide a link? *Lancet.* (1997) 349:1391–2. doi: 10.1016/S0140-6736(96)09424-X

23. Dinarello CA, Simon A, van der Meer JWM. Treating inflammation by blocking interleukin-1 in a broad spectrum of diseases. *Nat Rev Drug Discov.* (2012) 11:633–52. doi: 10.1038/nrd3800

24. Dinarello CA. Interleukin-1 in the pathogenesis and treatment of inflammatory diseases. *Blood.* (2011) 117:3720–32. doi: 10.1182/blood-2010-07-273417

25. Pedersen BK, Febbraio MA. Muscle as an endocrine organ: focus on muscle-derived interleukin-6. *Physiol Rev.* (2008) 88:1379–406. doi: 10.1152/physrev.90100.2007

26. Pedersen BK. Muscle as a secretory organ. *Compr Physiol.* (2013) 3:1337–62. doi: 10.1002/cphy.c120033

27. Woods JA, Wilund KR, Martin SA, Kistler BM. Exercise, inflammation and aging. *Aging Dis.* (2012) 3:130–40.

28. Fischer C. Interleukin-6 in acute exercise and training: what is the biological relevance. *Exerc Immunol Rev.* (2006) 12:6–33.

29. Christensen RH, Wedell-Neergaard AS, Lehrskov LL, Legaard GE, Dorph EB, Larsen MK, et al. Effect of aerobic and resistance exercise on cardiac adipose tissues: secondary analyses from a randomized controlled trial. *JAMA Cardiol.* (2019) 4:778–87. doi: 10.1001/jamacardio.2019.2074

30. Bay ML, Heywood S, Wedell-Neergaard A, Schauer T, Lehrskov LL, Christensen RH, et al. Human immune cell mobilization during exercise – effect of IL-6 receptor blockade. *Exp Physiol.* (2020) 105:2086–98. doi: 10.1113/EP088864

31. Ostrowski K, Rohde T, Asp S, Schjerling P, Pedersen BK. Pro- and anti-inflammatory cytokine balance in strenuous exercise in humans. *J Physiol.* (1999) 515(Pt 1):287–91. doi: 10.1111/j.1469-7793.1999.287ad.x

32. Starkie R, Ostrowski SR, Jauffred S, Febbraio M, Pedersen BK. Exercise and IL-6 infusion inhibit endotoxin-induced TNF-alpha production in humans. *FASEB J.* (2003) 17:884–6. doi: 10.1096/fj.02-0670fje

33. Pedersen BK. Anti-inflammatory effects of exercise: role in diabetes and cardiovascular disease. *Eur J Clin Invest.* (2017) 47:600–11. doi: 10.1111/eci.12781

34. Helge JW, Stallknecht B, Pedersen BK, Galbo H, Kiens B, Richter EA. The effect of graded exercise on IL-6 release and glucose uptake in human skeletal muscle. *J Physiol.* (2003) 546:299–305. doi: 10.1113/jphysiol.2002.030437

35. Cullen T, Thomas AW, Webb R, Hughes MG. Interleukin-6 and associated cytokine responses to an acute bout of high-intensity interval exercise: the effect of exercise intensity and volume. *Appl Physiol Nutr Metab.* (2016) 41:803–8. doi: 10.1139/apnm-2015-0640

36. Sawyer A, Cavalheri V, Hill K. Effects of high intensity interval training on exercise capacity in people with chronic pulmonary conditions: a narrative review. *BMC Sports Sci Med.* (2020) 12:22. doi: 10.1186/s13102-020-00167-y

37. de Souza DC, Matos VAF, dos Santos VOA, Medeiros IF, Marinho CSR, Nascimento PRP, et al. Effects of high-intensity interval and moderate-intensity continuous exercise on inflammatory, leptin, IgA, and lipid peroxidation responses in obese males. *Front Physiol.* (2018) 9:1–9. doi: 10.3389/fphys.2018.00567

38. Peake JM, Tan SJ, Markworth JF, Broadbent JA, Skinner TL, Cameron-Smith D. Metabolic and hormonal responses to isoenergetic high-intensity interval exercise and continuous moderate-intensity exercise. *Am J Physiol Endocrinol Metab.* (2014) 307:E539–52. doi: 10.1152/ajpendo.00276.2014

39. Kim JS, Lee YH, Kim JC, Ko YH, Yoon CS, Yi HK. Effect of exercise training of different intensities on anti-inflammatory reaction in streptozotocin-induced diabetic rats. *Biol Sport.* (2014) 31:73–9. doi: 10.5604/20831862.1093775

40. Li Y, Liu D, Wu H. HIIT: a potential rehabilitation treatment in COVID-19 pneumonia with heart disease. *Int J Cardiol.* (2020) 320:186. doi: 10.1016/j.ijcard.2020.07.030

41. Batacan RB, Duncan MJ, Dalbo VJ, Tucker PS, Fenning AS. Effects of high-intensity interval training on cardiometabolic health: a systematic review and meta-analysis of intervention studies. *Br J Sports Med.* (2017) 51:494–503. doi: 10.1136/bjsports-2015-095841

42. Pal S, Radavelli-Bagatini S, Ho S. Potential benefits of exercise on blood pressure and vascular function. *J Am Soc Hypertens.* (2013) 7:494–506. doi: 10.1016/j.jash.2013.07.004

43. Williams JS, Del Giudice M, Gurd BJ, Pyke KE. Reproducible improvement in endothelial function following two separate periods of high-intensity interval training in young men. *J Appl Physiol.* (2020) 129:725–31. doi: 10.1152/japplphysiol.00054.2020

44. Leandro CG, Ferreira E Silva WT, Lima-Silva AE. Covid-19 and exercise-induced immunomodulation. *Neuroimmunomodulation.* (2020) 27:75–8. doi: 10.1159/000508951

45. Baggish AL, Levine BD. Icarus and sports after COVID 19: too close to the sun? *Circulation.* (2020) 142:615–7. doi: 10.1161/CIRCULATIONAHA.120.048335

46. Wang M, Baker JS, Quan W, Shen S, Fekete G, Gu Y. A preventive role of exercise across the Coronavirus 2 (SARS-CoV-2) pandemic. *Front Physiol.* (2020) 11:1–8. doi: 10.3389/fphys.2020.572718

47. da Silveira MP, da Silva Fagundes KK, Bizuti MR, Starck É, Rossi RC, de Resende e Silva DT. Physical exercise as a tool to help the immune system against COVID-19: an integrative review of the current literature. *Clin Exp Med.* (2020) 21:15–28. doi: 10.1007/s10238-020-00650-3

48. Batatinha HAP, Krüger K, Neto JCR. Thromboinflammation and COVID-19 : the role of exercise in the prevention and treatment. *Front Cardiovasc Med.* (2020) 7:8–11. doi: 10.3389/fcvm.2020.582824

49. Hermann M, Pekacka-Egli A-M, Witassek F, Baumgaertner R, Schoendorf S, Spielmanns M. Feasibility and efficacy of cardiopulmonary rehabilitation after COVID-19. *Am J Phys Med Rehabil.* (2020) 99:865–9. doi: 10.1097/PHM.0000000000001549

50. Ellingsen Ø, Halle M, Conraads V, Støylen A, Dalen H, Delagardelle C, et al. High-intensity interval training in patients with heart failure with reduced ejection fraction. *Circulation.* (2017) 135:839–49. doi: 10.1161/CIRCULATIONAHA.116.022924

51. Rognmo O, Moholdt T, Bakken H, Hole T, Mølstad P, Myhr NE, et al. Cardiovascular risk of high-versus moderate-intensity aerobic exercise in coronary heart disease patients. *Circulation.* (2012) 126:1436–40. doi: 10.1161/CIRCULATIONAHA.112.123117

52. Keech A, Way K, Holgate K, Fildes J, Indraratna P, Yu J. HIIT for post-COVID patients within cardiac rehabilitation: response to letter to the editor. *Int J Cardiol.* (2020) 322:291–2. doi: 10.1016/j.ijcard.2020.08.086

53. Wewege MA, Ahn D, Yu J, Liou K, Keech A. High-intensity interval training for patients with cardiovascular disease-is it safe? A systematic review. *J Am Heart Assoc.* (2018) 7:1–19. doi: 10.1161/JAHA.118.009305

54. Alvarez Villela M, Chinnadurai T, Salkey K, Furlani A, Yanamandala M, Vukelic S, et al. Feasibility of high-intensity interval training in patients with left ventricular assist devices: a pilot study. *ESC Hear Fail.* (2020) 8:498–507. doi: 10.1002/ehf2.13106

55. Angadi SS, Mookadam F, Lee CD, Tucker WJ, Haykowsky MJ, Gaesser GA. High-intensity interval training vs. moderate-intensity continuous exercise training in heart failure with preserved ejection fraction: a pilot study. *J Appl Physiol.* (2015) 119:753–8. doi: 10.1152/japplphysiol.00518.2014

56. Guadalupe-Grau A, Aznar-Laín S, Mañas A, Castellanos J, Alcázar J, Ara I, et al. Short- and long-term effects of concurrent strength and HIIT training in octogenarians with COPD. *J Aging Phys Act.* (2017) 25:105–15. doi: 10.1123/japa.2015-0307

57. Trachsel LD, David LP, Gayda M, Henri C, Hayami D, Thorin-Trescases N, et al. The impact of high-intensity interval training on ventricular remodeling in patients with a recent acute myocardial infarction—A randomized training intervention pilot study. *Clin Cardiol.* (2019) 42:1222–31. doi: 10.1002/clc.23277

58. Gomes Neto M, Durães AR, Conceição LSR, Saquetto MB, Ellingsen Ø, Carvalho VO. High intensity interval training versus moderate intensity continuous training on exercise capacity and quality of life in patients with heart failure with reduced ejection fraction: a systematic review and meta-analysis. *Int J Cardiol.* (2018) 261:134–41. doi: 10.1016/j.ijcard.2018.02.076

59. Villelabeitia-Jaureguizar K, Vicente-Campos D, Senen AB, Jiménez VH, Garrido-Lestache MEB, Chicharro JL. Effects of high-intensity interval versus continuous exercise training on post-exercise heart rate recovery in coronary heart-disease patients. *Int J Cardiol.* (2017) 244:17–23. doi: 10.1016/j.ijcard.2017.06.067

9

Prognostic Value of Coronary Artery Calcium Score in Hospitalized COVID-19 Patients

Maria-Luiza Luchian [1†], Stijn Lochy [1†], Andreea Motoc [1*], Dries Belsack [2], Julien Magne [3,4], Bram Roosens [1], Johan de Mey [2], Kaoru Tanaka [2], Esther Scheirlynck [1], Sven Boeckstaens [1], Karen Van den Bussche [1], Tom De Potter [5], Berlinde von Kemp [1], Xavier Galloo [1], Clara François [1], Caroline Weytjens [1], Steven Droogmans [1] and Bernard Cosyns [1]

[1] Department of Cardiology, University Hospital of Brussels (Centrum voor Hart-en Vaat ziekten, Universitair Ziekenhuis Brussel), Brussels, Belgium, [2] Department of Radiology, University Hospital of Brussels, Brussels, Belgium, [3] CHU Limoges, Hôpital Dupuytren, Service Cardiologie, Limoges, France, [4] INSERM 1094, Faculté de médecine de Limoges, 2, rue Marcland, Limoges, France, [5] Faculty of Medicine and Pharmacy, Vrije Universiteit Brussel, Brussels, Belgium

*Correspondence:
Andreea Motoc
andreea.motoc@gmail.com

[†] These authors have contributed equally to this work

Background: The association of known cardiovascular risk factors with poor prognosis of coronavirus disease 2019 (COVID-19) has been recently emphasized. Coronary artery calcium (CAC) score is considered a risk modifier in the primary prevention of cardiovascular disease. We hypothesized that the absence of CAC might have an additional predictive value for an improved cardiovascular outcome of hospitalized COVID-19 patients.

Materials and methods: We prospectively included 310 consecutive hospitalized patients with COVID-19. Thirty patients with history of coronary artery disease were excluded. Chest computed tomography (CT) was performed in all patients. Demographics, medical history, clinical characteristics, laboratory findings, imaging data, in-hospital treatment, and outcomes were retrospectively analyzed. A composite endpoint of major adverse cardiovascular events (MACE) was defined.

Results: Two hundred eighty patients (63.2 ± 16.7 years old, 57.5% male) were included in the analysis. 46.7% patients had a CAC score of 0. MACE rate was 21.8% (61 patients). The absence of CAC was inversely associated with MACE (OR 0.209, 95% CI 0.052–0.833, $p = 0.027$), with a negative predictive value of 84.5%.

Conclusion: The absence of CAC had a high negative predictive value for MACE in patients hospitalized with COVID-19, even in the presence of cardiac risk factors. A semi-qualitative assessment of CAC is a simple, reproducible, and non-invasive measure that may be useful to identify COVID-19 patients at a low risk for developing cardiovascular complications.

Keywords: Corona virus, coronary artery calcium score, major adverse cardiac and cerebral event, chest computed tomography, risk stratification

INTRODUCTION

Coronavirus disease 2019 (COVID-19) has significantly impacted the healthcare system, due to the rapid spread of infection and unpredictable disease course. Studies have shown that advanced age and comorbidities including hypertension, diabetes mellitus, cardiovascular diseases, and cerebrovascular diseases are predictors of an unfavorable prognosis and mortality in COVID-19 infection (1–4). Coronary artery calcium (CAC) score assessed by computed tomography (CT) is considered a risk modifier in primary prevention of cardiovascular disease (5, 6).

The CAC score offers two main assets: (1) it has an independent additional value in the prediction of all-cause mortality and mortality due to coronary artery disease in asymptomatic individuals; (2) it may reclassify patients considered as being at low or intermediate risk according to the clinical risk scores at high risk of atherosclerotic coronary events (6–9).

However, data regarding the role of CAC score in the prediction of cardiovascular events and outcome in COVID-19 patients are still scarce.

We hypothesized that the absence of CAC might have an additional predictive value for an improved cardiovascular outcome of hospitalized COVID-19 patients.

MATERIALS AND METHODS

We prospectively included 310 consecutive hospitalized patients with confirmed COVID-19 by real-time reverse transcription polymerase chain reaction (RT-PCR) test, between March 2020 and April 2020. Thirty patients with a history of coronary artery disease (stable angina, unstable angina, history of acute coronary syndrome) were excluded from the analysis. Demographics, medical history, clinical characteristics, laboratory findings, imaging data, in-hospital treatment, and outcomes were retrospectively analyzed. A composite endpoint [major adverse cardiovascular events (MACE)] was defined as all-cause mortality, heart failure, acute coronary syndrome, atrial fibrillation, and stroke.

In the absence of widely available RT-PCR at the beginning of the pandemic, chest CT had been systematically performed in all suspected COVID-19 patients. All patients were scanned on an Apex Revolution CT (GE Healthcare, Milwaukee, WI, USA). The low-dose non-contrast CT thorax scan protocol consisted of a 128×0.625 mm spiral acquisition with pitch 1, rotation time 0.35 s, automated kVp selection and automated mA modulation. Images with 1.25 mm slice thickness were reconstructed with deep learning image reconstruction (DLIR) set at medium level. The average volume CT dose index (CTDIvol) and dose-length product (DLP) were 4.4 mGy (95% CI: 4.3–4.5) and 159 mGy·cm (95% CI: 157–162), respectively. Visual assessment of CAC was performed using ordinal scoring: each of the four main coronary arteries was identified (left main, left anterior descending, left circumflex, and right coronary artery). Calcium was scored as 0, 1, 2, or 3 for every artery, corresponding to absent, mild, moderate, or severe CAC. Mild CAC was defined as

involvement of less than one third of the vessel length, moderate as involvement of one to two thirds of the vessel length and severe CAC as involvement of more than two thirds of the vessel length. A total score was calculated by summing the score of each vessel. The total score was then categorized as 0 (undetectable), 1–3 (mild), 4–5 (moderate), and ≥ 6 (severe) (10) (**Figure 1**).

Intraobserver and interobserver reproducibility analyses of CAC score were performed by repeating the measurements in 20 random patients by the same primary investigator 2 weeks after the first assessment and by an additional investigator, respectively. During the repeated analysis, the investigators were blinded to any previous results.

The study was approved by the local Ethical Committee of the University Hospital of Brussels and was carried out in accordance with the ethical principles for medical research involving human subjects established by the Declaration of Helsinki, protecting the privacy of all participants as well as the confidentiality of their personal information. All data were fully anonymized. The need for consent in this study was waived by the ethical committee.

Statistical Analysis

Continuous variables were presented as means with standard deviations (SD) or median [interquartile range (IQR)] for skewed variables. Categorical variables were expressed as percentages. Normality of data was tested using Kolmogorov–Smirnov test. Comparisons of continuous variables were done using Student t-test or Mann–Whitney U-test and of binominal variables using chi-square or Fisher exact test, respectively. Intraobserver and interobserver variability for CAC score assessment was tested by Cohen's Kappa coefficient. The following criteria for Kappa coefficient were used to interpret the results: <0.00 = poor, $0.00–0.20$ = light, $0.21–0.40$ = fair, $0.41–0.60$ = moderate, $0.61–0.80$ = substantial, and $0.81–0.99$ = almost perfect (11). Univariate and multivariate logistic regression models were used to evaluate potential predictors of MACE. Variables included in the multivariate analysis were chosen based on their statistical significance in the univariate analysis ($p < 0.05$) and on their clinical significance. Specificity, sensitivity, and negative predictive value of CAC score = 0 were calculated using a cross-tabulation table. Specificity was defined as the probability that a test result will be negative when the disease is not present (true negative rate). Sensitivity was defined as the probability that a test result will be positive when the disease is present (true positive rate). Negative predictive value was defined as the probability that the disease is not present when the test is negative (12, 13). Statistical significance was considered for a $p < 0.05$. Statistical analyses were performed using IBM SPSS Statistic for Windows, Version 27.0 (IBM Corp., Armonk, NY, USA).

RESULTS

A total of 280 patients (63.2 ± 16.7 years old, 57.5% male) were included in the analysis.

Mean length of hospitalization was 13.6 ± 13.2 days. Sixty-one patients (21.8%) had at least one MACE: 16 (5.7%) patients presented acute heart failure, 15 (5.3%) patients had atrial

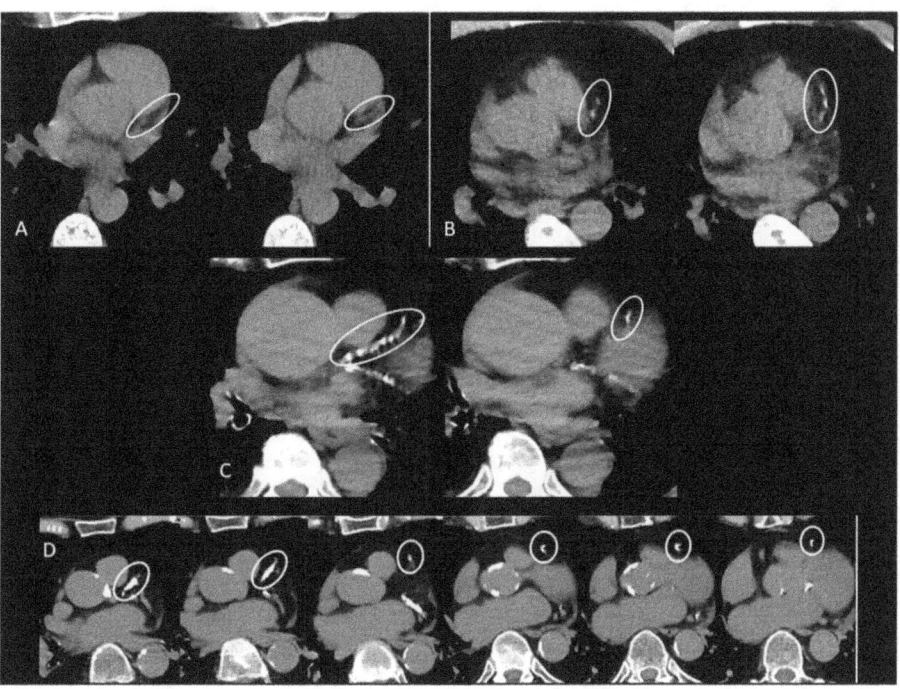

FIGURE 1 | (A) CAC score zero in left anterior descending (LAD) coronary artery. **(B)** Mild CAC in LAD. **(C)** Moderate CAC in LAD. **(D)** Severe CAC in LAD.

fibrillation, 4 (1.4%) patients presented acute coronary syndrome [2 (0.7%) patients had a non-ST elevation myocardial infarction and 2 (0.7%) patients had unstable angina], and 3 (1.0%) patients presented a stroke, respectively. In-hospital mortality rate was 16.1% (45 patients). CAC score = 0 was found in 46.7% (131) patients, vs. 53.2% (149) patients with CAC score ≥1. The baseline characteristics of the study population and the comparison between patients with a CAC score = 0 and CAC score ≥ 1 are shown in **Table 1**.

Univariate analysis for the prediction of MACE is shown in **Supplementary Table 1**.

Multivariate analysis (**Table 2**) showed that a CAC score of 0 was inversely associated with the occurrence of MACE [p = 0.027, odds ratio (OR) = 0.209, 95% confidence interval (CI) 0.052–0.833]. The negative predictive value of CAC score for MACE was 84.5% (sensitivity 72%, specificity 55%).

Reproducibility of CAC score assessment using Cohen's k showed substantial intraobserver and interobserver agreement for the total CAC score assessment (k = 0.859, 95% CI 0.678–1.000, p < 0.001 and k = 0.795, 95% CI 0.581–1.000, p < 0.001, respectively).

DISCUSSION

The main findings of this study were the following: (1) MACE rate in COVID-19 hospitalized patients was 21.8%; (2) the absence of CAC was independently associated with a lower rate of MACE in COVID-19 hospitalized patients.

COVID-19 promotes a rapid systemic inflammation and cytokine storm, which can cause vascular dysfunction, destabilization of atherosclerotic plaques, or myocardial infiltration, which are potential pathways for cardiovascular complications (14). The most commonly reported MACE in COVID-19 hospitalized patients include heart failure, arrhythmia, and acute coronary syndrome, similar to results from the present study (14–16). Moreover, patients with pre-existing cardiac disease are more predisposed to develop cardiac complications during hospitalization for COVID-19 (14, 15).

Similar to previous reports, in the present study, older age was independently associated with worse outcome of COVID-19 patients (17, 18). Moreover, an increased cardiac troponin independently predicted MACE, which is in line with recent studies showing evidence of myocardial injury in hospitalized COVID-19 patients and subsequently increased disease severity (2, 19).

Current guidelines consider CAC score to be a risk modifier in primary prevention of cardiovascular disease (5, 6). Moreover, CAC score has been shown to improve cardiovascular risk prediction in addition to classical risk factors (5, 6, 20) and to be a potential tool for risk reclassification (21–24). The Multi-Ethnic Study of Atherosclerosis (MESA) showed that CAC improved risk prediction at 10-year follow-up compared with traditional risk factors alone (25).

Interestingly, multiple studies have focused on the role of the absence of CAC as a potential downward cardiovascular risk reclassification (26–29). In the present study, the absence of CAC score independently predicted lower MACE rate in COVID-19 hospitalized patients.

TABLE 1 | Comparison between patients with CAC score 0 and those with CAC score ≥1.

	Total ($n = 280$)	CAC score = 0 ($n = 131$)	CAC score ≥ 1 ($n = 149$)	p-value
Age (years)	63.2 ± 16.7	53.7 ± 13.1	72.7 ± 13.2	<0.001
Weight (kg)	80.5 ± 16.7	84.4 ± 16.3	76.6 ± 15.8	<0.001
BMI (kg/m²)	27.8 ± 5.2	28.9 ± 5.2	26.8 ± 4.9	0.001
Male gender (n, %)	161 (57.5)	76 (58.0)	76 (60.3)	0.707
History				
Heart failure (n, %)	6 (2.1)	1 (0.8)	5 (4.0)	0.089
Valve disease (n, %)	6 (2.1)	1 (0.8)	5 (4.0)	0.089
Atrial fibrillation (n, %)	14 (5.0)	3 (2.2)	11 (7.3)	0.023
CKD (n, %)	32 (11.4)	9 (6.9)	23 (18.3)	0.006
Chronic pulmonary disease (n, %)	43 (15.3)	20 (15.2)	23 (15.4)	0.718
Cancer (n, %)	28 (10)	7 (5.3)	21 (16.7)	0.004
Risk factors				
Hypertension (n, %)	128 (45.7)	40 (30.5)	78 (61.9)	<0.001
DM (n, %)	64 (22.8)	33 (25.2)	31 (24.6)	0.913
Dyslipidemia (n, %)	89 (31.8)	39 (29.8)	50 (39.7)	0.095
Smoking (n, %)	30 (10.7)	13 (9.9)	17 (13.5)	0.373
Laboratory values				
Hemoglobin (g/dl)	13.5 ± 1.8	13.7 ± 1.7	13.4 ± 2.0	0.205
Platelets (10³/mm³)	218.4 ± 86.8	218.3 ± 84.1	212.2 ± 86.5	0.572
WBC (10³/mm³)	7.8 ± 4.4	7.2 ± 3.0	8.1 ± 5.0	0.072
CRP (mg/L)	135.7 ± 96.5	128.0 ± 97.9	140.1. 94.1	0.312
D-dimers (ng/ml)	1,638.6 ± 2,720.7	1,048.5 ± 1,442.4	1,830.9 ± 2,613.0	0.042
LDH (U/L)	968.4 ± 1,183.8	988.6 ± 608.8	1,000.3 ± 595.8	0.877
Lactate (mmol/L)	1.0 ± 0.6	1.0 ± 0.5	1.1 ± 0.6	0.659
cTnT (μg/L)	0.02 ± 0.04	0.01 ± 0.01	0.02 ± 0.01	<0.001
Creatinine (mg/dl)	1.2 ± 1.2	1.0 ± 0.9	1.3 ± 1.4	0.012
Chest CT				
Ground-glass opacity (n, %)	226 (80.7)	115 (87.7)	111 (74.4)	0.854
Interlobular septal thickening (n, %)	25 (8.9)	9 (6.8)	17 (11.4)	0.076
Pulmonary consolidation (n, %)	94 (33.5)	44 (33.5)	50 (33.5)	0.267
Pleural effusion (n, %)	14 (5.0)	4 (3.0)	10 (6.7)	0.068
ICU admission (n, %)	71 (18.2)	33 (25.1)	39 (26.1)	0.500

BMI, body mass index; CKD, chronic kidney disease; DM, diabetes mellitus; WBC, white blood cells; NLR, neutrophil to lymphocyte ratio; CRP, C-reactive protein; LDH, lactate dehydrogenase; cTnT, cardiac troponin T; CT, computed tomography; ICU, intensive care unit; CAC, coronary artery calcium.

Dillinger et al. (30) evaluated the role of CAC in COVID-19 patients hospitalized at the intensive care unit (ICU) and showed that the presence of CAC score was associated with the occurrence of mechanical ventilation, extracorporeal membrane oxygenation, or death. Compared to the present study and other previous series, mortality rate in the study of Dillinger et al. (30) was significantly lower, even if the authors reported only the mortality among ICU patients (2, 19, 31, 32). In our cohort, 71 (25.7%) patients were transferred to ICU, among whom 19 (26.7%) died. Surprisingly, the proportion of elevated CAC score in patients younger than 61 years old was higher in the study of Dillinger et al. (30) compared to the results from our cohort. For the same group of ethnicity, the MESA study showed that CAC score increased with age, which is comparable to data from the present study (33). In contrast to MESA, there was no significant difference in CAC score between genders in this study.

In another recent report by Nai Fovino et al. the presence of CAC in COVID-19 patients was associated with ICU admission and in-hospital mortality (34). However, this study had a small sample population in whom CAC score was evaluated as high or low-intermediate, and potential confounders were not included; therefore, the results cannot be compared to our cohort. Zimmerman et al. also evaluated the role of CAC in the prediction of ICU admission and death in COVID-19 patients (35). Nevertheless, in this study, patients with a history of coronary artery disease were not excluded from the analysis, and the potential relationship between CAC and inflammatory markers was not assessed.

Although recent studies focused on the power of CAC score 0 to predict an improved cardiovascular outcome, data regarding the role of CAC in COVID-19 patients with classical cardiac risk factors are still limited (27, 36). In this study, the absence of CAC translated into a low risk for MACE in COVID-19

TABLE 2 | Predictors of MACE.

	OR	95% CI	p
Age	1.067	1.009–1.129	0.024
Male gender	0.702	0.221–2.228	0.548
Atrial fibrillation	1.175	0.182–7.595	0.865
Creatinine	1.018	0.49–2.090	0.962
CRP	1.009	1.004–1.015	0.001
cTnT	1.072	1.026–1.120	0.002
CAC score = 0	0.209	0.052–0.833	0.027

CRP, C-reactive protein; cTnT, cardiac troponin T; CAC, coronary artery calcium; OR, odds ratio; CI, confidence interval; MACE, major adverse cardiovascular events.

patients, independent of age and the presence of risk factors or inflammation, reinforcing the idea that the assessment of CAC score in hospitalized COVID-19 patients could be a useful marker for patients' risk stratification and management.

At the beginning of the pandemic, RT-PCR tests were not widely available; therefore, a systematic chest CT was performed in almost all COVID-19 patients. The ability to assess CAC score on non-gated chest CT allows the application of CAC to the risk evaluation of COVID-19 patients with no additional cost or time consumption. Moreover, most studies report a low-dose radiation for chest CT in COVID-19 patients (37). The semi-qualitative assessment of CAC on routine chest CT has proved to be accurate and reproducible when compared to Agatston scoring (10). Similarly, in our study intraobserver and interobserver reproducibility of CAC score was very good.

Evidence that viral infections represent a trigger for cardiovascular events is increasing, but data regarding long-term follow-up of patients admitted with respiratory viral diseases are still scarce (38, 39). Future directions should focus on the implementation of CAC score into mid-term and long-term follow-up of this particular population, to provide a more precise and earlier estimation of cardiovascular risk.

STUDY LIMITATIONS

This was a single-center study, the sample size was relatively small, and no comparison with a control group was performed; therefore, the extrapolation of these results is limited. The method used to assess CAC is a semi-qualitative scoring system using a non-gated chest CT. The absence of triggering, the lower temporal resolution, and larger field of view which alters the voxel size might modify CAC score assessment. However, this method has been previously validated against quantitative CAC assessment, and its accuracy to predict Agatston score was demonstrated (10).

CONCLUSION

In this study, the absence of CAC had a high negative predictive value for MACE in patients hospitalized with COVID-19, independent of the presence of cardiac risk factors. A semi-qualitative assessment of CAC is a simple, reproducible, and non-invasive measure that may be useful for the risk stratification of COVID-19 patients.

AUTHOR CONTRIBUTIONS

M-LL, SL, AM, and BC contributed to the conception and design of the study. M-LL, AM, and SL wrote the first draft of the manuscript. AM and JMa performed the statistical analysis. DB, JMe, SB, and KT performed CT analysis. ES, BR, KV, TD, BK, XG, and CF participated to the investigation, clinical assessment and database. CW, SD, and BC contributed to project administration, supervision and validation. All authors contributed to manuscript revision, read, and approved the submitted version.

REFERENCES

1. Madjid M, Safavi-Naeini P, Solomon SD, Vardeny O. potential effects of coronaviruses on the cardiovascular system: a review. *JAMA Cardiol.* (2020) 5:831–40. doi: 10.1001/jamacardio.2020.1286
2. Shi S, Qin M, Shen B, Cai Y, Liu T, Yang F, et al. Association of cardiac injury with mortality in hospitalized patients with COVID-19 in Wuhan, China. *JAMA Cardiol.* (2020) 5:802–10. doi: 10.1001/jamacardio.2020.0950
3. Wang Y, Lu X, Li Y, Chen H, Chen T, Su N, et al. Clinical course and outcomes of 344 intensive care patients with COVID-19. *Am J Respir Crit Care Med.* (2020) 201:1430–4. doi: 10.1164/rccm.202003-0736LE
4. Zhou F, Yu T, Du R, Fan G, Liu Y, Liu Z, et al. Clinical course and risk factors for mortality of adult inpatients with COVID-19 in Wuhan, China: a retrospective cohort study. *Lancet.* (2020) 395:1054–62. doi: 10.1016/S0140-6736(20)30566-3
5. Arnett DK, Blumenthal RS, Albert MA, Buroker AB, Goldberger ZD, Hahn EJ, et al. 2019 ACC/AHA guideline on the primary prevention of cardiovascular disease: executive summary: a report

of the American college of cardiology/American heart association task force on clinical practice guidelines. *J Am Coll Cardiol.* (2019). 74:1376–414. doi: 10.1161/CIR.0000000000000677
6. Piepoli MF, Hoes AW, Agewall S, Albus C, Brotons C, Catapano AL, et al. 2016 European guidelines on cardiovascular disease prevention in clinical practice: the sixth joint task force of the european society of cardiology and other societies on cardiovascular disease prevention in clinical practice (constituted by representatives of 10 societies and by invited experts)developed with the special contribution of the European association for cardiovascular prevention & rehabilitation (EACPR). *Eur Heart J.* (2016). 37:2315–81. doi: 10.1016/j.atherosclerosis.2016.05.037
7. Akram K, O'Donnell RE, King S, Superko HR, Agatston A, Voros S. Influence of symptomatic status on the prevalence of obstructive coronary artery disease in patients with zero calcium score. *Atherosclerosis.* (2009) 203:533–7. doi: 10.1016/j.atherosclerosis.2008.07.008
8. Hussain A, Ballantyne CM, Nambi V. Zero coronary artery calcium score: desirable, but enough? *Circulation.* (2020) 142:917–9. doi: 10.1161/CIRCULATIONAHA.119.045026
9. Knez A, Becker A, Leber A, White C, Becker CR, Reiser MF, et al. Relation of coronary calcium scores by electron beam tomography to obstructive

disease in 2,115 symptomatic patients. *Am J Cardiol.* (2004) 93:1150–2. doi: 10.1016/j.amjcard.2004.01.044

10. Azour L, Kadoch MA, Ward TJ, Eber CD, Jacobi AH. Estimation of cardiovascular risk on routine chest CT: ordinal coronary artery calcium scoring as an accurate predictor of agatston score ranges. *J Cardiovasc Comput Tomogr.* (2017) 11:8–15. doi: 10.1016/j.jcct.2016.10.001

11. Landis JR, Koch GG. The measurement of observer agreement for categorical data. *Biometrics.* (1977) 33:159–74. doi: 10.2307/2529310

12. Antonelli P, Chiumello D, Cesana BM. Statistical methods for evidence-based medicine: the diagnostic test. Part II. *Minerva Anestesiol.* (2008) 74:481–8.

13. Cesana BM, Antonelli P, Chiumello D. Statistical methods for evidence-based medicine: the diagnostic test. Part I. *Minerva Anestesiol.* (2008) 74:431–7.

14. Guzik TJ, Mohiddin SA, Dimarco A, Patel V, Savvatis K, Marelli-Berg FM, et al. COVID-19 and the cardiovascular system: implications for risk assessment, diagnosis, and treatment options. *Cardiovasc Res.* (2020) 116:1666–87. doi: 10.1093/cvr/cvaa106

15. Linschoten M, Peters S, van Smeden M, Jewbali LS, Schaap J, Siebelink HM, et al. Cardiac complications in patients hospitalised with COVID-19. *Eur Heart J Acute Cardiovasc Care.* (2020) 9:817–23. doi: 10.1177/2048872620974605

16. Huang C, Wang Y, Li X, Ren L, Zhao J, Hu Y, et al. Clinical features of patients infected with 2019 novel coronavirus in Wuhan, China. *Lancet.* (2020) 395:497–506. doi: 10.1016/S0140-6736(20)30183-5

17. Guan WJ, Liang WH, Zhao Y, Liang HR, Chen ZS, Li YM, et al. Comorbidity and its impact on 1590 patients with COVID-19 in China: a nationwide analysis. *Eur Respir J.* (2020) 55:2001227. doi: 10.1183/13993003.01227-2020

18. Yang J, Zheng Y, Gou X, Pu K, Chen Z, Guo Q, et al. Prevalence of comorbidities and its effects in patients infected with SARS-CoV-2: a systematic review and meta-analysis. *Int J Infect Dis.* (2020) 94:91–5. doi: 10.1016/j.ijid.2020.03.017

19. Lala A, Johnson KW, Januzzi JL, Russak AJ, Paranjpe I, Richter F, et al. Prevalence and impact of myocardial injury in patients hospitalized with COVID-19 infection. *J Am Coll Cardiol.* (2020) 76:533–46. doi: 10.1101/2020.04.20.20072702

20. Hadamitzky M, Freissmuth B, Meyer T, Hein F, Kastrati A, Martinoff S, et al. Prognostic value of coronary computed tomographic angiography for prediction of cardiac events in patients with suspected coronary artery disease. *JACC Cardiovasc Imaging.* (2009) 2:404–11. doi: 10.1016/j.jcmg.2008.11.015

21. Budoff MJ, Achenbach S, Blumenthal RS, Carr JJ, Goldin JG, Greenland P, et al. Assessment of coronary artery disease by cardiac computed tomography: a scientific statement from the American heart association committee on cardiovascular imaging and intervention, council on cardiovascular radiology and intervention, and committee on cardiac imaging, council on clinical cardiology. *Circulation.* (2006) 114:1761–91. doi: 10.1161/CIRCULATIONAHA.106.178458

22. Greenland P, Bonow RO, Brundage BH, Budoff MJ, Eisenberg MJ, Grundy SM, et al. ACCF/AHA 2007 clinical expert consensus document on coronary artery calcium scoring by computed tomography in global cardiovascular risk assessment and in evaluation of patients with chest pain: a report of the American college of cardiology foundation clinical expert consensus task force (accf/aha writing committee to update the 2000 expert consensus document on electron beam computed tomography) developed in collaboration with the society of atherosclerosis imaging and prevention and the society of cardiovascular computed tomography. *J Am Coll Cardiol.* (2007) 49:378–402. doi: 10.1016/j.jacc.2006.10.001

23. Peters SAE, den Ruijter HM, Bots ML, Moons KGM. Improvements in risk stratification for the occurrence of cardiovascular disease by imaging subclinical atherosclerosis: a systematic review. *Heart.* (2012) 98:177–84. doi: 10.1136/heartjnl-2011-300747

24. Radford NB, DeFina LF, Barlow CE, Lakoski SG, Leonard D, Paixao AR, et al. Progression of CAC score and risk of incident CVD. *JACC Cardiovasc Imaging.* (2016) 9:1420–9. doi: 10.1016/j.jcmg.2016.03.010

25. Budoff MJ, Young R, Burke G, Jeffrey Carr J, Detrano RC, Folsom AR, et al. Ten-year association of coronary artery calcium with atherosclerotic cardiovascular disease (ASCVD) events: the multi-ethnic study of atherosclerosis (MESA). *Eur Heart J.* (2018) 39:2401–8. doi: 10.1093/eurheartj/ehy217

26. Piepoli MF, Abreu A, Albus C, Ambrosetti M, Brotons C, Catapano AL, et al. Update on cardiovascular prevention in clinical practice: a position paper of the European association of preventive cardiology of the European society of cardiology. *Eur J Prev Cardiol.* (2020) 27:181–205. doi: 10.1177/2047487319893035

27. Blaha MJ, Cainzos-Achirica M, Greenland P, McEvoy JW, Blankstein R, Budoff MJ, et al. Role of coronary artery calcium score of zero and other negative risk markers for cardiovascular disease: the multi-ethnic study of atherosclerosis (MESA). *Circulation.* (2016) 133:849–58. doi: 10.1161/CIRCULATIONAHA.115.018524

28. Mortensen MB, Fuster V, Muntendam P, Mehran R, Baber U, Sartori S, et al. Negative risk markers for cardiovascular events in the elderly. *J Am Coll Cardiol.* (2019) 74:1–11. doi: 10.1016/j.jacc.2019.04.049

29. Sarwar A, Shaw LJ, Shapiro MD, Blankstein R, Hoffmann U, Cury RC, et al. Diagnostic and prognostic value of absence of coronary artery calcification. *JACC Cardiovasc Imaging.* (2009) 2:675–88. doi: 10.1016/j.jcmg.2008.12.031

30. Dillinger JG, Benmessaoud FA, Pezel T, Voicu S, Sideris G, Chergui N, et al. Coronary artery calcification and complications in patients with COVID-19. *JACC Cardiovasc Imaging.* (2020) 13:2468–70. doi: 10.1016/j.jcmg.2020.07.004

31. Chen FF, Zhong M, Liu Y, Zhang Y, Zhang K, Su DZ, et al. The characteristics and outcomes of 681 severe cases with COVID-19 in China. *J Crit Care.* (2020) 60:32–7. doi: 10.1016/j.jcrc.2020.07.003

32. Du RH, Liang LR, Yang CQ, Wang W, Cao TZ, Li M, et al. Predictors of mortality for patients with COVID-19 pneumonia caused by SARS-CoV-2: a prospective cohort study. *Eur Respir J.* (2020) 55:2000524. doi: 10.1183/13993003.00524-2020

33. McClelland RL, Chung H, Detrano R, Post W, Kronmal RA. Distribution of coronary artery calcium by race, gender, and age: results from the multi-ethnic study of atherosclerosis (MESA). *Circulation.* (2006) 113:30–7. doi: 10.1161/CIRCULATIONAHA.105.580696

34. Nai Fovino L, Cademartiri F, Tarantini G. Subclinical coronary artery disease in COVID-19 patients. *Eur Heart J Cardiovasc Imaging.* (2020) 21:1055–6. doi: 10.1093/ehjci/jeaa202

35. Zimmermann GS, Fingerle AA, Muller-Leisse C, Gassert F, von Schacky CE, Ibrahim T, et al. Coronary calcium scoring assessed on native screening chest CT imaging as predictor for outcome in COVID-19: an analysis of a hospitalized German cohort. *PLoS ONE.* (2020) 15:e0244707. doi: 10.1371/journal.pone.0244707

36. Arbas Redondo E, Tebar Marquez D, Poveda Pinedo ID, Dalmau Gonzalez-Gallarza R, Valbuena Lopez SC, Guzman Martinez G, et al. Diagnostic and prognostic value of coronary artery calcium score of zero: is it time for guidelines to change? *European Heart Journal.* (2020) 41 (Suppl. 2):1383. doi: 10.1093/ehjci/ehaa946.1383

37. Kalra MK, Homayounieh F, Arru C, Holmberg O, Vassileva J. Chest CT practice and protocols for COVID-19 from radiation dose management perspective. *Eur Radiol.* (2020) 30:1–7. doi: 10.1007/s00330-020-07034-x

38. Siriwardena AN. Increasing evidence that influenza is a trigger for cardiovascular disease. *J Infect Dis.* (2012) 206:1636–8. doi: 10.1093/infdis/jis598

39. Xiong TY, Redwood S, Prendergast B, Chen M. Coronaviruses and the cardiovascular system: acute and long-term implications. *Eur Heart J.* (2020) 41:1798–800. doi: 10.1093/eurheartj/ehaa231

10

COVID-19: The Cause of the Manifested Cardiovascular Complications during the Pandemic

Audditiya Bandopadhyay[1]*, Alok Kumar Singh[2] and Gyaneshwer Chaubey[1]*

[1] Cytogenetics Laboratory, Department of Zoology, Banaras Hindu University, Varanasi, India, [2] M.D.D.M. (Cardiology), Senior Intervention Cardiologist, Lifeline Hospital, Varanasi, India

*Correspondence:
Audditiya Bandopadhyay
audditiyab@gmail.com
Gyaneshwer Chaubey
gyaneshwer.chaubey@bhu.ac.in

In the course of human history, we encountered several devastating waves of pandemics, affecting millions of lives globally and now the rapid and progressive spread of the novel SARS-CoV-2, causing Coronavirus disease (COVID-19) has created a worldwide wave of crisis. Profoundly straining national health care systems, it also significantly impacted the global economic stability. With the introduction of COVID-19 measures, mainly driven by immunization drives, casualties due to the virus were reported to decrease considerably. But then comes into play the post-Covid morbidities, along with their short and long-term effects on the elderly and the co-morbid population. Moreover, the pediatric population and the otherwise healthy cohort of the young athletes were also reported being largely affected by the varying amount of post-recovery virus-induced Cardiac manifestations, in the subsequent waves of the pandemic. Therefore, here we thrived to find answers to the seemingly unending series of questions that popped up with the advent of the disease, nevertheless, there still lies a blind spot in understanding the impacts of the disease on the Cardiovascular Health of an individual, even after the clinical recovery. Thus, along with the current data related to the diverse cardiovascular complications due to SARS-COV-2 infection, we suggest long-term 'Cardiac surveillance' for the COVID-19 recovered individuals.

Keywords: SARS-CoV-2, inflammation, myocardial damage, heart, CVD

INTRODUCTION

In late 2019, a cluster of cases of "pneumonia of unknown origin," emerged, the epicenter of which was linked to the seafood wholesale market in Wuhan, China, that heralded the onset of Coronavirus disease (1). However, there are further reports suggesting that this virus was already circulating in China before the seafood market cluster event (https://www.sciencemag.org/news/2020/01/wuhan-seafood-market-may-not-be-source-novel-virus-spreading-globally). The disease spread rapidly to several countries around the globe and was already declared a pandemic by WHO. To date, a total of 187,086,096 confirmed cases of COVID−19 with a mortality of 4,042,921 have been reported (2). COVID−19 questioned the existence of mankind in the twenty-first century not just by crippling the global healthcare system but also contributing to the psychological and socio-economic burden on the entire humanity.

The family of seven known human Coronaviruses has long been associated with emerging respiratory distress syndromes and flu-like outbreaks. This is the reason behind the high occurrence of cases of pneumonia and bronchitis in patients with a severe COVID-19 infection. In the past two decades, two recorded epidemics were caused by the same family of the virus—Severe Acute Respiratory Syndrome Coronavirus (SARS-CoV), in 2002–2003, and more recently, the Middle East Respiratory Coronavirus (MERS-CoV) in 2012, has widely been mentioned. Previously known human coronavirus variants, which were associated with the common cold—HCoV-229E, HCoV-NL63, HCoV-OC43, and HCoV-HKU1, have not yet been found to be associated with heart abnormalities. But there are few reports of the patients suffering from the Middle East respiratory syndrome (MERS; caused by MERS-CoV) with myocarditis and a few cases of cardiac disease in the patients who suffered from SARS (caused by SARS-CoV) (3, 4). However, recent literature reported serious cardiovascular complications occurring in about 10–20% of hospitalized patients, apart from the respiratory effects of COVID-19; and the patients who suffered from pre-existing heart ailments may suffer either a heart attack or congestive heart failure (5). This deciphers distinct characteristics of SARS-CoV-2 in its comprehensive cardiac involvement, which could also be a consequence of the exposure of the virus to millions due to the pandemic. Reports also stated that COVID-19 triggered inflammation of the heart muscle—Myocarditis (6). The most recent severe acute respiratory syndrome coronavirus 2 (SARS-CoV-2), displayed tropism for the heart and can lead to myocarditis (inflammation of the heart), necrosis of its cells, mimicking heart attacks, arrhythmias, and acute or protracted heart failure (muscle dysfunction) (3). These complications, which at times are the sole features of COVID-19 clinical presentation, have occurred even in the cases with milder symptoms and in people who did not experience any symptoms. Unsuspected cardiac involvement including sudden cardiac death, in such healthy and young athlete groups, has further elevated the concerns regarding our current knowledge about the impact of the disease on heart health.

STRUCTURAL ASPECTS OF COVID-19 VIRUS

The difference between SARS-CoV-2 and SARS is apparently a furin polybasic site that alters their structure, and when cleaved, broadens the types of cells (tropism) that the virus can infect (7). It is a large family of single positive-stranded, enveloped RNA virus that finds its host in several animals, and by methods not yet explained, they can pass from one species to another. The virus targets the angiotensin-converting enzyme 2 (ACE2) receptor throughout the body, which facilitates the entry of viral genetic material by the means of its spike protein, along with the assistance of the cellular serine protease transmembrane protease serine 2 (TMPRSS2), heparan sulfate, and other proteases, which cleaves the viral spikes protein and make the entry pathway for the viral genetic contents (8). So, the higher the ACE2 receptor's number of receptors in any cell, the higher the susceptibility for the viral entry and greater viral load possibility. The involvement of ACE2 in the regulation of blood volume, systemic vascular resistance, and thus cardiovascular homeostasis is monumental (**Figure 1**). Previous studies have shown its association with hypertension, stroke, dyslipidemia, and cardiovascular diseases,

and kidney diseases (9–12). The heart also has a high level of ACE2 expression which makes it more susceptible to the SARS-COV-2 infection. The affinity of SARS-CoV-2 to ACE2 is significantly higher than that of SARS (13), and thus it may perturb the angiotensin-renin pathway severely.

COVID-19 AND ITS SYSTEMIC IMPLICATIONS

The tropism to other organs beyond the lungs has been quoted in some studies from the autopsy specimens. It was found that the SARS-CoV-2 genomic RNA was the highest in the lungs. However, in the heart, kidney, and liver, considerable amounts of viral load were detected in 16 out of 22 deceased patients (14). In a report from (15), out of a series of an autopsy of 39 deceased COVID-19 patients, only 31% had a high viral load, i.e., above 1,000 copies, in the heart while ~38% of the deceased was not found to possess a detectable viral load in the myocardium. Accordingly, SARS-CoV-2 infection can damage the heart in both direct and indirect ways. In-vitro studies have shown the ability of SARS-CoV-2 to infect the induced pluripotent stem cells (iPSCs) derived cardiomyocytes, causing the distinctive pattern of cell fragmentation along with the complete dissolution of the contractile machinery (16). In another iPSC study, SARS-CoV-2 infection leads to apoptosis, and ultimately the heartbeat ceases within 72 h of the viral exposure (17). Besides the direct involvement of the viral infection in the heart muscles, its entry into the endothelial lining of the blood vessels of the heart and multiple vesicular beds has also been reported. Another potential threat is the effects of secondary immune response in the infected heart and endothelial cells (endothelitis) which may include the dysregulation of the renin-angiotensin-aldosterone system modulating blood pressure; activation of pro-inflammatory responses including platelets, neutrophils, macrophages, and lymphocytes, the cytokine storm and a prothrombotic state (**Figure 1**).

There is a varying level of cardiovascular manifestations, oscillating from limited necrosis of cardiac cells leading to myocarditis to an often-fatal failure of the heart to pump sufficient blood leading to cardiogenic shock (18). One out of every five hospitalized COVID-19 patients suffering from cardiac injury reflects an accumulation of troponin (a cardiac muscle-specific marker) in blood and the same happens with those having pre-existing heart ailments. Also, for this kind of myocardial injury in-hospital mortality, troponin accumulation is an indicator of morbidity risk (19). Moreover, it has been observed that patients with higher troponin amounts also have increased levels of many inflammatory markers [including interleukin-6(IL-6), C- reactive protein, ferritin, lactate dehydrogenase (LDH), and an increased neutrophil count] and heart dysfunction (amino-terminal pro-B–type natriuretic peptide) (20). Conversely, an immunologic basis is likely as there is a possibility of myocarditis results from the hyperimmune response in order to tackle coronavirus by releasing excess cytokines. Cytokines could result in inflammation that damages the lungs and the heart alike. This

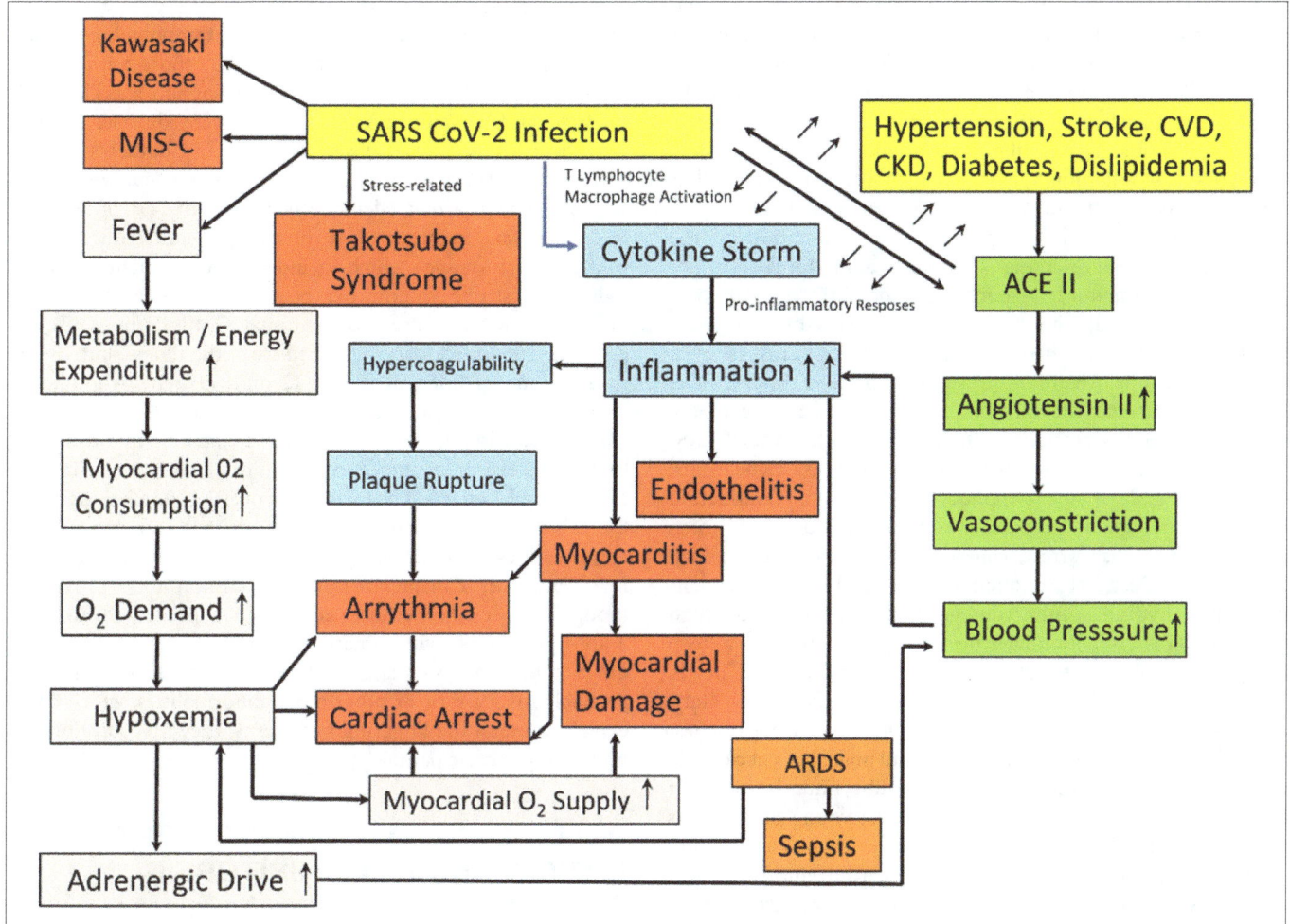

FIGURE 1 | Schematic representation of the pathways leading to post-COVID Heart conditions. The Yellow boxes represent the causes, whereas the Red and the Orange boxes depict the consequences of the infection on the heart and the lungs. The Pink, Blue, and the Green boxes depict the various systemic pathways involved, leading to the development of the conditions.

condition, known as a cytokine storm, is more serious in the elderly and the co-morbid population. However, it was also seen to affect the middle-aged population largely during the subsequent waves of the pandemic in India. It is the primary reason for the severe respiratory complications which lead to death in patients suffering from coronavirus (21). Cytokines promote blood coagulation and thus, interfere with the body's clot-busting system. Blood clots in coronary arteries in turn can block blood flow and cause heart attacks. A tendency for clotting, both in the microvasculature and large vessels, has been reported in multiple autopsy reports and in young COVID-19 patients with a history of stroke. Another relevant possibility could be the development of cardiac complications in some coronavirus patients, as a consequence of infections in their lungs. Insufficient oxygen increases the risk of arrhythmias. At the same time, fever caused by the virus increases the body's metabolism, thus the cardiac output. As a result, the patient's heart struggles with an elevated oxygen demand along with a reduced supply, causing an imbalance that leads to a myocardial injury. The causes of death might involve multiple

organ dysfunctions in most cases, and therefore it is difficult to differentiate the myocardial injury as the sole reason for such cases. Schematic representation of the different pathways leading to the post-COVID conditions has been depicted in **Figure 1**.

CARDIOVASCULAR HEALTH WITH THE RISE OF COVID-19

With an ascent in the number of COVID-19 confirmed cases and the accumulating clinical data, in addition to the common presentation of respiratory failure, the cardiovascular manifestations induced by this viral infection have generated considerable concern (22). Huang et al. (23) reported that 12% of the patients with COVID-19 were diagnosed to have an acute myocardial injury, manifested due to the elevated levels of high-sensitive troponin I. This was further supported by reports stating 16.7% out of 138 hospitalized patients with COVID-19 had suffered from arrhythmias and 7.2% had an acute myocardial injury (24). However, the plausible cause of the COVID-19 infection in the development of myocardial injury in the hospitalized patients suffering from underlying cardiovascular disease (CVD) is still unknown and it requires extensive study. Although still unclear, whether it is an after-effect of a hyperactive immune response against the virus or the virus itself leading to myocardial inflammation which is associated with cardiac function impairment and ventricular tachyarrhythmias.

Myocarditis is a diffuse pattern of inflammation of the heart, typically representing a variable admixture of injury and an inflammatory response to the injury, and may extend through all the three layers of the human heart to the pericardium, encompassing the heart. This is even more worrisome than the restricted pattern injury. The immunological and the inflammatory response is one of the most common observations at the autopsy studies after SARS-CoV-2 infections, unlike the SARS-associated myocarditis, which didn't show any lymphocyte infiltration. Conduction block and malignant ventricular arrhythmias, both of which can lead to cardiac arrest, can occur when myocytes, which synchronize electrical conduction, are involved. Besides in-hospital arrhythmias, numerous geographic regions with high COVID-19 dissemination have been reported to observe a steep increase in out-of-hospital cardiac arrest and sudden death. There has been a rise of 77% in the cases in Lombardy, Italy, as compared to the previous year (25). Due to a cluster of chest pain-like sensations, an irregular EKG, and high levels of cardiac-specific enzymes in the blood, myocarditis imitating a heart attack has been reported in individuals as young as 16 years old (3). Heart failure, acute cor pulmonale (right heart failure with potential pulmonary emboli), and cardiogenic shock can occur when there is significant and diffuse heart muscle injury. Other pathways that could also be responsible for COVID-19-related heart dysfunction, such as Takotsubo syndrome or the Broken heart syndrome (a transient stress-related illness that causes apical ballooning), ischemia caused by endocarditis, and related atherosclerotic plaque rupture with thrombosis were reported (3). Other causes included the multisystem inflammatory syndrome of children (MIS-C), although MIS-C reported here, was not only exclusive to children but also the same clinical features have been the subject of case reports in adults, such as in a 45-year-old (3).

Although the children were thought to be less susceptible to COVID-19, as compared to the adults, and while the majority of them with COVID-19 were asymptomatic or presented with only milder forms of the symptoms, the reports of COVID-19 associated severe inflammatory symptoms among the pediatric patients were not null (26–28). An unexpected cluster of eight children (aged 4–14 years) presenting with a hyperinflammatory syndrome with symptoms of Kawasaki Disease was reported in a case series from the United Kingdom (26). COVID-19 patients who underwent magnetic resonance imaging (MRI) or echocardiogram of the heart have recently revealed some fresh information concerning some cardiac involvement (29–31). In one such study, the left and the right ventricular abnormalities were reported in 479 out of 1,216 patients, and 397 patients, respectively, with evidence of new myocardial infarction in 36 of them. Myocarditis was reported in 35 and Takotsubo

Cardiomyopathy in 19 patients in the same study. Severe cardiac disease (severe ventricular dysfunction or tamponade) was also observed in 15% of the patients. And in those without any pre-existing cardiac disease, the echocardiogram was abnormal in 46%, and 13% of the cases had severe disease. Patients were between 52 and 78 years old (30). In another study, 15 patients had abnormal CMR findings on conventional CMR sequences: myocardial edema was found in 54% of patients, and LGE was found in 31% of the patients reduced right ventricle performance which includes ejection fraction, cardiac index, and stroke volume per body surface area were found in patients with positive conventional CMR findings (31). A group of 100 individuals recovered from the illness, but 78 had cardiac abnormalities, including 12 of 18 patients who had no symptoms, and 60 showed continuing myocardial inflammation, which is consistent with myocarditis (29). These findings point to the necessity for more research on covid-19's long-term cardiovascular effects. The majority of over 1,200 individuals with COVID-19 in a large prospective cohort had echocardiographic abnormalities (30). This raises questions about whether heart involvement is considerably more common than previously thought, especially because at least 30–40% of SARS-CoV-2 infections are asymptomatic. Because all of these patients did not have a systematic cardiovascular assessment for any probable myocarditis or other heart abnormalities, which could explain some of the lingering symptoms, they may have hidden underlying cardiac pathology.

ROLE OF ANGIOTENSIN-CONVERTING ENZYME AND IT'S INHIBITORS IN COVID-19

Angiotensin-converting enzyme inhibitors (ACEIs) and angiotensin receptor blockers (ARBs), both of which are known to block the renin-angiotensin system (RAS), also might affect an individual's susceptibility to COVID-19 and further worsen its severity (32–35). Angiotensin II, the main effector molecule in the renin-angiotensin-aldosterone system (RAAS), is upregulated in many clinical conditions, for which inhibition of angiotensin II by RAAS inhibitors is a common therapeutic strategy. Angiotensin-converting enzyme (ACE) produces angiotensin II from angiotensin I, whereas ACE2 inactivates angiotensin II by converting it to angiotensin (1–7) (34). Therefore, ACE2 has been assumed to have a protective effect against cardiovascular disease and lung injury. It has been shown that the RAAS inhibitors may increase the ACE2 expression, thus raise concern among COVID-19 positive patients (33).

On the other hand, a study reported significant interactions between ethnicity and ACE inhibitors and ARBs for COVID-19 disease. The risk of COVID-19 disease associated with ACE inhibitors was shown to be higher in the Caribbean and Black African groups than the white group. Variations among the ethnic groups raise the possibility of ethnic-specific effects of ACE inhibitors/ARBs on COVID-19 disease susceptibility and severity (36). Another study found that the administration of ACEI/ARB drugs had a positive effect on reducing D-dimer and the number of people with fever (37). As a result of such paradoxical issues of using ACEIs/ARBs during COVID-19, it is still an area requiring extended investigation to prove. However, in the setting of coronavirus disease, downregulation of ACE2 by severe acute respiratory syndrome coronavirus 2 (SARS-CoV-2) infection might be involved in mediating cardiovascular damage, besides, the medications that have been proposed as treatments for COVID-19 such as hydroxychloroquine and azithromycin have pro-arrhythmic effects, AF, atrial fibrillation; VF, ventricular fibrillation; VT, ventricular tachycardia (38).

PRESENT SCENARIO

Previous studies have depicted the overall clinical attributes and epidemiological findings of patients with COVID-19, and a portion of it has shown that the condition of some patients with COVID-19 deteriorates rapidly. In contrast to the asymptomatic, a substantial proportion of people suffer a long-standing, often incapacitating illness, called long-COVID. Typical symptoms of this include fatigue, difficulty in breathing, chest pain, and abnormal heart rhythm (39, 40). While the patients with underlying Cardiovascular pathology, but without myocardial injury put up with a relatively favorable prognosis, myocardial injury is much more common in patients with COVID-19 and has been found to have a significant association with the fatalities due to COVID-19.

The most intriguing question that stirred up in this while is that why do certain individuals have a propensity for heart involvement after the SARS-CoV-2 infection? Studies deciphered that the infected patients who get myocarditis do not necessarily have any more virus in their bodies than those who do not foster the condition. The prediction once recognized a few months into the pandemic, was that the cardiac involvement would chiefly occur in patients with severe COVID-19. Clearly, it is found to be much more common than anticipated. However, the true incidence is unknown. Primarily, it is vital to determine any cause that drives the pathogenesis. Whether it represents an individual's inflammatory response, an autoimmune phenomenon or some other explanations are yet to be clarified.

Beyond the prevention of COVID-19 infections, the goal of averting cardiovascular involvement is paramount. The marked heterogeneity of the disease, ranging from lack of symptoms to fatality, is poorly understood. A newly emerged virus, widely circulating throughout the human population, with a panoply of manifestations, has made this especially daunting to untangle. It wouldn't surprise much in the future if the patients present with cardiomyopathy of unknown etiology and test positive for SARS-CoV-2 antibodies. However, attributing all such cardiomyopathy solely to the virus may be difficult, given the high prevalence of infections. A biopsy might be a necessity to identify any virus particles to support any causality.

These sudden after-effects could be attributed and studied to be validated at two different levels. First is the entry point for the virus, that is the ACE2 receptors and their variations among the individuals of certain ethnicities, which makes them more susceptible or resistant toward the virus. There have been studies concluding the polymorphism within the ACE2 gene within the populations that explains the outcome, on comparing

the Western and the Indian populations, and their affinity with the East Asians (41).

The other points to be considered include the immunity of the individual and its effects after the entry of the virus. The reaction of the immunity toward the non-self determines its activity, and thus results in a hyperactive state of immune responses, that leads to systemic inflammation, which prevails for a much longer time, as compared to the symptoms themselves. The classification of asymptomatic people for COVID-19 is vague. And in many cases, the asymptomatic individuals are sometimes just the result of the symptoms getting masked due to ignorance or the socio-economic background of those individuals. They may have underlying inflammation-related pneumonia due to the disease and still not experience any level of hypoxia and thus, be considered asymptomatic. On the other hand, the body of the athletes, in practice, may demand more oxygen and experience the symptoms of hypoxia and thus, can lead to cardiac arrest due to pulmonary thromboembolism, as a consequence of dilated arteries due to the disease-related inflammation (42). The same demographic group of young and healthy, that is most common to lack the symptoms after SARS-CoV-2 infections, raises the question of how many athletes have an occult cardiac disease. Systematic assessment through some form of cardiac imaging and arrhythmia screening of athletes, who test positive for SARS-CoV-2, irrespective of symptoms, seems prudent until more is perceived. The authors in a study reported on a cohort, consisting of a large sample size of 2,461 athletes, of whom 1,597 (64.9%) had the complete comprehensive screening testing, including CMR imaging without prior selection, where they found that 37 (2.3%) of these athletes demonstrated diagnostic criteria for myocarditis by CMR imaging, including 20 without cardiovascular symptoms and with normal ECG, echocardiography, and troponin test results, who would not have been identified without CMR imaging (43). However, another subsequent study was published, where a cohort of 145 competitive athletes, who had tested positive for COVID-19 with either mild to moderate or, no symptoms, were evaluated approximately 15 days post-positive test result, using cardiac MRI, EEG, and serum markers of cardiac pathology, and only two were found to have MRI findings consistent with myocarditis. This led to conclude that its incidence following COVID-19 was much less prevalent than previously thought (44). Controversies remain until the results are validated further, on larger cohorts, considering ethnicity (ancestry) as a parameter, as that could play a vital role in the risk prediction of an individual.

FUTURE DIRECTION AND CONCLUSION

Long-term observation and prospective study design (Cardiac Surveillance) on the viability of treatments, explicit for myocardial injury are of utmost significance. Further, aggressive treatment may be considered for patients with myocardial injury. Therefore, monitoring of myocardial injury markers and cardiac function is of extreme importance, and attention should be paid to the early identification and comprehensive management of myocardial injury in such patients. But what has so far driven populations to be more vulnerable to post-COVID morbidities?

We hypothesize it as the genetic variability among the individuals at these two tiers, making them more or less susceptible toward the mentioned long-standing ailments, which are probably more severe than the disease itself. There comes into play the role of genetic mapping. Genome-wide analysis (GWAS) and Whole-genome analysis (WGA) study designs would reveal and map a particular population at risk, would categorize the vulnerable groups to prioritize them at first, and thus manage the casualties due to the disease burden.

AUTHOR CONTRIBUTIONS

GC and AB conceived and designed the study. AB, GC, and AS constituted the manuscript. All authors contributed to the article and approved the submitted version.

REFERENCES

1. Pradhan RR, Yadav AK, Mandal S. Cardiovascular implications of coronavirus disease 2019 (COVID-19): a systematic review. (2020). doi: 10.21203/rs.3.rs-39929/v1
2. Cascella M, Rajnik M, Aleem A, Dulebohn S, Di Napoli R. Features, evaluation, and treatment of coronavirus (COVID-19). In: StatPearls. Treasure Island, FL: StatPearls Publishing (2021). Available online at: https://www.ncbi.nlm.nih.gov/books/NBK554776/
3. Topol EJ. COVID-19 can affect the heart. Science. (2020) 370:408–9. doi: 10.1126/science.abe2813
4. Xiong TY, Redwood S, Prendergast B, Chen M. Coronaviruses and the cardiovascular system: acute and long-term implications. Eur Heart J. (2020) 41:1798–800. doi: 10.1093/eurheartj/ehaa231
5. Lewis DKL. How Does Cardiovascular Disease Increase the Risk of Severe Illness and Death From COVID-19. Harvard Health Blog (2020).
6. Basu-Ray I, Adeboye A, Soos MP. Cardiac manifestations of coronavirus (COVID-19). In: StatPearls. Treasure Island, FL: StatPearls Publishing (2021). Available online at: https://www.ncbi.nlm.nih.gov/books/NBK556152/
7. Matheson NJ, Lehner PJ. How does SARS-CoV-2 cause COVID-19? Science. (2020) 369:510–1. doi: 10.1126/science.abc6156
8. Hikmet F, Méar L, Edvinsson Å, Micke P, Uhlén M, Lindskog C. The protein expression profile of ACE2 in human tissues. Mol Syst Biol. (2020) 16:e9610. doi: 10.15252/msb.20209610
9. Wu X, Zhu B, Zou S, Shi J. The association between ACE2 gene polymorphism and the stroke recurrence in Chinese population. J Stroke Cerebrovasc Dis. (2018) 27:2770–80. doi: 10.1016/j.jstrokecerebrovasdis.2018.06.001
10. Zhang Q, Cong M, Wang N, Li X, Zhang H, Zhang K, et al. Association of angiotensin-converting enzyme 2 gene polymorphism and enzymatic activity with essential hypertension in different gender: a case-control study. Medicine. (2018) 97:e12917. doi: 10.1097/MD.0000000000012917
11. Pan Y, Wang T, Li Y, Guan T, Lai Y, Shen Y, et al. Association of ACE2 polymorphisms with susceptibility to essential hypertension and dyslipidemia in Xinjiang, China. Lipids Health Dis. (2018) 17:1–9. doi: 10.1186/s12944-018-0890-6
12. Wang M, Zhang W, Zhou Y, Zhou X. Association between serum angiotensin-converting enzyme 2 levels and postoperative myocardial infarction following coronary artery bypass grafting. Exp Ther Med. (2014) 7:1721–7. doi: 10.3892/etm.2014.1640
13. Gupta A, Madhavan MV, Sehgal K, Nair N, Mahajan S, Sehrawat TS, et al. Extrapulmonary manifestations of COVID-19. Nat Med. (2020) 26:1017–32. doi: 10.1038/s,41591-020-0968-3
14. Puelles VG, Lütgehetmann M, Lindenmeyer MT, Sperhake JP, Wong MN, Allweiss L, et al. Multiorgan and renal tropism of SARS-CoV-2. N Engl J Med. (2020) 383:590–2. doi: 10.1056/NEJMc2011400
15. Lindner D, Fitzek A, Bräuninger H, Aleshcheva G, Edler C, Meissner K, et al. Association of cardiac infection with SARS-CoV-2 in confirmed COVID-19 autopsy cases. JAMA Cardiol. (2020) 5:1281–5. doi: 10.1001/jamacardio.2020.3551
16. Perez-Bermejo JA, Kang S, Rockwood SJ, Simoneau CR, Joy DA, Silva AC, et al. SARS-CoV-2 infection of human iPSC-derived cardiac cells reflects cytopathic features in hearts of patients with COVID-19. Sci Transl Med. (2021) 13:eabf7872. doi: 10.1126/scitranslmed.abf7872
17. Sharma A, Garcia G Jr, Wang Y, Plummer JT, Morizono K, Arumugaswami V, et al. Human iPSC-derived cardiomyocytes are susceptible to SARS-CoV-2 infection. Cell Rep Med. (2020) 1:100052. doi: 10.1016/j.xcrm.2020.100052
18. Shafi AM, Shaikh SA, Shirke MM, Iddawela S, Harky A. Cardiac manifestations in COVID-19 patients-A systematic review. J Card Surg. (2020) 35:1988–2008. doi: 10.1111/jocs.14808
19. Gomila-Grange A, Espasa M, Moglia E. Cardiogenic shock caused by SARS-CoV-2 in a patient with serial negative nucleic acid amplification tests. Case Report SN Comprehens Clin Med. (2020) 2:1903–5. doi: 10.1007/s42399-020-00496-6
20. Bonow RO, Fonarow GC, O'Gara PT, Yancy CW. Association of coronavirus disease 2019 (COVID-19) with myocardial injury and mortality. JAMA Cardiol. (2020) 5:751–3. doi: 10.1001/jamacardio.2020.1105
21. Tay MZ, Poh CM, Rénia L, MacAry PA, Ng LF. The trinity of COVID-19: immunity, inflammation and intervention. Nat Rev Immunol. (2020) 20:363–74. doi: 10.1038/s41577-020-0311-8
22. Kwenandar F, Japar KV, Damay V, Hariyanto TI, Tanaka M, Lugito NPH, et al. Coronavirus disease 2019 and cardiovascular system: a narrative review. IJC Heart Vascul. (2020) 2020:100557. doi: 10.1016/j.ijcha.2020.100557
23. Huang C, Wang Y, Li X, Ren L, Zhao J, Hu Y, et al. Clinical features of patients infected with 2019 novel coronavirus in Wuhan, China. Lancet. (2020) 395:497–506. doi: 10.1016/S0140-6736(20)30183-5
24. Guo T, Fan Y, Chen M, Wu X, Zhang L, He T, et al. Cardiovascular implications of fatal outcomes of patients with coronavirus disease 2019 (COVID-19). JAMA Cardiol. (2020) 5:811–8. doi: 10.1001/jamacardio.2020.1017
25. Baldi E, Sechi GM, Mare C, Canevari F, Brancaglione A, Primi R, et al. Out-of-hospital cardiac arrest during the Covid-19 outbreak in Italy. N Engl J Med. (2020) 383:496–8. doi: 10.1056/NEJMc2010418
26. Qiu H, Wu J, Hong L, Luo Y, Song Q, Chen D. Clinical and epidemiological features of 36 children with coronavirus disease 2019 (COVID-19) in Zhejiang, China: an observational cohort study. Lancet Infect Dis. (2020) 20:689–96. doi: 10.1016/S1473-3099(20)30198-5
27. Riphagen S, Gomez X, Gonzalez-Martinez C, Wilkinson N, Theocharis P. Hyperinflammatory shock in children during COVID-19 pandemic. Lancet. (2020) 395:1607–8. doi: 10.1016/S0140-6736(20)31094-1
28. Verdoni L, Mazza A, Gervasoni A, Martelli L, Ruggeri M, Ciuffreda M, et al. An outbreak of severe Kawasaki-like disease at the Italian epicentre of the SARS-CoV-2 epidemic: an observational cohort study. Lancet. (2020) 395:1771–8. doi: 10.1016/S0140-6736(20)31103-X
29. Puntmann VO, Carerj ML, Wieters I. Outcomes of cardiovascular magnetic resonance imaging in patients recently recovered from coronavirus disease 2019 (COVID-19). JAMA Cardiol. (2020) 5:1265–73. doi: 10.1001/jamacardio.2020.3557
30. Dweck MR, Bularga A, Hahn RT, Bing R, Lee KK, Chapman AR, et al. Global evaluation of echocardiography in patients with COVID-19. Eur Heart J Cardiovasc Imaging. (2020) 21:949–58. doi: 10.1093/ehjci/jeaa178
31. Huang L, Zhao P, Tang D, Zhu T, Han R, Zhan C, et al. Cardiac involvement in patients recovered from COVID-2019 identified using

magnetic resonance imaging. *JACC Cardiovasc Imaging.* (2020) 13:2330–9. doi: 10.1016/j.jcmg.2020.05.004

32. Morales DR, Conover MM, You SC, Pratt N, Kostka K, Duarte-Salles T, et al. Renin-angiotensin system blockers and susceptibility to COVID-19: an international, open science, cohort analysis. *Lancet Digit Health.* (2021) 3:e98–114. doi: 10.1016/S2589-7500(20)30289-2

33. Vaduganathan M, Vardeny O, Michel T, McMurray JJ, Pfeffer MA, Solomon SD. Renin-angiotensin-aldosterone system inhibitors in patients with Covid-19. *New England Journal of Medicine.* (2020) 382:1653–9. doi: 10.1056/NEJMsr2005760

34. Nishiga M, Wang DW, Han Y, Lewis DB, Wu JC. COVID-19 and cardiovascular disease: from basic mechanisms to clinical perspectives. *Nat Rev Cardiol.* (2020) 17:543–58. doi: 10.1038/s41569-020-0413-9

35. Li W, Moore MJ, Vasilieva N, Sui J, Wong SK, Berne MA, et al. Angiotensin-converting enzyme 2 is a functional receptor for the SARS coronavirus. *Nature.* (2003) 426:450–4. doi: 10.1038/nature02145

36. Hippisley-Cox J, Young D, Coupland C, Channon KM, San Tan P, Harrison DA, et al. Risk of severe COVID-19 disease with ACE inhibitors and angiotensin receptor blockers: cohort study including 8.3 million people. *Heart.* (2020) 106:1503–11. doi: 10.1136/heartjnl-2020-3 17393

37. Xue Y, Sun S, Cai J, Zeng L, Wang S, Wang S, et al. Effects of ACEI and ARB on COVID-19 patients: a meta-analysis. *J Renin-Angioten Aldosterone Syst.* (2020) 21:1470320320981321. doi: 10.1177/14703203209 81321

38. Sanders JM, Monogue ML, Jodlowski TZ, Cutrell JB. Pharmacologic treatments for coronavirus disease 2019 (COVID-19): a review. *JAMA.* (2020) 323:1824–36. doi: 10.1001/jama.2020.6019

39. Del Rio C, Collins LF, Malani P. Long-term health consequences of COVID-19. *JAMA.* (2020) 324:1723–4. doi: 10.1001/jama.2020.19719

40. Nalbandian A, Sehgal K, Gupta A, Madhavan MV, McGroder C, Stevens JS, et al. Post-acute COVID-19 syndrome. *Nat Med.* (2021) 27:601–15. doi: 10.1038/s41591-021-01283-z

41. Srivastava A, Pandey RK, Singh PP, Kumar P, Rasalkar AA, Tamang R, et al. Most frequent South Asian haplotypes of ACE2 share identity by descent with East Eurasian populations. *PLoS ONE.* (2020) 15:e0238255. doi: 10.1371/journal.pone.0238255

42. Davey MS, Davey MG, Hurley R, Hurley ET, Pauzenberger L. Return to play following COVID-19 infection-A systematic review of current evidence. *J Sport Rehabil.* (2021) 25:1–6. doi: 10.1123/jsr.2021-0028

43. Udelson JE, Rowin EJ, Maron BJ. Return to play for athletes after COVID-19 infection: the fog begins to clear. *JAMA Cardiol.* (2021) 6:997–9. doi: 10.1001/jamacardio.2021.2079

44. Starekova J, Bluemke DA, Bradham WS, Eckhardt LL, Grist TM, Kusmirek JE, et al. Evaluation for myocarditis in competitive student athletes recovering from coronavirus disease 2019 with cardiac magnetic resonance imaging. *JAMA Cardiol.* (2021) 6:945–50. doi: 10.1001/jamacardio.2020.7444

11

Association of ACEi/ARB use and Clinical Outcomes of COVID-19 Patients with Hypertension

Jing Ma [1,2,3†], Xiaowei Shi [1,2†], Jiong Yu [1,2†], Feifei Lv [3], Jian Wu [1,4], Xinyu Sheng [1,2], Qiaoling Pan [1,2], Jinfeng Yang [1,2], Hongcui Cao [1,2*] and Lanjuan Li [1,2]

[1] State Key Laboratory for the Diagnosis and Treatment of Infectious Diseases, National Clinical Research Center for Infectious Diseases, The First Affiliated Hospital, Zhejiang University School of Medicine, Hangzhou, China, [2] Collaborative Innovation Center for Diagnosis and Treatment of Infectious Diseases, Hangzhou, China, [3] Department of Laboratory Medicine, The First Affiliated Hospital, Zhejiang University School of Medicine, Hangzhou, China, [4] Department of Laboratory Medicine, The First People's Hospital of Yancheng City, Yancheng, China

*Correspondence:
Hongcui Cao
hccao@zju.edu.cn

† These authors have contributed equally to this work

Objectives: Evidence has shown that angiotensin-converting enzyme 2 (ACE2), which can be upregulated after angiotensin-converting enzyme inhibitor (ACEi) and angiotensin receptor blocker (ARB) treatment, may play a dual role in the pathogenesis and progression of coronavirus disease 2019 (COVID-19). We aimed to assess the association between the use of ACEi/ARB and the outcome of COVID-19 patients with preexisting hypertension in non-endemic areas.

Methods: From January 17, 2020, to February 19, 2020, 286 patients with hypertension were enrolled in this retrospective study out of 1,437 COVID-19 patients from 47 centers in Zhejiang and Jiangsu Province. The composite endpoints consisted of mechanical ventilation, intensive care unit (ICU) admission, or death. Cox proportional hazards analysis was performed to assess the association between ACEi/ARB and clinical outcomes of COVID-19 patients with hypertension.

Results: In the main analysis, 103 patients receiving ACEi/ARB were compared with 173 patients receiving other regimens. Overall, 44 patients (15.94%) had an endpoint event. The risk probability of crude endpoints in the ACEi/ARB group (12.62%) was lower than that in the non-ACEi/ARB group (17.92%). After adjusting for confounding factors by inverse probability weighting, the results showed that the use of ACEi/ARB reduced the occurrence of end events by 47% [hazard ratio (HR) = 0.53; 95% CI, 0.34–0.83]. Similar results were obtained in multiple sensitivity analyses.

Conclusions: In this retrospective study, among COVID-19 patients with hypertension, the use of ACEi/ARB is not associated with an increased risk of disease severity compared with patients without ACEi/ARB. The trends of beneficial effects of ACEi/ARB need to be further evaluated in randomized clinical trials.

Keywords: angiotensin-converting enzyme inhibitors, angiotensin receptor blockers, COVID-19, hypertension, SARS-CoV-2

INTRODUCTION

The novel coronavirus disease 2019 (COVID-19) is spreading worldwide, with an increasing number of confirmed cases and deaths, and has received widespread attention from the World Health Organization. It is currently known that COVID-19 patients with hypertension are prone to have poor clinical outcomes (1). Angiotensin-converting enzyme inhibitors (ACEis) and angiotensin receptor blockers (ARBs) are widely used in the treatment of hypertension. In animal studies, the expression of angiotensin-converting enzyme 2 (ACE2) is upregulated after ACEi and ARB treatment (2). Intriguingly, ACE2 plays a dual role in COVID-19 progression. On one hand, severe acute respiratory syndrome coronavirus 2 (SARS-CoV-2) binds with ACE2 to enter the host cell during invasion (3), resulting in a decrease in ACE2 and subsequently causing vasoconstriction. Based on this, patients with a medical history of ACEi/ARB may be more likely to suffer from SARS-COV-2 infection and severe progression due to elevated ACE2 expression, and it has proposed that alternative treatments be sought for those with a high risk of infection (4). On the other hand, evidence from various acute respiratory distress syndrome (ARDS) animal models showed that exogenous ACE2 supplementation can reduce inflammation and increase oxygenation (2). The absence of the protective role of ACE2 may lead to renin–angiotensin system (RAS) dysregulation and potentially give rise to extensive endothelial dysfunction and acute lung injury (5). Thus, ACEi/ARB may, in turn, be beneficial as it prevents RAS overactivation by increasing ACE2 expression, reducing the risk of acute lung injury and acute respiratory distress syndrome.

Several studies have indicated that ACEi/ARB use was associated with decreased mortality in patients with COVID-19 (6–8), but most studies supported that ACEi/ARB use was not related to disease severity (1, 8–12). A recent meta-review of ours also concluded that ACEi/ARB therapy was associated with a lower risk of mortality compared to those who have non-ACEi/ARB antihypertensive drugs but not associated with a higher risk of COVID-19 severity (13). Indeed, the use of ACEi/ARB in patients with COVID-19 remains controversial. And very few large-sample studies are conducted outside the pandemic area in China (14, 15). Therefore, the present study aimed to assess the association between ACEi/ARB use and its impact on the risk of severity in COVID-19 patients with hypertension in non-endemic areas by inverse probability of treatment weighting (IPTW) analysis.

METHODS

Patients

Patients diagnosed with COVID-19 were recruited for this multicenter retrospective study from 47 centers in Zhejiang and Jiangsu Province between January 17, 2020, and February 19, 2020. All patients enrolled in this study were diagnosed with hypertension and COVID-19 according to the diagnostic criteria of the National Health Commission. This study was approved by the Ethics Committee of the First Affiliated Hospital,

College of Medicine, Zhejiang University (No. IIT20200005C), and complied with the ethical guidelines of the Declaration of Helsinki. Written informed consent was waived, as this study was conducted on an emerging infectious disease and the researchers analyzed only anonymous data.

Data Collection

Epidemiological, demographic, comorbidities, clinical, laboratory, time from illness onset to hospital admission, time to the first dose of antiviral delivery, chest radiological findings at admission, and outcome data were collected from patients' electronic medical records, with verification by independent doctors. The COVID-19 cases were all confirmed by throat swab specimens from the upper respiratory tract using sequencing or RT-PCR assay. Clinical outcomes were followed up to March 15, 2020.

Definition

The patients were classified into four types: mild, moderate, severe, and critical type according to the guidelines on the Diagnosis and Treatment of COVID-19 by the National Health Commission (16). All patients taking ACEi and ARB antihypertensive drugs, whether combined or not, were classified in the ACEi/ARB group based on their main complaint at admission. In principle, the antihypertensive regimens remained the same as the drugs used by patients before admission. Hypertension grades were defined as Grade 1, Grade 2, and Grade 3 according to 2018 guidelines of the European Society of Hypertension (ESH). The onset of COVID-19 was defined as the time when symptoms were first noticed. The endpoint of this study was defined as a composite measure consisting of mechanical ventilation, intensive care unit (ICU) admission, or death. Briefly, the endpoint represented at least one criterion: respiratory failure occurs and mechanical ventilation is required, develops other organ failures and needs ICU monitoring and treatment, or death (17). If the patient met several criteria for the event, the calculation will be based on the time of the first criterion appearance and follow-up until the patient was discharged.

Statistical Analysis

Continuous variables were expressed as medians and interquartile range (IQR) 25–75% and were compared by t-test or Mann–Whitney U-test. Categorical variables were expressed as percentages and tested with chi-square test or Fisher's exact test. To assess the association between ACEi/ARB use and clinical outcomes of COVID-19 patients, our main analysis compared the 103 participants who received ACEi/ARB with the 173 who received other regimens. Cox proportional hazards regression models were used to assess the association between ACEi/ARB use and the composite endpoint of intubation, ICU admission, or death. The primary analyses adjusted for benchmark covariates, including sex, age, body mass index (BMI), smoking status, duration from onset to admission, C-reactive protein (CRP), treatment of antivirus drugs, clinical type on admission, grade of hypertension, and comorbidities. The main analysis was performed by IPTW to minimize

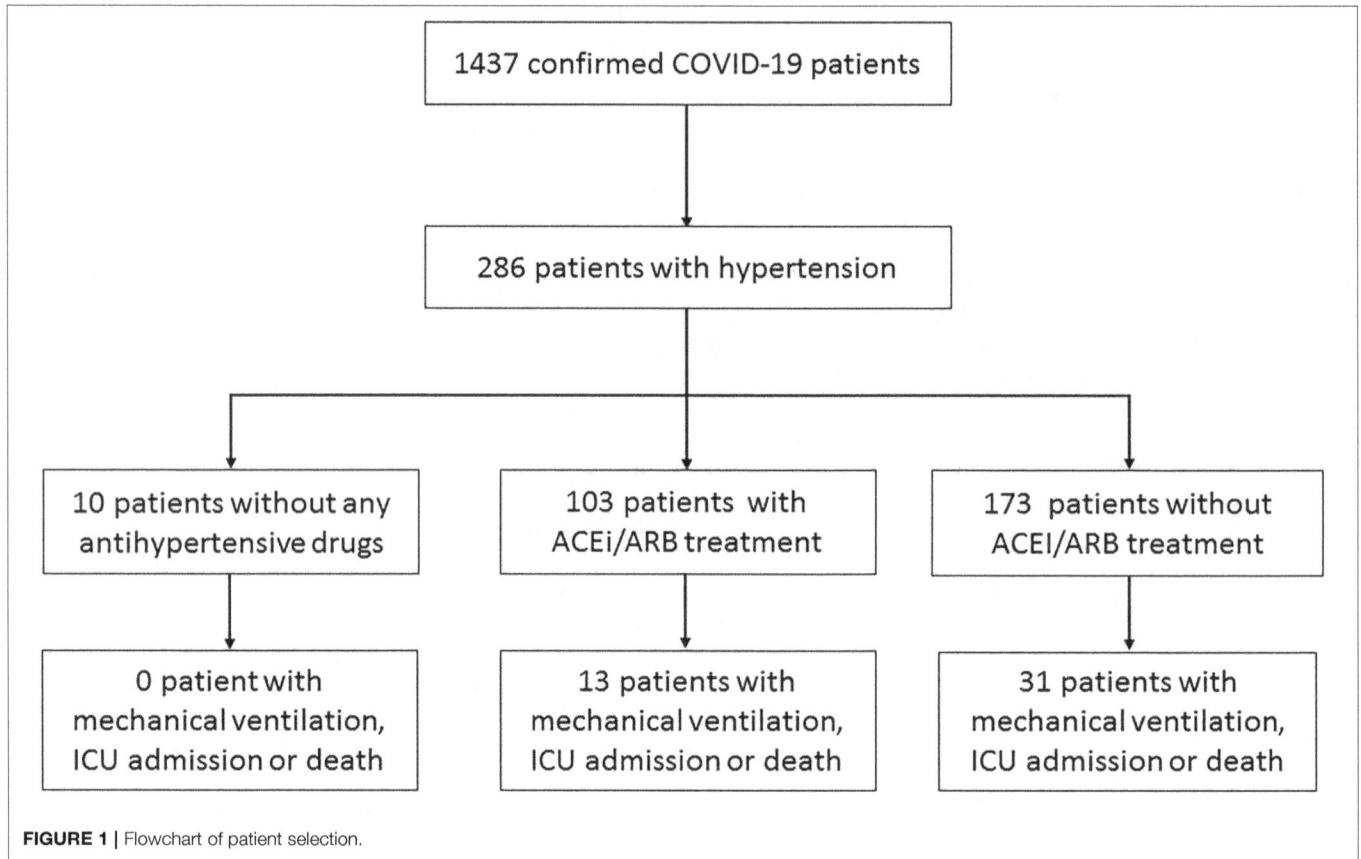

FIGURE 1 | Flowchart of patient selection.

the effect of ACEi/ARB use selection bias and to control for potential confounding factors (18), which included the same covariates as the Cox regression model (19). The estimated propensity score was obtained as the predicted probability of each subject treated with ACEi/ARB. The standardized differences were examined to assess the covariates included in estimating propensity scores before and after weighting, with a statistic <10% indicating a clinically meaningful balance between the two groups (19). Missing data were performed through multiple imputations by chained equations using the other variables available (20). All statistical analyses were performed by Statistical Package for the Social Sciences version 19.0 (International Business Machines Corporation, Armonk, NY) and R version 3.4 (R Foundation, Vienna, Austria). All tests were two–tailed, and $p < 0.05$ was considered to indicate statistical significance.

Other Sensitivity Analyses

In addition, we conducted eight prespecified subgroups and sensitivity analyses to evaluate the robustness of the composite endpoint: (1) age (age <60 vs. ≥60 years), (2) sex (male vs. female), (3) median value of onset to admission (<4 vs. ≥4 days), (4) CRP (<8 vs. ≥8 mg/L), (5) BMI (<25 vs. ≥25 kg/m^2), (6) presence of diabetes (yes vs. no), (7) clinical type on admission (mild/moderate vs. severe), (8) grade of hypertension (1 vs. 2 vs. 3).

Second, all patients eligible for the study were analyzed, and those without any antihypertensive drugs were analyzed in the control group.

RESULTS

Clinical Characteristics and Symptoms on Admission

From January 17, 2020, to February 19, 2020, 286 patients with hypertension were enrolled in this study out of 1,437 COVID-19 patients in 47 centers of Zhejiang and Jiangsu Province (**Figure 1**). Among the patients, 103 patients received ACEi/ARB therapy, including 12 with ACEi, 91 with ARB, and 46 combined with other types of drugs. Besides, 173 patients were treated with other regimens, including 143 (82.66%) with calcium channel blockers, 20 (11.56%) with beta-blockers, 40 (22.73%) with diuretics, and three (1.73%) with centrally acting agents (**Table 2**) and 10 without any antihypertensive drugs.

Clinical characteristics of patients from the ACEi/ARB group and other regimens group are shown in **Table 1**. There were no significant differences in either age or sex between the two groups ($p > 0.05$). Fever and cough were the main symptoms in the ACEi/ARB group and other regimens group, and the proportion in the two groups had no significant differences. In addition to hypertension, 97 (35.14%) patients had at least one comorbidity other than hypertension. The ACEi/ARB group included 22 cases

TABLE 1 | Characteristics of COVID-19 patients with hypertension with or without ACEi/ARB therapy.

Characteristic	Non-ACEi/ARB (n = 173)	ACEi/ARB (n = 103)	p-value
Age (years)	62 (52–68)	59 (52–67)	0.450
BMI (kg/m^2)*	25.53 (23.52–27.28)	24.84 (22.58–27.30)	0.190
Duration from onset to admission (days)	4 (2–7)	5 (3–7)	0.928
Temperatures (°C)	38.00 (37.50–38.50)	38.00 (37.40–38.50)	0.211
Female (%)	76 (43.93%)	55 (53.40%)	0.128
Current smoker (%)	15 (8.67%)	9 (8.74%)	1
Exposure history			
Contact with patients (%)	91 (52.60%)	54 (52.43%)	0.978
Cluster (%)	31 (17.92%)	19 (18.45%)	0.912
From Wuhan (%)	50 (28.90%)	34 (33.01%)	0.473
Symptoms			
Fever (%)	139 (80.35%)	79 (76.70%)	0.472
Cough (%)	107 (61.85%)	69 (66.99%)	0.390
Expectoration (%)	52 (30.06%)	25 (24.27%)	0.300
Sore throat (%)	15 (8.67%)	13 (12.62%)	0.293
Muscle ache (%)	19 (10.98%)	10 (9.71%)	0.739
Fatigue (%)	43 (24.86%)	26 (25.24%)	0.943
Shortness of breath (%)	19 (10.98%)	12 (11.65%)	0.865
Diarrhea (%)	15 (8.67%)	6 (5.83%)	0.485
Sick (%)	6 (3.47%)	3 (2.91%)	1
Headache (%)	6 (3.47%)	4 (3.88%)	1
Coexisting comorbidity			
Cardiovascular diseases (%)	21 (12.14%)	5 (4.85%)	0.055
Diabetes (%)	32 (18.50%)	22 (21.36%)	0.562
COPD (%)	2 (1.16%)	0 (0.00%)	0.530
Asthma (%)	2 (1.16%)	0 (0.00%)	0.530
Cancer (%)	6 (3.47%)	1 (0.97%)	0.263
Chronic liver disease (%)	13 (7.51%)	9 (8.74%)	0.819
Chronic renal disease (%)	3 (1.73%)	3 (2.91%)	0.674
Chest x-ray/CT findings			0.520
Normal	12 (6.94%)	3 (2.97%)	
Unilateral pneumonia (%)	20 (11.56%)	10 (9.90%)	
Bilateral pneumonia (%)	96 (55.49%)	59 (58.42%)	
Multiple mottling and ground-glass opacity (%)	45 (26.01%)	29 (28.71%)	
Grade of hypertension			0.003
Grade 1 (%)	109 (63.01%)	54 (52.43%)	
Grade 2 (%)	33 (19.08%)	38 (36.89%)	
Grade 3 (%)	31 (17.92%)	11 (10.68%)	
Severe/critical type on admission (%)	14 (8.09%)	10 (9.71%)	0.663
C-reactive protein (mg/L)**	15.53 (4.54–43.11)	15.80 (5.42–34.16)	0.164

ACEi, angiotensin-converting enzyme inhibitor; ARB, angiotensin receptor blocker; BMI, body mass index; COPD, chronic obstructive pulmonary disease; COVID-19, coronavirus disease 2019.
*21 patients with missing data of BMI.
**2 patients with missing data of C-reactive protein.

of diabetes, five cases of cardiovascular diseases, and nine cases of chronic liver disease. And there were 32 with diabetes, 21 with cardiovascular disease, and 13 with chronic liver disease in the non-ACEi/ARB group. There are significant differences in the

TABLE 2 | In-hospital management and outcomes of ACEi/ARB and non-ACEi/ARB groups.

Variable	Non-ACEi/ARB (n = 173)	ACEi/ARB (n = 103)	p-value
Interferon-α	110 (63.58%)	64 (63.37%)	0.971
Oseltamivir	3 (1.73%)	5 (4.95%)	0.149
Fapiravir	6 (3.47%)	5 (5.00%)	0.535
Arbidol	127 (73.41%)	71 (70.30%)	0.579
Lopinavir/ritonavir	96 (55.49%)	61 (60.40%)	0.428
Darunavir	3 (1.84%)	2 (2.27%)	1
Chloroquine phosphate	2 (1.23%)	1 (1.14%)	0.95
Glucocorticoids	60 (34.68%)	33 (32.04%)	0.653
IVIGt	47 (27.17%)	25 (24.27%)	0.596
Antibiotics drug	80 (46.24%)	45 (43.69%)	0.68
Antihypertensive agents			
Calcium channel blockers	137 (82.66%)	47 (45.63%)	<0.001
ACEi	0 (0.00%)	12 (11.65%)	<0.001
ARB	0 (0.00%)	91 (88.35%)	<0.001
Beta-blockers	20 (11.56%)	7 (6.80%)	0.198
Diuretics	34 (19.65%)	12 (11.65%)	0.084
Centrally antihypertensive agents	3 (1.73%)	0 (0.00%)	0.296
Shock	1 (0.55%)	1 (0.97%)	1
Admission to ICU	24 (13.87%)	10 (9.71%)	0.309
Mechanical Ventilation	22 (12.72%)	9 (8.74%)	0.311
Venovenous hemofiltration	3 (1.73%)	1 (0.97%)	1
ECMO	6 (3.47%)	2 (1.94%)	0.714
Lung transplantation	1 (0.97%)	0 (0.00%)	1
Composite endpoint	31 (17.92%)	13 (12.62%)	0.245

ACEi, angiotensin-converting enzyme inhibitor; ARB, angiotensin receptor blocker; ICU, intensive care unit; ECMO, extracorporeal membrane oxygenation; IVIGt, intravenous immunoglobulin treatment.

grade of hypertension: the proportion of grade 1 hypertension was 54 (52.43%) in the ACEi/ARB group vs. 109 (63.01%) in the non-ACEi/ARB group; grade 2, 38 (36.89%) vs. 33 (19.08%); and grade 3, 11 (10.68%) vs. 31 (17.92%), respectively (p = 0.003) (**Table 1**). The results of the remaining laboratory tests were shown in **Supplementary Table 1**.

The Association of Angiotensin-Converting Enzyme Inhibitor/Angiotensin Receptor Blocker Use With the Composite Endpoints

With a median time of 9 days, 44 patients had disease progression or death in the entire cohort. In detail, two had septic shock and were given vasoactive medications, 34 (12.32%) were admitted to the ICU, 31 (11.23%) received mechanical ventilation, one patient died after intubation, one had lung transplantation, and eight (2.90%) received extracorporeal membrane oxygenation (ECMO) (**Table 2**). Until March 15, 2020, nine patients had not been discharged, and one of them was in the ACEi/ARB group. The composite endpoints were documented in 13 of 103 (12.62%) patients who received ACEi/ARB therapy compared with 31 of 173 (17.92%) patients in the non-ACEi/ARB group. The rate of events was numerically lower in the ACEi/ARB group than in the non-ACEi/ARB group, but the difference was not significant. The median progression event time was significantly different in the ACEi/ARB group compared with the non-ACEi/ARB group (12 vs. 9 days, $p = 0.003$). In the crude unadjusted analysis, Kaplan–Meier curves for events-free survival showed a hazard ratio (HR) of 0.65 (95% CI, 0.34–1.25; $p = 0.2002$); after adjusting the benchmark covariate, the HR was 0.41 (95% CI, 0.19–0.88; $p = 0.0211$) in the primary multivariable analysis (**Figure 2A**).

In the IPTW analysis, baseline characteristics were balanced in the two groups (**Supplementary Figure 1**, **Supplementary Table 2**). Among the 276 patients in the two groups, the events-free survival was 89.48% in the ACEi/ARB group and 81.85% in the non-ACEi/ARB group; the weighted HR was 0.53 (95% CI, 0.34–0.83; $p = 0.006$; **Figure 2B**).

Other Sensitivity Analyses

To further confirm whether the observed findings were robust to potential confounders, we performed stratified analyses by prespecified subgroups; all analyses were adjusted for all variables as the Cox regression model except for the stratification variable itself. Compared with the non-ACEi/ARB group, the risk of composite endpoint events probability did not increase in the ACEi/ARB group, with HRs ranging from 0.07 to 0.80 (**Figure 3**), and no statistically significant interaction was found. In addition, adding the 10 patients who were not taking any antihypertensive drugs in the control group did not change the result; the weighted HR was 0.48 (95% CI, 0.30–0.77; $p = 0.0022$; **Supplementary Figure 2**). The results of the sensitivity analyses support our main findings.

DISCUSSION

In this multicenter retrospective study, our results suggest that chronic treatment with ACEi/ARB is not associated with an increased severity of clinical outcome in COVID-19 patients with hypertension. The values of HRs were below 1 in all subgroups considered and after careful adjustments, including an IPTW analysis. In addition, the median progression event time of the ACEi/ARB group was significantly longer than that of the non-ACEi/ARB group (12 vs. 9 days, $p < 0.001$). This finding supported the continued use of RAS inhibitors in COVID-19 patients with hypertension, which provides clinical evidence for the recommendations of international societies.

RAS plays an important role in the pathogenesis and development of hypertension. ACEis and ARBs are commonly used in hypertensive patients as two targeted RAS system inhibitors. There is evidence demonstrating that activation of RAS is associated with acute lung injury in the SARS-CoV-infected model with downregulated ACE2 expression in the lungs, but the lung failure in this setting could be attenuated by treatment with ACEi/ARB (21–23). Furthermore, a systematic meta-study showed that ACEi/ARB can reduce the incidence of community-acquired pneumonia and pneumonia-related mortality (24). A recent study found that angiotensin II was significantly elevated in COVID-19 patients and was in a positive linear correlation with viral load and lung injury (25). Another study also supported the use of ACEi/ARB in improving clinical

outcomes of COVID-19 patients with hypertension, as they found that using ACEi/ARB could significantly reduce the level of interleukin 6 while increasing the level of peripheral blood T cells (26).

To assess the potential effects of ACEi/ARB use on these in-hospital patients with COVID-19, we limited our analysis to a cohort of patients with coexisting hypertension and excluded those without hypertension. Several previous studies included the patients without hypertension in the non-ACEi/ARB group and concluded that the use of ACEi/ARB was not related to the severity of the disease (27–30), which may underestimate the effect of ACEi/ARB on patients with COVID-19, since hypertension itself was a risk factor for disease progression (31).

To the best of our knowledge, several observational studies have evaluated the impact of ACEi/ARB use on clinical outcomes in patients with COVID-19 (1, 6–11) and have offered different perspectives. Observational studies may be prone to bias and cannot provide robust results because interventions are not randomly assigned. Despite such shortcomings, observational data represent current clinical practice and apply modern methods to minimize selection bias to assess the effectiveness of clinical interventions and may help guide clinical decision-making. Two recent systematic reviews and meta-analyses concluded that the use of ACEi/ARB is significantly associated with decreased mortality in COVID-19 patients with hypertension but not associated with disease severity (13, 32). These systematic reviews recognized similar limitations, such as research heterogeneity, all studies included were observational, and most studies only adjusted for age and gender without considering other potential confounders and selection bias. Therefore, it is impossible to determine whether ACEi/ARB use is actually effective in SARS-COV-2-infected patients.

Feng et al. (33) first reported from Wuhan that there was a significant difference in ACEi/ARB usage among patients of different severities; the number of severe or critical patients was significantly lower in the ACEi/ARB group than in the non-ACEi/ARB group, but this research did not consider confounding factors, as other studies have done (8, 10). Another multicenter retrospective study performed an analysis among 1,128 COVID-19 patients with preexisting hypertension, which included 188 patients on treatment with ACEi/ARB (7). The effect of ACEi/ARB treatment was analyzed using a multivariate adjustment for confounding variables and propensity score (PS) matching. And results stated that ACEi/ARB was associated with a lower rate of severe outcomes with SARS-CoV-2 infection. These data are in concordance with our results, but the mortality rate in our patients was substantially lower. This discrepancy might result from several factors, i.e., delayed hospitalization after symptom onset in Hubei may lead to disease progression (34). In addition, in every five death cases of COVID-19, only one received invasive mechanical ventilation or further active respiratory support, suggesting that ventilation equipment was limited and intubation was delayed for many patients (35). But the authors did not provide many details about the duration between the onset of symptoms to admission (36) and the grade of hypertension like another study from Korea (9), which were

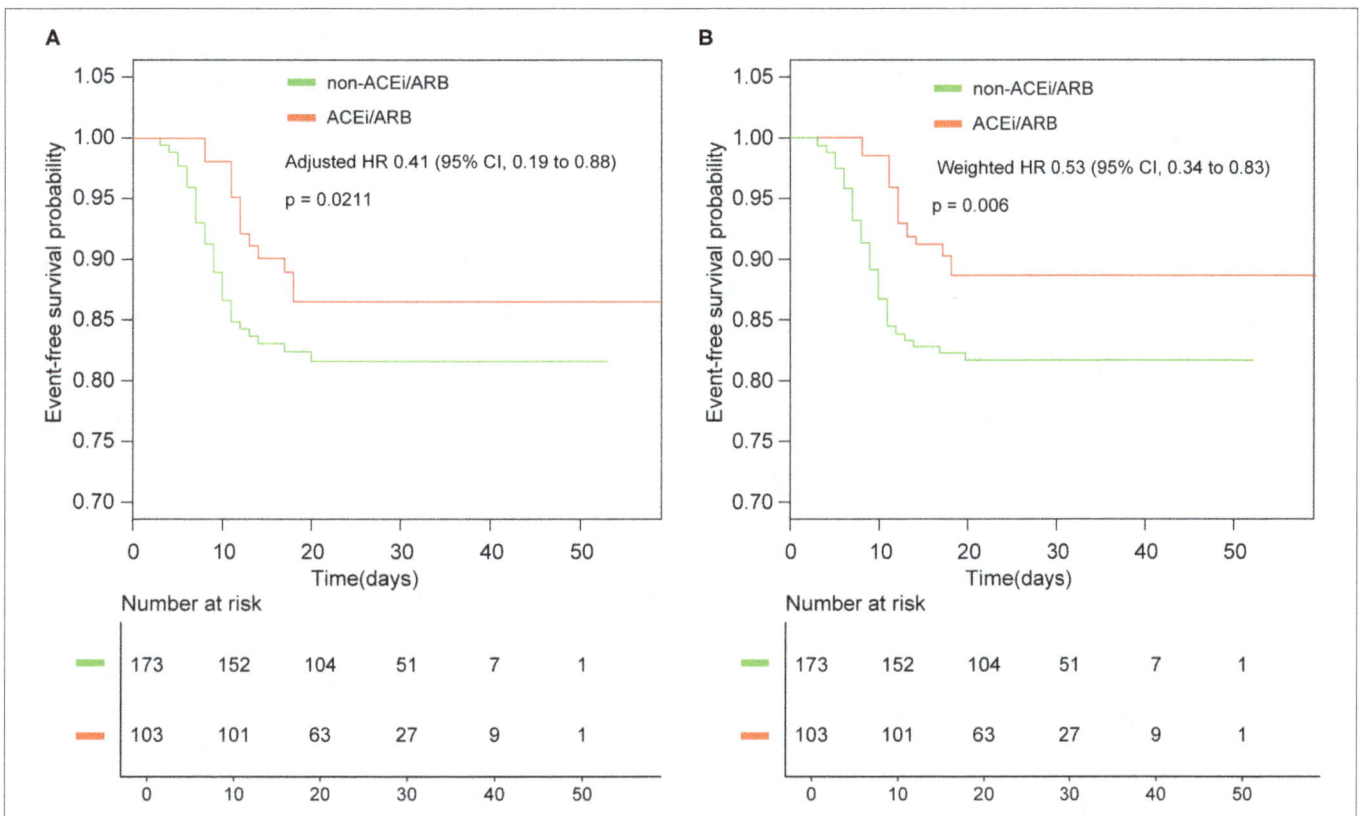

FIGURE 2 | Kaplan–Meier curves for survival without events. **(A)** Kaplan–Meier curves for event-free survival without weighted; **(B)** Kaplan–Meier curves for event-free survival after inverse probability of treatment weighting. ACEi, angiotensin-converting enzyme inhibitor; ARB, angiotensin receptor blocker; HR, hazard ratio.

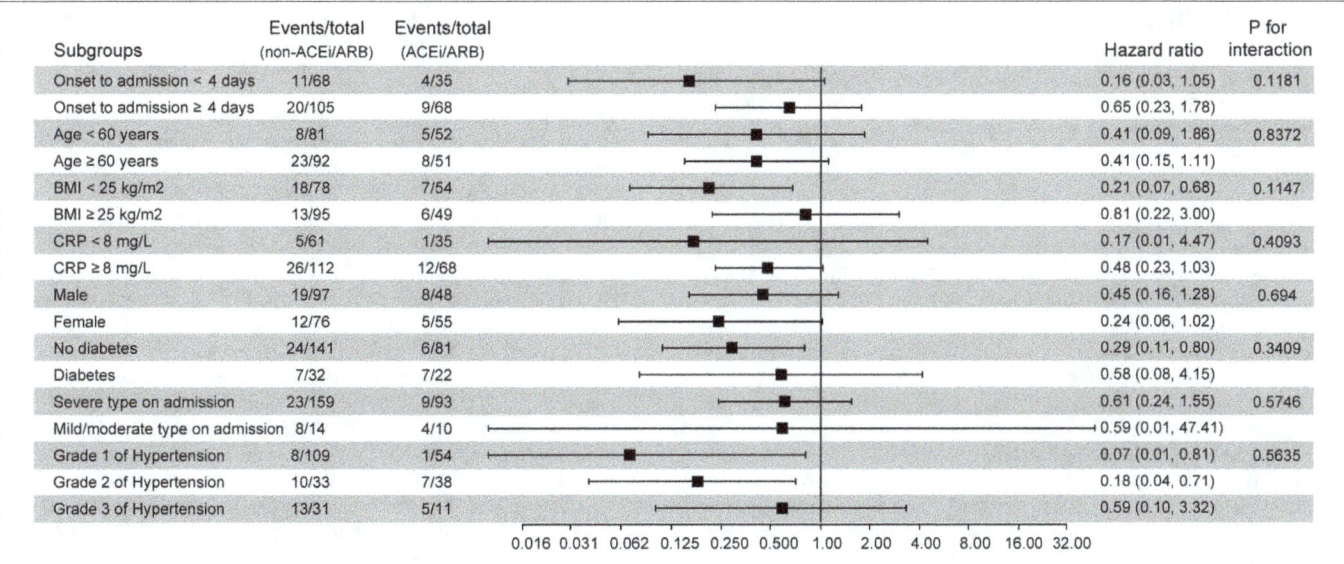

FIGURE 3 | Subgroup analysis of component endpoints according to ACEi/ARB treatment. ACEi, angiotensin-converting enzyme inhibitor; ARB, angiotensin receptor blocker; BMI, body mass index; CRP, C-reactive protein; HR, hazard ratio.

found to be significantly associated with the severity of COVID-19 in our study (**Supplementary Table 3**). After controlling important confounding factors through multivariate adjustment and IPTW analysis, the results suggested a favorable association

of using ACEi/ARB and less severity in COVID-19 patients. Furthermore, sensitivity analyses supported our main finding.

The main advantage of this study is exploring the association between chronic treatment with ACEi/ARB and COVID-19 progression after adjusting the major confounding factors such as the interval between symptom onset to admission and grade of hypertension, and our sample size is relatively larger compared with studies conducted in non-endemic areas in China (14, 15). However, we recognize some limitations. First, due to the relatively lower mortality rate, we could not assess the association between ACEi/ARB use and mortality in COVID-19 patients with hypertension. Since the study was conducted in a non-epidemic pandemic area and there were sufficient medical resources to support the treatment of patients with COVID-19, this study can better reduce confounding factors caused by a shortage of medical resources. Second, the sample size in this study is not big enough. This study included 103 patients receiving ACEi/ARB therapy; only 12 of whom received ACEi. Therefore, subgroup analysis of the differences between the two drugs could not be performed. Third, since patients were not randomly allocated to ACEi/ARB therapy or other regimens, the results may be affected by selection/collider bias. IPTW analysis was used to minimize selection bias, which is a powerful and flexible approach to adjust for collider bias and reduce observational bias and is the best evidence available in observational studies. But IPTW analysis may also have limitations, as this approach may not reflect possible biases in observational studies, and some residual confounding may persist. Fourth, our results were obtained from patients with COVID-19 in non-endemic areas of China. Due to policy reasons, the impact of using ACEi/ARB in other countries/regions on SARS-CoV-2-infected patients needs further study. Whether the current results are applicable to other global populations, long-term prospective studies and randomized clinical trials are still needed to investigate the effects of these treatments.

CONCLUSION

In a group of hospitalized COVID-19 patients with preexisting hypertension, chronic treatment with ACEi/ARB does not seem to increase the risk of disease severity after adequate adjustment by IPTW. ACEi/ARB could be continued as antihypertensive therapy for COVID-19 patients with hypertension according to the recommendations of international societies.

AUTHOR CONTRIBUTIONS

HC and LL: concept and study design. JYu, XShi, JM, FL, JW, XShe, QP, and JYa: data acquisition. JYu and XShi: data analyses. JYu and JM: statistics. JYu: manuscript preparation. JYu, XShi, JM, FL, JW, QP, JYa, HC, and LL: review of the manuscript. All authors approved the final version of the manuscript.

REFERENCES

1. Li J, Wang X, Chen J, Zhang H, Deng A. Association of renin-angiotensin system inhibitors with severity or risk of death in patients with hypertension hospitalized for coronavirus disease 2019 (COVID-19) infection in Wuhan, China. *JAMA Cardiol.* (2020) 5:825–30. doi: 10.1001/jamacardio.2020.1624

2. Zhang H, Baker A. Recombinant human ACE2: acing out angiotensin II in ARDS therapy. *Crit Care.* (2017) 21:305. doi: 10.1186/s13054-017-1882-z

3. Zhou P, Yang XL, Wang XG, Hu B, Zhang L, Zhang W, et al. A pneumonia outbreak associated with a new coronavirus of probable bat origin. *Nature.* (2020) 579:270–3. doi: 10.1038/s41586-020-2012-7

4. Fang L, Karakiulakis G, Roth M. Are patients with hypertension and diabetes mellitus at increased risk for COVID-19 infection? *Lancet Respir Med.* (2020) 8:e21. doi: 10.1016/S2213-2600(20)30116-8

5. Kuba K, Imai Y, Rao S, Gao H, Guo F, Guan B, et al. Penninger: a crucial role of angiotensin converting enzyme 2 (ACE2) in SARS coronavirus-induced lung injury. *Nat Med.* (2005) 11:875–9. doi: 10.1038/nm1267

6. Zhou F, Liu YM, Xie J, Li H, Lei F, Yang H, et al. Comparative impacts of angiotensin converting enzyme inhibitors versus angiotensin II receptor blockers on the risk of COVID-19 mortality. *Hypertension.* (2020) 76:e15–7. doi: 10.1161/HYPERTENSIONAHA.120.15622

7. Zhang P, Zhu L, Cai J, Lei F, Qin J, Xie J, et al. Association of inpatient use of angiotensin converting enzyme inhibitors and angiotensin ii receptor blockers with mortality among patients with hypertension hospitalized with COVID-19. *Circ Res.* (2020) 126:e142–3. doi: 10.1161/CIRCRESAHA.120.317242

8. Tan ND, Qiu Y, Xing XB, Ghosh S, Chen MH, Mao R. Associations between angiotensin converting enzyme inhibitors and angiotensin ii receptor blocker use, gastrointestinal symptoms, and mortality among patients with COVID-19. *Gastroenterology.* (2020) 159:1170–2.e1. doi: 10.1053/j.gastro.2020.05.034

9. Jung SY, Choi JC, You SH, Kim Y. Association of renin-angiotensin-aldosterone system inhibitors with COVID-19-related outcomes in Korea: a nationwide population-based cohort study. *Clin Infect Dis.* (2020) 71:2121–8. doi: 10.1093/cid/ciaa624

10. Yang G, Tan Z, Zhou L, Yang M, Peng L, Liu J, et al. Effects of ARBs and ACEIs on virus infection, inflammatory status and clinical outcomes in COVID-19 patients with hypertension: a single center retrospective study. *Hypertension.* (2020) 76:51–8. doi: 10.1161/HYPERTENSIONAHA.120.15143

11. Mehta N, Kalra A, Nowacki AS, Anjewierden S, Han Z, Bhat P, et al. Association of use of angiotensin-converting enzyme inhibitors and angiotensin II receptor blockers with testing positive for coronavirus disease 2019 (COVID-19). *JAMA Cardiol.* (2020) 5:1020–6. doi: 10.1001/jamacardio.2020.1855

12. Ren L, Yu S, Xu W, Overton JL, Chiamvimonvat N, Thai N. Lack of association of antihypertensive drugs with the risk and severity of COVID-19: a meta-analysis. *J Cardiol.* (2020) 77:482–91. doi: 10.1016/j.jjcc.2020.10.015

13. Zhang X, Yu J, Pan LY, Jiang HY. ACEI/ARB use and risk of infection or severity or mortality of COVID-19: a systematic review and meta-analysis. *Pharmacol Res.* (2020) 158:104927. doi: 10.1016/j.phrs.2020.104927

14. Hu J, Zhang X, Zhang X, Zhao H, Lian J, Hao S, et al. Sheng: COVID-19 is more severe in patients with hypertension; ACEI/ARB treatment does not influence clinical severity and outcome. *J Infect.* (2020) 81:979–97. doi: 10.1016/j.jinf.2020.05.056

15. Liu X, Liu Y, Chen K, Yan S, Bai X, Li J, et al. Efficacy of ACEIs/ARBs vs CCBs on the progression of COVID-19 patients with hypertension in Wuhan: a hospital-based retrospective cohort study. *J Med Virol.* (2021) 93:854–62. doi: 10.1002/jmv.26315

16. Wu J, Liu J, Zhao X, Liu C, Wang W, Wang D, et al. Clinical characteristics of imported cases of COVID-19 in Jiangsu Province: a multicenter descriptive study. *Clin Infect Dis.* (2020) 71:706–12. doi: 10.1093/cid/ciaa199

17. Guan WJ, Ni ZY, Hu Y, Liang WH, Ou CQ, He JX, et al. China medical treatment expert group for: clinical characteristics of coronavirus disease 2019 in China. *N Engl J Med.* (2020) 382:1708–20. doi: 10.1101/2020.02.06.20020974

18. Griffith GJ, Morris TT, Tudball MJ, Sterne J, Palmer TM, Davey Smith G, et al. Collider bias undermines our understanding of COVID-19 disease risk and severity. *Nat Commun.* (2020) 11:5749. doi: 10.1038/s41467-020-19478-2

19. McCaffrey DF, Griffin BA, Almirall D, Slaughter M, Ramchand R, Burgette LF. A tutorial on propensity score estimation for multiple treatments using generalized boosted models. *Stat Med.* (2013) 32:3388–414. doi: 10.1002/sim.5753

20. Su YS, Gelman A, Hill J, Yajima M. Multiple imputation with diagnostics (mi) in R: opening windows into the black box. *J Stat Softw.* (2011) 45:1–31. doi: 10.1007/s10822-011-9505-2

21. Imai Y, Kuba K, Penninger JM. The discovery of angiotensin-converting enzyme 2 and its role in acute lung injury in mice. *Exp Physiol.* (2008) 93:543–8. doi: 10.1113/expphysiol.2007.040048

22. Guo J, Huang Z, Lin L, Lv J. Coronavirus disease 2019 (COVID-19) and cardiovascular disease: a viewpoint on the potential influence of angiotensin-converting enzyme inhibitors/angiotensin receptor blockers on onset and severity of severe acute respiratory syndrome coronavirus 2 infection. *J Am Heart Assoc.* (2020) 9:e016219. doi: 10.1161/JAHA.120.016219

23. Li Y, Zeng Z, Li Y, Huang W, Zhou M, Zhang X, et al. Angiotensin-converting enzyme inhibition attenuates lipopolysaccharide-induced lung injury by regulating the balance between angiotensin-converting enzyme and angiotensin-converting enzyme 2 and inhibiting mitogen-activated protein kinase activation. *Shock.* (2015) 43:395–404. doi: 10.1097/SHK.0000000000000302

24. Caldeira D, Alarcao J, Vaz-Carneiro A, Costa J. Risk of pneumonia associated with use of angiotensin converting enzyme inhibitors and angiotensin receptor blockers: systematic review and meta-analysis. *BMJ.* (2012) 345:e4260. doi: 10.1136/bmj.e4260

25. Liu Y, Yang Y, Zhang C, Huang F, Wang F, Yuan J, et al. Clinical and biochemical indexes from 2019-nCoV infected patients linked to viral loads and lung injury. *Sci China Life Sci.* (2020) 63:364–74. doi: 10.1007/s11427-020-1643-8

26. Meng J, Xiao G, Zhang J, He X, Ou M, Bi J, et al. Renin-angiotensin system inhibitors improve the clinical outcomes of COVID-19 patients with hypertension. *Emerg Microbes Infect.* (2020) 9:757–60. doi: 10.1080/22221751.2020.1746200

27. Tedeschi S, Giannella M, Bartoletti M, Trapani F, Tadolini M, Borghi C, et al. Clinical impact of renin-angiotensin system inhibitors on in-hospital mortality of patients with hypertension hospitalized for COVID-19. *Clin Infect Dis.* (2020) 155:473–81. doi: 10.1093/cid/ciaa492

28. Reynolds HR, Adhikari S, Pulgarin C, Troxel AB, Hausvater A, Newman JD, et al. Renin-angiotensin-aldosterone system inhibitors and risk of covid-19. *N Engl J Med.* (2020) 382:2441–8. doi: 10.1056/NEJMoa2008975

29. de Abajo FJ, Rodriguez-Martin S, Lerma V, Mejia-Abril G, Aguilar M, Angeles Galvez M, et al. Use of renin-angiotensin-aldosterone system inhibitors and risk of COVID-19 requiring admission to hospital: a case-population study. *Lancet.* (2020) 395:1705–14. doi: 10.1016/S0140-6736(20)31030-8

30. Mancia G, Rea F, Ludergnani M, Apolone G, Corrao G. Renin-angiotensin-aldosterone system blockers and the risk of Covid-19. *N Engl J Med.* (2020) 382:2431–40. doi: 10.1056/NEJMoa2006923

31. Guan WJ, Liang WH, Zhao Y, Liang H, Chen ZS, Li YM, et al. China medical treatment expert group for: comorbidity and its impact on 1590 patients with Covid-19 in China: a nationwide analysis. *Eur Respir J.* (2020) 55:2000547. doi: 10.1183/13993003.00547-2020

32. Guo X, Zhu Y, Hong Y. Decreased mortality of COVID-19 with renin-angiotensin-aldosterone system inhibitors therapy in patients with hypertension: a meta-analysis. *Hypertension.* (2020) 76:e13–4. doi: 10.1161/HYPERTENSIONAHA.120.15572

33. Feng Y, Ling Y, Bai T, Xie Y, Huang J, Li J, et al. COVID-19 with different severity: a multi-center study of clinical features. *Am J Respir Crit Care Med.* (2020) 201:1380–8. doi: 10.1164/rccm.202002-0445OC

34. Liang WH, Guan WJ, Li CC, Liang HR, Zhao Y, Liu XQ, et al. Clinical characteristics and outcomes of hospitalised patients with COVID-19 treated in Hubei (epicenter) and outside Hubei (non-epicenter): a nationwide analysis of China. *Eur Respir J.* (2020) 55:2000562. doi: 10.1183/13993003.00562-2020

35. Xie J, Tong Z, Guan X, Du B, Qiu H. Clinical characteristics of patients who died of coronavirus disease 2019 in China. *JAMA Netw Open.* (2020) 3:e205619. doi: 10.1001/jamanetworkopen.2020.5619

36. Wu J, Li W, Shi X, Chen Z, Jiang B, Liu J, et al. Early antiviral treatment contributes to alleviate the severity and improve the prognosis of patients with novel coronavirus disease (COVID-19). *J Intern Med.* (2020) 288:128–38. doi: 10.1111/joim.13063

12

Evaluation of Endothelial Dysfunction and Inflammatory Vasculopathy after SARS-CoV-2 Infection

Philipp Jud[1]*, Paul Gressenberger[1], Viktoria Muster[1], Alexander Avian[2], Andreas Meinitzer[3], Heimo Strohmaier[4], Harald Sourij[5], Reinhard B. Raggam[1], Martin Helmut Stradner[6], Ulrike Demel[6], Harald H. Kessler[7], Kathrin Eller[8] and Marianne Brodmann[1]

[1] Division of Angiology, Department of Internal Medicine, Medical University of Graz, Graz, Austria, [2] Institute for Medical Informatics, Statistics and Documentation, Medical University of Graz, Graz, Austria, [3] Clinical Institute of Medical and Chemical Laboratory Diagnostics, Medical University of Graz, Graz, Austria, [4] Department Center of Medical Research, Medical University of Graz, Graz, Austria, [5] Division of Endocrinology, Department of Internal Medicine, Medical University of Graz, Graz, Austria, [6] Division of Rheumatology and Immunology, Department of Internal Medicine, Medical University of Graz, Graz, Austria, [7] Diagnostic and Research Institute of Hygiene, Microbiology and Environmental, Medical University of Graz, Graz, Austria, [8] Division of Nephrology, Department of Internal Medicine, Medical University of Graz, Graz, Austria

*Correspondence:
Philipp Jud
philipp.jud@medunigraz.at

Background: Rising data suggest that COVID-19 affects vascular endothelium while the underlying mechanisms promoting COVID-19-associated endothelial dysfunction and inflammatory vasculopathy are largely unknown. The aim was to evaluate the contribution of COVID-19 to persisting vascular injury and to identify parameters linked to COVID-19-associated endothelial dysfunction and inflammatory vasculopathy.

Methods: In a cross-sectional design, flow-mediated dilation (FMD), nitroglycerine-related dilation (NMD), pulse-wave velocity (PWV), augmentation index, intima-media thickness (IMT), compounds of the arginine and kynurenine metabolism, homocysteine, von Willebrand factor (vWF), endothelial microparticles (EMP), antiendothelial cell antibodies, inflammatory, and immunological parameters, as well as nailfold capillary morphology were measured in post-COVID-19 patients, patients with atherosclerotic cardiovascular diseases (ASCVD) and healthy controls without prior or recent SARS-CoV-2 infection.

Results: Post-COVID-19 patients had higher values of PWV, augmentation index, IMT, asymmetric and symmetric dimethylarginine, vWF, homocysteine, CD31+/CD42b− EMP, C-reactive protein, erythrocyte sedimentation rate, interleukin-6, and β-2-glycoprotein antibodies as well as lower levels of homoarginine and tryptophan compared to healthy controls (all with $p < 0.05$). A higher total number of pathologically altered inflammatory conditions and higher rates of capillary ramifications, loss, caliber variability, elongations and bushy capillaries with an overall higher microangiopathy evolution score were also observed in post-COVID-19 patients (all with $p < 0.05$). Most parameters of endothelial dysfunction and inflammation were comparably altered in post-COVID-19 patients and patients with ASCVD, including FMD and NMD.

Conclusion: COVID-19 may affect arterial stiffness, capillary morphology, EMP and selected parameters of arginine, kynurenine and homocysteine metabolism as well as of inflammation contributing to COVID-19-associated endothelial dysfunction and inflammatory vasculopathy.

Keywords: COVID-19, endothelial dysfunction, inflammation, vasculopathy, capillary changes

INTRODUCTION

COVID-19 caused by the severe acute respiratory syndrome coronavirus 2 (SARS-CoV-2) has evolved into a pandemic since it was detected in the end of 2019. A higher mortality rate was reported among patients with preexisting cardiovascular diseases compared to patients without an underlying disease and cardiovascular diseases seem to be risk factors for severe SARS-CoV-2 infection (1–3). Additionally, there are rising data suggesting that SARS-CoV-2 affects directly and indirectly endothelial cells, thus leading to endothelial injury and dysfunction thereby contributing to thromboembolism, vasculitic changes and abnormal nailfold capillaroscopy (4–9). The underlying mechanisms promoting COVID-19-associated endothelial dysfunction and inflammatory vasculopathy are yet still largely unknown while potential dysregulation of the renin-angiotensin-aldosterone system, immunothrombosis, and direct endothelial infection have been proposed (10–12).

Endothelial dysfunction may be a key contributor of vasculopathy due to underlying functional and structural changes of endothelial cells, and numerous parameters have been attributed to endothelial dysfunction. Flow-mediated dilation (FMD), pulse-wave velocity (PWV), and intima-media thickness (IMT) represent widely used, non-invasive indicators of vascular reactivity, arterial stiffness, and morphological changes of large arteries (13–15). All have been thoroughly evaluated in atherosclerotic cardiovascular diseases (ASCVD) as predictors for cardiovascular events and mortality (16–18). Additionally, homocysteine, kynurenine and compounds of the arginine metabolism, like homoarginine, asymmetric dimethylarginine (ADMA) and symmetric dimethylarginine (SDMA), are important mediators of endothelial dysfunction representing further predictors of cardiovascular mortality (19–22). Moreover, endothelial microparticles (EMP), which are released during apoptosis or activation of endothelial cells, as well as antiendothelial cell antibodies (AECA) may be associated with endothelial injury and activation, thus contributing to vasculopathy and endothelial dysfunction (23, 24).

Data about the respective parameters of endothelial dysfunction and inflammatory vasculopathy are largely lacking in COVID-19. Furthermore, data investigating if SARS-CoV-2 infection may cause persistent endothelial and vascular immunopathologic changes are also very limited. The aim of this study was to investigate if previous SARS-CoV-2 infection contributes to persisting endothelial dysfunction, inflammatory vasculopathy, macro-, and microvascular changes and to compare these findings to patients with ASCVD and healthy controls without SARS-CoV-2 infection.

MATERIALS AND METHODS

Study Population and Design

Post-COVID-19 patients diagnosed between March and April 2020 and inpatient treatment at the division of Angiology of the Medical University of Graz were screened *via* charts review for study inclusion and invited to participate. For every COVID-19 subject, one sex-matched healthy volunteer was recruited as well as one age—(± 1 year) and sex-matched subject with known ASCVD was also screened for study inclusion and invited to participate in the study (**Figure 1**). Overall, 42 subjects participated that study which were subdivided into three respective groups with 14 subjects per group. Inclusion criterion for the group of patients with COVID-19 was a known prior SARS-CoV-2 infection. Inclusion criterion for the ASCVD group was the presence of at least one detected, asymptomatic or symptomatic ASCVD, either coronary artery disease, or cerebrovascular disease, or lower extremity arterial disease (LEAD) or upper extremity arterial disease (UEAD). Exclusion criteria for all three cohorts were age < 18 years, any type of preexisting connective tissues disease or vasculitis, existing autoimmune diseases, recent pregnancy, recent malignancies and any acute infections, including foot ulcers or necrosis, at time of enrollment. For the group of COVID-19 subjects, preexisting history of diabetes mellitus, asymptomatic and symptomatic ASCVD, including angina pectoris, myocardial infarction, stroke, intermittent claudication, rest pain, and/or necrosis or ulcers of the lower or upper extremity, were additional exclusion criteria. All subjects were instructed to withhold potentially vasodilatory medications, including calcium channel blockers, phosphodiesterase-5 inhibitors, or prostanoids, and anticoagulation at least 24 h prior to study measurements. All participating patients with ASCVD and healthy controls underwent measurement of COVID-19 immunoglobulin (Ig) G

Abbreviations: ACP, anti-citrullinated protein; ADMA, asymmetric dimethylarginine; AECA, antiendothelial cell antibodies; ANA, antinuclear antibodies; ANCA, anti-neutrophil cytoplasmic antibodies; ASCVD, atherosclerotic cardiovascular diseases; CRP, C-reactive protein; CSURI, capillaroscopic skin ulcer risk index; ELISA, enzyme-linked immunosorbent assay; EMP, endothelial microparticles; ENA, extractable nuclear antigen; ESR, erythrocyte sedimentation rate; FMD, flow-mediated dilation; GAB, global arginine bioavailability; Ig, immunoglobulin; IL-6, interleukin 6; IMT, intima-media thickness; LEAD, lower extremity arterial disease; MES, microangiopathy evolution score; NMD, nitroglycerine-related dilation; NVC, nailfold video capillaroscopy; PCR, polymerase chain reaction; PWV, pulse-wave velocity; SAA, serum amyloid A; SARS-CoV-2, severe acute respiratory syndrome coronavirus 2; SD, standard deviation; SDMA, symmetric dimethylarginine; UEAD, upper extremity arterial disease; vWF, von Willebrand factor.

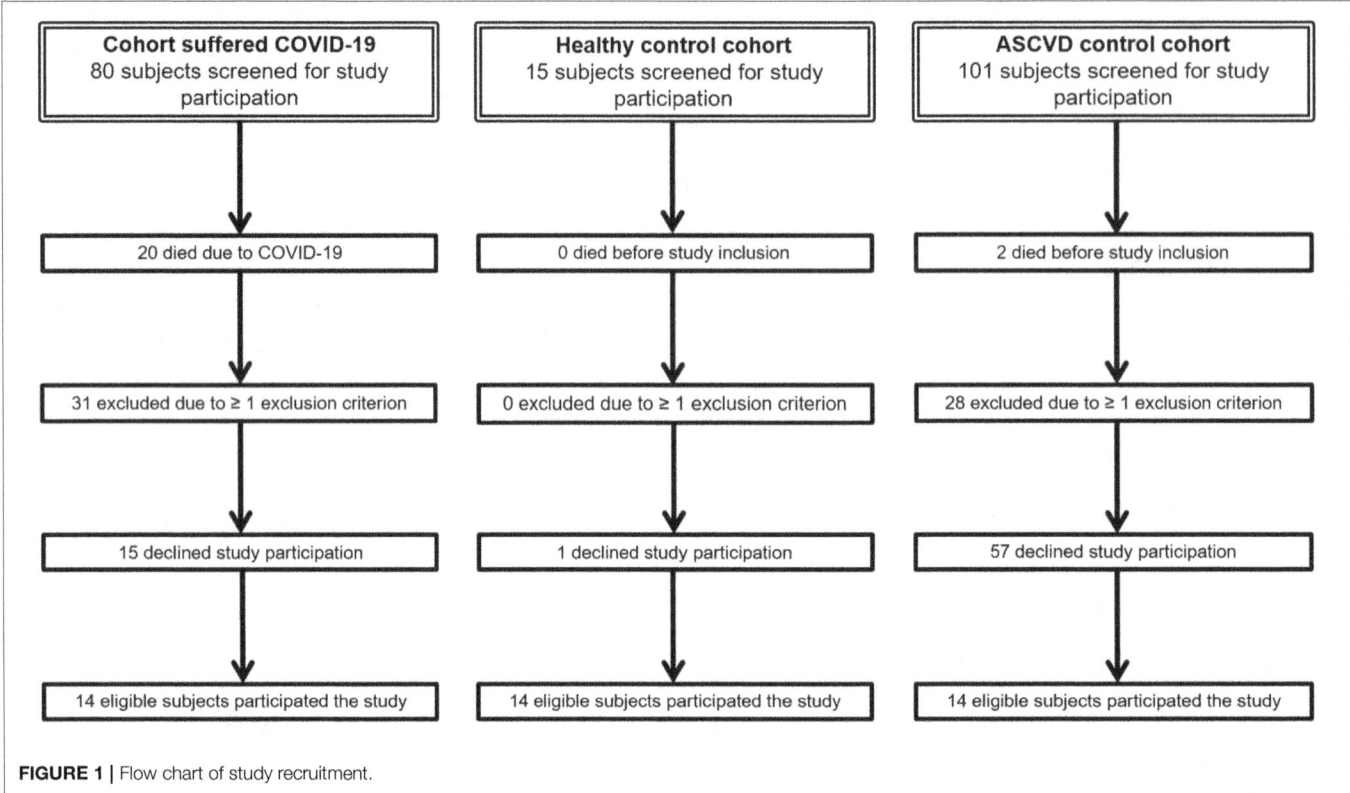

FIGURE 1 | Flow chart of study recruitment.

antibodies and detection of SARS-CoV-2 RNA by polymerase chain reaction (PCR) testing within 3 days prior to start of the study in order to exclude a preexisting or recent SARS-CoV-2 infection. SARS-CoV-2 IgG antibodies were measured by the LIAISON® SARS-CoV-2 S1/S2 IgG (DiaSorin, Saluggia, Italy). This fully automated test allows detection and quantitation of IgG antibodies against S1/S2 antigens of SARS-CoV-2. For detection of SARS-CoV-2 RNA, oropharyngeal swabs were collected by using the Copan ESwab collection system containing 1 ml of transport medium. Samples were tested for SARS-CoV-2 RNA at the Molecular Diagnostics Laboratory, Medical University of Graz, within 12 h of arrival. Presence of SARS-CoV-2 RNA was determined by real-time PCR using the SARS-CoV-2 Test for use on the cobas® 6800/8800 Systems (Roche Molecular Diagnostics, Pleasanton, USA). With this assay, selective amplification of target nucleic acid from the sample is achieved by the use of target-specific forward and reverse primers for ORF1a/b nonstructural region that is unique to SARS-CoV-2. In addition, a conserved region in the structural protein envelope E-gene is chosen for pan-Sarbecovirus detection. The pan-Sarbecovirus detection set also detects SARS-CoV-2 virus. No study subject had received COVID-19 vaccines prior to study measurements.

Between September 2020 and March 2021, parameters of endothelial dysfunction, immune-inflammatory parameters, and capillary morphology of the nailfold were investigated. Primary endpoint was the difference of FMD between post-COVID-19 patients, patients with ASCVD and healthy controls. Secondary endpoints were differences of nitroglycerine-related dilation

(NMD), PWV, IMT, homocysteine, compounds of the arginine metabolism, kynurenine, tryptophan, von Willebrand factor (vWF), EMP, AECA, immune-inflammatory parameters and capillary morphology of the nailfold between patients with previous SARS-CoV-2 infection, ASCVD and healthy controls. After signing the informed consent form, blood sampling or biochemical analysis were obtained followed by medical history evaluating cardiovascular risk factors. Subsequently, pulse-wave analysis and measurements of IMT, FMD, NMD and capillary changes by nailfold video capillaroscopy (NVC) were performed. Measurements of pulse-wave analysis, IMT, FMD, NMD, laboratory parameters, and NVC were performed in the morning between 7:00 a.m. and 9:00 a.m. after an overnight fast in a temperature-controlled (22–24°C) and quiet room.

Pulse-Wave Analysis, Intima-Media Thickness, and Flow-Mediated Dilation

Pulse-wave analysis including aortic PWV, augmentation index and pulse pressure was measured and calculated *via* the oscillometric device Mobil-O-Graph® (I.E.M., Aachen, Germany) by automated analysis. After obtainment of blood samples and a rest of 5 min, size-adjusted cuff was placed on the right upper arm about 2–4 cm above the ante-cubital fossa in supine position and subsequent pulse-wave analysis was performed. The patients were requested not to speak and not to move over the whole pulse-wave analysis. PWV of >10 m/s was defined as pathologic PWV (17).

Measurement of the IMT of the common carotid, axillary and superficial femoral artery was assessed in supinely positioned patients. After further rest of 5 min, both common carotid, axillary, and femoral arteries were examined in a longitudinal plane using a high-resolution linear array probe with 8–13 MHz (Siemens ACUSON S2000^{TM}, Siemens Healthcare Corp., Erlangen, Germany). The thickness of the intimal and medial layers of the vascular wall was measured on frozen longitudinal images in at least 1-cm-long segment of the artery. Three IMT measurements were performed per subject and per anatomic location while the mean value of the three measurements of the respective location was recorded.

All FMD measurements were performed by the same trained technician according to recent guidelines (13). All recommendations of those guidelines were fulfilled regarding subject preparation, protocol, and operator-dependent factors while sublingual administration of 0.4 mg glyceryl trinitrate was used instead of recommended 25 μg glyceryl trinitrate. Guideline recommendations for technique and analysis, including continuous measurement of velocity and diameter using simultaneous live duplex ultrasound and the use of continuous edge-detection and wall tracking software calculating peak diameter and shear rate stimulus, could not be fulfilled since such a software was not available during the study. Instead, offline analysis by a blinded observer was performed. A blood pressure cuff was placed below the antecubital fossa on the forearm and the baseline diameter of brachial artery was examined in a longitudinal plane between 2 and 7 cm proximal to the antecubital fossa. Three end-diastolic diameters between two intimal layers were measured ECG-gated during image acquisition in a one-centimeter-long segment of the brachial artery. Afterwards, the cuff was inflated >50 mmHg above the resting systolic pressure for 5 min and then deflated. The postischemic diameter of the brachial artery was measured 60 s after cuff release. FMD was defined as the change in postischemic diameter as a percentage of the baseline diameter. After a rest of 15 min, NMD was performed. Diameter of the brachial artery was recorded similar to the technique described for FMD before and 5 min after sublingual administration of 0.4 mg glyceryl trinitrate spray. All FMD and NMD measurements were performed using a conventional ultrasound scanner (Siemens ACUSON S2000^{TM}, Siemens Healthcare Corp., Erlangen, Germany) with an 8–13 MHz linear array transducer. Additionally, values of FMD < 7% and of NMD < 15.6% were defined as pathologic FMD and NMD values according to proposed reference values (25, 26).

Biochemical Analyses

Fasting blood samples for evaluation of L-arginine, homoarginine, citrulline, ornithine, ADMA, and SDMA, kynurenine, tryptophan, vWF, homocysteine, AECA, and EMP and immune-inflammatory parameters were obtained. Present leukocytosis, lymphopenia, hypocomplementemia, elevated levels of C-reactive protein (CRP), erythrocyte sedimentation rate (ESR), serum amyloid A (SAA), interleukin 6 (IL-6), antinuclear antibodies (ANA), extractable nuclear antigen (ENA) antibodies, antiphospholipid antibodies, anti-neutrophil cytoplasmic antibodies (ANCA), anti-citrullinated protein (ACP)

TABLE 1 | Immune-inflammatory parameters and cut-off values indicating potentially inflammatory conditions.

White blood cells (WBC)	Antinuclear antibodies (ANA)
C-reactive protein (CRP)	Extractable nuclear antigen (ENA) antibodies
Erythrocyte sedimentation rate (ESR)	Lupus anticoagulant
Serum amyloid A (SAA)	Cardiolipin and β-2-glycoprotein antibodies
Complement factors C3 and C4	Anti-neutrophil cytoplasmic antibodies (ANCA)
Interleukin 6 (IL-6)	Anti-citrullinated protein (ACP) antibodies
Immunoglobulin (Ig) A, G, M	Rheumatoid factor
IgG subclasses 1–4	Cytoplasmic antibodies

Definitions of pathologically altered inflammatory conditions

Leucocytosis > 11.3 × 10^9/L	Elevated antiphospholipid antibodies: Lupus anticoagulant > 45 s
Lymphopenia < 20%	Cardiolipin antibodies > 10 U/mL
Elevated CRP > 5 mg/L	β-2-glycoprotein antibodies > 10 U/mL
Elevated ESR > 20 mm/h	Elevated ANCA:
	MPO-ANCA > 5 U/mL
Elevated SAA > 6.4 mg/L	PR3-ANCA > 10 U/mL
Hypocomplementemia	c-ANCA ≥ 1:80
C3 < 0.9 g/L	p-ANCA titer ≥ 1:80
C4 < 0.1 g/L	x-ANCA ≥ 1:80
Elevated IL-6 > 7.0 pg/mL	Elevated ACP antibodies > 10 U/mL
Elevated ANA titer ≥ 1:80	Elevated rheumatoid factor > 20 U/mL
Elevated ENA antibodies > 1 U/mL	Positive cytoplasmic antibodies
Decreased Ig	Elevated Ig
IgA < 0.7 g/L	IgA > 4 g/L
IgG < 7 g/L	IgG > 16 g/L
IgM < 0.4 g/L	IgM > 2.3 g/L
IgG$_1$ < 4.05 g/L	IgG$_1$ > 10.11 g/L
IgG$_2$ < 1.69 g/L	IgG$_2$ > 7.86 g/L
IgG$_3$ < 0.11 g/L	IgG$_3$ > 0.85 g/L
IgG$_4$ < 0.03 g/L	IgG$_4$ > 2.01 g/L

antibodies, rheumatoid factor, and cytoplasmic antibodies, as well as decreased and increased levels of Ig were additionally recorded. Detailed list of the respective immune-inflammatory parameters is shown in **Table 1**.

Blood sample for measurement of parameters of the arginine and kynurenine metabolism as well as AECA were centrifuged at 4,000 × g for 10 min at 15°C temperature within 1 h after blood sampling obtainment. The supernatant was collected and divided into aliquots of 1 ml, which were stored at −80°C until final analysis. Amino acids and metabolites were measured by high-performance liquid chromatography as described elsewhere (27–29). L-arginine/ADMA, L-arginine/SDMA, homoarginine/ADMA, homoarginine/SDMA, L-arginine/ornithine, citrulline/L-arginine, citrulline/ornithine, global arginine bioavailability (GAB) ratio, defined as ratio of L-arginine over ornithine plus citrulline, and kynurenine/tryptophan were calculated by division of the respective parameter. AECA were measured by enzyme-linked immunosorbent assay (ELISA) method using a qualitative ELISA kit (Cusabio Technology, Wuhan, China) according to the user manual.

EMP were measured according to the recommendations for the analysis of extracellular vesicles published by Cossarizza et al. (30). Blood samples were collected in 5 ml citrate tubes after discarding the first 2 ml of blood without venous stasis and kept in upright position. Within 1 h after obtaining blood sampling, the plasma was centrifuged at 2,500 × g for 15 min at room temperature to obtain platelet-poor plasma. One milliliter of the supernatant was centrifuged again at 2,500 × g for 15 min at room temperature to obtain platelet-free plasma. The supernatant was collected and divided into aliquots of 0.1 ml, which were snap-frozen in liquid nitrogen and stored at −80°C until further analysis. A platelet-free plasma aliquot was thawed in a water bath at 37°C and immediately processed for fluorescence staining. Twenty-five microliters of platelet-free plasma was mixed with fluorochrome-labeled anti-human CD31, CD42b, CD51, CD54, CD62E, CD105, and CD144 antibodies (Biolegend, San Diego, USA) and incubated for 1.5 h at 4°C in the dark, followed by incubation with fluorescein-isothiocyanate-labeled lactadherin (CellSystems, Troisdorf, Germany) for another 30 min. Lactadherin binds specifically to phosphatidylserine on the outer surface of extracellular vesicles. Corresponding fluorochrome-labeled isotype antibodies were used as negative controls. After incubation, the samples were diluted 1:50 with 0.22 μm filtered phosphate buffered saline prior to flow cytometric analysis. EMP were identified as events that are positive for the above-mentioned markers and negative for CD42b. CD42b was used to distinguish EMP from platelet-derived microparticles (31). A microparticle gate was established using fluorescent 1 μm silica beads (Kisker Biotech, Steinfurt, Germany) for size calibration.

The remaining laboratory parameters were measured in sera and plasma samples of the patients at a single central lab of the Medical University of Graz.

Nailfold Video Capillaroscopy and Capillary Changes

NVC of the second to the fifth finger on both hands was performed in sitting position after pulse-wave analysis (Skinview, Optometron Ltd., Ismaning, Germany). Morphological changes of the capillaries, including microhemorrhages, capillary edema, capillary ramifications, bushy capillaries, capillary loss, giant capillaries, capillary ectasia, tortuous capillaries, capillary caliber variability, elongated capillaries, capillary thrombosis and disorganization of the microvascular array were recorded and a semi-quantitative rating scale to score each capillary abnormality was adopted (0 = no changes; 1 = <33% of capillary changes; 2 = 33–66% of capillary changes; 3 = more than 66% of capillary changes, per linear millimeter). The score values from the eight digits were added together and divided by eight resulting in the final score values. Microvascular disease activity was assessed by capillaroscopic skin ulcer risk index (CSURI) and microangiopathy evolution score (MES) (32, 33). Microvascular changes were also quantified

into early, active and late pattern, as defined by Cutolo et al. (34).

Statistical Analysis

Categorical variables were represented by frequency and percentages. Continuous variables were given as median and interquartile range or as mean ± standard deviation (SD). Normal distribution was examined *via* Shapiro–Wilk test. In case of normally distributed data, two-sided *t*-test was used and for non-normally distributed data Mann–Whitney *U*-test was utilized. $P < 0.05$ were assumed as statistically significant and statistical analyses were executed *via* SPSS version 26.0.

Ethical Approval

The study was approved by the Institutional Review Board of the Medical University Graz, Austria (EK 32-502 ex 19/20). All patients gave their written informed consent.

RESULTS

Fourteen post-COVID-19 patients (7 male, 50%) with a mean age (± SD) of 68.7 (±12.0) years, 14 sex-matched healthy controls with a mean age (± SD) of 30.7 (±4.2) years, and 14 sex- and age-matched patients with ASCVD and a mean age (± SD) of 66.9 (±10.9) years participated in that study. Age-matching was impossible for two patients with ASCVD due to a high refusal rate of study participation (**Figure 1**). No subject of the healthy controls and ASCVD controls had a positive COVID-19 PCR or COVID-19 antibody testing. Patients characteristics are shown in **Table 2**.

Endothelial Dysfunction and Macrovascular Changes

No difference between all three groups were found for FMD and NMD. Post-COVID-19 patients had a higher rate of pathologic aortic PWV with >10 m/s ($p = 0.001$) and higher values of aortic PWV, augmentation index, IMT of the common carotid, axillary and superficial femoral artery, ADMA, SDMA, kynurenine/tryptophan ratio, vWF antigen and activity, homocysteine and CD31+/CD42b− EMP compared to healthy controls ($p < 0.001$; $p = 0.009$; $p < 0.001$; $p < 0.001$; $p < 0.001$; $p = 0.001$; $p = 0.043$; $p = 0.001$; $p = 0.002$; $p = 0.004$; $p = 0.004$; $p = 0.020$, respectively). In the group of post-COVID-19 patients, values of those respective parameters were comparable to patients with ASCVD without significant differences, except for IMT of the axillary artery, which was lower ($p = 0.017$), and for CD31+/CD42b− EMP, which were higher ($p = 0.012$) in the COVID-19 group. Significantly lower values of homoarginine, tryptophan, L-arginine/ADMA, homoarginine/ADMA, and homoarginine/SDMA ratio were found in post-COVID-19 patients compared to healthy controls ($p = 0.004$; $p = 0.027$; $p < 0.001$; $p < 0.001$; $p = 0.002$, respectively), which were again comparable to the values of patients with established ASCVD. Ornithine was lower and L-arginine/ornithine and GAB ratio were higher in post-COVID-19 patients compared to patients with ASCVD ($p = 0.001$; $p = 0.020$; $p = 0.022$, respectively). AECA, CD54+/CD42b−,

TABLE 2 | Patients' characteristics.

	COVID-19 (*n* = 14)	ASCVD (*n* = 14)	Controls (*n* = 14)
Patients, *n* (%)			
Female	7 (50.0%)	7 (50.0%)	7 (50.0%)
Male	7 (50.0%)	7 (50.0%)	7 (50.0%)
Age (years), mean (± SD)	68.7 ± 12.0*	66.9 ± 10.9[†]	30.7 ± 4.2
Duration after SARS-CoV-2 infection (weeks), mean (± SD)	28.6 ± 3.0	–	–
COVID-19 phenotype, *n* (%)			
COVID-19 pneumonia	14 (100.0)	–	–
COVID-19 ARDS	3 (21.4)	–	–
Disease duration of ASCVD (weeks), median (25th–75th percentile)	–	293.3 (62.1–529.9)	–
Prior familial ASCVD, *n* (%)	5 (35.7)	9 (64.3)	4 (28.6)
BMI (kg/m², mean (± SD)	29.4 ± 8.3*	27.6 ± 4.5[†]	23.8 ± 3.2
HbA$_{1c}$ (mmol/mol), median (25th–75th percentile)	39 (33–42)*	41 (37–47)[†]	33 (32–34)
eGFR (ml/min/1.73 m²), median (25th–75th percentile)	84.4 (72.2–90.7)*	76.7 (65.1–89.1)[†]	103.4 (97.6–115.7)
Current sport activity, *n* (%)	8 (57.1)*	5 (35.7)[†]	13 (92.9)
Times per week (*n*), median (25th–75th percentile)	2 (0–3)*	0 (0–3)[†]	4 (2–5)
Duration per week (min), median (25th–75th percentile)	30 (0–60)[‡]	0 (0–45)[†]	50 (30–60)
Previous history, *n* (%)			
COPD	1 (7.1%)	3 (21.4)	0 (0.0)
Smoking			
Current	0 (0.0)*[‡]	5 (35.7)	4 (28.6)
Ex	6 (42.9)	6 (42.9)	4 (28.6)
Non-smokers	8 (57.1)	3 (21.4)	6 (42.9)
Bronchial asthma	0 (0.0)	0 (0.0)	0 (0.0)
Arterial hypertension	6 (42.9)*[‡]	13 (92.9)[†]	0 (0.0)
Diabetes mellitus	0 (0.0)[‡]	4 (28.6)[†]	0 (0.0)
Atrial fibrillation	1 (7.1)	2 (14.3)	0 (0.0)
Hypercholesterolemia	6 (42.9)*[‡]	12 (85.7)[†]	0 (0.0)
Hypertriglyceridemia	2 (14.3)[‡]	7 (50.0)[†]	0 (0.0)
CKD	1 (7.1)	3 (21.4)	0 (0.0)
Inactive malignancy	4 (28.6)*	1 (7.1)	0 (0.0)
Coronary artery disease	0 (0.0)[‡]	8 (57.1)[†]	0 (0.0)
Myocardial infarction	0 (0.0)[‡]	4 (28.6)[†]	0 (0.0)
Cerebrovascular disease	0 (0.0)[‡]	11 (78.6)[†]	0 (0.0)
Stroke	0 (0.0)	2 (14.3)	0 (0.0)
Upper extremity arterial disease	0 (0.0)	3 (21.4)	0 (0.0)
Lower extremity arterial disease	0 (0.0)[‡]	13 (92.9)[†]	0 (0.0)
Renal artery disease	0 (0.0)	1 (7.1)	0 (0.0)
Mesenteric artery disease	0 (0.0)	1 (7.1)	0 (0.0)
PCI/PTA	0 (0.0)[‡]	11 (78.6)[†]	0 (0.0)
Drug therapy, *n* (%)			
ACE inhibitors	3 (21.4)	4 (28.6)[†]	0 (0.0)
ARB	2 (14.3)	5 (35.7)[†]	0 (0.0)
Beta blockers	3 (21.4)[‡]	9 (64.3)[†]	0 (0.0)
Calcium antagonists	2 (14.3)	5 (35.7)[†]	0 (0.0)
Diuretics	1 (7.1)	4 (28.6)[†]	0 (0.0)
Other antihypertensives	0 (0.0)	0 (0.0)	0 (0.0)
Antiplatelet therapy	0 (0.0)[‡]	9 (64.3)[†]	0 (0.0)
Oral anticoagulation	2 (14.3)	3 (21.4)	0 (0.0)
Statins	0 (0.0)[‡]	10 (71.4)[†]	0 (0.0)
PCSK-9 inhibitors	0 (0.0)	2 (14.3)	0 (0.0)
Metformin	0 (0.0)[‡]	4 (28.6)[†]	0 (0.0)

(Continued)

TABLE 2 | Continued

	COVID-19 (*n* = 14)	ASCVD (*n* = 14)	Controls (*n* = 14)
Other oral antihyperglycemic agents	0 (0.0)	2 (14.3)	0 (0.0)
Insulin	0 (0.0)	0 (0.0)	0 (0.0)

ACE, angiotensin-converting enzyme; ARB, Angiotensin receptor blockers; ARDS, acute respiratory distress syndrome; ASCVD, atherosclerotic cardiovascular diseases; BMI, body mass index; CKD, chronic kidney disease; COPD, chronic obstructive pulmonary disease; eGFR, estimated glomerular filtration rate; PCI, percutaneous coronary intervention; PCSK-9, proprotein convertase subtilisin/kexin type 9; PTA, percutaneous transluminal angioplasty.
*p < 0.05 between group with previous COVID-19 and healthy controls.
†p < 0.05 between group with ASCVD and healthy controls.
‡p < 0.05 between group with previous COVID-19 and group with ASCVD.

CD62E+/CD42b−, CD105+/CD42b−, and CD144+/CD42b− EMP were undetectable in all three groups (**Table 3**).

Inflammation

Higher values of CRP, ESR, IL-6, and β-2-glycoprotein antibodies as well as higher frequencies of CRP elevation and any Ig decrease were observed for post-COVID-19 patients compared to healthy controls ($p = 0.009$; $p = 0.007$; $p = 0.004$; $p = 0.031$; $p = 0.007$; $p = 0.015$, respectively). Again, these parameters were comparable between the ASCVD und the COVID-19 cohort, without statistically significant differences. Post-COVID-19 patients revealed higher levels of PR3-ANCA, IgM, and IgG_2 compared to patients with ASCVD ($p = 0.016$; $p = 0.011$; $p = 0.036$, respectively), but not to healthy controls. Healthy controls had lower levels of C3 and C4 and higher rates of hypocomplementemia than patients with previous COVID-19 and with ASCVD (all with $p < 0.05$). Post-COVID-19 patients had a higher total number of pathologically altered inflammatory conditions compared to healthy controls ($p = 0.016$), but not to patients with ASCVD ($p = 0.385$) (**Table 4**).

Microvascular Changes

Capillary ramifications, loss, caliber variability, and elongations were more frequently observed in post-COVID-19 patients compared to patients with ASCVD ($p = 0.015$; $p = 0.034$; $p = 0.047$; $p = 0.020$, respectively) and capillary ramifications, loss, caliber variability and bushy capillaries were more frequently compared to healthy controls ($p = 0.015$; $p = 0.034$; $p = 0.003$; $p = 0.014$, respectively). Using a semi-quantitative rating scale, significantly higher score values were achieved for capillary ramifications, capillary loss and elongated capillaries in the group with previous COVID-19 compared to the group with ASCVD ($p = 0.016$; $p = 0.035$; $p = 0.028$, respectively). Higher score values were also observed for capillary ramifications, loss, caliber variability, elongation and bushy capillaries compared to healthy controls ($p = 0.016$; $p = 0.035$; $p = 0.003$; $p = 0.028$; $p = 0.018$, respectively). Total MES was higher in post-COVID-19 patients compared to patients with ASCVD ($p = 0.048$) and to healthy controls ($p = 0.040$) (**Table 5**).

DISCUSSION

We could demonstrate substantial differences of selected pathways contributing to endothelial dysfunction in patients 6 months after SARS-CoV-2 infection. Although no differences were observed for markers of vascular reactivity, post-COVID-19 patients had an increased arterial stiffness, distinct alterations of the arginine and kynurenine metabolism, and higher values of IMT, vWF, homocysteine, and CD31+/CD42b− EMP compared to healthy controls. Additionally, many of the respective parameters, including also FMD and NMD, were altered to an extent comparable with the values of patients with clinically relevant ASCVD; 78.6% of those had a prior endovascular intervention. Furthermore, capillary changes have been observed more frequently in post-COVID-19 patients compared to healthy controls and the group of ASCVD including also a higher MES. Changes for most of the respective parameters have previously been described in patients mainly with acute COVID-19 while data about persistent changes after suffered COVID-19 are very limited (9, 35–40).

Pathophysiological mechanisms contributing to endothelial dysfunction in COVID-19 are largely unknown. Direct and indirect endothelial damage due to SARS-CoV-2 by binding to the angiotensin-converting-enzyme-2 receptor and by acute systemic inflammation have been proposed (4, 41). While direct infection of endothelial cells by SARS-CoV-2 may be unlikely, as there is lacking evidence of expression of angiotensin-converting-enzyme-2 receptor on human endothelial cells, indirect endothelial damage by release of inflammatory mediators may affect several pathways contributing to endothelial dysfunction, including nitric oxide or kynurenine metabolism, resulting subsequently in impaired FMD and increased arterial stiffness (22, 42–45). Our findings support the hypothesis of indirect endothelial damage caused by systemic inflammation. On the one hand, post-COVID-19 patients revealed numerous altered parameters of endothelial dysfunction, and subclinical inflammation expressed by elevated levels of CRP, ESR, and IL-6 as well as by a higher total number of pathologically altered inflammatory conditions (17, 25, 26). Respective inflammatory changes of post-COVID-19 patients were again similar to those observed in patients with ASCVD. Furthermore, although FMD and NMD did not differ between the three cohorts, post-COVID-19 patients had similar values of FMD and NMD compared to patients with ASCVD and

TABLE 3 | Parameters of endothelial dysfunction.

	COVID-19 ($n = 14$)	ASCVD ($n = 14$)	Controls ($n = 14$)
FMD (%), mean (± SD)	4.44 ± 2.90	3.17 ± 2.95	4.58 ± 3.48
<7%, n (%)	10 (71.4%)	11 (78.6%)	10 (71.4%)
NMD (%), mean (± SD)	16.78 ± 6.32	17.11 ± 9.23	20.60 ± 8.46
<15.6%, n (%)	5 (38.5%)	7 (50.0%)	3 (21.4%)
Aortic PWV (m/s), median (25th–75th percentile)	10.75 (8.10–11.45)*	9.95 (8.40–11.60)[†]	5.70 (5.38–6.05)
>10m/s, n (%)	8 (57.1%)*	7 (50.0%)[†]	0 (0.0%)
Augmentation index (%), median (25th–75th percentile)	22 (10–40)*	33 (24–39)[†]	4 (1–11)
Pulse pressure (mmHg), median (25th–75th percentile)	47 (35–50)	52 (48–67)	49 (41–53)
IMT (mm), median (25th–75th percentile)			
IMT common carotid artery average	0.59 (0.52–0.68)*	0.72 (0.60–1.01)[†]	0.44 (0.40–0.45)
IMT axillary artery average	0.58 (0.45–0.64)*[‡]	0.71 (0.59–0.88)[†]	0.40 (0.39–0.46)
IMT superficial femoral artery average	0.54 (0.47–0.62)*	0.55 (0.43–0.61)[†]	0.40 (0.36–0.40)
ADMA (μmol/L), median (25th–75th percentile)	0.76 (0.65–0.79)*	0.80 (0.72–0.83)[†]	0.60 (0.62–0.65)
SDMA (μmol/L), median (25th–75th percentile)	0.73 (0.65–0.86)*	0.84 (0.65–1.07)[†]	0.65 (0.62–0.70)
L-arginine (μmol/L), median (25th–75th percentile)	119.74 (113.40–142.29)	136.64 (120.34–149.80)	132.50 (107.62–143.44)
Homoarginine (μmol/L), median (25th–75th percentile)	1.59 (1.16–2.31)*	1.59 (1.41–2.21)[†]	2.36 (1.90–3.45)
Citrulline (μmol/L), median (25th–75th percentile)	34.59 (31.13–38.69)	39.21 (32.46–50.94)	32.11 (25.91–40.24)
Ornithine (μmol/L), median (25th–75th percentile)	66.17 (63.33–73.63)[‡]	94.30 (80.98–114.48)[†]	64.25 (38.44–78.30)
L-arginine/ADMA ratio, median (25th–75th percentile)	173.33 (143.28–188.47)*	165.88 (151.23–192.94)[†]	207.22 (200.43–224.48)
L-arginine/SDMA ratio, median (25th–75th percentile)	167.33 (132.87–188.57)	153.82 (125.35–201.30)[†]	190.40 (167.97–220.01)
Homoarginine/ADMA ratio, median (25th–75th percentile)	2.16 (1.47–2.90)*	2.02 (1.75–2.82)[†]	3.75 (2.99–5.67)
Homoarginine/SDMA ratio, median (25th–75th percentile)	2.01 (1.39–3.20)*	2.04 (1.38–2.93)[†]	3.79 (2.89–5.19)
L-arginine/ornithine ratio, median (25th–75th percentile)	1.88 (1.53–2.11)[‡]	1.49 (1.10–1.78)[†]	2.22 (1.46–2.82)
Citrulline/L-arginine ratio, median (25th–75th percentile)	0.28 (0.21–0.31)	0.31 (0.22–0.38)	0.27 (0.22–0.28)
Citrulline/ornithine ratio, median (25th–75th percentile)	0.50 (0.39–0.56)	0.43 (0.40–0.46)	0.59 (0.39–0.66)
GAB ratio, median (25th–75th percentile)	1.20 (1.06–1.42)[‡]	0.95 (0.77–1.17)[†]	1.38 (1.07–1.71)
Kynurenine (μmol/L), median (25th–75th percentile)	2.45 (2.00–3.14)	2.96 (2.37–3.23)[†]	2.21 (2.00–2.39)
Tryptophan (μmol/L), median (25th–75th percentile)	54.40 (49.97–59.15)*	59.52 (54.33–66.96)	61.76 (56.25–70.70)
Kynurenine/tryptophan ratio, median (25th–75th percentile)	0.050 (0.040–0.053)*	0.045 (0.040–0.050)[†]	0.030 (0.030–0.040)
vWF antige n (%), mean (± SD)	138.6 ± 14.1*	137.8 ± 11.1[†]	109.3 ± 25.3
vWF activity (%), mean (± SD)	168.5 ± 60.8*	177.9 ± 55.3[†]	110.5 ± 31.5
Homocysteine (μmol/L), median (25th–75th percentile)	12.3 (10.5–14.8)*	9.7 (6.6–14.8)	9.0 (8.6–10.4)
AECA, n (%)			
Positive	0 (0.0)	0 (0.0)	0 (0.0)
Negative	14 (100.0)	14 (100.0)	14 (100.0)
EMP (U/μl)			
CD31+/CD42b–	201.25 (158.88–279.50)*[‡]	115.50 (90.88–169.75)	137.50 (73.00–171.38)
CD51+/CD42b–	13.50 (5.25–49.25)	27.75 (19.38–39.63)	22.25 (17.88–28.50)
CD54+/CD42b–	–[§]	–[§]	–[§]
CD62E+/CD42b–	–[§]	–[§]	–[§]
CD105+/CD42b–	–[§]	–[§]	–[§]
CD144+/CD42b–	–[§]	–[§]	–[§]

ADMA, asymmetric dimethylarginine; AECA, antiendothelial cell antibodies; ASCVD, atherosclerotic cardiovascular diseases; EMP, endothelial microparticles; FMD, flow-mediated dilation; GAB, global arginine bioavailability; IMT, intima-media thickness; NMD, nitroglycerine-related dilation; PWV, pulse-wave velocity; SDMA, symmetric dimethylarginine; vWF, von Willebrand factor.
*p < 0.05 between group with previous COVID-19 and healthy controls.
[†]p < 0.05 between group with ASCVD and healthy controls.
[‡]p < 0.05 between group with previous COVID-19 and group with ASCVD.
[§]not detectable.

also the number of post-COVID-19 with pathologic FMD and NMD values according to proposed reference values were similar compared to patients with ASCVD (25, 26).

Interestingly, FMD and NMD values of our healthy control cohort were also comparable to FMD and NMD values of post-COVID-19 and ASCVD patients, which may be attributed

TABLE 4 | Immune-inflammatory parameters.

	COVID-19 ($n = 14$)	ASCVD ($n = 14$)	Controls ($n = 14$)
WBC (10^9/L), median (25th–75th percentile)	6.0 (5.7–6.6)	6.8 (5.1–8.2)	5.3 (3.9–7.0)
Leukocytosis, n (%)	0 (0.0%)	0 (0.0%)	0 (0.0%)
Lymphocytes (10^9/L), median (25th–75th percentile)	1.5 (1.1–1.7)	1.5 (1.3–2.2)	1.6 (1.2–1.9)
Lymphopenia, n (%)	3 (21.4%)	5 (35.7%)	1 (7.1%)
CRP (mg/dL), median (25th–75th percentile)	2.5 (0.8–7.8)*	1.9 (0.8–3.8)[†]	0.7 (0.5–1.3)
CRP elevation, n (%)	6 (42.9%)*	3 (21.4%)	0 (0.0%)
ESR (mm/h), median (25th–75th percentile)	7 (5–10)*	9 (4–15)[†]	2 (2–5)
ESR elevation > 20, n (%)	1 (7.1%)	0 (0.0%)	0 (0.0%)
SAA (mg/L), median (25th–75th percentile)	4.5 (2.2–9.3)	5.7 (3.3–8.2)	4.5 (1.1–6.0)
SAA elevation > 6.4, n (%)	5 (35.7%)	5 (35.7%)	3 (21.4%)
Complement factors (g/L), median (25th–75th percentile)			
C3	1.136 (1.086–1.302)*	1.245 (1.102–1.336)[†]	1.001 (0.858–1.190)
C4	0.193 (0.170–0.243)*	0.216 (0.146–0.245)[†]	0.158 (0.140–0.197)
Hypocomplementemia, n (%)	0 (0.0)*	0 (0.0)[†]	4 (28.6)
IL-6 (pg/mL), median (25th–75th percentile)	2.5 (1.8–4.0)*	3.1 (1.6–4.7)[†]	1.4 (1.4–1.7)
Elevated IL-6, n (%)	0 (0.0)	0 (0.0)	0 (0.0)
Positive ANA titer ≥ 1:80, n (%)	5 (35.7)	4 (28.6)	4 (28.6)
ENA (U/mL), median (25th–75th percentile)	0.0 (0.0–0.1)	0.1 (0.0–0.1)	0.1 (0.0–0.2)
Elevated ENA, n (%)	0 (0.0)	0 (0.0)	0 (0.0)
Antiphospholipid antibodies			
Lupus anticoagulant (sec), median (25th–75th percentile)	32.8 (31.2–38.5)	35.3 (33.8–37.4)	33.7 (31.6–35.3)
Elevated lupus anticoagulant, n (%)	0 (0.0)	1 (7.1)	0 (0.0)
Total level of cardiolipin antibodies including IgA, IgG, IgM cardiolipin antibodies (U/mL), median (25th–75th percentile)	1.7 (0.1–3.9)	3.1 (2.5–4.4)[†]	0.5 (0.3–1.1)
Elevated cardiolipin antibodies, n (%)	2 (14.3)	0 (0.0)	0 (0.0)
Total level of β-2-glycoprotein antibodies including IgA, IgG, IgM β-2-glycoprotein antibodies (U/mL), median (25th–75th percentile)	2.2 (1.6–2.7)*	2.3 (1.9–2.4)[†]	1.6 (1.5–1.8)
Elevated β-2-glycoprotein antibodies, n (%)	1 (7.1)	0 (0.0)	0 (0.0)
Any elevated antiphospholipid antibody, n (%)	2 (14.3)	1 (7.1)	0 (0.0)
ANCA			
MPO-ANCA (U/mL), median (25th–75th percentile)	0.8 (0.6–1.1)	0.8 (0.8–1.0)[†]	1.2 (0.8–1.3)
Elevated MPO-ANCA, n (%)	0 (0.0)	0 (0.0)	0 (0.0)
PR3-ANCA (U/mL), median (25th–75th percentile)	0.4 (0.4–1.9)[‡]	0.4 (0.4–0.4)[†]	0.5 (0.4–2.4)
Elevated PR3-ANCA, n (%)	0 (0.0)	0 (0.0)	0 (0.0)
Positive c-ANCA titer ≥ 1:80, n (%)	0 (0.0)	1 (7.1)	0 (0.0)
Positive p-ANCA titer ≥ 1:80, n (%)	0 (0.0)	0 (0.0)	0 (0.0)
Positive x-ANCA titer ≥ 1:80, n (%)	0 (0.0)	0 (0.0)	0 (0.0)
ACP antibodies (U/mL), median (25th–75th percentile)	0.9 (0.5–1.1)	0.8 (0.5–1.1)	0.9 (0.6–1.1)
Elevated ACP antibodies, n (%)	0 (0.0)	0 (0.0)	0 (0.0)
Rheumatoid factor (U/mL), median (25th–75th percentile)	0 (0–7)	0 (0–1)	0 (0–8)
Elevated rheumatoid factor, n (%)	0 (0.0)	0 (0.0)	1 (7.1)
Positive cytoplasmic antibodies, n (%)	1 (7.1)	1 (7.1)	0 (0.0)
Ig (g/L), median (25th–75th percentile)			
IgA	1.88 (1.07–2.82)	1.77 (1.60–2.42)	1.52 (1.18–2.00)
<0.7, n (%)	1 (7.1)	1 (7.1)	0 (0.0)
> 4, n (%)	1 (7.1)	1 (7.1)	1 (7.1)
IgG	10.55 (8.47–12.10)	9.13 (8.25–10.30)	9.61 (9.13–10.80)
<7, n (%)	1 (7.1)	1 (7.1)	0 (0.0)
> 16, n (%)	0 (0.0)	0 (0.0)	0 (0.0)

(Continued)

TABLE 4 | Continued

	COVID-19 ($n = 14$)	ASCVD ($n = 14$)	Controls ($n = 14$)
IgM	1.03 (0.72–1.24)[‡]	0.55 (0.49–0.76)[†]	0.83 (0.57–1.04)
<0.4, n (%)	0 (0.0)	1 (7.1)	0 (0.0)
> 2.3, n (%)	0 (0.0)	1 (7.1)	0 (0.0)
IgG$_1$	6.44 (5.02–8.14)	6.11 (5.33–7.72)	5.99 (5.41–7.45)
<4.05, n (%)	0 (0.0)	1 (7.1)	0 (0.0)
> 10.11, n (%)	0 (0.0)	0 (0.0)	1 (7.1)
IgG$_2$	3.00 (2.12–4.31)[‡]	2.27 (1.77–2.72)[†]	3.46 (2.5–3.88)
<1.69, n (%)	0 (0.0)	2 (14.3)	0 (0.0)
> 7.86, n (%)	0 (0.0)	0 (0.0)	0 (0.0)
IgG$_3$	0.35 (0.17–0.41)	0.28 (0.25–0.43)	0.32 (0.27–0.41)
<0.11, n (%)	2 (14.3)	0 (0.0)	0 (0.0)
> 0.85, n (%)	0 (0.0)	0 (0.0)	0 (0.0)
IgG$_4$	0.41 (0.13–1.04)	0.23 (0.11–1.02)	0.45 (0.27–0.54)
<0.03, n (%)	2 (14.3)	0 (0.0)	0 (0.0)
>2.01, n (%)	1 (7.1)	0 (0.0)	0 (0.0)
Any Ig elevation, n (%)	2 (14.3)	2 (14.3)	2 (14.3)
Any Ig decrease, n (%)	5 (35.7)*	4 (28.6)[†]	0 (0.0)
Total number of pathologically altered inflammatory conditions, median (25th–75th percentile)	2 (1–3)*	2 (1–2)	1 (0–2)

ACP, anti-citrullinated protein; ANA, antinuclear antibodies; ANCA, anti-neutrophil cytoplasmic antibodies; ASCVD, atherosclerotic cardiovascular diseases; CRP, C-reactive protein; ENA, extractable nuclear antigen; ESR, erythrocyte sedimentation rate; Ig, immunoglobulin; IL-6, interleukin 6; SAA, serum amyloid A; WBC, white blood cells.
$p < 0.05$ between group with previous COVID-19 and healthy controls.
[†]*$p < 0.05$ between group with ASCVD and healthy controls.*
[‡]*$p < 0.05$ between group with previous COVID-19 and group with ASCVD.*

to other subject-related factors influencing vascular reactivity, like smoking, physical activity, mental stress, alcohol intake or hormonal changes during physiological menstrual cycle (13). The association between inflammation and atherosclerosis is well-established and it may be possible that persisting changes of inflammatory parameters caused by SARS-CoV-2 may affect endothelial cells similarly (46). On the other hand, the occurrence of persisting capillary changes in post-COVID-19 patients also suggests an interaction *via* inflammation and immunological pathways. Capillary changes have mainly been described in autoimmune disorders, especially in systemic sclerosis (32–34). Interestingly, post-COVID-19 patients had a higher prevalence of capillary ramifications and capillary loss, which are typically seen in long-lasting systemic sclerosis, while no capillary pattern suggestive for systemic sclerosis were observed. Compared to the study of Natalello et al. (9), we could observe less capillary edema, thrombosis and ectasia but higher rates of capillary ramifications, bushy capillaries and capillary loss. Additionally, higher rates of capillary caliber variability and elongations were observed and higher scores using semi-quantitative rating scale of respective capillary changes and total MES were found in post-COVID-19 patients. As connective tissues diseases or vasculitides were an exclusion criterion, it can be assumed that SARS-CoV-2 affects substantially and persistently microvasculature. Finally, endothelial damage caused by SARS-CoV-2 *per se* without interaction *via* inflammatory pathways may also be a potential pathophysiologic explanation for COVID-19-associated endothelial dysfunction and vasculopathy. Associations between

EMP and parameters of the arginine metabolism to other viruses, like parvovirus B19 or human immunodeficiency virus, have previously been described (47, 48). Furthermore, ADMA and CD31+/CD42b– EMP have been associated with capillary changes in systemic sclerosis (49, 50). Therefore, direct but yet unknown interactions of SARS-CoV-2 to nitric oxide metabolism or endothelial homeostasis may also contribute to the persistent endothelial dysfunction and vasculopathy observed in our study.

Limitations of our study are that this study included a limited number of patients and the fact that we did not measure the above-named parameters before, during and after SARS-CoV-2 infection to evaluate potential changes. Therefore, it can be only hypothesized that persisting endothelial damage is caused directly or indirectly due to COVID-19. However, measuring endothelial function in people before COVID-19 is challenging, given that one would need to assess a large number of people to ascertain that a subgroup will have a SARS-CoV-2 infection. Additionally, while no post-COVID-19 patient had any preexisting ASCVD, most of them had at least one atherosclerotic cardiovascular risk factor. Although those cardiovascular risk factors were not significantly different or overrepresented in post-COVID-19 patients, a potential bias affecting the results on endothelial dysfunction due to present cardiovascular risk factors cannot be definitely excluded. Furthermore, the large age difference between the control group and the two patient groups need to be mentioned which may affect several measured parameters. However, the aim of this study was to compare parameters of endothelial

TABLE 5 | Capillary changes.

	COVID-19 (*n* = 14)	ASCVD (*n* = 14)	Controls (*n* = 14)
Microhemorrhages			
n, (%)	8 (57.1)	6 (42.9)	3 (21.4)
Points, median (25th–75th percentile)	0.125 (0.000–0.250)	0.000 (0.000–0.125)	0.000 (0.000–0.031)
Capillary edema			
n, (%)	0 (0.0)	0 (0.0)	0 (0.0)
Points, median (25th–75th percentile)	0.000 (0.000–0.000)	0.000 (0.000–0.000)	0.000 (0.000–0.000)
Capillary ramifications			
n, (%)	5 (35.7)*‡	0 (0.0)	0 (0.0)
Points, median (25th–75th percentile)	0.000 (0.000–0.125)*‡	0.000 (0.000–0.000)	0.000 (0.000–0.000)
Bushy capillaries			
n, (%)	7 (50.0)*	3 (21.4)	1 (7.1)
Points, median (25th–75th percentile)	0.063 (0.000–0.156)*	0.000 (0.000–0.031)	0.000 (0.000–0.000)
Capillary loss			
n, (%)	4 (28.6)*‡	0 (0.0)	0 (0.0)
Points, median (25th–75th percentile)	0.000 (0.000–0.469)*‡	0.000 (0.000–0.000)	0.000 (0.000–0.000)
Giant capillaries (≥50 μm)			
n, (%)	0 (0.0)	0 (0.0)	0 (0.0)
Points, median (25th–75th percentile)	0.000 (0.000–0.000)	0.000 (0.000–0.000)	0.000 (0.000–0.000)
Capillary ectasia (≥25 μm)			
n, (%)	1 (7.1)	2 (14.3)	0 (0.0)
Points, median (25th–75th percentile)	0.000 (0.000–0.000)	0.000 (0.000–0.000)	0.000 (0.000–0.000)
Tortuous capillaries			
n, (%)	12 (85.7)	8 (57.1)	9 (64.3)
Points, median (25th–75th percentile)	0.500 (0.125–1.375)	0.375 (0.000–1.063)	0.125 (0.000–0.531)
Capillary caliber variability			
n, (%)	7 (50.0)*‡	2 (14.3)	0 (0.0)
Points, median (25th–75th percentile)	0.063 (0.000–0.281)*	0.000 (0.000–0.000)	0.000 (0.000–0.000)
Elongated capillaries			
n, (%)	8 (57.1)‡	2 (14.3)	3 (21.4)
Points, median (25th–75th percentile)	0.125 (0.000–0.469)*‡	0.000 (0.000–0.000)	0.000 (0.000–0.031)
Capillary thrombosis			
n, (%)	0 (0.0)	1 (7.1)	0 (0.0)
Points, median (25th–75th percentile)	0.000 (0.000–0.000)	0.000 (0.000–0.000)	0.000 (0.000–0.000)
Disorganization of microvascular array			
n, (%)	12 (85.7)	8 (57.1)	8 (57.1)
Points, median (25th–75th percentile)	1.063 (0.250–2.156)	0.375 (0.000–1.313)	0.313 (0.000–1.125)
Early pattern, *n* (%)	0 (0.0)	0 (0.0)	0 (0.0)
Active pattern, *n* (%)	0 (0.0)	0 (0.0)	0 (0.0)
Late pattern, *n* (%)	0 (0.0)	0 (0.0)	0 (0.0)
CSURI (points)	–§	–§	–§
MES (points), median (25th–75th percentile)	1.630 (0.250–2.438)*‡	0.375 (0.000–1.313)	0.315 (0.00–1.125)

ASCVD, atherosclerotic cardiovascular diseases; CSURI, capillaroscopic skin ulcer risk index; MES, microangiopathy evolution score.
*p < 0.05 between group with previous COVID-19 and healthy controls.
†p < 0.05 between group with ASCVD and healthy controls.
‡p < 0.05 between group with previous COVID-19 and group with ASCVD.
§not detectable.

dysfunction and inflammation in post-COVID-19 patients between a healthy group without suspected alterations and a group of patients with suspected altered parameters to rank the potential influence of COVID-19 on endothelial dysfunction and inflammatory vasculopathy. Therefore, young, healthy and sex-matched controls were used instead of age-matched controls.

Strengths of our study are that all parameters were measured together in one study cohort with balanced sex and age distribution and a quite homogenous COVID-19 phenotype.

Another strength of our study is that we included a healthy control and a sex- and age-matched ASCVD control group to discriminate the impact of COVID-19 on endothelial dysfunction and inflammatory vasculopathy, which has not been done before in studies investigating endothelial function in people who had COVID-19. In previous studies, different COVID-19 phenotypes and COVID-19 subjects with several cardiovascular comorbidities were commonly included (9, 34–39). A further strength is that all controls had no proven recent or prior SARS-CoV-2 infection at study measurement.

In conclusion, COVID-19 may contribute to enhanced endothelial dysfunction and disturbed vascular homeostasis *via* influence of EMP, inflammatory pathways as well as of arginine, kynurenine and homocysteine metabolism. Thus, changes of arterial stiffness, vascular reactivity and microvasculature may be promoted after SARS-CoV-2 infection. Further studies are needed to elucidate the underlying pathways of COVID-19 associated endothelial dysfunction and to clarify if those vascular changes are long-lasting and if COVID-19 may be even a potential risk factor for the development of atherosclerotic or inflammatory vascular diseases.

AUTHOR CONTRIBUTIONS

PJ contributed to conception of the manuscript, subject recruitment, data acquisition, data interpretation, and writing of the manuscript. PG contributed to conception of the manuscript and data acquisition. VM and HSo contributed to subject recruitment. AA contributed to statistical analysis. AM, HSt, RR, MS, UD, and HK contributed to data analysis and interpretation. KE contributed to data acquisition. MB contributed to conception and supervision of the manuscript. All authors revised the manuscript and gave their final approval of the manuscript version to be published.

ACKNOWLEDGMENTS

We thank Gudrun Dimsity, Eva-Maria Pock, Cornelia Missbrenner, Sabrina Teschl, and Verena Zrim for their assistance in the measurements of parameters of endothelial dysfunction.

REFERENCES

1. Dou Q, Wei X, Zhou K, Yang S, Jia P. Cardiovascular manifestations and mechanisms in patients with COVID-19. *Trends Endocrinol Metab.* (2020) 31:893–904. doi: 10.1016/j.tem.2020.10.001
2. Figliozzi S, Masci PG, Ahmadi N, Tondi L, Koutli E, Aimo A, et al. Predictors of adverse prognosis in COVID-19: a systematic review and meta-analysis. *Eur J Clin Invest.* (2020) 50:e13362. doi: 10.1111/eci.13362
3. Fathi M, Vakili K, Sayehmiri F, Mohamadkhani A, Hajiesmaeili M, Rezaei-Tavirani M, et al. The prognostic value of comorbidity for the severity of COVID-19: a systematic review and meta-analysis study. *PLoS One.* (2021) 16:e0246190. doi: 10.1371/journal.pone.0246190
4. Varga Z, Flammer AJ, Steiger P, Haberecker M, Andermatt R, Zinkernagel AS, et al. Endothelial cell infection and endotheliitis in COVID-19. *Lancet.* (2020) 395:1417–8. doi: 10.1016/S0140-6736(20)30937-5
5. Ackermann M, Verleden SE, Kuehnel M, Haverich A, Welte T, Laenger F, et al. Pulmonary vascular endothelialitis, thrombosis, and angiogenesis in Covid-19. *N Engl J Med.* (2020) 383:120–8. doi: 10.1056/NEJMoa2015432
6. Ren B, Yan F, Deng Z, Zhang S, Xiao L, Wu M, et al. Extremely high incidence of lower extremity deep venous thrombosis in 48 patients with severe COVID-19 in Wuhan. *Circulation.* (2020) 142:181–3. doi: 10.1161/CIRCULATIONAHA.120.047407
7. Schaller T, Hirschbühl K, Burkhardt K, Braun G, Trepel M, Märkl B, et al. Postmortem examination of patients with COVID-19. *JAMA.* (2020) 323:2518–20. doi: 10.1001/jama.2020.8907
8. McGonagle D, Bridgewood C, Ramanan AV, Meaney JFM, Watad A. COVID-19 vasculitis and novel vasculitis mimics. *Lancet Rheumatol.* (2021) 3:e224–e33. doi: 10.1016/S2665-9913(20)30420-3
9. Natalello G, De Luca G, Gigante L, Campochiaro C, De Lorenzis E, Verardi L, et al. Nailfold capillaroscopy findings in patients with coronavirus disease 2019: Broadening the spectrum of COVID-19 microvascular involvement. *Microvasc Res.* (2021) 133:104071. doi: 10.1016/j.mvr.2020.104071
10. Gheblawi M, Wang K, Viveiros A, Nguyen Q, Zhong JC, Turner AJ, et al. Angiotensin-converting enzyme 2: SARS-CoV-2 receptor and regulator of the renin-angiotensin system: celebrating the 20th anniversary of the discovery of ACE2. *Circ Res.* (2020) 126:1456–474. doi: 10.1161/CIRCRESAHA.120.317015
11. Iba T, Connors JM, Levy JH. The coagulopathy, endotheliopathy, and vasculitis of COVID-19. *Inflamm Res.* (2020) 69:1181–9. doi: 10.1007/s00011-020-01401-6
12. Teuwen LA, Geldhof V, Pasut A, Carmeliet P. COVID-19: the vasculature unleashed. *Nat Rev Immunol.* (2020) 20:389–91. doi: 10.1038/s41577-020-0343-0
13. Thijssen DHJ, Bruno RM, van Mil ACCM, Holder SM, Faita F, Greyling A, et al. Expert consensus and evidence-based recommendations for the assessment of flow-mediated dilation in humans. *Eur Heart J.* (2019) 40:2534–47. doi: 10.1093/eurheartj/ehz350
14. Stoner L, Young JM, Fryer S. Assessments of arterial stiffness and endothelial function using pulse wave analysis. *Int J Vasc Med.* (2012) 2012:903107. doi: 10.1155/2012/903107
15. Naqvi TZ, Lee MS. Carotid intima-media thickness and plaque in cardiovascular risk assessment. *JACC Cardiovasc Imaging.* (2014) 7:1025–1038. doi: 10.1016/j.jcmg.2013.11.014
16. Benjamin EJ, Larson MG, Keyes MJ, Mitchell GF, Vasan RS, Keaney JF Jr, et al. Clinical correlates and heritability of flow-mediated dilation in the community: the Framingham Heart Study. *Circulation.* (2004) 109:613–9. doi: 10.1161/01.CIR.0000112565.60887.1E
17. Williams B, Mancia G, Spiering W, Agabiti Rosei E, Azizi M, Burnier M, et al. 2018 ESC/ESH Guidelines for the management of arterial hypertension. *Eur Heart J.* (2018) 39:3021–104. doi: 10.1093/eurheartj/ehy339
18. Baldassarre D, Hamsten A, Veglia F, de Faire U, Humphries SE, Smit AJ, et al. Measurements of carotid intima-media thickness and of interadventitia common carotid diameter improve prediction of cardiovascular events: results of the IMPROVE (Carotid Intima Media Thickness [IMT] and IMT-Progression as Predictors of Vascular Events in a High Risk European Population) Study. *J Am Coll Cardiol.* (2012) 60:1489–99. doi: 10.1016/j.jacc.2012.06.034

19. Zhu M, Mao M, Lou X. Elevated homocysteine level and prognosis in patients with acute coronary syndrome: a meta-analysis. *Biomarkers.* (2019) 24:309–16. doi: 10.1080/1354750X.2019.1589577

20. Vogl L, Pohlhammer J, Meinitzer A, Rantner B, Stadler M, Peric S, et al. Serum concentrations of L-arginine and L-homoarginine in male patients with intermittent claudication: a cross-sectional and prospective investigation in the CAVASIC Study. *Atherosclerosis.* (2015) 239:607–14. doi: 10.1016/j.atherosclerosis.2015.02.019

21. Schlesinger S, Sonntag SR, Lieb W, Maas R. Asymmetric and symmetric dimethylarginine as risk markers for total mortality and cardiovascular outcomes: a systematic review and meta-analysis of prospective studies. *PLoS One.* (2016) 11:e0165811. doi: 10.1371/journal.pone.0165811

22. Zuo H, Ueland PM, Ulvik A, Eussen SJ, Vollset SE, Nygård O, et al. Plasma biomarkers of inflammation, the kynurenine pathway, and risks of all-cause, cancer, and cardiovascular disease mortality: the Hordaland Health Study. *Am J Epidemiol.* (2016) 183:249–58. doi: 10.1093/aje/kwv242

23. Werner N, Wassmann S, Ahlers P, Kosiol S, Nickenig G. Circulating CD31+/annexin V+ apoptotic microparticles correlate with coronary endothelial function in patients with coronary artery disease. *Arterioscler Thromb Vasc Biol.* (2006) 26:112–6. doi: 10.1161/01.ATV.0000191634.13057.15

24. Aslim E, Hakki Akay T, Bastürk B, Ozkan S, Gültekin B, Ozcobanoglu S, et al. The role of antiendothelial cell antibodies in the development and follow-up of coronary and peripheral arterial diseases. *Angiology.* (2008) 59:209–13. doi: 10.1177/0003319707304537

25. Maruhashi T, Kajikawa M, Kishimoto S, Hashimoto H, Takaeko Y, Yamaji T, et al. Diagnostic criteria of flow-mediated vasodilation for normal endothelial function and nitroglycerin-induced vasodilation for normal vascular smooth muscle function of the brachial artery. *J Am Heart Assoc.* (2020) 9:e013915. doi: 10.1161/JAHA.119.013915

26. Moens AL, Goovaerts I, Claeys MJ, Vrints CJ. Flow-mediated vasodilation: a diagnostic instrument, or an experimental tool? *Chest.* (2005) 127:2254–63. doi: 10.1378/chest.127.6.2254

27. Hervé C, Beyne P, Jamault H, Delacoux E. Determination of tryptophan and its kynurenine pathway metabolites in human serum by high-performance liquid chromatography with simultaneous ultraviolet and fluorimetric detection. *J Chromatogr B Biomed Appl.* (1996) 675:157–61. doi: 10.1016/0378-4347(95)00341-X

28. Schwarz EL, Roberts WL, Pasquali M. Analysis of plasma amino acids by HPLC with photodiode array and fluorescence detection. *Clin Chim Acta.* (2005) 354:83–90. doi: 10.1016/j.cccn.2004.11.016

29. Meinitzer A, Puchinger M, Winklhofer-Roob BM, Rock E, Ribalta J, Roob JM, et al. Reference values for plasma concentrations of asymmetrical dimethylarginine (ADMA) and other arginine metabolites in men after validation of a chromatographic method. *Clin Chim Acta.* (2007) 384:141–8. doi: 10.1016/j.cca.2007.07.006

30. Cossarizza A, Chang HD, Radbruch A, Acs A, Adam D, Adam-Klages S, et al. Guidelines for the use of flow cytometry and cell sorting in immunological studies (second edition). *Eur J Immunol.* (2019) 49:1457–973. doi: 10.1002/eji.201970107

31. Deng F, Whang S, Zang L. Endothelial microparticles act as novel diagnostic and therapeutic biomarkers of circulatory hypoxia-related diseases: a literature review. *J Cell Mol Med.* (2017) 21:1698–710. doi: 10.1111/jcmm.13125

32. Sebastiani M, Manfredi A, Colaci M, D'amico R, Malagoli V, Giuggioli D, et al. Capillaroscopic skin ulcer risk index: a new prognostic tool for digital skin ulcer development in systemic sclerosis patients. *Arthritis Rheum.* (2009) 61:688–94. doi: 10.1002/art.24394

33. Sulli A, Secchi ME, Pizzorni C, Cutolo M. Scoring the nailfold microvascular changes during capillaroscopic analysis in systemic sclerosis patients. *Ann Rheum Dis.* (2008) 67:885–7. doi: 10.1136/ard.2007.079756

34. Cutolo M, Sulli A, Pizzorni C, Accardo S. Nailfold videocapillaroscopy assessment of microvascular damage in systemic sclerosis. *J Rheumatol.* (2000) 27:155–60.

35. Riou M, Oulehri W, Momas C, Rouyer O, Lebourg F, Meyer A, et al. Reduced flow-mediated dilatation is not related to COVID-19 severity three months after hospitalization for SARS-CoV-2 infection. *J Clin Med.* (2021) 10:1318. doi: 10.3390/jcm10061318

36. Schnaubelt S, Oppenauer J, Tihanyi D, Mueller M, Maldonado-Gonzalez E, Zejnilovic S, et al. Arterial stiffness in acute COVID-19 and potential associations with clinical outcome. *J Intern Med.* (2021) 290:437–43. doi: 10.1111/joim.13275

37. Szeghy RE, Province VM, Stute NL, Augenreich MA, Koontz LK, Stickford JL, et al. Carotid stiffness, intima-media thickness and aortic augmentation index among adults with SARS-CoV-2. *Exp Physiol.* (2021). doi: 10.1113/EP089481. [Epub ahead of print].

38. Hannemann J, Balfanz P, Schwedhelm E, Hartmann B, Ule J, Müller-Wieland D, et al. Elevated serum SDMA and ADMA at hospital admission predict in-hospital mortality of COVID-19 patients. *Sci Rep.* (2021) 11:9895. doi: 10.1038/s41598-021-89180-w

39. Hoechter DJ, Becker-Pennrich A, Langrehr J, Bruegel M, Zwissler B, Schaefer S, et al. Higher procoagulatory potential but lower DIC score in COVID-19 ARDS patients compared to non-COVID-19 ARDS patients. *Thromb Res.* (2020) 196:186–92. doi: 10.1016/j.thromres.2020.08.030

40. Ponti G, Roli L, Oliva G, Manfredini M, Trenti T, Kaleci S, et al. Homocysteine (Hcy) assessment to predict outcomes of hospitalized Covid-19 patients: a multicenter study on 313 Covid-19 patients. *Clin Chem Lab Med.* (2021) 59:e354–e7. doi: 10.1515/cclm-2021-0168

41. Mehta P, McAuley DF, Brown M, Sanchez E, Tattersall RS, Manson JJ, et al. COVID-19: consider cytokine storm syndromes and immunosuppression. *Lancet.* (2020) 395:1033–4. doi: 10.1016/S0140-6736(20)30628-0

42. McCracken IR, Saginc G, He L, Huseynov A, Daniels A, Fletcher S, et al. Lack of evidence of angiotensin-converting enzyme 2 expression and replicative infection by SARS-CoV-2 in human endothelial cells. *Circulation.* (2021) 143:865–8. doi: 10.1161/CIRCULATIONAHA.120.052824

43. Hingorani AD, Cross J, Kharbanda RK, Mullen MJ, Bhagat K, Taylor M, et al. Acute systemic inflammation impairs endothelium-dependent dilatation in humans. *Circulation.* (2000) 102:994–9. doi: 10.1161/01.CIR.102.9.994

44. Vlachopoulos C, Dima I, Aznaouridis K, Vasiliadou C, Ioakeimidis N, Aggeli C, et al. Acute systemic inflammation increases arterial stiffness and decreases wave reflections in healthy individuals. *Circulation.* (2005) 112:2193–200. doi: 10.1161/CIRCULATIONAHA.105.535435

45. Wang Q, Liu D, Song P, Zou MH. Tryptophan-kynurenine pathway is dysregulated in inflammation, and immune activation. *Front Biosci (Landmark Ed).* (2015) 20:1116–43. doi: 10.2741/4363

46. Baldassarre D, De Jong A, Amato M, Werba JP, Castelnuovo S, Frigerio B, et al. Carotid intima-media thickness and markers of inflammation, endothelial damage and hemostasis. *Ann Med.* (2008) 40:21–44. doi: 10.1080/07853890701645399

47. Bachelier K, Biehl S, Schwarz V, Kindermann I, Kandolf R, Sauter M, et al. Parvovirus B19-induced vascular damage in the heart is associated with elevated circulating endothelial microparticles. *PLoS One.* (2017) 12:e0176311. doi: 10.1371/journal.pone.0176311

48. Kurz K, Teerlink T, Sarcletti M, Weiss G, Zangerle R, Fuchs D. Asymmetric dimethylarginine concentrations decrease in patients with HIV infection under antiretroviral therapy. *Antivir Ther.* (2012) 17:1021–7. doi: 10.3851/IMP2304

49. Silva I, Teixeira A, Oliveira J, Almeida I, Almeida R, Águas A, et al. Endothelial dysfunction and nailfold videocapillaroscopy pattern as predictors of digital ulcers in systemic sclerosis: a Cohort Study and Review of the Literature. *Clin Rev Allergy Immunol.* (2015) 49:240–52. doi: 10.1007/s12016-015-8500-0

50. Michalska-Jakubus M, Kowal-Bielecka O, Smith V, Cutolo M, Krasowska D. Plasma endothelial microparticles reflect the extent of capillaroscopic alterations and correlate with the severity of skin involvement in systemic sclerosis. *Microvasc Res.* (2017) 110:24–31. doi: 10.1016/j.mvr.2016.11.006

13

Biomarkers of Cardiac Injury, Renal Injury and Inflammation are Strong Mediators of Sex-Associated Death in COVID-19

Heidi S. Lumish [1]*, Eunyoung Kim [1], Caitlin Selvaggi [2,3,4], Tingyi Cao [2,3,4], Aakriti Gupta [5], Andrea S. Foulkes [2,3,4†] and Muredach P. Reilly [1,6*†]

[1] Division of Cardiology, Columbia University, New York, NY, United States, [2] Biostatistics Center, Massachusetts General Hospital, Boston, MA, United States, [3] Department of Medicine, Harvard Medical School, Boston, MA, United States, [4] Department of Biostatistics, Harvard T. H. Chan School of Public Health, Boston, MA, United States, [5] Division of Interventional Cardiology, Cedars-Sinai Medical Center, Los Angeles, CA, United States, [6] Irving Institute for Clinical and Translational Research, Columbia University, New York, NY, United States

*Correspondence:
Heidi S. Lumish
hl2738@cumc.columbia.edu
Muredach P. Reilly
mpr2144@cumc.columbia.edu

† These authors have contributed equally to this work and share senior authorship

Background: Studies examining outcomes among individuals with COronaVIrus Disease 2019 (COVID-19) have consistently demonstrated that men have worse outcomes than women, with a higher incidence of myocardial injury, respiratory failure, and death. However, mechanisms of higher morbidity and mortality among men remain poorly understood. We aimed to identify mediators of the relationship between sex and COVID-19-associated mortality.

Methods: Patients hospitalized at two quaternary care facilities, New York Presbyterian Hospital (CUIMC/NYPH) and Massachusetts General Hospital (MGH), for SARS-CoV-2 infection between February and May 2020 were included. Five independent biomarkers were identified as mediators of sex effects, including high-sensitivity cardiac troponin T (hs-cTNT), high sensitivity C-reactive protein (hs-CRP), ferritin, D-dimer, and creatinine.

Results: In the CUIMC/NYPH cohort ($n = 2,626$, 43% female), male sex was associated with significantly greater mortality (26 vs. 21%, $p = 0.0146$) and higher peak hs-cTNT, hs-CRP, ferritin, D-dimer, and creatinine ($p < 0.001$). The effect of male sex on the primary outcome of death was partially mediated by peak values of all five biomarkers, suggesting that each pathophysiological pathway may contribute to increased risk of death in men. Hs-cTnT, creatinine, and hs-CRP were the strongest mediators. Findings were highly consistent in the MGH cohort with the exception of D-dimer.

Conclusions: This study suggests that the effect of sex on COVID-19 outcomes is mediated by cardiac and kidney injury, as well as underlying differences in inflammation and iron metabolism. Exploration of these specific pathways may facilitate sex-directed diagnostic and therapeutic strategies for patients with COVID-19 and provides a framework for the study of sex differences in other complex diseases.

Keywords: biomarkers, myocardial injury, SARS-CoV-2, sex differences, inflammation

INTRODUCTION

Across numerous studies of COronaVIrus Disease 2019 (COVID-19), men have had consistently worse rates of severe outcomes than women, with higher rates of cardiac injury, respiratory failure, shock, intensive care unit (ICU) admission, and death (1–3). This sex-related difference in outcomes has been confirmed in cohorts from China (4), Italy (5), and the United States (2, 6). There are multiple mechanisms hypothesized to contribute to this sex difference in COVID-19 outcomes – for example, sex-related factors that affect disease susceptibility, including differences in smoking and drinking habits, rates of handwashing, and social obligations (7). Men are also known to have higher rates of baseline co-morbidities, including hypertension and cardiovascular disease (8), and they may be more susceptible to the effects of age and co-morbidities than women (9). However, prior studies have demonstrated that the sex-related difference in outcomes is not entirely accounted for by a difference in baseline co-morbidities (10). Hormonal and genetic factors are also thought to play a role in disease pathogenesis. Sex hormones have been shown to modify inflammatory pathways and affect the regulation of angiotensin converting enzyme 2 (ACE2), which mediates Severe Acute Respiratory Syndrome Coronavirus-2 (SARS-CoV-2) entry into cells (11–13). Genes conferring immunity are located on the X chromosome, some of which escape X-inactivation leading to a dose-related difference in the gene effect between men and women (11, 12). There are likely other important pathophysiological determinants of sex differences that are incompletely understood.

Downstream of social, clinical, hormonal and genetic processes, there are multiple biological pathways driving COVID-19 outcomes that may be mechanistically important and therapeutically tractable in the described sex differences. Several studies have demonstrated a sex difference in the relationship between various biomarkers and COVID-19 outcomes. Candidate biomarkers are implicated in immune response, inflammatory pathways, and coagulation pathways, as well as end organ dysfunction (9, 11, 14, 15). Specifically, men have been shown to have higher incidence of myocardial injury, as measured by troponin elevation (3). However, to date there has been no systematic examination of biomarkers of these pathophysiological processes and their relative effects as mediators of the sex difference in COVID-19 outcomes. Mediation analysis, our novel focus in this paper, aims to inform whether a biomarker (of a pathologic process) is in the causal pathway between an exposure (e.g., sex) and outcome (e.g., death) whereas the assessment of modification, a focus of prior studies (15–17), examines whether the exposure interacts with a biomarker in its association with the outcome.

In this study, we investigated potential pathophysiological biomarker mediators of the effect of sex on COVID-19 outcomes, to better understand the potential mechanisms and therapeutic implications for increased risk of poor outcomes in men. We evaluated 15 candidate blood biomarkers of biological pathways perturbed in COVID-19 as potential mediators of sex differences in COVID-19 outcomes, including markers of cardiac injury, inflammation, iron metabolism and coagulation, as well as renal and liver injury.

METHODS

Study Populations

The study population included a total of 4,017 patients hospitalized for SARS-CoV-2 infection between February and May 2020 at two independent quaternary care facilities, Columbia University Irving Medical Center/New York Presbyterian Hospital (CUIMC/NYPH) and Massachusetts General Hospital (MGH).

CUIMC/NYPH COVID-19 Cohort

The CUIMC/NYPH COVID-19 cohort includes 2,626 adult patients (≥18 years of age) who were hospitalized at CUIMC and the Allen Hospital sites of NYPH between February 1 and May 12, 2020, with positive SARS-CoV-2 reverse transcriptase-polymerase chain reaction testing of nasopharyngeal or oropharyngeal specimens (18). Patients who were admitted for <24 h were excluded from the analysis. Patients were followed until discharge, death, or the end of study follow-up on June 11, 2020. Patient data were identified in the electronic health record (EHR) by using the institution's clinical data warehouse, which included information on individuals who receive care at CUIMC/NYPH. Analysis was based on index hospitalization. Clinical comorbidities including hypertension, diabetes, coronary artery disease (CAD), heart failure, stroke or transient ischemic attack, atrial arrhythmias (atrial fibrillation, atrial flutter, and supraventricular tachycardia), chronic lung disease, chronic kidney disease, and chronic liver disease, were identified using ICD-10 medical billing codes (**Supplementary Table S1**). Cancer was defined by an automated search of the EHR for the terms "cancer," "carcinoma," "malignancy," "malignant," "neoplasm," "-noma," or "blastoma," excluding those with the terms "screen" or "hypertension." Obesity was defined as body mass index (BMI) ≥30 at the time of index hospitalization. The primary outcome was in-hospital mortality within 30 days of admission. Peak biomarker values were defined over the duration of hospitalization.

MGH COVID-19 Patient Registry

A replication analysis was performed using retrospective data on 1,391 individuals from the MGH COVID-19 Patient Registry (19, 20). All patients were hospitalized between March 11, 2020 and May 31, 2020 and tested positive for SARS-CoV2. Demographic information, comorbid conditions, medications, laboratory tests, and clinical outcomes at index hospitalization were manually extracted from electronic health records. The primary outcome was death within 28 days of presentation to care, defined as first contact with a health care provider due to COVID-19-related symptoms. Peak biomarker values were defined over the duration of hospitalization within 28 days of index date.

Statistical Methods

Baseline characteristics were summarized for the overall cohort and stratified by sex for both the CUIMC/NYP and MGH

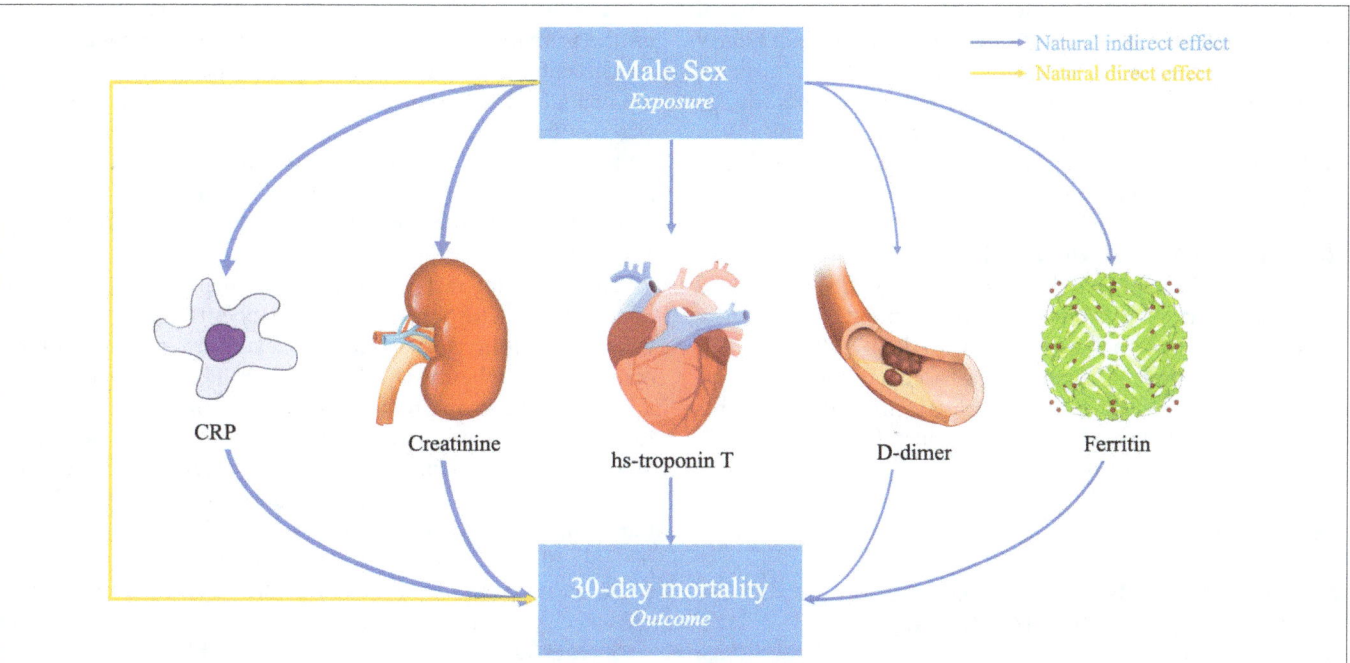

FIGURE 1 | Causal mediation model. This study assessed the degree to which peak serum biomarkers mediated the association between male sex and death due to SARS-CoV-2 infection in hospitalized patients. Of the fifteen biomarkers tested, five were significant mediators of the association between male sex and 30-day mortality, with varying proportion mediated as represented by the arrow thickness. Potential confounders accounted for in the primary analysis included age, sex, race/ethnicity, and number of biomarker measurements. The proportion mediated is given by the Natural Indirect Effect (NIE) divided by the Total Effect [NIE + Natural Direct Effect (NDE)].

registries. Unadjusted two-sided tests of proportions (or means) were used to compare baseline characteristics for male and female patients.

In the CUIMC/NYPH data, we evaluated 15 biomarkers of pathways perturbed in COVID-19 as potential mediators of sex differences in COVID-19 outcomes. Of these, two (IL-6, lactate) were excluded because of >50% missing data, and four (albumin, ALC, ESR, platelets) were excluded because their peak values were not associated with sex. Although associated with sex, WBC and automated lymphocytes were not reported as main findings because they were correlated and redundant with hs-CRP, which had stronger mediation effects (**Supplementary Table S2**). Hepatic injury markers (AST and ALT) were excluded because of race/ethnicity interactions in their association with death, limiting statistical power for race/ethnicity-specific mediation effects (**Supplementary Table S2**). Details on all additional biomarkers that were screened but not presented as primary findings are given in **Supplementary Table S2**. Thus, five biomarkers representing distinct biological pathways – hs-cTNT, hs-CRP, ferritin, creatinine, and D-dimer – were analyzed and presented here for their mediation of sex effects on death during index hospitalization. Each of these had peak values that were significantly associated with sex, had observed data in >50% of individuals, and represented distinct pathophysiological processes. Peak biomarker values were natural log transformed and standardized prior to inclusion in models.

We applied the causal mediation analysis approach described by Imai et al. (21) and as we applied in Foulkes et al. (22) which uses the results of three models to determine the proportion of the association between sex and severe outcomes that is mediated by the biomarker: (1) A Total Effect Model using a logit link with death (Y) as the outcome and sex (T) as a predictor variable, where the biomarker (M) is not included in the model; (2) A Mediator Model using an identify link with peak biomarker as the outcome and sex as a predictor; and (3) An Outcome Model using a logit link with death as the outcome and both sex and peak biomarker as predictor variables. All models were initially conditioned on age, sex, obesity, race/ethnicity and number of biomarker measurements. The reported odds ratios (ORs) are computed in the same way as using standard statistical model fitting procedures.

The average proportion mediated and corresponding p-value were reported for each biomarker. Models were fitted overall based on data from adult patients (≥ 18 years of age) using the peak biomarker value for each patient. Analysis used a complete case analysis for each biomarker separately assuming data were missing completely at random. Summary level data on characteristics of patients with and without missing data are provided (**Supplementary Table S3**). Primary analysis was based on data derived from the CUIMC/NYP cohort. Replication analysis was based on the MGH cohort. To explore mediation effects that might differ by menopausal status in women, we performed secondary analyses of age strata (≥ 50 vs. <50 years of age) designed as a surrogate for pre- and post-menopausal status in women. Additional sensitivity analyses in the CUIMC/NYP cohort were performed to check the consistency of our conclusions when (1) adjusting for additional potential confounders (coronary artery disease, chronic kidney disease, lung disease, hypertension, type 2 diabetes mellitus, cancer, heart failure, and stroke) in the multivariable models, (2) restricting to individuals with complete data for all variables ($N = 1,688$). Analyses were completed using R version 3.5.0. Mediation analysis was performed using the R package "mediation."

Human Subjects and IRB Approvals

The CUIMC IRB approved this study (#AAAS9835) and waived the requirement for obtaining informed consent. The Partners HealthCare Institutional Review Board (IRB) (#2020P000829) approved collection of curated data based on comprehensive manual chart reviews and data extractions from EHRs on patients who receive care through the Mass General Brigham (MGB, formerly Partners) system.

RESULTS

Baseline Characteristics of the CUIMC/NYP COVID-19 Cohort

Baseline clinical, demographic, and laboratory findings, overall and stratified by sex, are shown in **Table 1**. Median age was 66 (IQR 54, 77) years. Women accounted for 43% of the study cohort, and women were older (69 [57, 80] vs. 64 [53, 75], $p < 0.001$) and more obese (BMI 29.0 [24.9, 34.1] vs. 27.5 [24.4, 31.5], $p < 0.001$) than men. There were no significant differences in baseline statin and angiotensin-converting enzyme inhibitors (ACEi) or angiotensin receptor blocker (ARB) use between men and women. Men had a trend toward higher rates of baseline CAD, though this was not statistically significant, and women had significantly higher rates of hypertension (58 vs. 52%, $p = 0.0047$) and lung disease (23 vs. 14%, $p < 0.001$). There were no sex differences in the baseline proportions of patients with diabetes mellitus, chronic kidney disease (CKD), cancer, heart failure or stroke (**Table 1**). On admission, compared to women, men had significantly higher hs-CRP, creatinine, hs-cTnT levels and especially ferritin. There was no sex difference in D-dimer levels at the time of admission (**Table 1**).

Unadjusted Analyses of Biomarkers and Outcome by Sex in the CUIMC/NYP COVID-19 Cohort

Peak values for all five biomarkers were significantly higher in men than in women, as shown in **Table 2**. The most notable sex difference was in median peak ferritin level, which was 1184.5 (IQR 621, 2,269) in men as compared to 615.5 (IQR 295, 1,307) in women. Mortality at 30 days was significantly higher in men than in women (26 vs. 21%, $p = 0.0146$, **Table 2**).

Mediation Effects in the CUIMC/NYP COVID-19 Cohort

In adjusted models, male sex was a significant predictor of death at 30 days (OR ~2.0 depending on the specific sample of patients with available biomarker data, $p < 0.001$, **Table 3**). Male sex was also a significant predictor of the peak hs-CRP, ferritin, D-dimer,

hs-cTnT, and creatinine ($p < 0.001$, **Table 3**). The effect of sex on the primary outcome of death was partially attenuated after adjustment for each of the five peak biomarker values, suggesting a potential mediation effect for each. The proportion mediated was significantly different than 0 for all of the biomarkers. The estimated proportion mediated was greatest for hs-cTnT (0.45, $p < 0.001$), hs-CRP (0.42, $p < 0.001$), and creatinine (0.35, $p < 0.001$) and lowest for D-dimer (0.22, $p < 0.001$, **Table 3**, **Figure 1**).

There were interaction effects with biomarkers in the outcome model for hs-CRP and ferritin with obesity and for D-dimer with age, and therefore stratified analyses are included in these cases. In the obesity (BMI >30) stratified analyses for hs-CRP, the estimated proportion mediated remained the same for obese and non-obese patients (0.42, $p < 0.001$ for each). While ferritin remained a significant mediator of the effect of sex on COVID-19 outcomes after stratifying by obesity, the estimated proportion mediated was larger among obese patients (0.51, $p = 0.010$) as compared to non-obese patients (0.24, $p < 0.001$). For D-dimer, the estimated proportion mediated was slightly lower in the older strata (0.18 for >65 years vs. 0.25 for age <65 years, **Table 3**). In secondary age-stratified analyses ($\geq$ or < age 50), a surrogate for menopausal status in women, the mediation effects of each biomarker were largely consistent across younger vs. older age categories. However, hs-CRP had a greater proportion mediated for age <50 years (0.59) as compared to those with age $\geq$ 50 years (0.35), and ferritin had a trend toward a greater proportion mediated in those aged <50 (0.57 vs. 0.42, **Supplementary Table S4**).

Replication Analyses in the MGH COVID-19 Patient Registry

Replication analysis was performed in the MGH registry. The clinical characteristics, laboratory values, and outcomes overall and by sex in the MGH cohort are shown in **Supplementary Tables S5, S6**. Similar to the CUIMC/NYP cohort, women were more obese than men (BMI 29.8 [25.6, 35.0] vs. 28.6 [25.2, 32.9], $p = 0.016$) and had significantly more lung disease (33 vs. 27%, $p = 0.030$). While in the CUIMC/NYP cohort men had a trend toward higher rates of CAD, in the MGH cohort men had significantly more CAD and were also more likely to be smokers. In unadjusted analysis, peak values for all five biomarkers were significantly higher in men than in women, consistent with the CUIMC/NYP cohort. Also in unadjusted analysis and similar to the CUIMC/NYP cohort, men in the MGH cohort had significantly higher rates of the primary endpoint of death.

The results of the mediation analysis of the five candidate biomarkers in the MGH cohort are shown in **Table 4**. CRP, ferritin, creatinine, and hs-cTnT were all significant mediators of the effect of sex on COVID-19-related mortality. Stratified analyses by obesity for CRP and ferritin had similar patterns to the CUIMC/NYP cohort with no difference in proportion mediated between obese and non-obese for CRP but a greater proportion mediated for obese with ferritin (0.51 vs. 0.24). While

TABLE 1 | Clinical characteristics and admission labs overall and by sex in the CUIMC/NYP COVID-19 cohort.

	Overall (*N* = 2,626)	Male (*N* = 1,497)	Female (*N* = 1,129)	*P*-value*
Presentation to care				
Age in years (median [IQR])	66 (54, 77)	64 (53, 75)	69 (57, 80)	<0.001
Age ≥65 years	1,420/2,626 (0.54)	748/1,497 (0.50)	672/1,129 (0.60)	<0.001
White/non-Hispanic	237/2,626 (0.09)	139/1,497 (0.09)	98/1,129 (0.09)	0.6406
Black/non-Hispanic	320/2,626 (0.12)	180/1,497 (0.12)	140/1,129 (0.12)	0.8169
Hispanic	1,314/2,626 (0.50)	747/1,497 (0.50)	567/1,129 (0.50)	0.9015
Other	755/2,626 (0.29)	431/1,497 (0.29)	324/1,129 (0.29)	0.9932
Fever	604/2,624 (0.23)	371/1,497 (0.25)	233/1,127 (0.21)	0.0152
Body mass index (Median [IQR])	28.02 (24.60, 32.66)	27.46 (24.36, 31.46)	28.96 (24.89, 34.13)	<0.001
On statins	951/2,626 (0.36)	519/1,497 (0.35)	432/1,129 (0.38)	0.0634
On ACEi or ARBs[†]	442/2,626 (0.17)	238/1,497 (0.16)	204/1,129 (0.18)	0.1559
Co-morbidities				
Obesity[‡]	794/2,113 (0.38)	393/1,219 (0.32)	401/894 (0.45)	<0.001
Coronary artery disease	329/2,626 (0.13)	204/1,497 (0.14)	125/1,129 (0.11)	0.0576
Hypertension	1,430/2,626 (0.54)	779/1,497 (0.52)	651/1,129 (0.58)	0.0047
Diabetes mellitus type 2	968/2,626 (0.37)	553/1,497 (0.37)	415/1,129 (0.37)	0.9561
Chronic kidney disease	370/2,626 (0.14)	219/1,497 (0.15)	151/1,129 (0.13)	0.3908
Lung disease	463/2,626 (0.18)	207/1,497 (0.14)	256/1,129 (0.23)	<0.001
Cancer	261/2,626 (0.10)	155/1,497 (0.10)	106/1,129 (0.09)	0.4517
Heart failure	275/2,626 (0.10)	149/1,497 (0.10)	126/1,129 (0.11)	0.3494
Stroke	225/2,626 (0.09)	130/1,497 (0.09)	95/1,129 (0.08)	0.8620
Admission labs (median [IQR])[§]				
hs-CRP (mg/L; *n* = 2,414)	118.46 (56.79, 205.18)	130.48 (63.66, 215.36)	105.79 (45.40, 184.04)	<0.001
D-Dimer (ng/mL; *n* = 2,179)	1,510 (830, 3,290)	1,490 (800, 3,440)	1,520 (873, 3,170)	0.6767
Ferritin (ng/mL; *n* = 2,391)	702.6 (345.40, 1,293)	870.4 (457.80, 1584.50)	479.4 (238.80, 929.60)	<0.001
Creatinine (mg/dL; *n* = 2,609)	1.07 (0.81, 1.64)	1.17 (0.91, 1.75)	0.92 (0.70, 1.48)	<0.001
hs-cTnT (ng/L; *n* = 2,402)	17 (8, 42)	19 (9, 43)	16 (8, 39)	0.0028

*P-values correspond to a two-sample test of proportions (for categorical variables) or Wilcoxon rank sum tests (for numeric variables) comparing corresponding characteristics of male vs. female patients; [†] ACEi, angiotensin-converting enzyme inhibitors; ARB, angiotensin receptor blockers; [‡] Obesity is defined as BMI ≥30 and is missing for 513 patients; §Admission labs - recorded within +/-3 days of hospital admission.
IQR, interquartile range; hs-CRP, high sensitivity C-reactive protein; hs-cTNT, high sensitivity cardiac Troponin T.

TABLE 2 | Peak laboratory values and outcomes overall and by sex in the CUIMC/NYP COVID-19 cohort.

	Overall (*N* = 2,626)	Male (*N* = 1,497)	Female (*N* = 1,129)	*P*-value*
Peak labs (median [IQR])[†]				
hs-CRP (mg/L; *n* = 2,416)	167.12 (83.80, 281.45)	185.11 (101.11, 293.01)	143.99 (65.80, 261.38)	<0.001
D-Dimer (ng/ml; *n* = 2,180)	2,565 (1060, 9805)	2,790 (1060, 12260)	2,230 (1050, 7463)	0.0016
Ferritin (ng/ml; *n* = 2,393)	931.40 (437.90, 1,934)	1,184.5 (620.70, 2,269)	615.5 (295.40, 1,307)	<0.001
Creatinine (mg/dL; *n* = 2,609)	1.34 (0.92, 2.71)	1.49 (1.05, 3.07)	1.11 (0.80, 2.28)	<0.001
hs-cTnT (ng/L; *n* = 2,402)	26 (10, 79)	29 (11, 84)	24 (9, 67)	<0.001
Follow-up (30 day) outcomes				
Ventilator or death	908/2,626 (0.35)	555/1,497 (0.37)	353/1,129 (0.31)	0.0022
Ventilator[‡]	559/2,626 (0.21)	365/1,497 (0.24)	194/1,129 (0.17)	<0.001
Death	623/2,626 (0.24)	382/1,497 (0.26)	241/1,129 (0.21)	0.0146

*P-values correspond to a two-sample test of proportions (for categorical variables) or Wilcoxon rank sum tests (for numeric variables) comparing corresponding characteristics of male vs. female patients; [†] Peak labs – high sensitivity C-reactive protein (hs-CRP), high sensitivity cardiac Troponin T (hs-cTnT) [‡] 349 patients died without being on ventilator.
IQR, interquartile range; hs-CRP, high sensitivity C-reactive protein; hs-cTNT, high sensitivity cardiac Troponin T.

TABLE 3 | Primary mediation analyses of peak values* of biomarkers in CUIMC/NYP COVID-19 cohort.

	Total effect model[†] outcome: death	Mediator model[†] outcome: biomarker	Outcome model[†] outcome: death		Proportion mediated
	OR (sex)	Estimate (sex)	OR (sex)	OR (biomarker)	
hs-CRP					
All (n = 1,978)	2.00 (p < 0.001)	0.285 (p < 0.001)	1.71 (p < 0.001)	-	0.42 (p < 0.001)
Obese (n = 748)	2.00 (p = 0.001)	0.204 (p = 0.002)	1.87 (p = 0.005)	8.24 (p < 0.001)	0.42 (p < 0.001)
Non-obese (n = 1,230)	2.00 (p < 0.001)	0.329 (p < 0.001)	1.62 (p = 0.003)	2.80 (p < 0.001)	0.42 (p < 0.001)
Ferritin					
All (n = 1,070)	2.33 (p < 0.001)	0.474 (p < 0.001)	2.04 (p = 0.002)	-[‡]	0.33 (p < 0.001)
Obese (n = 483)	1.96 (p = 0.046)	0.510 (p < 0.001)	1.57 (p = 0.204)	2.62 (p < 0.001)	0.51 (p = 0.010)
Non-obese (n = 587)	2.64 (p = 0.001)	0.456 (p < 0.001)	2.47 (p = 0.003)	1.92 (p < 0.001)	0.24 (p < 0.001)
D-dimer					
All (n = 1,814)	2.03 (p < 0.001)	0.207 (p < 0.001)	1.84 (p < 0.001)	-[‡]	0.22 (p < 0.001)
≥ 65 yrs (n = 945)	1.88 (p < 0.001)	0.165 (p = 0.010)	1.76 (p < 0.001)	2.13 (p < 0.001)	0.18 (p = 0.008)
< 65 yrs (n = 869)	2.44 (p = 0.001)	0.205 (p = 0.005)	2.17 (p = 0.007)	3.35 (p < 0.001)	0.25 (p = 0.006)
Creatinine					
All (n = 2,106)	1.98 (p < 0.001)	0.430 (p < 0.001)	1.52 (p=0.001)	2.24 (p < 0.001)	0.45 (p < 0.001)
hs-Troponin T					
All (n = 1,954)	2.05 (p < 0.001)	0.301 (p < 0.001)	1.70 (p < 0.001)	2.55 (p < 0.001)	0.35 (p < 0.001)

*Peak biomarker level was determined based on all measurements. All values were natural log transformed and standardized for analysis; [†] All models included terms for sex and were adjusted for age, obesity, race/ethnicity, and the number of biomarker measurements. The outcome model included both sex and the biomarker as predictor variables; [‡] The outcome model included a biomarker by obesity/age interaction and therefore the main effect of the biomarker was not reported here.
OR, odds ratio; hs-CRP, high sensitivity C-reactive protein; hs-Troponin T, high sensitivity cardiac Troponin T.

D-dimer was a significant mediator in the CUIMC/NYP cohort, it was not a significant mediator in the MGH registry data.

Sensitivity Analyses

Additional analyses in the CUIMC/NYP COVID-19 Cohort tested the robustness of findings. In mediation analyses that adjusted for additional covariates and potential confounders (CAD, CKD, lung disease, hypertension, type 2 diabetes mellitus, cancer, heart failure, and stroke), the findings for each biomarker were highly consistent with the primary findings (**Supplementary Table S7**). Similarly, in models that restricted data to patients that had complete data for all biomarkers and covariates (N = 1,688), mediation findings were also consistent with the main analyses (**Supplementary Table S8**).

DISCUSSION

In this study of 4,017 patients with COVID-19 at two tertiary care centers, we confirm that compared to female sex, male sex was associated with higher mortality at 30 days. Further, we report the novel finding that specific biomarkers of pathophysiological processes mediate the effect of sex on COVID-19 outcomes. These include hs-cTnT, hs-CRP, D-dimer, ferritin and creatinine – with proportion mediated estimated to be greatest for cardiac injury (hs-cTnT), intermediate for inflammation (hs-CRP) and kidney function (creatinine), and least for thrombosis (D-dimer). Additional evaluated biomarkers were excluded because their

peak values were not associated with sex (albumin, ALC, ESR, platelets), they were correlated and redundant with hs-CRP (WBC and automated lymphocytes) or because of excess missing data (IL-6 and lactate). Our findings suggest that biological pathways of inflammation, iron metabolism, and coagulation, as well as cardiac and kidney injury that may be downstream of these pathways, are implicated in the strong sex-related difference in COVID-19 outcomes.

Several prior small studies have looked at patterns of biomarker elevation by sex in association with COVID-19 outcomes, though none have performed rigorous analyses of these biomarkers as mediators. A study of 776 patients hospitalized in New Orleans with COVID-19 found that troponin and D-dimer were predictors of worse outcomes in men, while ferritin was associated with death only in women (16). In a retrospective review of 168 patients hospitalized with COVID-19 in Wuhan, China, there were five biomarkers identified that were higher among men who died than among women who died (NLR, CRP, AST, LDH, and creatinine) (9). Importantly, ours is the first study to report which biomarkers and pathways are potential causal mediators of sex effects. Our findings are robust even after adjusting for multiple baseline comorbidities, and our work is rigorous in providing replication of key findings at two independent major academic medical centers with large numbers of complex and severe COVID-19 cases.

TABLE 4 | Replication mediation analyses of peak values* of biomarkers in MGH cohort.

	Total effect model[†] outcome: death	Mediator model[†] outcome: biomarker	Outcome model[†] outcome: death		Proportion mediated
	OR (sex)	Estimate (sex)	OR (sex)	OR (biomarker)	
hs-CRP					
All ($n = 1,088$)	2.24 ($p < 0.001$)	0.102 ($p = 0.058$)	2.09 ($p = 0.002$)	–[‡]	0.20 ($p = 0.048$)
Obese ($n = 491$)	1.92 ($p = 0.051$)	0.080 ($p = 0.277$)	1.78 ($p = 0.123$)	9.07 (p<0.001)	0.22 ($p = 0.284$)
Non-obese ($n = 597$)	2.44 ($p = 0.002$)	0.144 ($p = 0.065$)	2.18 ($p = 0.012$)	4.64 ($p < 0.001$)	0.22 ($p = 0.062$)
Ferritin					
All ($n = 1,070$)	2.33 ($p < 0.001$)	0.474 (p<0.001)	2.04 ($p = 0.002$)	–[‡]	0.33 ($p < 0.001$)
Obese ($n = 483$)	1.96 ($p = 0.046$)	0.510 ($p < 0.001$)	1.57 ($p = 0.204$)	2.62 (p<0.001)	0.51 ($p = 0.010$)
Non-obese ($n = 587$)	2.64 ($p = 0.001$)	0.456 (p<0.001)	2.47 ($p = 0.003$)	1.92 ($p < 0.001$)	0.24 ($p < 0.001$)
D-dimer					
All ($n = 1,050$)	2.17 ($p < 0.001$)	0.022 ($p = 0.676$)	2.27 (p<0.001)	–[‡]	0.02 ($p = 0.700$)
$\geq$ 65 yrs ($n = 421$)	2.00 ($p = 0.005$)	0.025 ($p = 0.762$)	2.13 ($p = 0.003$)	1.99 ($p < 0.001$)	0.02 ($p = 0.732$)
< 65 yrs ($n = 629$)	3.21 ($p = 0.041$)	0.025 ($p = 0.718$)	3.29 ($p = 0.044$)	2.97 ($p < 0.001$)	0.02 (p=0.710)
Creatinine					
All ($n = 1,084$)	2.25 ($p < 0.001$)	0.568 ($p < 0.001$)	1.47 ($p = 0.104$)	2.44 ($p < 0.001$)	0.57 (p<0.001)
hs-Troponin T					
All ($n = 1,026$)	2.25 ($p < 0.001$)	0.194 ($p < 0.001$)	1.99 ($p = 0.003$)	2.26 ($p < 0.001$)	0.19 ($p = 0.002$)

*Peak biomarker level was determined based on all measurements. All values were natural log transformed and standardized for analysis; [†] All models included terms for sex and were adjusted for age, obesity, race/ethnicity, and the number of biomarker measurements. The outcome model included both sex and the biomarker as predictor variables; [‡] The outcome model included a biomarker by obesity interaction and therefore the main effect of the biomarker was not reported here.
OR, odds ratio; hs-CRP, high sensitivity C-reactive protein; hs-Troponin T, high sensitivity cardiac Troponin T.

Sex differences in inflammatory responses, as reflected by peak hs-CRP and ferritin, may amplify sex differences in cardiac and renal injury and thus contribute to our finding that biomarkers of cardiac and kidney end-organ damage mediate a substantial proportion of the effect of sex on COVID-19 outcomes. Although previous studies have identified sex differences in the rate of COVID-19-related myocardial injury (3) and an association between acute cardiac injury and death in COVID-19 (23) ours is the first to address cardiac injury as a mediator of sex effects on COVID-19 outcomes. Similarly, prior studies have demonstrated a sex difference in COVID-19-related kidney disease and acute kidney injury (24), yet biomarkers of renal function have never been tested as mediators. Further studies are required to determine the extent to which the effects of inflammation and cardiac and renal damage are independent contributors to sex-mediation of poor COVID-19 outcomes.

Of several markers (including WBC and ESR, see **Supplementary Table S2**), we focused on hs-CRP as representative of systemic inflammation and broad activation of innate and adaptive immunity in COVID-19. Prior studies, including our own (22), have demonstrated an association between elevated inflammatory markers and death or ICU admission, with a stronger association in men as compared to women (9, 15, 25). However, our study is the first to suggest that inflammation directly mediates the effect of sex on COVID-19-related mortality. This mediation could be due to established sex differences in both the innate and adaptive immune pathways (26). Many of the genes involved in innate and adaptive immunity are located on the X chromosome. Some of them may escape X inactivation,

leading to a more comprehensive immune response in women as compared to men (26, 27). Men and women also differ in the production of cytokines and chemokines by innate immune cells. During inflammatory stress, men have higher levels of pro-inflammatory cytokine production than females (26, 28), which could lead to a more severe cytokine storm associated with worse COVID-19 outcomes. Apart from genetics, there may be hormonal factors contributing to sex differences in the immune response to infection (29, 30). Testosterone is known to have an immunosuppressive effect (11, 26). At the same time, estradiol is thought to enhance cell-mediated and humoral immune responses, and progesterone has anti-inflammatory effects and may also contribute to differences in T cell populations (26). In secondary analyses, we found a trend toward a greater mediation effect of hs-CRP in patients age <50 years, which might support a role for the greater hormonal differences at pre-menopausal age in the contribution to sex differences in the inflammatory milieu and COVID-19.

Ferritin was a less potent mediator than hs-CRP of the effect of sex on COVID-19 outcomes, though the mediation effect was statistically significant and may be clinically important. In studies of patients with COVID-19, ferritin has been shown to correlate with disease severity in both men and women (31–33). In one study and in contrast to our findings, ferritin levels were found to be independently associated with death in women but not in men (16). Our larger CUIMC/NYPH data is the first to suggest that ferritin mediates the effect of male sex on worse outcomes in COVID-19 and this finding was highly consistent in the independent MGH registry. There are multiple possible explanations for the role of ferritin in mediating sex-related outcomes. Ferritin synthesis may increase as a result of the COVID-19 cytokine storm or inflammation may stimulate leakage of intracellular ferritin (33). This would suggest that peak ferritin levels, similar to hs-CRP, reflect systemic inflammation in mediating the effect of sex on outcomes. Alternatively, ferritin may play an independent causal role in the inflammatory cascade, acting as a mediator of immune dysregulation (33). Given that women of all ages have lower ferritin levels than men (34), lower baseline levels of ferritin could in fact be protective in women. Interestingly, when stratified by obesity, more of the effect of male sex on the primary outcome of death was explained by peak ferritin among obese patients as compared to non-obese patients. This finding may relate to differences in significance of ferritin levels in non-obese vs. obese patients. While in lean individuals ferritin may predominantly be a marker of iron stores, in obesity ferritin may correlate more with inflammation (35).

In the primary CUIMC/NYP cohort, we found that peak D-dimer levels were also mediators of the effect of sex on COVID-19 outcomes. In contrast, D-dimer levels were not found to be a mediator of the association between sex and COVID-19 outcomes in the MGH cohort. One possible explanation is that this might reflect differences in anticoagulation practice patterns for patients with COVID-19 across institutions, particularly early in the pandemic (36). Published work does suggest that microvascular dysfunction and thrombosis play a role in the pathogenesis of COVID-19, and studies have demonstrated an increased risk of severe outcomes and death in patients with elevated D-dimer (37). While there have been insufficient data to demonstrate a sex difference in the association between D-dimer and outcomes, sex differences in endothelial dysfunction have been well-established (38). Increased coagulation disorders may also cause more myocardial injury in men than in women, leading to worse outcomes (3). Prior studies have suggested that menopause is a risk factor for worse outcomes in women with COVID-19 (13, 39). In our age-stratified secondary analyses (≥ 50 vs. <50 years of age) designed as a surrogate for pre- and post-menopausal status in women, the proportion mediated by D-dimer was similar across younger vs. older age strata suggesting that thromboembolic mechanisms that drive higher risk in men are unlikely to reflect hormonal differences found in pre- or post-menopausal women. Future studies will need to focus more specifically on sex-related COVID-19 risks, including thromboembolic, in pre- and post-menopausal women.

Methodological strengths of this work include the novel application of mediation analysis to sex-related COVID-19 outcomes as well as a robust replication sample in which findings were highly consistent. Additional strengths include the sample size, the inclusion of a large percentage of under-represented minorities and the evaluation of 15 distinct biomarkers as potential mediators of sex effects on COVID-19 outcomes. There are several limitations of our study. First, the study used observational data extracted from the EHR in which missing data and measurement error are inherent and can result in biased findings (40). Second, the causal mediation framework assumes no unmeasured confounding (21). Third, despite robust replication across CUIMC/NYP and MGH cohorts, these two studies have differences in design and regional clinical contexts. Fourth, biomarkers are inherently limited as a markers of causal mechanisms and in therapeutic targeting, as they are surrogates for the underlying causal pathway. Indeed, serum creatinine has significant limitations as a measure of kidney function or as a surrogate for kidney injury, but data were missing for calculation of more reliable measures of acute kidney injury (e.g., using KDIGO recommendations) (41). Further, all validated equations for eGFR incorporate sex rendering invalid analyses of sex mediation through such a derived biomarker. However, ease in clinical use of these biomarkers means our findings are immediately translatable to clinical practice. There are also redundancies between clinically available biomarkers, e.g., we selected hsCRP over WBC and ESR because hsCRP had stronger sex-mediation effects than the other inflammatory markers (**Supplementary Table S2**). Moreover, given the complex relationships among sex, mediators and other factors in severe COVID-19 outcomes, future work on additional pathophysiological pathways is needed. Our analyses were limited to the 15 clinically available candidate blood biomarkers selected for our study, and therefore we cannot exclude other biomarkers and organs as mediators. Specifically, our initial analyses suggest that larger sample sizes than ours are required to study the effect of biomarkers of hepatic injury within racial and ethnic strata. Finally, future studies are needed to define optimal clinical translation including use of mediators in clinical trials stratifying for high-risk patients.

In summary, we identified several distinct biomarkers of pathophysiological processes, including cardiac injury, that are reproducible mediators of the effect of sex on COVID-19 outcomes. Each of these pathways is a downstream manifestation of genetic, hormonal, and socio-demographic differences between men and women. And each offers a unique opportunity for better risk stratification, resource utilization, and targeted clinical trials toward personalized interventions and therapies for subgroups of patients at highest risk for poor COVID-19 outcomes.

AUTHOR CONTRIBUTIONS

HL: literature search and writing—original draft preparation. EK and CS: database organization and statistical analysis. HL, AF, and MR: conceptualization and writing—draft revision. All authors contributed to manuscript revision, provided comments, and agreed to the published version of the manuscript.

ACKNOWLEDGMENTS

Support for the creation of the MGH Patient Registry was provided by the MGH Division of Clinical Research and the Department of Medicine.

REFERENCES

1. Galbadage T, Peterson BM, Awada J, Buck AS, Ramirez DA, Wilson J, et al. Systematic review and meta-analysis of sex-specific COVID-19 clinical outcomes. *Front Med.* (2020) 7:348. doi: 10.3389/fmed.2020.00348

2. Palaiodimos L, Kokkinidis DG Li W, Karamanis D, Ognibene J, Arora S, et al. Severe obesity, increasing age and male sex are independently associated with worse in-hospital outcomes, and higher in-hospital mortality, in a cohort of patients with COVID-19 in the Bronx, New York. *Metabolism.* (2020) 108:154262. doi: 10.1016/j.metabol.2020.154262

3. Cheng R, Liu C, Yang J, Yang Y, Chen R, Ding X, et al. Sex Differences in the incidence and risk factors of myocardial injury in covid-19 patients: a retrospective cohort study. *Front Physiol.* (2021) 12:632123. doi: 10.3389/fphys.2021.632123

4. Guan WJ Ni ZY, Hu Y, Liang WH, Ou CQ, He JX, et al. Clinical characteristics of coronavirus disease 2019 in China. *N Engl J Med.* (2020) 382:1708–20. doi: 10.1056/NEJMoa2002032

5. Grasselli G, Zangrillo A, Zanella A, Antonelli M, Cabrini L, Castelli A, et al. Baseline characteristics and outcomes of 1,591 patients infected with sars-Cov-2 admitted to icus of the lombardy region, Italy. *JAMA.* (2020) 323:1574–81. doi: 10.1001/jama.2020.5394

6. Rapp JL, Lieberman-Cribbin W, Tuminello S, Taioli E. Male sex, severe obesity, older age, and chronic kidney disease are associated with COVID-19 severity and mortality in New York City. *Chest.* (2021) 159:112–5. doi: 10.1016/j.chest.2020.08.2065

7. Gebhard C, Regitz-Zagrosek V, Neuhauser HK, Morgan R, Klein SL. Impact of sex and gender on COVID-19 outcomes in Europe. *Biol Sex Differ.* (2020) 11:29. doi: 10.1186/s13293-020-00304-9

8. Medzikovic L, Cunningham CM Li M, Amjedi M, Hong J, Ruffenach G, et al. Sex differences underlying preexisting cardiovascular disease and cardiovascular injury in COVID-19. *J Mol Cell Cardiol.* (2020) 148:25–33. doi: 10.1016/j.yjmcc.2020.08.007

9. Meng Y, Wu P, Lu W, Liu K, Ma K, Huang L, et al. Sex-specific clinical characteristics and prognosis of coronavirus disease-19 infection in Wuhan, China: a retrospective study of 168 severe patients. *PLoS Pathog.* (2020) 16:e1008520. doi: 10.1371/journal.ppat.1008520

10. Alkhouli M, Nanjundappa A, Annie F, Bates MC, Bhatt DL. Sex differences in case fatality rate of COVID-19: insights from a multinational registry. *Mayo Clin Proc.* (2020) 95:1613–20. doi: 10.1016/j.mayocp.2020.05.014

11. Haitao T, Vermunt JV, Abeykoon J, Ghamrawi R, Gunaratne M, Jayachandran M, et al. COVID-19 and sex differences: mechanisms and biomarkers. *Mayo Clin Proc.* (2020) 95:2189–203. doi: 10.1016/j.mayocp.2020.07.024

12. Viveiros A, Rasmuson J, Vu J, Mulvagh SL, Yip CYY, Norris CM, et al. Sex differences in COVID-19: candidate pathways, genetics of ACE2, and sex hormones. *Am J Physiol Heart Circ Physiol.* (2021) 320:H296–304. doi: 10.1152/ajpheart.00755.2020

13. Ding T, Zhang J, Wang T, Cui P, Chen Z, Jiang J, et al. Potential influence of menstrual status and sex hormones on female severe acute respiratory syndrome coronavirus 2 infection: a cross-sectional multicenter study in Wuhan, China. *Clin Infect Dis.* (2021) 72:e240–e8. doi: 10.1093/cid/ciaa1022

14. Ten-Caten F, Gonzalez-Dias P, Castro I, Ogava RLT, Giddaluru J, Silva JCS, et al. In-depth analysis of laboratory parameters reveals the interplay between sex, age, and systemic inflammation in individuals with COVID-19. *Int J Infect Dis.* (2021) 105:579–87. doi: 10.1016/j.ijid.2021.03.016

15. Lau ES, McNeill JN, Paniagua SM, Liu EE, Wang JK, Bassett IV, et al. Sex differences in inflammatory markers in patients hospitalized with COVID-19 infection: insights from the MGH COVID-19 patient registry. *PLoS ONE.* (2021) 16:e0250774. doi: 10.1371/journal.pone.0250774

16. Yoshida Y, Gillet SA, Brown MI, Zu Y, Wilson SM, Ahmed SJ, et al. Clinical characteristics and outcomes in women and men hospitalized for coronavirus disease 2019 in New Orleans. *Biol Sex Differ.* (2021) 12:20. doi: 10.1186/s13293-021-00359-2

17. Marik PE, DePerrior SE, Ahmad Q, Dodani S. Gender-based disparities in COVID-19 patient outcomes. *J Investig Med.* (2021). doi: 10.1136/jim-2020-001641

18. Gupta A, Madhavan MV, Poterucha TJ, DeFilippis EM, Hennessey JA, Redfors B, et al. Association between antecedent statin use and decreased mortality in hospitalized patients with COVID-19. *Nat Commun.* (2021) 12:1325. doi: 10.1038/s41467-021-21553-1

19. Bassett IV, Triant VA, Bunda BA, Selvaggi CA, Shinnick DJ, He W, et al. Massachusetts general hospital Covid-19 registry reveals two distinct populations of hospitalized patients by race and ethnicity. *PLoS ONE.* (2020) 15:e0244270. doi: 10.1371/journal.pone.0244270

20. Seiglie J, Platt J, Cromer SJ, Bunda B, Foulkes AS, Bassett IV, et al. Diabetes as a risk factor for poor early outcomes in patients hospitalized with COVID-19. *Diabetes Care.* (2020) 43:2938–44. doi: 10.2337/dc20-1506

21. Imai K, Keele L, Yamamoto T. Identification, inference and sensitivity analysis for causal mediation effects. *Statistical Science* (2010) 25:51–71. doi: 10.1214/10-STS321

22. Foulkes AS, Selvaggi C, Shinnick D, Lumish H, Kim E, Cao T, et al. Understanding the link between obesity and severe COVID-19 outcomes: causal mediation by systemic inflammatory response. *J Clin Endocrinol Metab.* (2021) 107:e698–e707. doi: 10.1210/clinem/dgab629

23. Li JW, Han TW, Woodward M, Anderson CS, Zhou H, Chen YD, et al. The impact of 2019 novel coronavirus on heart injury: a Systematic review and meta-analysis. *Prog Cardiovasc Dis.* (2020) 63:518–24. doi: 10.1016/j.pcad.2020.04.008

24. Cheng Y, Luo R, Wang K, Zhang M, Wang Z, Dong L, et al. Kidney disease is associated with in-hospital death of patients with COVID-19. *Kidney Int.* (2020) 97:829–38. doi: 10.1016/j.kint.2020.03.005

25. Qin L, Li X, Shi J, Yu M, Wang K, Tao Y, et al. Gendered effects on inflammation reaction and outcome of COVID-19 patients in Wuhan. *J Med Virol.* (2020) 92:2684–92. doi: 10.1002/jmv.26137

26. Klein SL, Flanagan KL. Sex differences in immune responses. *Nat Rev Immunol.* (2016) 16:626–38. doi: 10.1038/nri.2016.90

27. Libert C, Dejager L, Pinheiro I. The X chromosome in immune functions: when a chromosome makes the difference. *Nat Rev Immunol.* (2010) 10:594–604. doi: 10.1038/nri2815

28. Ferguson JF, Patel PN, Shah RY, Mulvey CK, Gadi R, Nijjar PS, et al. Race and gender variation in response to evoked inflammation. *J Transl Med.* (2013) 11:63. doi: 10.1186/1479-5876-11-63

29. Straub RH. The complex role of estrogens in inflammation. *Endocr Rev.* (2007) 28:521–74. doi: 10.1210/er.2007-0001

30. Taneja V. Sex hormones determine immune response. *Front Immunol.* (2018) 9:1931. doi: 10.3389/fimmu.2018.01931

31. Gandini O, Criniti A, Ballesio L, Giglio S, Galardo G, Gianni W, et al. Serum ferritin is an independent risk factor for acute respiratory distress syndrome in COVID-19. *J Infect.* (2020) 81:979–97. doi: 10.1016/j.jinf.2020.09.006

32. Gandini O, Criniti A, Gagliardi MC, Ballesio L, Giglio S, Balena A, et al. Sex-disaggregated data confirm serum ferritin as an independent predictor of disease severity both in male and female COVID-19 patients. *J Infect.* (2021) 82:414–51. doi: 10.1016/j.jinf.2020.10.012

33. Lin Z, Long F, Yang Y, Chen X, Xu L, Yang M. Serum ferritin as an independent risk factor for severity in COVID-19 patients. *J Infect.* (2020) 81:647–79. doi: 10.1016/j.jinf.2020.06.053

34. Ellidag HY, Eren E, Akdag M, Giray O, Kiraz K, Yilmaz N. The relationship between serum ferritin levels and serum lipids and HDL function with respect to age and gender. *Ukr Biochem J.* (2016) 88:76–86. doi: 10.15407/ubj88.06.076

35. Khan A, Khan WM, Ayub M, Humayun M, Haroon M. Ferritin is a marker of inflammation rather than iron deficiency in overweight and obese people. *J Obes.* (2016) 2016:1937320. doi: 10.1155/2016/1937320

36. Rosovsky RP, Sanfilippo KM, Wang TF, Rajan SK, Shah S, Martin KA, et al. Anticoagulation practice patterns in COVID-19: a global survey. *Res Pract Thromb Haemost.* (2020). doi: 10.1002/rth2.12414

37. Shah S, Shah K, Patel SB, Patel FS, Osman M, Velagapudi P, et al. Elevated D-dimer levels are associated with increased risk of mortality in coronavirus disease 2019: a systematic review and meta-analysis. *Cardiol Rev.* (2020) 28:295–302. doi: 10.1097/CRD.0000000000000330

38. Stanhewicz AE, Wenner MM, Stachenfeld NS. Sex differences in endothelial function important to vascular health and overall cardiovascular disease risk across the lifespan. *Am J Physiol Heart Circ Physiol.* (2018) 315:H1569–H88. doi: 10.1152/ajpheart.00396.2018

39. Wang XW, Hu H, Xu ZY, Zhang GK Yu QH, Yang HL, et al. Association of menopausal status with COVID-19 outcomes: a propensity score matching analysis. *Biol Sex Differ.* (2021) 12:16. doi: 10.1186/s13293-021-00363-6

40. Weber GM, Adams WG, Bernstam EV, Bickel JP, Fox KP, Marsolo

K, et al. Biases introduced by filtering electronic health records for patients with "complete data". *J Am Med Inform Assoc.* (2017) 24:1134–41. doi: 10.1093/jamia/ocx071

41. KDIGO. Clinical practice guideline for acute kidney injury. *Kidney Internat Suppl.* (2012) 2:8–12. doi: 10.1038/kisup.2012.1

14

Blood Glucose Control Strategy for Type 2 Diabetes Patients with COVID-19

Hiroyuki Futatsugi[1†], Masato Iwabu[1*†], Miki Okada-Iwabu[1,2], Koh Okamoto[3], Yosuke Amano[4], Yutaka Morizaki[5], Takashi Kadowaki[1,6,7] and Toshimasa Yamauchi[1]

[1] Department of Diabetes and Metabolic Diseases, Graduate School of Medicine, The University of Tokyo, Tokyo, Japan, [2] Laboratory for Advanced Research on Pathophysiology of Metabolic Diseases, The University of Tokyo, Tokyo, Japan, [3] Department of Infectious Diseases, The University of Tokyo Hospital, Tokyo, Japan, [4] Department of Respiratory Medicine, The University of Tokyo Hospital, Tokyo, Japan, [5] Department of Orthopaedic Surgery, The University of Tokyo Hospital, Tokyo, Japan, [6] Department of Prevention of Diabetes and Life-Style Related Diseases, The University of Tokyo, Tokyo, Japan, [7] Toranomon Hospital, Tokyo, Japan

*Correspondence:
Masato Iwabu
iwabu-tky@umin.ac.jp

[†] These authors have contributed equally to this work

Since December 2019, coronavirus disease 2019 (COVID-19) caused by a novel coronavirus has spread all over the world affecting tens of millions of people. Another pandemic affecting the modern world, type 2 diabetes mellitus is among the major risk factors for mortality from COVID-19. Current evidence, while limited, suggests that proper blood glucose control may help prevent exacerbation of COVID-19 even in patients with type 2 diabetes mellitus. Under current circumstances where the magic bullet for the disease remains unavailable, it appears that the role of blood glucose control cannot be stressed too much. In this review the profile of each anti-diabetic agent is discussed in relation to COVID-19.

Keywords: COVID-19, diabetes mellitus, antidiabetic agents, healthy diet, exercise

CORONAVIRUS DISEASE 2019 PANDEMIC

Coronavirus disease 2019 (COVID-19), caused by coronavirus SARS coronavirus 2 (SARS-CoV-2), was originally identified in Wuhan, China in December 2019 (1). Since then, the disease has spread all over the world at a tremendous rate and the number of confirmed cases already exceeded 13 million, killing more than 570 thousand people (2). Though measures are being taken in affected countries, such as lockdown of major cities, to control the pandemic, the numbers are still growing day by day (3, 4).

SARS-CoV-2 belongs to the Betacoronavirus genus as SARS coronavirus (SARS-CoV) and MERS coronavirus (MERS-CoV) do (5). As with SARS-CoV, SARS-CoV-2 spike glycoprotein interacts with and binds to human angiotensin-converting enzyme 2 (ACE2) when the virus enters into target cells (6). While ACE2, a type I transmembrane glycoprotein, serves as a functional receptor for SARS-CoV-2, ACE2 is also shown to play a protective role against acute respiratory distress syndrome (ARDS) and SARS pathogenesis by catalyzing angiotensin I and angiotensin II to angiotensin (1-9) and angiotensin (1-7), respectively (7). However, its overall impact on COVID-19 remains to be further elucidated.

A clue could be found with angiotensin-converting enzyme inhibitors (ACE inhibitors) and angiotensin II receptor blockers (ARBs). Since several data suggested that these agents can increase ACE2 expression through their influence on the level of angiotensin II, there was concern over their potential negative influence on COVID-19 morbidity, severity and mortality rates (8). However, multiple large-scaled studies show that their use affected none of these rates (9–11). Actually, at present, almost all medical associations, including the International Society of Hypertension, American College of Cardiology, American Heart Association and Heart Failure Society of America, have published statements recommending the continued use of ACE inhibitors and ARBs (12, 13).

COVID-19 is thought unlikely to become severe in a majority of cases. In fact, a recent meta-analysis of 47,344 patients with COVID-19 in China shows that the risks of severity and mortality were 18.0 and 3.2%, respectively, among these patients, while these rates increased if patients had comorbidities (14).

COVID-19 AND DIABETES

Diabetes mellitus is another global pandemic affecting 463 million people worldwide (15). In the face of the COVID-19 pandemic, two facts need to be taken to heart. First, nutrition and exercise therapy represent the cornerstone of diabetes management (16). However, the resultant need for home confinement to control the pandemic, as well as for a new lifestyle to reduce the risk of infection, is shown to reduce physical activity and increase sweet food consumption (17, 18), while, now more than ever, the importance of healthy diet and exercise needs to be stressed. Second, which concerns the main theme of this review, diabetes is among the comorbidities associated with increased risk of COVID-19 (19). According to a recent meta-analysis, COVID-19 patients who had diabetes at baseline had increased severity and mortality (HR, 2.11 [CI, 1.40–3.18], 1.69 [CI, 1.22–2.33], respectively), although the prevalence of diabetes in the affected population did not seem to differ from that in the non-affected population in Asia (20). Fortunately, however, it is indicated in a retrospective multicenter study conducted in China that proper blood glucose control may reduce not only the severity of COVID-19 but mortality from the disease in patients with pre-existing diabetes showing improvements in systemic inflammation as measured by serum inflammation markers (21). Actually, in the study, during the 28-day observation period, patients with favorable glycemic control (3.9–10 mmol/L) had a significantly lower mortality rate compared to those with poorly glycemic control (the lowest BG level, >3.9 mmol/L or the highest BG level, >10 mmol/L) (HR 0.14 [CI, 0.03–0.60])(21). In the current situation where COVID-19 and diabetes are so prevalent that they combine to affect a high proportion of patients and where there is no critical medicine or vaccine for COVID-19, the fact that blood glucose control has a role to play in reducing the severity of the disease as well as mortality from the disease, cannot be stressed too much (21).

STRATEGY FOR BLOOD GLUCOSE CONTROL

Then, how should we achieve blood glucose control? First, we would suggest that PCR-confirmed asymptomatic type 2 diabetic patients with COVID-19 or those with mild self-limiting COVID-19 should continue with their current prescription

because, to date, there is no evidence to suggest that certain glucose-lowering agents interact with or worsen the disease in patients with asymptomatic or mild COVID-19 (22). This strategy is supported by the fact that hyperglycemia itself is likely to lead to greater severity of COVID-19 and higher mortality from the disease (23, 24). In patients with moderate to severe symptoms who need hospital admission, however, given the pathophysiological and clinical characteristics of COVID-19, some drugs may not be deemed favorable, due to their side effects that could potentially adversely affect the course of the illness. In this review focused on biguanides, thiazolidinediones, sulfonylureas, dipeptidyl peptidase-4 (DPP4) inhibitors, glucagon-like peptide-1 receptor (GLP-1R) agonists, sodium-glucose cotransporter-2 (SGLT2) inhibitors and insulin, their profiles will be discussed in relation to COVID-19.

BIGUANIDES

Biguanides, represented by metformin, is one of the most frequently prescribed oral glucose-lowering agents. Metformin mainly functions by activating AMP-activated protein kinase (AMPK) through inhibition of the respiratory chain of mitochondria thereby subsequently reducing gluconeogenesis in the liver (25). In most situations, metformin is a well-tolerated drug with a relatively low rate of adverse effects. However, as it inhibits mitochondrial respiration and increases lactate production, it may induce lactic acidosis in some patients receiving it, with nearly half of all patients developing lactic acidosis dying from it. Of note, while the risk of lactic acidosis is increased in patients with renal or hepatic impairment, dehydration, shock, hypoxic states, sepsis and advanced age (26), these conditions are often found to be present in patients with severe COVID-19 (27). In addition, up to half of all hospitalized COVID-19 patients are shown to suffer deep venous thrombosis (DVT) thus often requiring the use of contrast-enhanced CT for DVT assessment (28). When transient renal impairment occurs following injection of an iodinated contrast agent in patients receiving a biguanide, however, the renal excretion of the drug is decreased, and their lactic acid levels increased, thus placing these patients at risk of lactic acidosis (29). On the contrary, a recent retrospective study performed in China showed that metformin-treated patients hospitalized for COVID-19 had a lower mortality rate compared to non-metformin-treated patients (30, 31). Thus, overall, while diabetic patients with asymptomatic or mild COVID-19 may continue current metformin therapy and further interventional studies should be conducted to prove or disprove this recommendation, it appears that, as a rule, metformin should be withdrawn in hospitalized patients.

THIAZOLIDINEDIONES

Thiazolidinediones are shown to achieve their blood glucose-lowering effect by activating peroxisome proliferator-activated receptor γ (PPARγ) thereby increasing insulin sensitivity (32). In addition to their glucose-lowering effects, thiazolidinediones are also shown to exert immunomodulatory effects (33). Given that immune hyperactivity is considered to be involved in the pathophysiology of COVID-19, it appears reasonable to assume that they may have some positive impact on the disease progression (33–36). However, there are also some concerns. First, while its clinical impact is not known, pioglitazone has the potential to enhance ACE2 expression in the liver, adipose tissue and skeletal muscle (37, 38), suggesting that the use of thiazolidinediones may affect not only the prevalence of COVID-19 but the mortality from the disease. Second, thiazolidinediones also act on the collecting tubule to increase water and sodium reabsorption by enhancing the expression of the epithelial Na^+ channel, thus causing edema and fluid retention (39, 40). This adverse effect may be enhanced in patients with COVID-19, given that the disease is sometimes shown to damage the kidneys and myocardium (41, 42). Therefore, it appears that, for the time being at least, it is advisable to avoid using thiazolidinediones in hospitalized patients.

SULFONYLUREAS AND GLINIDES

Sulfonylureas, the oldest oral antidiabetic drugs, are shown to promote insulin release from pancreatic β cells by binding to and closing the ATP-sensitive potassium channel resulting in depolarization of the plasma membrane and increased calcium influx thus leading to insulin exocytosis (43). Again, glinides represent viable options in managing postprandial hyperglycemia due to their rapid and short-lasting insulinotropic effects (44, 45). However, sulfonylureas are known to cause hypoglycemia at a non-negligible rate with the risk shown to increase in acute settings (46), thus making their use inappropriate in patients with severe COVID-19.

DIPEPTIDYL PEPTIDASE-4 INHIBITORS

DPP4 inhibitors exert their anti-diabetic effects by inhibiting DPP4, which degrades incretin hormones, gastric inhibitory polypeptide (GIP) and glucagon-like peptide-1 (GLP-1), thus elevating blood levels of these hormones. Since these hormones stimulate insulin release glucose-dependently, DPP4 inhibitors lower blood glucose levels with no significant risk of hypoglycemia (43). Although DPP4 is considered to be a functional receptor of MERS-CoV (47), a sibling of SARS-CoV-2, there is no evidence to date to show that it interacts with SARS-CoV-2. Actually, a case control study conducted in Italy showed no association between the exposure to DPP4 inhibitor and the risk of hospitalization due to COVID-19 (48). Of note, DPP4 inhibitors exert anti-inflammatory effects without increasing the risk of infectious disease and thus may prove protective against COVID-19-induced lung injury (49–51). To confirm these hypotheses, a phase 4 clinical trial of linagliptin vs. insulin is currently underway to compare their effectiveness not only in achieving glucose control but in preventing the progression of COVID-19 in type 2 diabetic patients with mild to moderate COVID-19 (52). While, given its glucose-dependent effects and the risk of hypoglycemia thought to be relatively low with this DPP-4 inhibitor, the use of DPP-4 inhibitors as a class

may be deemed relatively safe in these patients mild to moderate COVID-19, consideration should be given to switching to insulin in patients with severe COVID-19.

GLUCAGON-LIKE PEPTIDE-1 RECEPTOR AGONISTS

While the mechanism of action of GLP-1R agonists is not fully understood, it seems likely that it involves cAMP signaling pathways and intracellular glucose metabolism in restoring β-cell glucose sensitivity (53). Due to this mechanism, GLP-1R agonists are assumed to lower blood glucose with relatively low risk of hypoglycemia (54). In addition, they help reduce food intake and body weight and thus may often be beneficial for diabetic patients who tend to be overweight (53–55). Also, their cardio- and renoprotective profile may prove beneficial for patients with COVID-19 (56, 57). In addition, of the GLP-1 agonists, liraglutide has the potential to increase lung ACE2 expression, while the net effect of ACE2 on COVID-19 still remains unknown (58). Nevertheless, GLP-1R agonists may as well be withdrawn from diabetic patients requiring hospitalization with COVID-19, given that their frequent adverse events, gastrointestinal symptoms (e.g., nausea, diarrhea or vomiting) are likely to worsen dehydration and, as a consequence, cause renal failure, which often occur in patients with COVID-19 (27, 53).

SODIUM-GLUCOSE COTRANSPORTER-2 INHIBITORS

Unlike other oral glucose-lowering agents described above, this class of drugs exert their effects, independently of insulin, by blocking sodium-glucose cotransporter 2 (SGLT2) in the renal proximal tubules from reabsorbing filtered glucose, i.e., by increasing glucose excretion thereby decreasing levels of blood glucose (59). Moreover, SGLT2 inhibitors are known to have cardio- and renoprotective effects (60–62) and have the potential to improve systemic metabolism, thus possibly preventing respiratory failure and organ dysfunction associated with COVID-19. To test this speculation, a phase 3 international, multicenter, double-blind, randomized, placebo-controlled trial of dapagliflozin is now underway in hospitalized, mild-to-moderate COVID-19 patients with preexisting comorbidities (63). However, an international expert panel warns that increased glucose excretion may also lead to fluid loss, possibly resulting in worsening of dehydration and onset of diabetic ketoacidosis in diabetic patients with COVID-19 (22, 64). Based on these findings, therefore, consideration should be given to discontinuing SGLT2 inhibitors in diabetic patients with COVID-19 at high risk of respiratory failure and thrombosis.

INSULIN ANALOGS

The only hormone available to lower blood levels of glucose, insulin is released from pancreatic β cells sensitized by glucose influx through glucose transporter type 2 (GLUT2) and stimulates the uptake of carbohydrates, peptides and lipids by

TABLE 1 | Ongoing trials evaluating the antidiabetic drugs in COVID-19 patients.

Clinical trial number	Clinical phase/Multicenter	Arms	Target number of patients	Primary outcome	Estimated date of study completion
NCT04341935	4/No	• Experimental arm: linagliptin + standard of care insulin regimen as per hospital protocol during hospitalization for up to 14 days • Active comparator arm: standard of care insulin regimen as per hospital protocol during hospitalization for up to 14 days	20	1. Changes in glucose levels	March 30, 2021
NCT04371978	3/No	• Experimental arm: linagliptin + standard of care insulin regimen as per hospital protocol during their entire hospitalization • Nonintervention arm: standard of care insulin regimen as per hospital protocol during their entire hospitalization	100	1. Time to clinical change	September 30, 2021
NCT04365517	3/No	• Active comparator arm: sitagliptin + nutritional therapy with or without insulin treatment • Nonintervention arm: nutritional therapy with or without insulin treatment	170	1. Time for clinical improvement 2. Clinical parameters of acute lung disease 3. Biochemical parameter of acute lung disease	December 30, 2020
NCT04473274	4/No	• Experimental arm: pioglitazone 15–30 mg daily oral or enteral during hospitalization for up to 30 days + standard of care • Standard of care	20	1. Adverse events outcomes without attribution 2. Adverse events attributable	June 1, 2021
NCT04510194	2 (prevention), 3 (treatment)/No	Prevention • Experimental arm: metformin (500 mg; twice daily) • Comparator: placebo Treatment • Experimental: metformin (500 mg; twice daily) • Placebo	1,522	1. Rate of death due to COVID-19 2. Rate of hospitalization due to COVID-19 3. Rate of emergency department utilization 4. Rate of urgent care utilization	September 2021
NCT04350593	3/Yes	• Active comparator: dapagliflozin 10 mg daily • Placebo comparator arm: dapagliflozin matching placebo 10 mg daily	900	1. Time to first occurrence of either death from any cause or new/worsened organ dysfunction through 30 days of follow up	December 2020

other cells. Simultaneously, it inhibits hepatic gluconeogenesis and glycolysis, thus causing a rapid drop of blood glucose (65, 66). In normal settings, the goal of insulin therapy is to reproduce physiologic insulin secretion using long-acting analogs as basal insulin release and rapid-acting analogs as prandial insulin release (67). Unlike other oral antidiabetic agents, insulin has been used in critically ill patients whose prognosis is shown to improve to a greater extent with conventional insulin therapy than with intensive insulin therapy (68, 69). While insulin therapy prior to admission was shown to be associated with higher mortality in patients with COVID-19 (70, 71), there is a possibility that blood glucose control with insulin therapy during hospitalization leads to reductions in the risk of sever disease in these patients (72). Of course, when using insulin, close monitoring of blood glucose levels is essential, because it is sometimes associated with hypoglycemic events thus possibly raising mortality rates in critically ill patients (73, 74). However, given the current circumstances where there is no accumulated evidence to support the use of other agents, insulin appears to be the best choice for diabetic inpatients with COVID-19.

ONGOING STUDIES

While the possible harms and benefits of antidiabetic drugs have been summarized in the context of COVID-19, some of these recommendations remain rather hypothetical, because of the paucity of current evidence. Again, several clinical trials are now underway to investigate the actual effect of these drugs in controlling blood glucose diabetic patients with COVID-19, with some of these drugs expected to prevent exacerbation of COVID-19 even in non-diabetic patients. The characteristics of these trials are summarized in **Table 1**. These include NCT04341935 and NCT04371978, both randomized open label studies in diabetic patients with COVID-19, with the former intended to prove the efficacy of the investigational drugs in controlling blood glucose, and the latter aimed to reveal the efficacy of the study drugs in improving the severity of the disease (52, 75); NCT04365517, also a randomized controlled open label study designed to investigate the potential respiratory role of the DPP4 inhibitor sitagliptin in diabetic patients suffering from pneumonia due to COVID-19 (76). Through these studies, DPP4 inhibitors may be shown to be effective in controlling blood glucose in diabetic patients with COVID-19. Again, a non-randomized matching cohort study, NCT04473274 is intended to investigate the safety of the thiazolidinedione pioglitazone in patients with relative hyperglycemia requiring hospital admission due to COVID-19 (77) and may be able to address the speculative concern posed above. NCT04510194 is a large-scale, randomized, quadruple blinded study evaluating metformin not only for its therapeutic but for its preventive role against COVID-19 (78). Given the large sample size and the reliable study design, as well as the fact that, to date, virtually no drug has been proved to prevent the infection itself, the results of this study are worth paying attention to. Furthermore, another large-scale study, NCT04350593 should be of particular interest, given the unavailability of any established treatment for the disease (63). Again, overall, the outcomes of these trials may help further optimize blood glucose control strategy for diabetic patients with COVID-19.

CONCLUSION

The present review was an attempt to summarize the profiles of currently available antidiabetic agents and their role in maintaining blood glucose control in hospitalized diabetic patients with COVID-19. While it remains important to continue current regimens for glucose control in patients with mild, self-limiting COVID-19, it appears that insulin may be a good choice for patients with severe COVID-19, while DPP4 inhibitors may also prove to be a good choice, along with insulin, for patients with mild to moderate disease, pending the results of clinical trials currently underway. At any rate, given that the COVID-19 pandemic is unlikely to end any time soon and that diabetes is closely associated with disease progression, continued efforts need to be made to accumulate evidence that guides the use of antidiabetic agents in diabetic patients with COVID-19 and to establish the best possible approach to achieving blood glucose control in these patients.

AUTHOR CONTRIBUTIONS

HF, MI, MO-I, and TY wrote the manuscript. All authors reviewed the manuscript.

REFERENCES

1. Zhu N, Zhang D, Wang W, Li X, Yang B, Song J, et al. A novel coronavirus from patients with pneumonia in China, 2019. *N Engl J Med.* (2020) 382:727–33. doi: 10.1056/NEJMoa2001017
2. *Coronavirus Disease (COVID-19) Outbreak Situation.* World Health Organization (2020). Available online at: https://www.who.int/emergencies/diseases/novel-coronavirus-2019/ (accessed July 14, 2020).
3. Lopez L, Rodo X. The end of social confinement and COVID-19 re-emergence risk. *Nat Hum Behav.* (2020) 4:746–55. doi: 10.1038/s41562-020-0908-8
4. Scala A, Flori A, Spelta A, Brugnoli E, Cinelli M, Quattrociocchi W, et al. Time, space and social interactions: exit mechanisms for the Covid-19 epidemics. *Sci Rep.* (2020) 10:13764. doi: 10.1038/s41598-020-70631-9
5. Lu R, Zhao X, Li J, Niu P, Yang B, Wu H, et al. Genomic characterisation and epidemiology of 2019 novel coronavirus: implications for virus origins and receptor binding. *Lancet.* (2020) 395:565–74. doi: 10.1016/S0140-6736(20)30251-8
6. Lan J, Ge J, Yu J, Shan S, Zhou H, Fan S, et al. Structure of the SARS-CoV-2 spike receptor-binding domain bound to the ACE2 receptor. *Nature.* (2020) 581:215–20. doi: 10.1038/s41586-020-2180-5
7. Imai Y, Kuba K, Ohto-Nakanishi T, Penninger JM. Angiotensin-converting enzyme 2 (ACE2) in disease pathogenesis. *Circ J.* (2010) 74:405–10. doi: 10.1253/circj.CJ-10-0045
8. Vaduganathan M, Vardeny O, Michel T, McMurray JJV, Pfeffer MA, Solomon SD. Renin-angiotensin-aldosterone system inhibitors in patients with Covid-19. *N Engl J Med.* (2020) 382:1653–9. doi: 10.1056/NEJMsr2005760
9. Mancia G, Rea F, Ludergnani M, Apolone G, Corrao G. Renin-angiotensin-aldosterone system blockers and the risk of Covid-19. *N Engl J Med.* (2020) 382:2431–40. doi: 10.1056/NEJMoa2006923
10. Reynolds HR, Adhikari S, Pulgarin C, Troxel AB, Iturrate E, Johnson SB, et al. Renin-angiotensin-aldosterone system inhibitors and risk of Covid-19. *N Engl J Med.* (2020) 382:2441–8. doi: 10.1056/NEJMoa2008975
11. Fosbol EL, Butt JH, Ostergaard L, Andersson C, Selmer C, Kragholm K, et al. Association of angiotensin-converting enzyme inhibitor or angiotensin receptor blocker use with COVID-19 diagnosis and mortality. *JAMA.* (2020) 324:168–77. doi: 10.1001/jama.2020.11301

12. *A Statement From the International Society of Hypertension on COVID-19.* International Society of Hypertension (2020). Available online at: https://ish-world.com/news/a/A-statement-from-the-International-Society-of-Hypertension-on-COVID-19/ (accessed August 6, 2020).
13. *HFSA/ACC/AHA Statement Addresses Concerns Re: Using RAAS Antagonists in COVID-19.* American College of Cardiology (2020). Available online at: https://www.acc.org/latest-in-cardiology/articles/2020/03/17/08/59/hfsa-acc-aha-statement-addresses-concerns-re-using-raas-antagonists-in-covid-19 (accessed August 6, 2020).
14. Hu Y, Sun J, Dai Z, Deng H, Li X, Huang Q, et al. Prevalence and severity of corona virus disease 2019 (COVID-19): a systematic review and meta-analysis. *J Clin Virol.* (2020) 127:104371. doi: 10.1016/j.jcv.2020.104371
15. *IDF Diabetes Atlas Ninth Edition.* (2019). Available online at: https://www.diabetesatlas.org/en/ (accessed July 14, 2020).
16. American Diabetes A. 4. Lifestyle management: standards of medical care in diabetes-2018. *Diabetes Care.* (2018) 41(Suppl. 1):S38–50. doi: 10.2337/dc18-S004
17. Martinez-Ferran M, de la Guia-Galipienso F, Sanchis-Gomar F, Pareja-Galeano H. Metabolic impacts of confinement during the COVID-19 pandemic due to modified diet and physical activity habits. *Nutrients.* (2020) 12:1549. doi: 10.3390/nu12061549
18. Ruiz-Roso MB, de Carvalho Padilha P, Mantilla-Escalante DC, Ulloa N, Brun P, Acevedo-Correa D, et al. Covid-19 confinement and changes of adolescent's dietary trends in Italy, Spain, Chile, Colombia and Brazil. *Nutrients.* (2020) 12:1807. doi: 10.3390/nu12061807
19. Yan Y, Yang Y, Wang F, Ren H, Zhang S, Shi X, et al. Clinical characteristics and outcomes of patients with severe covid-19 with diabetes. *BMJ Open Diabetes Res Care.* (2020) 8:e001343. doi: 10.1136/bmjdrc-2020-001343
20. Singh AK, Gillies CL, Singh R, Singh A, Chudasama Y, Coles B, et al. Prevalence of co-morbidities and their association with mortality in patients with COVID-19: a systematic review and meta-analysis. *Diabetes Obes Metab.* (2020). doi: 10.1111/dom.14124. [Epub ahead of print].
21. Zhu L, She ZG, Cheng X, Qin JJ, Zhang XJ, Cai J, et al. Association of blood glucose control and outcomes in patients with COVID-19 and pre-existing type 2 diabetes. *Cell Metab.* (2020) 31:1068–77.e3. doi: 10.1016/j.cmet.2020.04.021

22. Bornstein SR, Rubino F, Khunti K, Mingrone G, Hopkins D, Birkenfeld AL, et al. Practical recommendations for the management of diabetes in patients with COVID-19. *Lancet Diabetes Endocrinol.* (2020) 8:546–50. doi: 10.1016/S2213-8587(20)30152-2

23. Bode B, Garrett V, Messler J, McFarland R, Crowe J, Booth R, et al. Glycemic characteristics and clinical outcomes of COVID-19 patients hospitalized in the United States. *J Diabetes Sci Technol.* (2020) 14:813–21. doi: 10.1177/1932296820924469

24. Iacobellis G, Penaherrera CA, Bermudez LE, Bernal Mizrachi E. Admission hyperglycemia and radiological findings of SARS-CoV2 in patients with and without diabetes. *Diabetes Res Clin Pract.* (2020) 164:108185. doi: 10.1016/j.diabres.2020.108185

25. Rena G, Hardie DG, Pearson ER. The mechanisms of action of metformin. *Diabetologia.* (2017) 60:1577–85. doi: 10.1007/s00125-017-4342-z

26. DeFronzo R, Fleming GA, Chen K, Bicsak TA. Metformin-associated lactic acidosis: current perspectives on causes and risk. *Metabolism.* (2016) 65:20–9. doi: 10.1016/j.metabol.2015.10.014

27. Guan WJ, Ni ZY, Hu Y, Liang WH, Ou CQ, He JX, et al. Clinical characteristics of coronavirus disease 2019 in China. *N Engl J Med.* (2020) 382:1708–20. doi: 10.1056/NEJMoa2002032

28. Zhang L, Feng X, Zhang D, Jiang C, Mei H, Wang J, et al. Deep vein thrombosis in hospitalized patients with COVID-19 in Wuhan, China: prevalence, risk factors, and outcome. *Circulation.* (2020) 142:114–28. doi: 10.1161/CIRCULATIONAHA.120.046702

29. Jain V, Sharma D, Prabhakar H, Dash HH. Metformin-associated lactic acidosis following contrast media-induced nephrotoxicity. *Eur J Anaesthesiol.* (2008) 25:166–7. doi: 10.1017/S026502150700097X

30. Luo P, Qiu L, Liu Y, Liu XL, Zheng JL, Xue HY, et al. Metformin treatment was associated with decreased mortality in COVID-19 patients with diabetes in a retrospective analysis. *Am J Trop Med Hyg.* (2020) 103:69–72. doi: 10.4269/ajtmh.20-0375

31. Scheen AJ. Metformin and COVID-19: from cellular mechanisms to reduced mortality. *Diabetes Metab.* (2020). doi: 10.1016/j.diabet.2020.07.006. [Epub ahead of print].

32. Soccio RE, Chen ER, Lazar MA. Thiazolidinediones and the promise of insulin sensitization in type 2 diabetes. *Cell Metab.* (2014) 20:573–91. doi: 10.1016/j.cmet.2014.08.005

33. Ciavarella C, Motta I, Valente S, Pasquinelli G. Pharmacological (or synthetic) and nutritional agonists of PPAR-gamma as candidates for cytokine storm modulation in COVID-19 disease. *Molecules.* (2020) 25:2076. doi: 10.3390/molecules25092076

34. Tay MZ, Poh CM, Renia L, MacAry PA, Ng LFP. The trinity of COVID-19: immunity, inflammation and intervention. *Nat Rev Immunol.* (2020) 20:363–74. doi: 10.1038/s41577-020-0311-8

35. Jagat JM, Kalyan KG, Subir R. Use of pioglitazone in people with type 2 diabetes mellitus with coronavirus disease 2019 (COVID-19): boon or bane? *Diabetes Metab Syndr.* (2020) 14:829–31. doi: 10.1016/j.dsx.2020.06.015

36. Carboni E, Carta AR, Carboni E. Can pioglitazone be potentially useful therapeutically in treating patients with COVID-19? *Med Hypotheses.* (2020) 140:109776. doi: 10.1016/j.mehy.2020.109776

37. Zhang W, Li F, Liu B, Wu R, Zou N, Xu YZ, et al. Pioglitazone upregulates hepatic angiotensin converting enzyme 2 expression in rats with steatohepatitis. *Ann Hepatol.* (2013) 12:892–900. doi: 10.1016/S1665-2681(19)31294-3

38. Zhang W, Xu YZ, Liu B, Wu R, Yang YY, Xiao XQ, et al. Pioglitazone upregulates angiotensin converting enzyme 2 expression in insulin-sensitive tissues in rats with high-fat diet-induced non-alcoholic steatohepatitis. *ScientificWorldJournal.* (2014) 2014:603409. doi: 10.1155/2014/603409

39. Guan Y, Hao C, Cha DR, Rao R, Lu W, Kohan DE, et al. Thiazolidinediones expand body fluid volume through PPARgamma stimulation of ENaC-mediated renal salt absorption. *Nat Med.* (2005) 11:861–6. doi: 10.1038/nm1278

40. Satirapoj B, Watanakijthavonkul K, Supasyndh O. Safety and efficacy of low dose pioglitazone compared with standard dose pioglitazone in type 2 diabetes with chronic kidney disease: a randomized controlled trial. *PLoS ONE.* (2018) 13:e0206722. doi: 10.1371/journal.pone.0206722

41. Ronco C, Reis T, Husain-Syed F. Management of acute kidney injury in patients with COVID-19. *Lancet Respir Med.* (2020) 8:738–42. doi: 10.1016/S2213-2600(20)30229-0

42. Zheng YY, Ma YT, Zhang JY, Xie X. COVID-19 and the cardiovascular system. *Nat Rev Cardiol.* (2020) 17:259–60. doi: 10.1038/s41569-020-0360-5

43. Tahrani AA, Barnett AH, Bailey CJ. Pharmacology and therapeutic implications of current drugs for type 2 diabetes mellitus. *Nat Rev Endocrinol.* (2016) 12:566–92. doi: 10.1038/nrendo.2016.86

44. Owens DR, McDougall A. Repaglinide: prandial glucose regulation in clinical practice. *Diabetes Obes Metab.* (2000) 2(Suppl. 1):S43–8. doi: 10.1046/j.1463-1326.2000.0022s.x

45. International Hypoglycaemia Study G. Minimizing hypoglycemia in diabetes. *Diabetes Care.* (2015) 38:1583–91. doi: 10.2337/dc15-0279

46. Pasquel FJ, Fayfman M, Umpierrez GE. Debate on insulin vs. non-insulin use in the hospital setting-is it time to revise the guidelines for the management of inpatient diabetes? *Curr Diab Rep.* (2019) 19:65. doi: 10.1007/s11892-019-1184-8

47. Raj VS, Mou H, Smits SL, Dekkers DH, Muller MA, Dijkman R, et al. Dipeptidyl peptidase 4 is a functional receptor for the emerging human coronavirus-EMC. *Nature.* (2013) 495:251–4. doi: 10.1038/nature12005

48. Fadini GP, Morieri ML, Longato E, Bonora BM, Pinelli S, Selmin E, et al. Exposure to dipeptidyl-peptidase-4 inhibitors and COVID-19 among people with type 2 diabetes: a case-control study. *Diabetes Obes Metab.* (2020). doi: 10.1111/dom.14097. [Epub ahead of print].

49. Varin EM, Mulvihill EE, Beaudry JL, Pujadas G, Fuchs S, Tanti JF, et al. Circulating levels of soluble dipeptidyl peptidase-4 are dissociated from inflammation and induced by enzymatic DPP4 inhibition. *Cell Metab.* (2019) 29:320–34.e5. doi: 10.1016/j.cmet.2018.10.001

50. Bassendine MF, Bridge SH, McCaughan GW, Gorrell MD. COVID-19 and comorbidities: a role for dipeptidyl peptidase 4 (DPP4) in disease severity? *J Diabetes.* (2020) 12:649–58. doi: 10.1111/1753-0407.13052

51. Goossen K, Graber S. Longer term safety of dipeptidyl peptidase-4 inhibitors in patients with type 2 diabetes mellitus: systematic review and meta-analysis. *Diabetes Obes Metab.* (2012) 14:1061–72. doi: 10.1111/j.1463-1326.2012.01610.x

52. *Effects of DPP4 Inhibition on COVID-19.* (2020). Available online at: clinicaltrials.gov/ct2/show/NCT04341935 (accessed July 14, 2020).

53. Drucker DJ. Mechanisms of action and therapeutic application of glucagon-like peptide-1. *Cell Metab.* (2018) 27:740–56. doi: 10.1016/j.cmet.2018.03.001

54. Aroda VR. A review of GLP-1 receptor agonists: evolution and advancement, through the lens of randomised controlled trials. *Diabetes Obes Metab.* (2018) 20(Suppl. 1):22–33. doi: 10.1111/dom.13162

55. Htike ZZ, Zaccardi F, Papamargaritis D, Webb DR, Khunti K, Davies MJ. Efficacy and safety of glucagon-like peptide-1 receptor agonists in type 2 diabetes: a systematic review and mixed-treatment comparison analysis. *Diabetes Obes Metab.* (2017) 19:524–36. doi: 10.1111/dom.12849

56. Bethel MA, Patel RA, Merrill P, Lokhnygina Y, Buse JB, Mentz RJ, et al. Cardiovascular outcomes with glucagon-like peptide-1 receptor agonists in patients with type 2 diabetes: a meta-analysis. *Lancet Diabetes Endocrinol.* (2018) 6:105–13. doi: 10.1016/S2213-8587(17)30412-6

57. Kristensen SL, Rorth R, Jhund PS, Docherty KF, Sattar N, Preiss D, et al. Cardiovascular, mortality, and kidney outcomes with GLP-1 receptor agonists in patients with type 2 diabetes: a systematic review and meta-analysis of cardiovascular outcome trials. *Lancet Diabetes Endocrinol.* (2019) 7:776–85. doi: 10.1016/S2213-8587(19)30249-9

58. Romani-Perez M, Outeirino-Iglesias V, Moya CM, Santisteban P, Gonzalez-Matias LC, Vigo E, et al. Activation of the GLP-1 receptor by liraglutide increases ACE2 expression, reversing right ventricle hypertrophy, and improving the production of SP-A and SP-B in the lungs of type 1 diabetes rats. *Endocrinology.* (2015) 156:3559–69. doi: 10.1210/en.2014-1685

59. Heerspink HJ, Perkins BA, Fitchett DH, Husain M, Cherney DZ. Sodium Glucose cotransporter 2 inhibitors in the treatment of diabetes mellitus: cardiovascular and kidney effects, potential mechanisms, and clinical applications. *Circulation.* (2016) 134:752–72. doi: 10.1161/CIRCULATIONAHA.116.021887

60. Wiviott SD, Raz I, Bonaca MP, Mosenzon O, Kato ET, Cahn A, et al. Dapagliflozin and cardiovascular outcomes in type 2 diabetes. *N Engl J Med.* (2019) 380:347–57. doi: 10.1056/NEJMoa1812389

61. Neuen BL, Young T, Heerspink HJL, Neal B, Perkovic V, Billot L, et al. SGLT2 inhibitors for the prevention of kidney failure in patients with type 2 diabetes: a systematic review and meta-analysis. *Lancet Diabetes Endocrinol.* (2019) 7:845–54. doi: 10.1016/S2213-8587(19)30256-6

62. Thomas MC, Cherney DZI. The actions of SGLT2 inhibitors on metabolism, renal function and blood pressure. *Diabetologia.* (2018) 61:2098–107. doi: 10.1007/s00125-018-4669-0

63. *Dapagliflozin in Respiratory Failure in Patients With COVID-19 (DARE-19).* (2020). Available online at: clinicaltrials.gov/ct2/show/NCT04350593 (accessed July 14, 2020).

64. Fralick M, Schneeweiss S, Patorno E. Risk of diabetic ketoacidosis after initiation of an SGLT2 inhibitor. *N Engl J Med.* (2017) 376:2300–2. doi: 10.1056/NEJMc1701990

65. Mathieu C, Gillard P, Benhalima K. Insulin analogues in type 1 diabetes mellitus: getting better all the time. *Nat Rev Endocrinol.* (2017) 13:385–99. doi: 10.1038/nrendo.2017.39

66. Tokarz VL, MacDonald PE, Klip A. The cell biology of systemic insulin function. *J Cell Biol.* (2018) 217:2273–89. doi: 10.1083/jcb.201802095

67. Cahn A, Miccoli R, Dardano A, Del Prato S. New forms of insulin and insulin therapies for the treatment of type 2 diabetes. *Lancet Diabetes Endocrinol.* (2015) 3:638–52. doi: 10.1016/S2213-8587(15)00097-2

68. Investigators N-SS, Finfer S, Chittock DR, Su SY, Blair D, Foster D, et al. Intensive versus conventional glucose control in critically ill patients. *N Engl J Med.* (2009) 360:1283–97. doi: 10.1056/NEJMoa0810625

69. Griesdale DE, de Souza RJ, van Dam RM, Heyland DK, Cook DJ, Malhotra A, et al. Intensive insulin therapy and mortality among critically ill patients: a meta-analysis including NICE-SUGAR study data. *CMAJ.* (2009) 180:821–7. doi: 10.1503/cmaj.090206

70. Cariou B, Hadjadj S, Wargny M, Pichelin M, Al-Salameh A, Allix I, et al. Phenotypic characteristics and prognosis of inpatients with COVID-19 and diabetes: the CORONADO study. *Diabetologia.* (2020) 63:1500–15. doi: 10.1007/s00125-020-05180-x

71. Chen Y, Yang D, Cheng B, Chen J, Peng A, Yang C, et al. Clinical characteristics and outcomes of patients with diabetes and COVID-19 in association with glucose-lowering medication. *Diabetes Care.* (2020) 43:1399–407. doi: 10.2337/dc20-0660

72. Sardu C, D'Onofrio N, Balestrieri ML, Barbieri M, Rizzo MR, Messina V, et al. Outcomes in patients with hyperglycemia affected by COVID-19: can we do more on glycemic control? *Diabetes Care.* (2020) 43:1408–15. doi: 10.2337/dc20-0723

73. Umpierrez G, Korytkowski M. Diabetic emergencies–ketoacidosis, hyperglycaemic hyperosmolar state and hypoglycaemia. *Nat Rev Endocrinol.* (2016) 12:222–32. doi: 10.1038/nrendo.2016.15

74. Investigators N-SS, Finfer S, Liu B, Chittock DR, Norton R, Myburgh JA, et al. Hypoglycemia and risk of death in critically ill patients. *N Engl J Med.* (2012) 367:1108–18. doi: 10.1056/NEJMoa1204942

75. *Efficacy and Safety of Dipeptidyl Peptidase-4 Inhibitors in Diabetic Patients With Established COVID-19.* (2020). Available online at: clinicaltrials.gov/ct2/show/NCT04371978 (accessed September 4, 2020).

76. *The Effect of Sitagliptin Treatment in COVID-19 Positive Diabetic Patients (SIDIACO).* (2020). Available online at: clinicaltrials.gov/ct2/show/NCT04365517 (accessed September 4, 2020).

77. *GlitazOne Treatment for Coronavirus HypoxiA, a Safety and Tolerability Open Label With Matching Cohort Pilot Study (GOTCHA).* (2020). Available online at: clinicaltrials.gov/ct2/show/NCT04473274 (accessed September 4, 2020).

78. *MET-Covid Trial–METformin for Prevention and Outpatient Treatment of COVID-19.* (2020). Available online at: clinicaltrials.gov/ct2/show/NCT04510194 (accessed September 4, 2020).

15

Are we Witnessing an Increase of Chronic Ascending Aortic Dissection as a Collateral Effect to the COVID-19 Pandemic?

Arnaud Lyon[1]*, Ziyad Gunga[2†], Lars Niclauss[2†], Valentina Rancati[3†] and Piergiorgio Tozzi[2]

[1] School of Medicine, University of Lausanne, Lausanne, Switzerland, [2] Service de Chirurgie Cardiaque, Centre Hospitalier Universitaire Vaudois, Lausanne, Switzerland, [3] Département d'anesthésiologie, Hôpital Universitaire de Lausanne (CHUV), Lausanne, Switzerland

Correspondence:
Arnaud Lyon
arnaud.lyon@unil.ch

[†] *These authors have contributed equally to this work*

Background: The COVID-19 (coronavirus disease 2019) pandemic is reducing health care accessibility to non–life-threatening diseases, thus hiding their real incidence. Moreover, the incidence of potentially fatal conditions such as acute type A aortic dissection seems to have decreased since the pandemic began, whereas the number of cases of chronic ascending aortic dissections dramatically increased. We present two patients whose management has been affected by the exceptional sanitary situation we are dealing with.

Case report: A 70-year-old man with chest pain and an aortic regurgitation murmur had his cardiac workup delayed (4 months) because of sanitary restrictions. He was then diagnosed with chronic type A aortic dissection and underwent urgent replacement of ascending aorta and aortic root. The delay in surgical treatment made the intervention technically challenging because the ascending aorta grew up to 80 mm inducing strong adhesions and chronic inflammation. The second case report concerns a 68-year-old woman with right lower-limb pain who was diagnosed with deep vein thrombosis. However, a CT scan to exclude a pulmonary embolism could not be realized until 5 months later because of sanitary restrictions. When she eventually got the CT scan, it fortuitously showed a chronic dissection of the ascending aorta. She underwent urgent surgery, and the intervention was challenging because of adhesions and severe inflammation.

Conclusion: Delayed treatment due to sanitary restrictions related to COVID-19 pandemic is having a significant impact on the management of potentially life-threatening conditions including type A aortic dissection. We should remain careful to avoid COVID-19 also hitting patients who are not infected with the virus.

Keywords: ascending aorta, chronic aortic dissection, COVID–19, aortic surgery, delayed management

BACKGROUND

Acute Stanford type A aortic dissections (ATAADs) constitute critical emergencies that require immediate surgical treatment. This is due to the high risk of fatal complications, such as aortic rupture, severe aortic regurgitation, pericardial tamponade, and cerebral and coronary malperfusion (1), which are responsible for 33% mortality after 24 h and 50% mortality after 48 h (2). However, a very limited number of patients remain stable, with only mild to absent symptoms, and may thus survive the acute phase (1). After a 14-day period, the aortic dissection is defined as chronic (1). The global incidence of aortic dissection is 5 to 30 cases per 1 million people per year (3). We recently published our experience with ATAADs from 2014 to 2019. During the considered period, we treated 117 ATAADs in our center, which represents 3 to 5 ATAAD cases per month and had no chronic cases (4). However, between February and May 2020, the COVID-19 (coronavirus disease 2019) pandemic temporarily reduced health care accessibility. As such, these statistics were noticeably altered, with only three confirmed ATAADs, which represented a decrease of ¾, compared to the usual volume. Nevertheless, we experienced two cases of chronic type A aortic dissection (CTAAD) in July 2020, which is a pathology we usually see only once every 5 years (4).

This report illustrates the clinical implications of CTAAD that occurred in two patients shortly after the peak phase of the COVID-19 pandemic in our country.

FIRST CASE PRESENTATION

In February 2020, a 70-year-old man with a previously treated arterial hypertension consulted his general practitioner (GP) because of mild chest pain, without any other symptoms. The physical examination revealed a diastolic heart murmur that predominated in the aortic area. The patient's electrocardiogram (ECG) was normal, and the GP asked for cardiology advice. However, because of the sanitary restrictions due to the COVID-19 pandemic, the cardiologist examined the patient only 4 months later. The echocardiography revealed an aneurysm of the ascending aorta with signs of aortic dissection and severe aortic regurgitation.

A contrast medium thoracic computed tomography (CT) scan was immediately performed, which demonstrated an 82 × 87 mm aneurysm of the ascending aorta with a longitudinal tear of the intima that originated in a partially thrombosed circulating false lumen. The lesion began just above the ostium of the right coronary artery and extended up to the middle of the aortic arch with a 2.2-cm opening that was compatible with a Stanford type A aortic dissection. A 17-mm pericardial effusion was also identified (**Figures 1A,B**).

The patient underwent replacement of the ascending aorta and aortic root (Bentall procedure with a 25-mm Carpentier–Edwards biological valve mounted on a Valsalva-type 28-mm Dacron tube). The intervention was technically difficult, as the heart was totally displaced into the left chest, and there were strong adhesions due to chronic inflammatory reactions (**Figures 2A,B**). The perioperative echocardiography showed a thickened dissection flap localized just above the origin of the right coronary artery (**Figure 3**). The right coronary reimplantation was therefore challenging because the ostium was fragilized by the dissection.

The post-operative period was uneventful, and the patient quickly recovered.

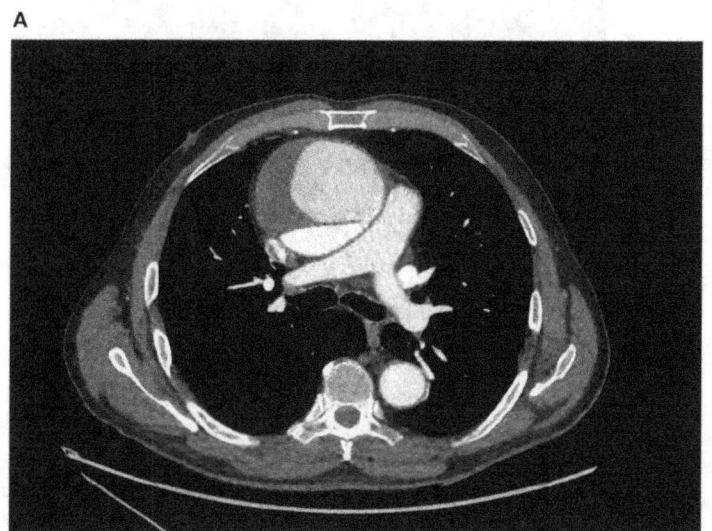
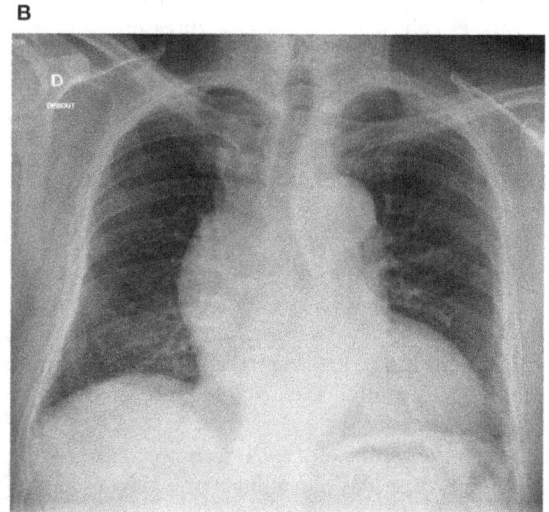

FIGURE 1 | (A) Contrast medium thoracic CT scan showing a CTAAD with a thick intimal tear (7 mm) and an enlarged ascending aorta (82 × 87 mm). The false lumen is partially thrombosed. **(B)** Chest X-ray showing an aortic aneurysm with a widening of the mediastinal silhouette, an enlargement of the aortic knob, and a displacement of the trachea from the midline. CT, computed tomography; CTAAD, chronic type A aortic dissection.

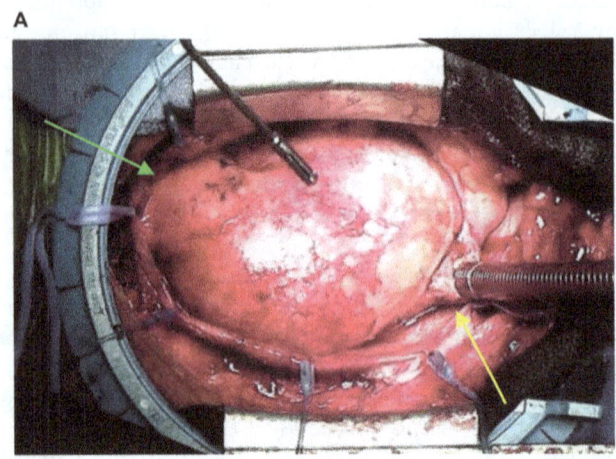
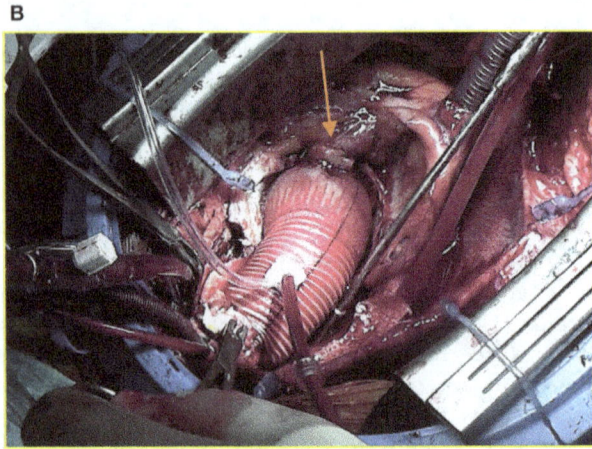

FIGURE 2 | (A) Surgical view of the mediastinum after sternotomy. The huge aneurysm of the ascending aorta (82 × 87 mm) filled the whole cavity, displacing the heart into the left chest. The yellow arrow indicates the right atrium, and the green arrow indicates the aortic arch. **(B)** The ascending aorta has been replaced by the Dacron tube, leaving a free space that was previously filled by the aneurysm. The orange arrow indicates the reimplantation of the right coronary ostium.

SECOND CASE PRESENTATION

A 68-year-old female active smoker with known hypercholesterolemia, who had been treated for arterial hypertension and had a history of stroke in 2010 and pulmonary embolism in 2016, consulted her GP on February 25, 2020. She complained about the spontaneous onset of acute right lower-limb pain. The patient did not present any chest pain or dyspnea. The clinical examination revealed a painful but mild pretibial edema on the left lower limb, whereas no heart murmur was documented. D-Dimer levels were 570 mg/L (reference, <500 mg/L). On the same day, the patient was referred to the angiology department where a diagnosis of unprovoked deep vein thrombosis (DVT) of the left lower limb was established. Her arterial pressure was 131/86 mm Hg in the right arm and 134/87 mm Hg in the left arm, and all peripheral pulses were palpable. The patient was discharged with a therapeutic anticoagulation treatment (rivaroxaban 20 mg, once daily), with a 3-month follow-up examination scheduled for May. The follow-up found a favorable development, so the rivaroxaban was stopped and replaced by cardioprotective aspirin.

In July, the patient's GP completed the diagnostic workup of her DVT with a CT scan. This examination unexpectedly showed an aneurysm of the ascending aorta (53 × 54 mm) with a chronic aortic dissection (**Figures 4A,B**). ECG was normal, and echocardiography found a ventricular function of 65% and a mild aortic insufficiency.

Based on the results of the CT scan, we performed an urgent repair of the dissected ascending aorta. We used a Gelweave 26-mm straight tube to replace the ascending aorta, just above the coronary ostia. The intervention was technically challenging, due to adhesions, but was ultimately uneventful, and the patient quickly recovered.

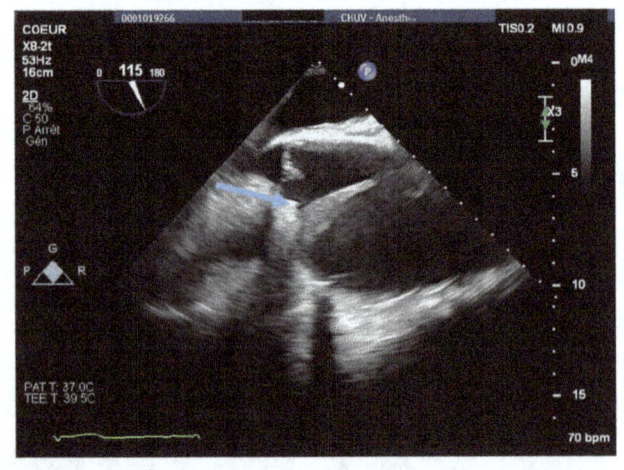

FIGURE 3 | Perioperative midesophageal long-axis view showing a thickened (5 mm) dissection flap localized in the proximal ascending aorta, immediately after the origin of the right coronary artery (blue arrow). The maximal diameter of the ascending aorta was 74 mm.

DISCUSSION

Delayed treatment of non–COVID-related diseases due to the COVID-19 pandemic is having a significant impact on patient safety even in developed countries such as Switzerland. Thousands of patients experience delayed management of potentially life-threatening conditions including type A aortic dissection. This is mainly due to a saturation of hospital capacity and patients' fear about becoming infected by the coronavirus in the hospital environment. We noticed a decrease in the number of ATAADs that were referred to our emergency department

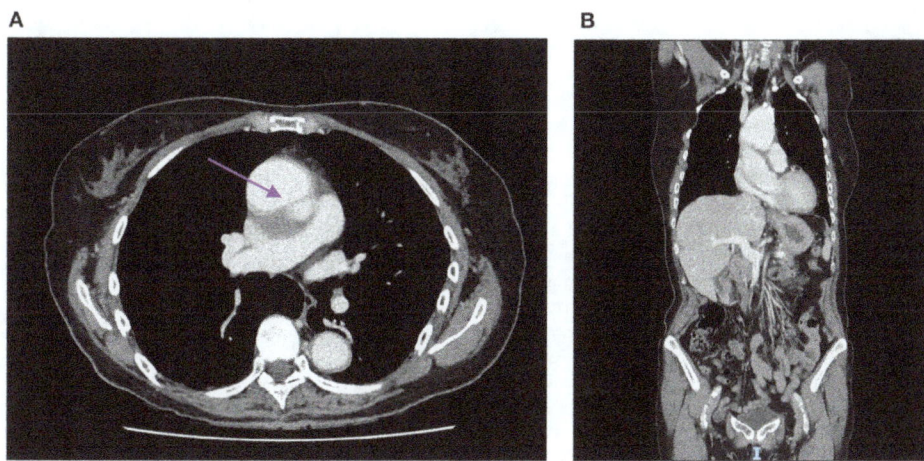

FIGURE 4 | (A) Contrast medium CT scan showing an aneurysm of the ascending aorta (53 × 54 mm) with a tear of the intima, creating a thick false lumen (4 mm), which is indicated by the purple arrow. **(B)** Sagittal section of the contrast medium CT scan, which also shows the aneurysm and thick tear of the intima. CT, computed tomography.

during the peak phase of the pandemic. This decrease of acute aortic syndromes was also highlighted by El-Hamamsy et al. who found the volume of ATAADs to be 76.5% lower than usual in New York City between March and April 2020 (5). Similar observations concerning myocardial infarctions and emergency department visits in general have also been reported (6, 7). Both of our patients exhibited atypical presentations with no specific symptoms or signs of ATAAD. We speculate that this played a role in their missed or delayed diagnoses. This may relate to the unexpected rise in CTAAD cases during the phase that followed the first peak of the pandemic. The absence of specific ATAAD symptoms in these patients was central to these delayed diagnoses. This phenomenon was reinforced by the pandemic, as patients altered their thresholds of symptoms that would normally compel them to seek medical advice. They waited longer before consulting a doctor than they would have before the pandemic.

CONCLUSION

The apparent decrease in acute aortic dissections during the COVID-19 pandemic does not appear to be real, and it only relied on many patients not consulting, and remaining unnoticed, thus preventing them to get the medical care they deserved. Most of these patients probably passed away due to the complications of their aortic dissections, while the acute aortic dissections of those with mild or atypical symptoms who survived may have evolved into a chronic state that was only discovered when normal accessibility to health care services resumed.

The surgical treatment of CTAADs is more challenging with respect to acute dissection because it is associated to strong adhesions and consistent inflammatory reaction, significantly increasing the surgical mortality and morbidity. Therefore,

delayed diagnosis also impacts the prognosis of patients with mild to absent symptoms (8).

The example of aortic dissections also illustrates the fact that patients affected by a wide range of diseases are directly impacted by the sanitary restrictions related to the COVID-19 pandemic. We thus conclude that more attention should be paid to avoid COVID-19 also hitting patients who are not infected with the virus.

Limitations

Our case report is an observational study on a limited number of patients aimed at highlighting one of the possible consequences of the sanitary restrictions imposed by the authorities during the COVID-19 pandemic on the natural history of aortic dissection. By being a case report, it is not intended to clearly prove or bring statistical evidence of an association between the pandemic and an apparent increase of chronic aortic dissection cases. However, it shows a tendency in our center, which we believe is worth sharing with the medical community and which should be further investigated in a future larger epidemiological study.

AUTHOR CONTRIBUTIONS

AL is responsible for the literature research as well as the writing of the manuscript. PT contributed to this work as senior author. All authors contributed to the article and approved the submitted version.

REFERENCES

1. Hynes CF, Greenberg MD, Sarin S, Trachiotis GD. Chronic type A aortic dissection two cases and a review of current management strategies. *Aorta*. (2016) 4:16–21. doi: 10.12945/j.aorta.2015.15.016

2. Fournier Y, Moix PA, Hugli O. Dissection aortique aiguë: utilité diagnostique des D-dimères. *Rev Med*. (2008) 4:1759–63.

3. Levy D, Goyal A, Grigorova Y. Aortic dissection. In: Abai B, editor. *StatPearls*. Treasure Island, FL: StatPearls publishing (2020). p. 1–14.

4. Tozzi P, Gunga Z, Niclauss L, Delay D, Roumy A, Pfisher R, et al. Type A aortic dissection in aneurysms having modelled pre-dissection maximum diameter below 45 mm: should we implement current guidelines to improve the survival benefit of prophylactic surgery? *Eur J Cardiothorac Surg*. (2021) 59:473–78. doi: 10.1093/ejcts/ezaa351

5. El-Hamamsy I, Brinster DR, DeRose JJ, Girardi LN, Hisamoto K, Imam MN, et al. The COVID-19 pandemic and acute aortic dissections in New York a matter of public health. *J Am Coll Cardiol*. (2020) 76:227–9. doi: 10.1016/j.jacc.2020.05.022

6. Zitelny E, Newman N, Zhaob D. STEMI during the COVID-19 pandemic - an evaluation of incidence. *Cardiovasc Pathol*. (2020) 48:107232. doi: 10.1016/j.carpath.2020.107232

7. Hartnett K, Kite-Powell A, DeVies J, Coletta MA, Boehmer TK, Adjemian J, et al. Impact of the COVID-19 pandemic on emergency department visits — United States. *MMWR Morb Mortal Wkly Rep*. (2020) 69:699–704. doi: 10.15585/mmwr.mm6923e1

8. Jault F, Rama A, Lievre L, Bonnet N, Leprince P, Pavie A, et al. Chronic dissection of the ascending aorta: surgical results during a 20-year period. *Eur J Cardiothorac Surg*. (2006) 29:1041–5. doi: 10.1016/j.ejcts.2006.02.034

16

An Unusual Case of Biventricular Thrombosis in a COVID-19 Patient with Ischemic Dilated Cardiomyopathy: Assessment of Mass Mobility and Embolic Risk by Tissue Doppler Imaging

Andrea Sonaglioni[1], Adriana Albini[2*], Gian Luigi Nicolosi[3], Elisabetta Rigamonti[1], Douglas M. Noonan[2,4] and Michele Lombardo[1]

[1] Department of Cardiology, Istituto di Ricovero e Cura a Carattere Scientifico (IRCCS) Multi Medica, Milan, Italy, [2] Scientific and Technological Pole, Istituto di Ricovero e Cura a Carattere Scientifico (IRCCS) Multi Medica, Milan, Italy, [3] Department of Cardiology, Policlinico San Giorgio, Pordenone, Italy, [4] Department of Biotechnology and Life Sciences, University of Insubria, Varese, Italy

*Correspondence:
Adriana Albini
albini.adriana@gmail.com

Severe acute respiratory syndrome coronavirus 2 (SARS-CoV-2) spike protein binds to angiotensin-converting enzyme 2 (ACE2) receptor on vascular cells. As a consequence, patients with COVID-19 have an increased incidence of thromboembolic complications of the SARS-CoV-2 infection and subsequent endothelial cell damage with consequence of development of systemic vasculitis and diffuse intravascular coagulation. The present case describes a COVID-19 female patient with ischemic dilated cardiomyopathy, who presented with congestive heart failure and echocardiographic evidence of biventricular apical thrombi. The peak antegrade longitudinal velocity (Va) of each thrombotic mass was measured by pulsed wave tissue Doppler imaging (PW-TDI). Both left ventricular and right ventricular apical thrombi were found with a TDI-derived mass peak Va < 10 cm/s. There was no clinical evidence of neither systemic nor pulmonary embolization, probably due to the hypomobility of both left and right ventricular masses.

Keywords: COVID-19, biventricular thrombosis, pulsed wave tissue Doppler imaging, ACE2, dilated cardiomyopathy

INTRODUCTION

Left ventricular (LV) thrombosis can complicate both ischemic and non-ischemic cardiomyopathies and can lead to arterial embolic complications such as stroke (1, 2). However, the occurrence of biventricular thrombi is very rare and only few cases have been previously described in literature (3–9). Here, we report the case of an 80-year-old woman infected by Coronavirus 2019 (COVID-19), presenting with congestive heart failure (CHF) due to ischemic dilated cardiomyopathy (DCM), who was diagnosed with biventricular apical thrombi by transthoracic echocardiography (TTE).

CLINICAL COURSE

An 80-year-old woman, BSA 1.62 m^2, body mass index (BMI) 22.6 Kg/m^2 with history of coronary artery disease presented to the Emergency Department (ED) with worsening dyspnea, non-productive cough, fatigue, and bilateral leg swelling. She had prior anterior myocardial infarction treated with percutaneous transluminal coronary angioplasty of the proximal left anterior descending coronary artery in 2019 and subsequent unfavorable evolution in DCM with severe systolic dysfunction (estimated left ventricular ejection fraction of 20%) and chronic renal failure (estimated glomerular filtration rate of 30 ml/min/1.73 m^2). She was in home-therapy with acetyl salicylic acid 75 mg/die, furosemide 50 mg/die, spironolactone 25 mg/die, and rosuvastatin 5 mg/die.

Parameters recorded at the admission were the following: body temperature 36.5°C, heart rate 82 beats per minute, blood pressure 150/90 mmHg, respiratory rate 28 times per minute, and oxygen saturation 90% on ambient air.

Blood tests showed a white blood cell count of 8,720/mmc (88.0% neutrophils and 8.0% lymphocytes), hemoglobin 16.5 g/dl, C-reactive protein at the level of 11.1 mg/dl (reference range 0.05–0.50 mg/dl), estimated glomerular filtration rate 25 ml/min/1.73 m^2, B-type natriuretic peptide level >20,000 pg/ml, D-dimer at the level of 17,108 ng/ml (reference range 1–500 ng/ml), and troponin I at the level of 0.08 ng/ml (reference range 0.00–0.04 ng/ml).

The electrocardiogram showed sinus rhythm, poor R wave progression in precordials, suggestive of old large anterior myocardial infarction and QRS voltage <5 mm in all limb leads.

Chest x-ray showed cardiomegaly, bilateral interstitial infiltrates and bilateral pleural effusions (**Figure 1**). A positive rapid antigen test for Severe Acute Respiratory Syndrome Coronavirus 2 (SARS-CoV2) was confirmed by the molecular test at hospital admission. Therefore, the patient was transferred from the ED to the semi-intensive care unit for COVID-19 patients.

A bedside TTE revealed the presence of large and roundish masses in the apex of both ventricles associated with severe biventricular dilatation (LV end-diastolic short axis diameter of 65 mm, right ventricular inflow tract of 45 mm) and dysfunction. Left ventricular ejection fraction (LVEF) estimated by modified Simpson's method was 15%, with dyskinesia/aneurism of the apex, and interventricular septum and marked hypokinesis of the other segments of the left ventricle. Right ventricular (RV) systolic function, measured by the tricuspid annular plane systolic excursion (TAPSE), was also severely impaired (TAPSE = 9 mm).

Both masses were acoustically distinct from underlying myocardium, with hypoechoic central space and hyperechoic border, well-circumscribed and sessile, attached to the apex of the left ventricle and of the right ventricle. The LV mass measured 23 mm × 21 mm, while the RV mass measured 18 mm × 15 mm. Both the masses were hypomobile and prominent in the apical 4-chamber view. Bilateral ventricular thrombi were diagnosed.

To precisely assess the mobility of the intracardiac thrombi, we employed pulsed-wave tissue Doppler imaging (PW-TDI) placing the sample volume at the level of the body of each mass. The peak antegrade longitudinal velocity (Va) of both LV and RV apical thrombi was measured.

Figure 2 illustrates the LV apical thrombus (**Figure 2A**) and the corresponding TDI-derived peak mass Va (**Figure 2B**), while **Figure 3** depicts the RV apical thrombus (**Figure 3A**) and the relative TDI-derived peak mass Va (**Figure 3B**). Moderate mitral and tricuspid regurgitation, dilatation of the inferior vena cava and moderate pulmonary hypertension (the estimated systolic pulmonary artery pressure was 60 mmHg) were also detected.

The above-mentioned echocardiographic examination was compared with a previous TTE performed in October 2020 that showed severe biventricular dilatation and dysfunction (LV ejection fraction of 20%, TAPSE of 13 mm), with no evidence of ventricular thrombi.

The diagnosis of CHF due to ischemic DCM complicated with biventricular thrombi in a COVID-19 patient was made. Thrombosis at other sites was excluded; no deep vein thrombosis of the abdomen and lower extremities was found by ultrasonography.

Conventional treatment for CHF with loop diuretics (intravenous furosemide 120 mg/die and canrenone 100 mg/die) and beta-blockers (bisoprolol 2.5 mg/die) was started. Moreover, the patient received antibiotic treatment (intravenous piperacillin and tazobactam three times daily) and oxygen therapy via nasal cannula (2 l/min). Low molecular weight heparin (enoxaparin sodium) was administered for the treatment of biventricular thrombosis (4,000 IU twice daily by subcutaneous injection).

During the hospitalization, the patient underwent diagnostic thrombophilia testing. Results showed that serum levels of protein C, protein S, antithrombin III, factor V Leiden, and antiphospholipid antibody were normal.

A subsequent TTE, performed after 10 days of anticoagulant treatment, showed the complete dissolution of both left and right ventricular thrombi (**Figure 4**). There was no clinical evidence of neither systemic nor pulmonary embolization, probably due to the hypomobility of both left, and right ventricular masses.

However, severe biventricular dysfunction persisted, and refractory CHF occurred, despite intensive diuretic therapy. The patient underwent serial chest x-ray which showed progressive increase of pulmonary congestion and interstitial infiltrates. Computed tomography scan was not performed due to the critical condition of the patient and the absence of clinical signs of pulmonary/systemic embolization. Finally, the patient's clinical conditions worsened, and she died 15 days after hospitalization.

DISCUSSION

Severe acute respiratory syndrome coronavirus 2 (SARS-CoV-2) spike protein binds to angiotensin-converting enzyme 2 (ACE2) receptor on vascular cells (10, 11). On endothelial cells from arterial and venous vessels there is ACE2 expression and there is evidence that endothelial cells are prone to SARS-CoV-2 infection which causes subsequent endothelial cell damage with development of systemic vasculitis and disseminated intravascular coagulation (DIC) (10). Since the

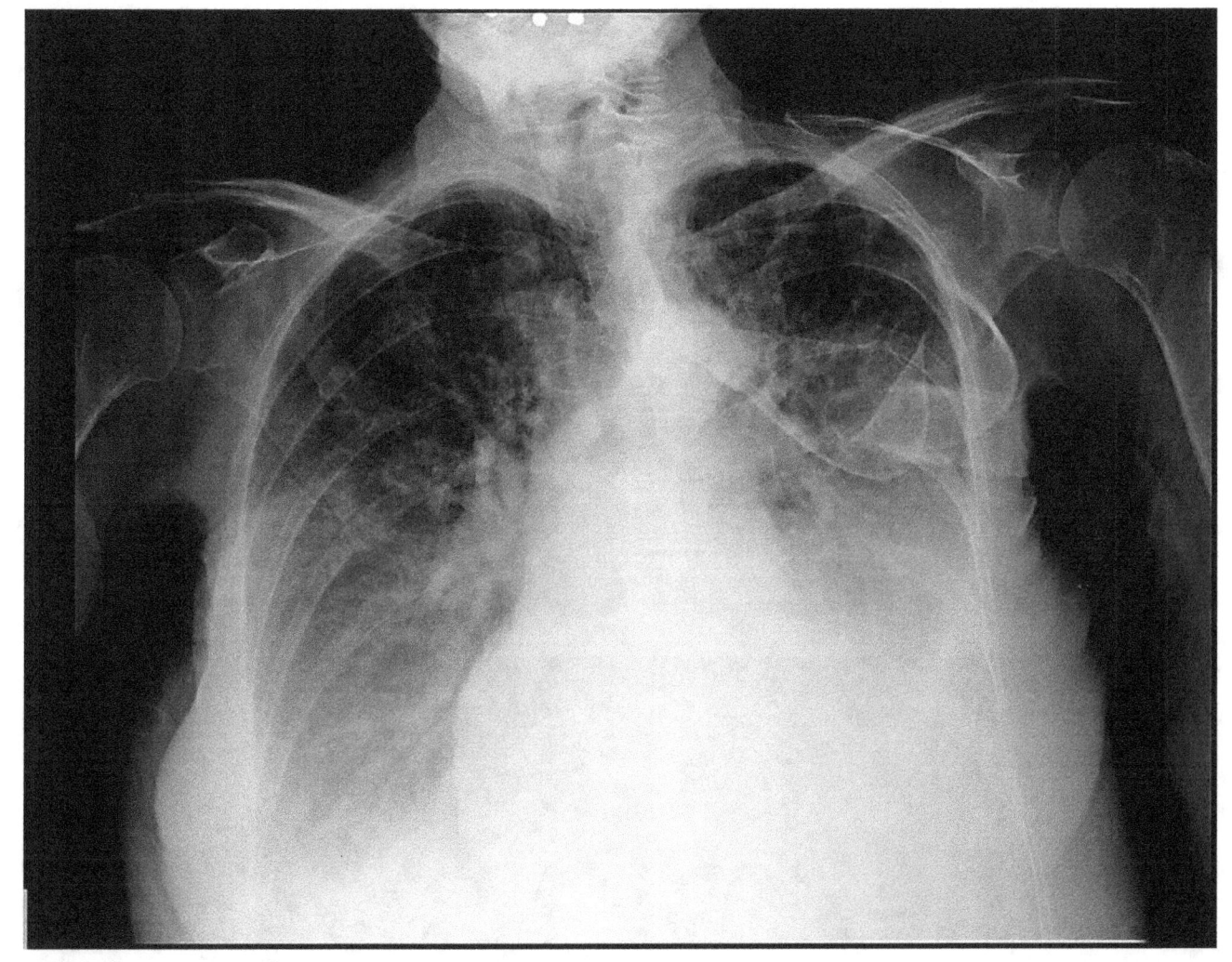

FIGURE 1 | Posteroanterior chest x-ray view revealing cardiomegaly, bilateral interstitial infiltrates and bilateral pleural effusions.

beginning of the COVID-19 pandemic, severe hypercoagulability and serious thrombotic complications have been reported in infected patients, especially in those patients who are admitted to intensive care unit (12–16). The most common thromboembolic complications detected in COVID-19 patients were deep vein thrombosis, acute pulmonary embolism, coronary and cerebral thrombosis, systemic arterial embolism, and placental thrombosis (17–21).

The occurrence of biventricular thrombi is a rare, but serious condition which may increase the risk of both systemic and pulmonary embolization. Previous cases of biventricular thrombosis have been described in patients with severe ventricular dysfunction, autoimmune disease, HIV infection, nephrotic syndrome, hypereosinophilic syndrome, heparin-induced thrombocytopenia, and antiphospholipid syndrome (3–9).

To date, there are only three case reports in literature who described biventricular thrombi in a COVID-19 patient (22–24).

One patient, a 63-year-old woman, with a known medical history of emphysema and active smoker, 2-week history of worsening dyspnea, nonproductive cough, and chills, she was positive for SARS-CoV-2 as detected by PCR (22). After, few hours from admission she had a cardiac arrest with successful cardiorespiratory resuscitation. The patient had 93% oxygen saturation, elevated troponin I, creatinine kinase, and lactate, with normal platelet count, coagulation parameters, and fibrinogen (22). Cardiac tomography revealed a right ventricular thrombus, measuring 4 mm by 10 mm, a left ventricular thrombus 12-mm in thickness extending over a 6-cm perimeter (22). The patient died of cardiogenic and pulmonary septic shock.

Another patient, a 58-year-old man, had obesity (BMI of 31 kg/m² on admission) and hypertension, he presented with intermittent fever and worsening shortness of breath on exertion he was positive for PCR SARS-CoV-2 (23). The patient initial clinical examination was normal except for an

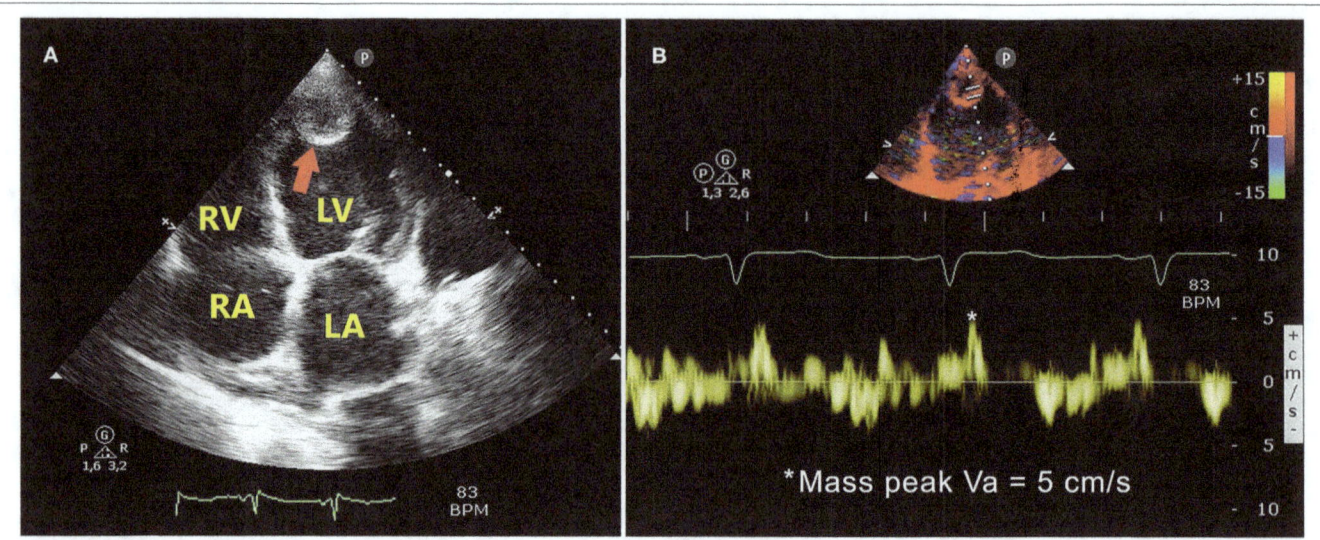

FIGURE 2 | Apical 4-chamber echocardiographic view showing a large and roundish LV apical thrombus with hypoechoic central space and hyperechoic border (**A**, red arrow). The LV thrombotic mass measured 23 mm × 21 mm. The TDI-derived LV mass peak Va was 5 cm/s, as depicted in panel (**B**). LA, left atrium; LV, left ventricular/left ventricle; TDI, tissue Doppler imaging; RA, right atrium; RV, right ventricle; Va, antegrade velocity.

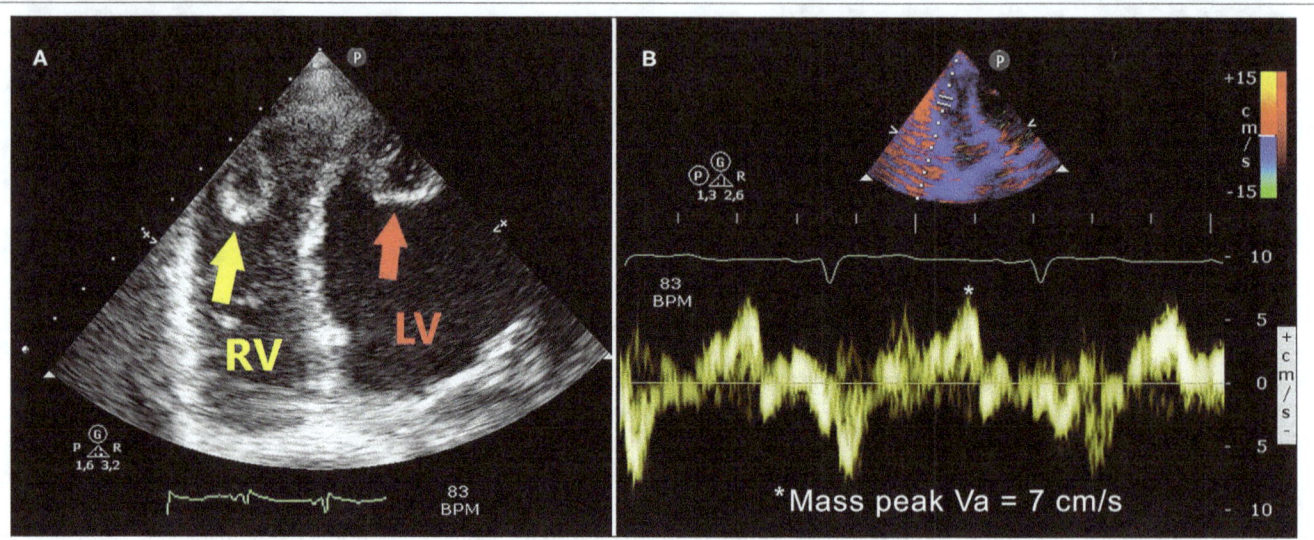

FIGURE 3 | Right ventricular focused 4-chamber echocardiographic view demonstrating RV (**A**, yellow arrow) and LV (**A**, red arrow) apical thrombi: both masses were found with hypoechoic central space and hyperechoic border. The RV thrombotic mass measured 18 mm × 15 mm. The TDI-derived RV mass peak Va was 7 cm/s, as depicted in panel (**B**). LV, left ventricular/left ventricle; TDI, tissue Doppler imaging; RV, right ventricular/right ventricle; Va, antegrade velocity.

outstanding oxygen requirement. The patient had high C-reactive protein (CRP) D-dimer was significantly elevated, with normal prothrombin time and activated partial thromboplastin time, no pulmonary thromboembolism appeared on CT pulmonary angiography (23). On day 4 the D-dimer levels were noted to have risen, and on day 9 they were steadily rising. On day 9, CT pulmonary angiography revealed simultaneous bilateral pulmonary thromboembolism, biventricular cardiac thrombi (23). The patient with multiple thromboses had appropriate prophylactic and therapeutic LMWH is this case (23). The patient was successfully discharged on day 19.

A 58-year-old African-American male, with a history of hypertension and diabetes mellitus, was brought to emergency room (24). He had 60% oxygen saturation the clinical laboratory test showed a hypercoagulable state (Fibrinogen was low and high D-dimer levels, PT 36 s, INR 3.6, and aPTT of 100 s) normal troponin I, CK, CK-MB at normal levels (24). He was taking care of parents, confirmed positive with COVID-19. In this patient transthoracic echocardiography has seen left ventricle extensive mural thrombus and highly mobile thrombus the in right atrium with extensive biventricular thrombi (24). The patient died of ventricular fibrillation within 24 h.

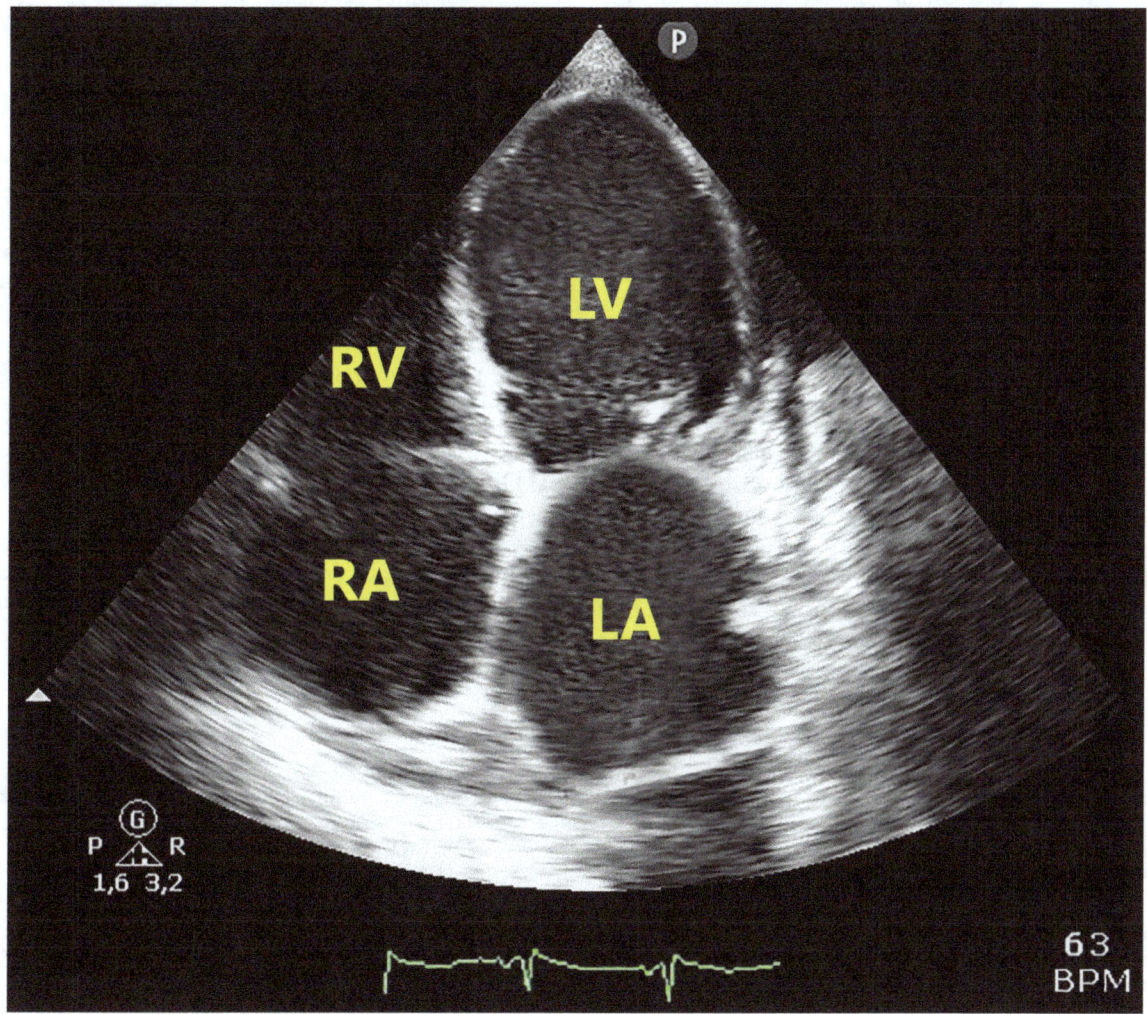

FIGURE 4 | Apical 4-chamber echocardiographic view showing disappearance of both RV and LV thrombotic masses after 10 days of anticoagulant treatment. LA, left atrium; LV, left ventricle; RA, right atrium; RV, right ventricle.

Obesity is one of the complications of the COVID-19 patients (25). The BMI of the African-American male, with a history of hypertension and diabetes mellitus, and 63-year-old woman active smoker and emphysema was not mentioned in these case reports (22, 24). In all the case reports of biventricular thrombi and COVID-19 the patients were ~60 years.

In this case report, a 80 years COVID-19 patient with CHF due to ischemic DCM was diagnosed with LV and RV apical thrombi. Our patient had severely depressed systolic biventricular function, suggesting a high risk of ventricular thrombi. However, she was never diagnosed with ventricular thrombi prior to admission and was tested negative for thrombophilia screening during hospitalization. As far as we know, this is the first case of biventricular thrombi described in a COVID-19 patient with ischemic dilated cardiomyopathy.

As proposed by Mehta et al. (26), the combination of a progressive dysregulated coagulative response to SARS-CoV-2 with consequent activation of a state of hypercoagulability and the blood stasis due to severe biventricular dilatation and contractile dysfunction might have contributed to the formation of LV and RV apical thrombi.

In the present case, the D-dimer level of the patient was 17,108 ng/ml, well-above reference values, and the patient was treated with low-molecular-weight heparin, while the surgical thrombectomy was not considered due to the patient's advanced age and the severe CHF. The 63 years woman patient coagulation parameters were normal, but the authors mention the D-dimer (22). In the two male cases D-dimers were highly elevated (23, 24).

In the present case, contrast echocardiography, which is particularly advantageous for detection of small or mural thrombi (27), was not performed to confirm the diagnosis of LV and RV apical thrombi, because both thrombotic masses were large in size and protuberant in shape. On the other hand, PW-TDI was useful to precisely assessing the mobility of the intracardiac thrombi. Therefore, the diagnosis of biventricular thrombosis was performed and confirmed by TTE, whereas PW-TDI provided a rapid characterization of mass-mobility. Differently from previous case reports which described biventricular thrombi detected by TTE in different clinical settings (3–9), our case is the only one that employed a TTE implemented with PW-TDI assessment of the thrombotic mass mobility in a COVID-19 patient.

Our previous prospective analysis performed on 72 patients with echocardiographically detected LV thrombi revealed that a TDI-derived mass peak Va $\geq$ 10 cm/s, was the most important and independent predictor of outcome at mid-term follow-up (28). Therefore, we demonstrated that the TDI-derived mass peak Va might represent a new objective marker of thrombotic mass motility and that a mass peak Va $\geq$ 10 cm/s might stratify the hospitalized patients with increased probability of embolic events in a mid-term follow-up, regardless of the mass dimension.

In this present case, both LV and RV apical thrombi were found with a mass peak Va < 10 cm/sec, as assessed by PW-TDI, and the clinical course was not clinically complicated by systemic nor pulmonary embolization. However, the patient's clinical conditions quickly worsened due to SARS-CoV-2 severe pneumonia.

CONCLUSION

This is a rare case of ischemic dilated cardiomyopathy complicated with biventricular apical thrombi early detected by TTE in a patient that was infected by COVID-19. The present case demonstrates the clinical usefulness of TTE implemented with PW-TDI for detecting ventricular thrombi and for measuring the thrombotic mass mobility. Although a biventricular thrombosis is a rare COVID-19 complication, performing appropriate diagnostic tests could decrease COVID-19 mortality in patients with dilated cardiomyopathy.

AUTHOR CONTRIBUTIONS

AS, ER, and ML performed the provided clinical procedures and collected the clinical data. AS, GN, ER, and ML analyzed the data and prepared the figures. AS, AA, DN, and ML discussed data and wrote the manuscript. All authors contributed to the article and approved the submitted version.

REFERENCES

1. Habash F, Vallurupalli S. Challenges in management of left ventricular thrombus. *Ther Adv Cardiovasc Dis.* (2017) 11:203–13. doi: 10.1177/1753944717711139

2. Lee JM, Park JJ, Jung HW, Cho YS, Oh IY, Yoon CH, et al. Left ventricular thrombus and subsequent thromboembolism, comparison of anticoagulation, surgical removal, antiplatelet agents. *J Atheroscler Thromb.* (2013) 20:73–93. doi: 10.5551/jat.13540

3. Missault L, Koch A, Colardyn F, Clement D. Biventricular thrombi in dilated cardiomyopathy: massive simultaneous pulmonary and systemic embolisation. *Eur Heart J.* (1994) 15:713–4. doi: 10.1093/oxfordjournals.eurheartj.a060574

4. Nishi I, Ishimitsu T, Ishizu T, Ueno Y, Suzuki A, Seo Y, et al. Peripartum cardiomyopathy and biventricular thrombi. *Circ J.* (2002) 66:863–5. doi: 10.1253/circj.66.863

5. Goncalves LF, Souto FM, Faro FN, Oliveira JL, Barreto-Filho JA, Sousa AC. Biventricular thrombus and endomyocardial fibrosis in antiphospholipid syndrome. *Arq Bras Cardiol.* (2012) 99:e162–5. doi: 10.1590/S0066-782X2012001400017

6. Hatanaka N, Ueda T. [Removal of biventricular thrombi for dilated cardiomyopathy in a patient with acute heart failure]. *Kyobu Geka.* (2014) 67:895–8.

7. Nkoke C, Kuate LM, Luchuo EB, Edie SD, Boombhi J, Menanga A. Biventricular thrombi in dilated cardiomyopathy in a patient with human immunodeficiency virus infection: a case report. *BMC Res Notes.* (2015) 8:168. doi: 10.1186/s13104-015-1140-x

8. Iwano T, Yunoki K, Tokunaga N, Shigetoshi M, Sugiyama H, Yamamoto H, et al. A case of biventricular thrombi in a patient with dilated cardiomyopathy: utility of multimodality imaging for diagnosis and management of treatment strategy. *J Cardiol Cases.* (2017) 15:91–4. doi: 10.1016/j.jccase.2016.10.013

9. Kammari CB, Rallabandi S, Rallabandi H, Daggubati SR, Adapa S, Naramala S, et al. Case report: dilated cardiomyopathy with biventricular thrombus secondary to impaired coagulation in a patient with HIV. *F1000Res.* (2020) 9:610. doi: 10.12688/f1000research.24016.2

10. Albini A, Di Guardo G, Noonan DM, Lombardo M. The SARS-CoV-2 receptor, ACE-2, is expressed on many different cell types: implications for ACE-inhibitor- and angiotensin II receptor blocker-based cardiovascular therapies. *Intern Emerg Med.* (2020) 15:759–66. doi: 10.1007/s11739-020-02364-6

11. Yang J, Petitjean SJL, Koehler M, Zhang Q, Dumitru AC, Chen W, et al. Molecular interaction and inhibition of SARS-CoV-2 binding to the ACE2 receptor. *Nat Commun.* (2020) 11:4541. doi: 10.1038/s41467-020-18319-6

12. Akel T, Qaqa F, Abuarqoub A, Shamoon F. Pulmonary embolism: a complication of COVID 19 infection. *Thromb Res.* (2020) 193:79–82. doi: 10.1016/j.thromres.2020.05.033

13. Klok FA, Kruip M, van der Meer NJM, Arbous MS, Gommers D, Kant KM, et al. Incidence of thrombotic complications in critically ill ICU patients with COVID-19. *Thromb Res.* (2020) 191:145–7. doi: 10.1016/j.thromres.2020.04.013

14. Middeldorp S, Coppens M, van Haaps TF, Foppen M, Vlaar AP, Muller MCA, et al. Incidence of venous thromboembolism in hospitalized patients with COVID-19. *J Thromb Haemost.* (2020) 18:1995–2002. doi: 10.1111/jth.14888

15. Paterson RW, Brown RL, Benjamin L, Nortley R, Wiethoff S, Bharucha T, et al. The emerging spectrum of COVID-19 neurology: clinical, radiological and laboratory findings. *Brain.* (2020) 143:3104–20. doi: 10.1093/brain/awaa240

16. Poissy J, Goutay J, Caplan M, Parmentier E, Duburcq T, Lassalle F, et al. Pulmonary embolism in patients with COVID-19: awareness of an increased prevalence. *Circulation.* (2020) 142:184–6. doi: 10.1161/CIRCULATIONAHA.120.047430

17. Helms J, Tacquard C, Severac F, Leonard-Lorant I, Ohana M, Delabranche X, et al. High risk of thrombosis in patients with severe SARS-CoV-2 infection: a multicenter prospective cohort study. *Intensive Care Med.* (2020) 46:1089–98. doi: 10.1007/s00134-020-06062-x

18. Kollias A, Kyriakoulis KG, Stergiou GS, Syrigos K. Heterogeneity in reporting venous thromboembolic phenotypes in COVID-19: methodological issues and clinical implications. *Br J Haematol.* (2020) 190:529–32. doi: 10.1111/bjh.16993

19. Marietta M, Ageno W, Artoni A, De Candia E, Gresele P, Marchetti M, et al. COVID-19 and haemostasis: a position paper from Italian Society on Thrombosis and Haemostasis (SISET). *Blood Transfus.* (2020) 18:167–9. doi: 10.2450/2020.0083-20

An Unusual Case of Biventricular Thrombosis in a COVID-19 Patient with Ischemic Dilated...

137

20. Oxley TJ, Mocco J, Majidi S, Kellner CP, Shoirah H, Singh IP, et al. Large-vessel stroke as a presenting feature of Covid-19 in the young. *N Engl J Med.* (2020) 382:e60. doi: 10.1056/NEJMc2009787

21. Wise J. Covid-19 and thrombosis: what do we know about the risks and treatment? *BMJ.* (2020) 369:m2058. doi: 10.1136/bmj.m2058

22. Soltani M, Mansour S. Biventricular thrombi associated with myocardial infarction in a patient with COVID-19. *Can J Cardiol.* (2020) 36:1326.e9–1326.e11. doi: 10.1016/j.cjca.2020.06.016

23. Ferguson K, Quail N, Kewin P, Blyth KG. COVID-19 associated with extensive pulmonary arterial, intracardiac and peripheral arterial thrombosis. *BMJ Case Rep.* (2020) 13:e237460. doi: 10.1136/bcr-2020-237460

24. Ozer M, Abbasi F, Mahdi M, Goksu SY, Struble E. Massive biventricular thrombi complicating new-onset heart failure in a patient with suspected COVID-19. *J Cardiol Cases.* (2021). doi: 10.1016/j.jccase.2021.02.016. [Epub ahead of print].

25. Caci G, Albini A, Malerba M, Noonan DM, Pochetti P, Polosa R. COVID-19 and obesity: dangerous liaisons. *J Clin Med.* (2020) 9:2511. doi: 10.3390/jcm9082511

26. Mehta JL, Calcaterra G, Bassareo PP. COVID-19, thromboembolic risk, and Virchow's triad: lesson from the past. *Clin Cardiol.* (2020) 43:1362–7. doi: 10.1002/clc.23460

27. Aggeli C, Dimitroglou Y, Raftopoulos L, Sarri G, Mavrogeni S, Wong J, et al. Cardiac masses: the role of cardiovascular imaging in the differential diagnosis. *Diagnostics (Basel).* (2020) 10:1088. doi: 10.3390/diagnostics10121088

28. Sonaglioni A, Nicolosi GL, Lombardo M, Anza C, Ambrosio G. Prognostic relevance of left ventricular thrombus motility: assessment by pulsed wave tissue doppler imaging. *Angiology.* (2021) 72:355–63. doi: 10.1177/0003319720974882

17

COVID-19 Management and Arrhythmia: Risks and Challenges for Clinicians Treating Patients Affected by SARS-CoV-2

Alexander Carpenter[1]*, Owen J. Chambers[2], Aziza El Harchi[1], Richard Bond[3], Oliver Hanington[1], Stephen C. Harmer[1], Jules C. Hancox[1] and Andrew F. James[1]

[1] *School of Physiology, Pharmacology and Neuroscience, University of Bristol, Bristol, United Kingdom,* [2] *Liverpool Heart and Chest Hospital NHS Foundation Trust, Liverpool, United Kingdom,* [3] *Gloucestershire Hospitals NHS Foundation Trust, Gloucester, United Kingdom*

*Correspondence:
Alexander Carpenter
alexander.carpenter@bristol.ac.uk

The COVID-19 pandemic is an unprecedented challenge and will require novel therapeutic strategies. Affected patients are likely to be at risk of arrhythmia due to underlying comorbidities, polypharmacy and the disease process. Importantly, a number of the medications likely to receive significant use can themselves, particularly in combination, be pro-arrhythmic. Drug-induced prolongation of the QT interval is primarily caused by inhibition of the hERG potassium channel either directly and/or by impaired channel trafficking. Concurrent use of multiple hERG-blocking drugs may have a synergistic rather than additive effect which, in addition to any pre-existing polypharmacy, critical illness or electrolyte imbalance, may significantly increase the risk of arrhythmia and Torsades de Pointes. Knowledge of these risks will allow informed decisions regarding appropriate therapeutics and monitoring to keep our patients safe.

Keywords: COVID-19, QT, arrhythmia, hERG, drug safety, QTc

INTRODUCTION

The novel coronavirus disease of 2019 (COVID-19) pandemic is uncharted territory for clinicians and healthcare systems alike. The potential for a high volume of severely unwell patients creates a significant challenge. In particular, the combination of severe infection, respiratory dysfunction, sepsis, shock, and/or haemodynamic instability (1–3) present significant potential for myocardial injury and potentially dangerous arrhythmia. Not only do these pathophysiological states promote the formation of arrhythmia, but unstable arrhythmia could present a significant threat to this cohort of patients who are at risk of haemodynamic instability.

Due to the potential strain on healthcare systems, it is likely that non-specialists will be involved in the management of COVID-19 patients including those experiencing arrhythmia. Similarly, clinicians may face situations where they are using multiple concurrent medications with which they may not be entirely familiar. Here, we attempt to summarize how the use of multiple different types of medication could contribute (synergistically, in some instances) to increase arrhythmic risk. In particular, we focus on the risk of drug-induced QT interval prolongation (commonly referred to as acquired long QT syndrome; aLQTS) which is a serious issue for many of the medications which are likely to be used.

While the use of drugs known to prolong the QT interval may well be necessary and unavoidable, an awareness and understanding of this risk should guide additional safety measures such as monitoring of the corrected QT interval (QTc) on 12-lead electrocardiogram (ECG) measurement. For cases of a prolonged QT interval there is a risk, particularly with a rate-corrected QT interval (QTc) of >500 ms (4), of dangerous arrhythmia including Torsades de Pointes (TdP); close monitoring and involvement of specialist cardiology input should be sought, as well as minimizing, where possible, the use of other known QT-prolonging medication.

INCREASED BASELINE ARRHYTHMIC RISK IN COVID-19 PATIENTS

From the data available, COVID-19 seems to cause more serious disease in older patients and those with comorbidities (1–3, 5–7). Zhou et al. (3) described hypertension, diabetes and coronary heart disease as the three most prevalent comorbidities in COVID-19 patients from two hospitals at the epicenter of the initial outbreak in Wuhan. Not only were these comorbidities associated with a significantly worse outcome, they are also, in combination with advanced age, significant risk factors for arrhythmia. Increasing age and co-morbidities also increase the likelihood of pre-existing polypharmacy, which may prove problematic in the context of additional potentially QT-prolonging medication. Unfortunately, published data of COVID-19 patient cohorts to date do not seem to include any ECG or specific arrhythmia data, although no doubt we will gain a better picture as our understanding of the disease and its management evolves.

INCREASED ARRHYTHMIC RISK OF COVID-19 INFECTION

SARS-CoV-2 is thought to gain entry to human host cells via the angiotensin converting enzyme 2 (ACE2) receptor, which is highly expressed in the heart and lungs and to which the viral spike protein has high affinity (8, 9). Interestingly, data during the previous SARS-CoV outbreak demonstrated ACE2-dependent cardiac infection and inflammation in both mouse and human hearts (10). The down-regulation of affected ACE2 receptors was suggested as a potential contributory factor to SARS-associated myocarditis and subsequent cardiomyopathy, with inflammation and fibrosis likely to provide a substrate for arrhythmia.

The risk of arrhythmia is likely to increase with the development of significant infection, and increase as the severity of the infection and/or systemic inflammatory response increases (11). Significant myocardial damage and fulminant myocarditis have been described (2, 3, 5), and cardiac arrest associated with ventricular arrhythmia (as well as non-shockable rhythms) is reported (7). Du et al. reported some form of arrhythmia present in 60% of a group of fatal cases, with cardiac arrest or malignant arrhythmia listed as the cause of death for over 10% of cases (12).

There is increasing awareness of the development in severely unwell patients of a hyperinflammatory state or cytokine storm (13) which can lead to multi-organ failure. Recent work strongly suggests this hypercytokinemia (in particular elevated levels of interleukin-6) further increases arrhythmic risk via multiple mechanisms, including, notably, hERG blockade (14) and QT prolongation (15, 16). Myocarditis itself is a heterogenous condition associated with a number of arrhythmic states including bradyarrhythmia and atrial or ventricular tachyarrhythmia (17). Data are urgently needed to describe the unique arrhythmic challenges of COVID-19 myocarditis.

Additionally, the multiple medications likely to receive significant use (antibiotics, anesthetic agents, anti-arrhythmic agents, and potentially specific agents to target COVID-19 such as anti-malarial or anti-viral medications) may indeed contribute to a pro-arrhythmic state in a patient group already at risk. Importantly, the additional risk of QT prolongation with some potential combinations of these medications may be synergistic rather than simply additive, due largely to their unique mechanisms of ion channel blockade. Finally, significant electrolyte disturbances, common in unwell patients, will further exacerbate arrhythmic risk (18).

CLINICAL MANAGEMENT OF COVID-19: SIGNIFICANT POTENTIAL FOR hERG BLOCKADE AND QT PROLONGATION

The hERG (or "Kv11.1") potassium channel (encoded by *human Ether-à-go-go Related Gene;* alternative nomenclature *KCNH2*) mediates the rapid component of cardiac delayed rectifier K^+ current (also known as I_{Kr}). Briefly, this channel is crucial to the repolarization phase of the cardiac action potential; we recommend an excellent review article (19). Inhibition of hERG is considered to be the most common and important mechanism of drug-induced QT prolongation (20, 21) and occurs through direct pharmacological channel block and/or impaired trafficking of hERG channels to the cell membrane. Consequently, hERG testing is a requirement during novel drug development: indeed, prolongation of the QT interval (and its association with dangerous TdP) has been the biggest cause of restriction or withdrawal of drugs already on the market (21–23).

Importantly, recent data including work from our group suggests that the effect on hERG (and thus on QT-prolongation) of multiple drugs may not be simply additive but synergistic (24, 25) (i.e., an effect in excess of the sum of their individual parts). This is particularly relevant when considering an older patient group who may already be taking hERG-blocking medication. In particular, the antimalarial medications chloroquine and hydroxychloroquine (26, 27) are receiving particular attention as antiviral agents: these drugs are multichannel blockers with particular effects on hERG and Kir2.1 and are likely to cause significant QT prolongation at the concentrations effective against SARS-CoV-2 *in vitro* (28–30), especially when combined with other antivirals (such as lopinavir/ritonavir) or antibiotics (macrolides and fluroquinolones being particularly notable) (26). Further information should be sought regarding novel antiviral agents (31) currently undergoing clinical trials; for example,

TABLE 1 | A list of medications which could be used in the management of COVID-19 which are also associated with risk of QT prolongation.

Type of medication	Drugs
Anesthetic agents	Propofol, sevoflurane
Antibiotic, antiviral or antifungal medication	Macrolides, fluoroquinolones, fluconazole, pentamidine, lopinavir/ritonavir*, favipiravir*
Anti-emetics	Domperidone, levomepromazine, ondansetron
Anti-arrhythmics	Amiodarone, flecainide, ibutilide, procainamide, quinidine, sotalol
Anti-psychotics (used for delirium)	Haloperidol, quetiapine, risperidone
Other potential therapies under consideration	Antimalarials such as chloroquine, hydroxychloroquine or mefloquine

*List intended to be illustrative as to risks and is not exhaustive. Further up to date information can be found online from trusted sources (www.crediblemeds.org). *possible rather than established risk.*

favipiravir has been associated with QT interval prolongation in a case report (32) and remdesivir awaits comprehensive testing.

Combination therapy with azithromycin and hydroxychloroquine is undergoing testing at present (33, 34). Notably, part of a Brazilian study comparing low vs. high dose chloroquine, in combination with ceftriaxone and azithromycin with or without oseltamivir, was terminated early due to safety concerns; with 25% of those in the high-dose arm showing QT prolongation (vs. 11% in the low-dose arm) and two patients in the high-dose arm experiencing ventricular tachycardia prior to death (35). Similarly, the head of a French cardiology unit reported they had prematurely terminated their hydroxychloroquine-azithromycin COVID-19 trial due to unacceptable QT prolongation (36). The randomized DisCoVeRy (NCT04315948), SOLIDARITY (EudraCT Number 2020-000982-18), and RECOVERY (EudraCT Number 2020-001113-21) studies will provide important evidence regarding the effectiveness and safety of various antiviral and antimalarial drugs in the treatment of COVID-19 patients (37).

Online resources can be consulted to clarify which drugs are associated with QT prolongation (see www.crediblemeds.org). **Table 1** lists medications associated with QT prolongation which

may be commonly used in the management of COVID-19 [as taken from the updated WHO management guidance (38) with additions from authors' clinical experience from UK practice]. The list is not exhaustive but attempts to highlight potential areas of risk when using these medications, as well as their use in combination.

DISCUSSION

The recent publication by Ackerman et al. of urgent guidance and a practical flow-chart regarding safe use of QT-prolonging medication is very welcome, and should be consulted as an aid to manage risk in the setting of QT prolongation (39), as should the Heart Rhythm Society (HRS) Task Force update (40). Other resources provide valuable guidance for clinicians dealing with specific patient populations: those with congenital heart disease (41) or inherited arrhythmia syndromes (42). Of note, a case report has reported significant QT prolongation (620 ms) in a patient with COVID-19 treated with multiple hERG blocking medications (including levofloxacin, hydroxychloroquine and azithromycin), which was successfully managed with drug cessation and intravenous lignocaine (43). Separately, mexiletine has also been suggested to be effective in treating TdP associated with acquired long QT syndrome (44).

COVID-19 represents a step into the unknown: not only are we grappling to come to terms with effective management of this new disease, but so too with safe use of these treatments. Effective therapy will be welcome, but the use of multiple drugs in combination has to be exercised with caution as it may increase the risk of QT prolongation and Torsades de Pointes, largely via pharmacological hERG blockade. Knowledge of this risk enables clinicians to ensure adequate monitoring of the QT interval and management of arrhythmic risk, maximizing safety for our patients in this challenging time.

AUTHOR CONTRIBUTIONS

All authors contributed to the concept, planning and writing of this mini-review, and approved the manuscript prior to submission.

REFERENCES

1. Guan W, Ni Z, Hu Y, Liang W, Ou C, He J, et al. Clinical characteristics of coronavirus disease 2019 in China. *N Engl J Med.* (2020). doi: 10.1101/2020.02.06.20020974. [Epub ahead of print].

2. Yang X, Yu Y, Xu J, Shu H, Xia A, Liu H, et al. Clinical course and outcomes of critically ill patients with SARS-CoV-2 pneumonia in Wuhan, China: a single-centered, retrospective, observational study. *Lancet Respir.* (2020). doi: 10.1016/S2213-2600(20)30079-5. [Epub ahead of print].

3. Zhou F, Yu T, Du R, Fan G, Liu Y, Liu Z, et al. Clinical course and risk factors for mortality of adult inpatients with COVID-19 in Wuhan, China: a retrospective cohort study. *Lancet.* (2020). doi: 10.1016/S0140-6736(20)30566-3. [Epub ahead of print].

4. Gibbs C, Thalamus J, Kristoffersen DT, Svendsen MV, Holla ØL, Heldal K, et al. QT prolongation predicts short-term mortality independent of comorbidity. *Europace.* (201) 21:1254–60. doi: 10.1093/europace/euz058

5. Ruan Q, Yang K, Wang W, Jiang L, Song J. Clinical predictors of mortality due to COVID-19 based on an analysis of data of 150 patients from Wuhan, China. *Intens Care Med.* (2020) 1–3. doi: 10.1007/s00134-020-05991-x. [Epub ahead of print].

6. Young BE, Ong SWX, Kalimuddin S, Low JG, Tan SY, Loh J, et al. Epidemiologic features and clinical course of patients infected with SARS-CoV-2 in Singapore. *JAMA.* (2020) 323:1488–94. doi: 10.1001/jama.2020.3204

7. Chen N, Zhou M, Dong X, Qu J, Gong F, Han Y, et al. Epidemiological and clinical characteristics of 99 cases of 2019 novel coronavirus pneumonia in Wuhan, China: a descriptive study. *Lancet.* (2020) 395:507–13. doi: 10.1016/S0140-6736(20)30211-7

8. Zhang H, Penninger JM, Li Y, Zhong N, Slutsky AS. Angiotensin-converting enzyme 2 (ACE2) as a SARS-CoV-2 receptor: molecular mechanisms and potential therapeutic target. *Intens Care Med.* (2020) 46:586–90. doi: 10.1007/s00134-020-05985-9

9. Crackower MA, Sarao R, Oliveira-dos-Santos AJ, Da Costa J, Zhang L. Angiotensin-converting enzyme 2 is an essential regulator of heart function. *Nature.* (2002) 417:822–8. doi: 10.1038/nature00786

10. Oudit GY, Kassiri Z, Jiang C, Liu PP, Poutanen SM, Penninger JM, et al. SARS-coronavirus modulation of myocardial ACE2 expression and inflammation in patients with SARS. *Eur J Clin Invest.* (2009) 39:618–25. doi: 10.1111/j.1365-2362.2009.02153.x

11. Shahreyar M, Fahhoum R, Akinseye O, Bhandari S, Dang G, Khouzam RN. Severe sepsis and cardiac arrhythmias. *Ann Transl Med.* (2018) 6:6. doi: 10.21037/atm.2017.12.26

12. Du Y, Tu L, Zhu P, Mu M, Wang R, Yang P, et al. Clinical features of 85 fatal cases of COVID-19 from Wuhan: a retrospective observational study. *Am J Respir Crit Care Med.* (2020). doi: 10.1164/rccm.202003-0543OC. [Epub ahead of print].

13. Mehta P, McAuley DF, Brown M, Sanchez E, Tattersall RS, Manson JJ. COVID-19: consider cytokine storm syndromes and immunosuppression. *Lancet.* (2020) 395:1033–4. doi: 10.1016/S0140-6736(20)30628-0

14. Aromolaran AS, Srivastava U, Alí A, Chahine M, Lazaro D, El-Sherif N, et al. Interleukin-6 inhibition of hERG underlies risk for acquired long QT in cardiac and systemic inflammation. *PLoS ONE.* (2018) 13:e0208321. doi: 10.1371/journal.pone.0208321

15. Lazzerini PE, Boutjdir M, Capecchi PL. COVID-19, arrhythmic risk and inflammation: mind the gap! *Circulation.* (2020). doi: 10.1161/CIRCULATIONAHA.120.047293. [Epub ahead of print].

16. Lazzerini PE, Laghi-Pasini F, Boutjdir M, Capecchi PL. Cardioimmunology of arrhythmias: the role of autoimmune and inflammatory cardiac channelopathies. *Nat Rev Immunol.* (2019) 19:63–4. doi: 10.1038/s41577-018-0098-z

17. Peretto G, Sala S, Rizzo S, De Luca G, Campochiaro C, Sartorelli S, et al. Arrhythmias in myocarditis: state of the art. *Heart Rhythm.* (2019) 16:793–801. doi: 10.1016/j.hrthm.2018.11.024

18. Zeltser D, Justo D, Halkin A, Prokhorov V, Heller K, Viskin S. Torsade de Pointes due to noncardiac drugs. *Medicine.* (2003) 82:282–90. doi: 10.1097/01.md.0000085057.63483.9b

19. Vandenberg JI, Perry MD, Perrin MJ, Mann SA, Ke Y, Hill AP. hERG K$^+$ channels: structure, function, and clinical significance. *Physiol Rev.* (2012) 92:1393–478. doi: 10.1152/physrev.00036.2011

20. Recanatini M, Poluzzi E, Masetti M, Cavalli A, De Ponti F. QT prolongation through hERG K$^+$ channel blockade: current knowledge and strategies for the early prediction during drug development. *Med Res Rev.* (2005) 25:133–66. doi: 10.1002/med.20019

21. Hancox JC, McPate MJ, El Harchi A, Zhang Y. The hERG potassium channel and hERG screening for drug-induced torsades de pointes. *Pharmacol Ther.* (2008) 119:118–32. doi: 10.1016/j.pharmthera.2008.05.009

22. Lasser KE, Allen PD, Woolhandler SJ, Himmelstein DU, Wolfe SM, Bor DH. Timing of new black box warnings and withdrawals for prescription medications. *J Am Med Assoc.* (2002) 287:2215–20. doi: 10.1001/jama.287.17.2215

23. Roden DM. Drug-induced prolongation of the QT interval. *N Engl J Med.* (2004) 350:1013–22. doi: 10.1056/NEJMra032426

24. Wiśniowska B, Lisowski B, Kulig M, Polak S. Drug interaction at hERG channel: *In vitro* assessment of the electrophysiological consequences of drug combinations and comparison against theoretical models. *J Appl Toxicol.* (2018) 38:450–8. doi: 10.1002/jat.3552

25. El Harchi A, Butler AS, Zhang Y, Dempsey CE, Hancox JC. The macrolide drug erythromycin does not protect the hERG channel from inhibition by thioridazine and terfenadine. *Physiol Rep.* (2020) 8:e14385. doi: 10.14814/phy2.14385

26. Cortegiani A, Ingoglia G, Ippolito M, Giarratano A, Einav S. A systematic review on the efficacy and safety of chloroquine for the treatment of COVID-19. *J Crit Care.* (2020). doi: 10.1016/j.jcrc.2020.03.005. [Epub ahead of print].

27. Colson P, Rolain J-M, Lagier J-C, Brouqui P, Raoult D. Chloroquine and hydroxychloroquine as available weapons to fight COVID-19. *Int J Antimicrob Agents.* (2020) 105932. doi: 10.1016/j.ijantimicag.2020.105932. [Epub ahead of print].

28. Rodríguez-Menchaca AA, Navarro-Polanco RA, Ferrer-Villada T, Rupp J, Sachse FB, Tristani-Firouzi M, et al. The molecular basis of chloroquine block of the inward rectifier Kir2.1 channel. *Proc Natl Acad Sci USA.* (2008) 105:1364–8. doi: 10.1073/pnas.0708153105

29. Traebert M, Dumotier B, Meister L, Hoffmann P, Dominguez-Estevez M, Suter W. Inhibition of hERG K$^+$ currents by antimalarial drugs in stably transfected HEK293 cells. *Eur J Pharmacol.* (2004) 484:41–8. doi: 10.1016/j.ejphar.2003.11.003

30. Vincent MJ, Bergeron E, Benjannet S, Erickson BR, Rollin PE, Ksiazek TG, et al. Chloroquine is a potent inhibitor of SARS coronavirus infection and spread. *Virol J.* (2005) 2:69. doi: 10.1186/1743-422X-2-69

31. Dong L, Hu S, Gao J. Discovering drugs to treat coronavirus disease 2019 (COVID-19). *Drug Discov Ther.* (2020) 14:58–60. doi: 10.5582/ddt.2020.01012

32. Chinello P, Petrosillo N, Pittalis S, Biava G, Ippolito G, Nicastri E. QTc interval prolongation during favipiravir therapy in an Ebolavirus-infected patient. *PLoS Negl Trop Dis.* (2017) 11:e0006034. doi: 10.1371/journal.pntd.0006034

33. Gautret P, Lagier J-C, Parola P, Hoang VT, Meddeb L, Mailhe M, et al. Hydroxychloroquine and azithromycin as a treatment of COVID-19: results of an open-label non-randomized clinical trial. *Int J Antimicrob Agents.* (2020) 105949. doi: 10.1016/j.ijantimicag.2020.105949. [Epub ahead of print].

34. Molina JM, Delaugerre C, Le Goff J, Mela-Lima B, Ponscarme D, Goldwirt L, et al. No evidence of rapid antiviral clearance or clinical benefit with the combination of hydroxychloroquine and azithromycin in patients with severe COVID-19 infection. *Médecine Mal Infect.* (2020). doi: 10.1016/j.medmal.2020.03.006. [Epub ahead of print].

35. Borba M, de Val FA, Sampaio VS, Alexandre MA, Melo GC, Brito M, et al. Chloroquine diphosphate in two different dosages as adjunctive therapy of hospitalized patients with severe respiratory syndrome in the context of coronavirus (SARS-CoV-2) infection: preliminary safety results of a randomized, double-blinded, phase IIb cl. *medRxiv.* (2020). doi: 10.1101/2020.04.07.20056424. [Epub ahead of print].

36. NEWSWEEK. *French Hospital Stops Hydroxychloroquine Treatment for COVID-19 Patient Over Major Cardiac Risk.* Available online at: https://www.newsweek.com/hydroxychloroquine-coronavirus-france-heart-cardiac-1496810 (accessed April 19, 2020).

37. Taccone FS, Gorham J, Vincent J-L. Hydroxychloroquine in the management of critically ill patients with COVID-19: the need for an evidence base. *Lancet.* (2020) doi: 10.1016/S2213-2600(20)30172-7. [Epub ahead of print].

38. World Health Organization. *Clinical Management of Severe Acute Respiratory Infection (SARI) When COVID-19 Disease Is Suspected: Interim Guidance* (2020).

39. Giudicessi JR, Noseworthy PA, Friedman PA, Ackerman MJ. Urgent guidance for navigating and circumventing the QTc-prolonging and torsadogenic potential of possible pharmacotherapies for Coronavirus Disease 19 (COVID-19). *Mayo Clin Proc.* (2020). doi: 10.1016/j.mayocp.2020.03.024. [Epub ahead of print].

40. Heart Rhythm Society. *HRS COVID-19 Task Force Update.* Heart Rhythm Society. Available online at: https://www.hrsonline.org/COVID19-Challenges-Solutions/hrs-covid-19-task-force-message-qtc-guidance (accessed April 16, 2020).

41. Tan W, Aboulhosn J. The cardiovascular burden of coronavirus disease 2019 (COVID-19) with a focus on congenital heart disease. *Int J Cardiol.* (2020). doi: 10.1016/j.ijcard.2020.03.063. [Epub ahead of print].

42. Wu C-I, Postema PG, Arbelo E, Behr ER, Bezzina CR, Napolitano C, et al. SARS-CoV-2, COVID-19 and inherited arrhythmia syndromes. *Heart Rhythm.* (2020). doi: 10.1016/j.hrthm.2020.03.024. [Epub ahead of print].

43. Mitra RL, Greenstein SA, Epstein LM. An algorithm for managing QT prolongation in Coronavirus Disease 2019 (COVID-19) patients treated with either chloroquine or hydroxychloroquine in conjunction with azithromycin: possible benefits of intravenous lidocaine. *Heart Case Rep.* (2020). doi: 10.1016/j.hrcr.2020.03.016. [Epub ahead of print].

44. Badri M, Patel A, Patel C, Liu G, Goldstein M, Robinson VM, et al. Mexiletine prevents recurrent torsades de pointes in acquired long QT syndrome refractory to conventional measures. *JACC Clin Electrophysiol.* (2015) 1:315–22. doi: 10.1016/j.jacep.2015. 05.008

18

Pre-Existing Health Conditions and Epicardial Adipose Tissue Volume: Potential Risk Factors for Myocardial Injury in COVID-19 Patients

Zhi-Yao Wei[1†], Rui Qiao[2†], Jian Chen[3†], Ji Huang[4†], Wen-Jun Wang[5†], Hua Yu[6†], Jing Xu[7†], Hui Wu[8,9†], Chao Wang[10†], Chong-Huai Gu[2†], Hong-Jiang Li[11], Mi Li[12], Cong Liu[13], Jun Yang[8,9], Hua-Ming Ding[14], Min-Jie Lu[15], Wei-Hua Yin[16], Yang Wang[17], Kun-Wei Li[18], Heng-Feng Shi[19], Hai-Yan Qian[1*], Wei-Xian Yang[1*] and Yong-Jian Geng[20*†]

[1] State Key Laboratory of Cardiovascular Disease, Department of Cardiology, Center for Coronary Heart Disease, National Center for Cardiovascular Diseases of China, Fu Wai Hospital, Peking Union Medical College, Chinese Academy of Medical Sciences, Beijing, China, [2] Department of Cardiology, Anqing Hospital, Anhui Medical University, Anqing, China, [3] Guangdong Provincial Key Laboratory of Biomedical Imaging, Department of Cardiovascular Medicine, Fifth Affiliated Hospital of Sun Yat-sen University, Zhuhai, China, [4] Department of Cardiology, Beijing Anzhen Hospital, Capital Medical University, Beijing, China, [5] Department of Cardiology, Daye Chinese Medicine Hospital, Daye, China, [6] Division of Life Sciences and Medicine, Department of Cardiology, The First Affiliated Hospital of University of Science and Technology of China, Hefei, China, [7] Division of Life Sciences and Medicine, Department of Infectious Diseases, The First Affiliated Hospital of University of Science and Technology of China, Hefei, China, [8] Institute of Cardiovascular Disease, China Three Gorges University, Yichang, China, [9] Department of Cardiology, Yichang Central People's Hospital, Yichang, China, [10] Coronary Care Unit, Baoding No.1 Central Hospital, Baoding, China, [11] Sixth Department of Hepatopathy, Baoding People's Hospital, Baoding, China, [12] Department of Gastroenterology, Yingcheng Chinese Medicine Hospital, Yingcheng, China, [13] Department of Otolaryngology, Daye People's Hospital, Daye, China, [14] Department of Radiology, Infection Hospital of Anhui Provincial Hospital (Hefei Infectious Diseases Hospital), Hefei, China, [15] State Key Laboratory of Cardiovascular Disease, Department of Magnetic Resonance Imaging, National Center for Cardiovascular Diseases of China, Fu Wai Hospital, Peking Union Medical College, Chinese Academy of Medical Sciences, Beijing, China, [16] State Key Laboratory of Cardiovascular Disease, Department of Radiology, National Center for Cardiovascular Diseases of China, Fu Wai Hospital, Peking Union Medical College, Chinese Academy of Medical Sciences, Beijing, China, [17] State Key Laboratory of Cardiovascular Disease, Medical Research and Biometrics Center, National Center for Cardiovascular Diseases of China, Fu Wai Hospital, Peking Union Medical College, Chinese Academy of Medical Sciences, Beijing, China, [18] Department of Radiology, Fifth Affiliated Hospital of Sun Yat-sen University, Zhuhai, China, [19] Department of Radiology, Anqing Hospital, Anhui Medical University, Anqing, China, [20] Division of Cardiology, Department of Internal Medicine, The Center for Cardiovascular Biology and Atherosclerosis Research, McGovern Medical School, University of Texas Health Science Center at Houston, Houston, TX, United States

*Correspondence:
Hai-Yan Qian
ahqhy712@163.com
Wei-Xian Yang
wxyang2009@sina.com
Yong-Jian Geng
yong-jian.geng@uth.tmc.edu

† These authors have contributed
equally to this work

Background: Myocardial injury is a life-threatening complication of coronavirus disease 2019 (COVID-19). Pre-existing health conditions and early morphological alterations may precipitate cardiac injury and dysfunction after contracting the virus. The current study aimed at assessing potential risk factors for COVID-19 cardiac complications in patients with pre-existing conditions and imaging predictors.

Methods and Results: The multi-center, retrospective cohort study consecutively enrolled 400 patients with lab-confirmed COVID-19 in six Chinese hospitals remote to the Wuhan epicenter. Patients were diagnosed with or without the complication of myocardial injury by history and cardiac biomarker Troponin I/T (TnI/T) elevation above the 99th percentile upper reference limit. The majority of COVID-19 patients with myocardial injury exhibited pre-existing health conditions, such as hypertension, diabetes, hypercholesterolemia, and coronary disease. They had increased levels of the inflammatory cytokine interleukin-6 and more in-hospital adverse events (admission to an intensive care unit, invasive mechanical ventilation, or death). Chest CT scan on admission demonstrated that COVID-19 patients with myocardial injury had higher epicardial adipose tissue volume ([EATV] 139.1 (83.8–195.9) vs. 92.6 (76.2–134.4) cm^2; $P = 0.036$). The optimal EATV cut-off value (137.1 cm^2) served as a useful factor for assessing myocardial injury, which yielded sensitivity and specificity of 55.0% (95%CI, 32.0–76.2%) and 77.4% (95%CI, 71.6–82.3%) in adverse cardiac events, respectively. Multivariate logistic regression analysis showed that EATV over 137.1 cm^2 was a strong independent predictor for myocardial injury in patients with COVID-19 [OR 3.058, (95%CI, 1.032–9.063); $P = 0.044$].

Conclusions: Augmented EATV on admission chest CT scan, together with the pre-existing health conditions (hypertension, diabetes, and hyperlipidemia) and inflammatory cytokine production, is associated with increased myocardial injury and mortality in COVID-19 patients. Assessment of pre-existing conditions and chest CT scan EATV on admission may provide a threshold point potentially useful for predicting cardiovascular complications of COVID-19.

Keywords: COVID-19, SARS-CoV-2, pandemic (COVID-19), CT imaging findings, cardiac complication

INTRODUCTION

Coronavirus disease 2019 (COVID-19) is a highly contagious disease caused by severe acute respiratory syndrome coronavirus 2 (SARS-CoV-2). Since its first breakout in Wuhan, China, the COVID-19 pandemic has triggered a worldwide health crisis. According to WHO, globally, as of September 20, 2020, COVID-19 has caused nearly one million deaths (1). SARS-CoV-2 mainly attacks the respiratory system, clinically characterized by rapidly progressive pneumonia and acute respiratory distress syndrome (ARDS) (2). However, the virus may damage other tissues and organs directly or indirectly, in particular, the cardiovascular system. Indeed, individuals with pre-existing health conditions are highly vulnerable to the pathological insults from the viral infection (3, 4). COVID-19 patients display not only the manifestations of pulmonary injury but also multiple organ damage and dysfunction. The viral injury to various tissue or organs constitutes a complex clinical syndrome with a broad spectrum of pathophysiological characteristics, which contribute to the severity and mortality of COVID-19 (5–8).

Currently, COVID-19 patients with myocardial injury are diagnosed when the serum levels of troponin I/T (TnI/T) increase above the 99th percentile upper reference limit, after excluding TnI/T elevation and other evidence related to pre-existing obstructive coronary artery disease. Thus, the abnormal levels of myocardial biomarkers constitute the main criteria to identify COVID-19 patients with myocardial injury. However, TnI/T changes may occur in other pathological conditions, such as infection, hypoxia, and renal insufficiency, commonly observed during the development of COVID-19. Hence, assessment of myocardial injury should be performed using a comprehensive approach, including non-invasive imaging, electrocardiography, and laboratory examination for proper clinical judgment

in patients with abnormal TnI/T levels. Regarding cardiac morphological examination or image analysis, echocardiography or cardiovascular magnetic resonance (CMR) is not routine examination for COVID-19 patients, and generates non-specific images that may be lagging in early detection of myocardial injury (9). Conversely, chest computed tomography (CT) is routinely performed in patients suspected for COVID-19, usually as soon as hospital admission, to evaluate the severity of pneumonia. Therefore, an early imaging indicator based on chest CT is valuable for timely assessment and diagnosis of myocardial injury morphologically. Epicardial adipose tissue volume (EATV) has been used to evaluate the adipose tissue between the epicardial surface and pericardium, and reportedly associated with heart inflammation (10). In this multi-center, retrospective study, we explored the pre-existing health conditions and chest CT EATV as potential risk factors for myocardial injury in COVID-19 patients.

METHODS

Study Design, Participants, and Data Recording

The current multi-centered, retrospective study of laboratory-confirmed COVID-19 patients was conducted in six independent hospitals, located in the Eastern, Southern, Northern, and Central regions of China. All the cases of COVID-19 were confirmed positively in SARS-CoV-2 detection of respiratory specimens by real-time reverse-transcriptase–polymerase-chain-reaction (RT-PCR), according to the guidelines of the World Health Organization and the National Health Commission of China (11, 12). A total of 549 consecutive patients with confirmed COVID-19 were admitted from January 3 to February 26, 2020.

Except for 43 patients who remain hospitalized and 106 patients with no record of TnI/T, all other 400 patients were enrolled in the final analysis.

The epidemiological, demographic, clinical, laboratory, imaging, treatment, and outcome data of enrolled patients were collected by experienced local clinicians, and entered into a computerized database and cross-checked. The time from the onset of symptoms to hospital admission was 5 (3–7) days. All the patients underwent at least one TnI/T test, 285/400 (96.3%) patients had TnI/T data available within the first 24 h of hospital admission, and 373/400 (93.3%) patients had more than one test result of TnI/T during hospitalization. Myocardial injury was diagnosed and confirmed according to the highest level of TnI/T during hospitalization.

Study Definitions

Myocardial injury was diagnosed when the highest level of Troponin I/T (TnI/T) was above the 99th percentile upper reference limit (reference range of each hospital is available at **Supplementary Table 1**), after excluding the possibility of acute coronary syndrome (13). Fever was defined as an axillary temperature of 37.3°C or higher. Hypertension was defined as systolic blood pressure over 140 mmHg or diastolic blood pressure over 90 mmHg. In-hospital adverse events included admission to an intensive care unit (ICU), the use of invasive mechanical ventilation, or death (14, 15). The injury was further confirmed by reviewing admission logs and histories from electronic medical care records.

Analysis of Epicardial Adipose Tissue Volume (EATV) by CT Scan

Chest CT scan was performed within the first 24 h of hospital admission in accordance with the guidance for COVID-19 from the Chinese National Health Commission (12). Chest CT images were collected, and measured using breath-hold electrocardiogram-gated CT scanners with 256 or 64 detector rows (uCT 760, uMI 780 scanners, United Imaging, Shanghai, China; Precision 32, CAMPO Imaging, Shenyang, China; NeuViz 64 In/En, Neusoft, Liaoning, China; SOMATOM Emotion 16, Siemens, Germany; SOMATOM definition AS, Siemens, Germany; Optima CT680, GE Healthcare, USA). The scan conditions were set as 120–140 kV, 300–320 mA, 512 × 512 matrix, and the field of view was 240 mm with a slice thickness of 1–3 mm. Images were reconstructed using a soft-tissue algorithm. EATV was calculated and established from mediastinal window images according to the standardized operation protocol by trained radiologists blinded to the study protocol. The baseline characteristics of patients with and without EATV were roughly the same (**Table 1**). Epicardial adipose tissue was identified on the CT scan as a hypodense rim surrounding the myocardium and limited to the pericardium. The visceral pericardium was traced manually from the aortic arch to the left ventricular apex, and all extra-pericardial tissue was excluded. The individual EATV measurement within the manually traced epicardium in each slice was detected by assigning a threshold CT value of −200 and −30 HU and

then was automatically summed with the software of Siemens Syngo.via (Siemens, Germany) to determine the total EATV.

Statistical Analyses

Data were presented as mean ± standard deviation (SD) or median with quartiles for continuous variables and number (%) for categorical variables. Differences between patients with and without myocardial injury were assessed with the two-tail t-test or Wilcoxon rank-sum test for continuous variables and Chi-square or Fisher's exact test for categorical variables. The receiver operating characteristic (ROC) curve analysis was used to select a cut-off value for EATV, and sensitivity and specificity for predicting myocardial injury incidence were calculated. Multivariate logistic regression analysis was applied to control confounding factors that might be associated with EATV (age, weight, history of hyperlipidemia, and coronary heart disease) when identifying the predicting value of EATV for the incidence of myocardial injury. Multivariate logistic regression analysis was also applied to control baseline confounders (age, history of hypertension, diabetes, and coronary heart disease) when exploring the association of myocardial injury with severe COVID-19. The consistency of the results was confirmed in patients with EATV value in subgroup analysis. Tests were two-sided with significance set at $\alpha < 0.05$. SPSS for Windows (Version 22.0, IBM) and Graphpad Prism 8.0 software were used for statistical analysis.

RESULTS

Baseline Characteristics and Pre-existing Health Conditions

The current cohort study enrolled 549 patients consecutively who suffered from laboratory-confirmed COVID-19 and admitted to six hospitals outside of the Wuhan epicenter as of March 8, 2020. Among them, there were 43 patients remained hospitalized and 106 patients with no record of TnI/T and thereby excluded from the study. All other 400 patients were entering into the final analysis, and the enrolling process was shown in **Figure 1**. There were 46 hospitalized COVID-19 patients were diagnosed suffering from myocardial injury. COVID-19 patients with myocardial injury were slightly older than those without [52.5 (42.8–68.0) vs. 49.0 (36.0–60.0) years]. The incidence of myocardial injury was much higher in patients with pre-existing health conditions, such as hypertension [12/46 (26.1%) vs. 50/354 (14.1%); $P = 0.035$], hyperlipidemia [4/46 (8.7%) vs. 7/354 (2.0%); $P = 0.028$], and chronic kidney disease [3/46 (6.5%) vs. 2/354 (0.6%); $P = 0.012$] as compared with non-myocardial injury COVID-19 patients.

There were no differences in the percentage of patients having the signs and symptoms between the myocardial and non-myocardial injury groups, except for fatigue and dyspnea (**Table 2**). Although no significant difference in pulse was found on admission, the incidence of tachycardia during hospitalization was significantly increased in patients undergoing myocardial injury.

TABLE 1 | Baseline comparison between general population ($n = 400$) and patients with EATV value ($n = 272$).

	Patients with EATV value	Patients without EATV value	P-value[a]
Age (yrs)	48.7 ± 15.4	48.0 ± 16.6	0.666
Female	137/272 (50.4%)	54/128 (42.2%)	0.127
Hypertension	45/272 (16.5%)	18/128 (14.1%)	0.525
Diabetes	26/272 (9.6%)	11/128 (8.6%)	0.756
White blood cells, × 10^9/L	5.0 (4.0–5.7)	5.0 (4.0–6.4)	0.553
Platelets, × 10^9/L ($n = 388$)	176.0 ± 60.6	167.7 ± 56.0	0.209
Alanine aminotransferase, U/L ($n = 392$)	24.0 (15.0–38.0)	23.0 (15.0–41.0)	0.922
Creatinine, μmol/L ($n = 391$)	54.9 (46.0–67.1)	64.0 (55.0–79.0)	<0.001
C-reactive protein, mg/L ($n = 393$)	17.0 (4.1–69.0)	23.0 (5.7–49.5)	0.082

[a]Significant difference ($p < 0.05$) was determined between patients with EATV value and patients without EATV value.

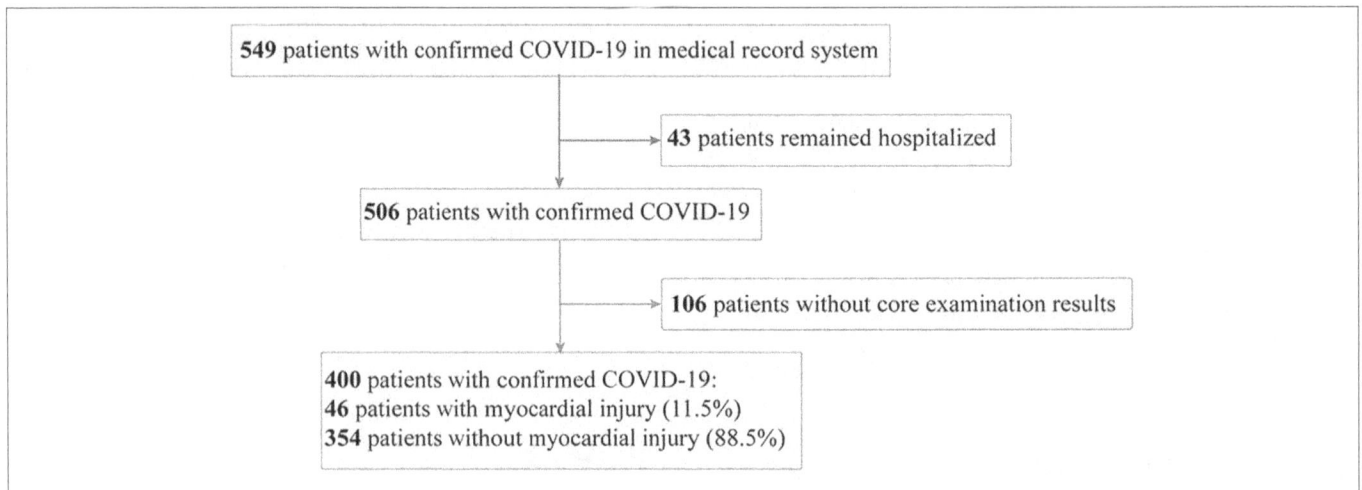

FIGURE 1 | Flowchart of patient recruitment. COVID-19 cases confirmed by RT-PCR assays were enrolled in this cohort study from six hospitals or regional medical centers remote to the Wuhan epicenter from January 3 to February 26, 2020.

Laboratory and Electrocardiographic Findings Showing Cardiac Dysfunction

COVID-19 patients with myocardial injury showed markedly increased levels of interleukin-6 [6.5 (5.2–17.9) vs. 2.3 (1.5–6.3) pg/mL; $P < 0.001$]. However, there was no significant difference on the levels of CRP, an acute phase protein known to arise during inflammation, between the cardiac injury and non-injury groups. We observed that patients with elevated TnI/T also had increased blood levels of other types of biomarkers for cardiac injury and dysfunction [e.g., lactate dehydrogenase, creatine kinase, and N-terminal pro-B-type natriuretic peptide (NT-proBNP)]. Compared with non-myocardial injury patients, the abnormality of lipid metabolites in peripheral blood occurred at a higher frequency in myocardial injury patients, with raising levels of total cholesterol (4.7 ± 1.1 vs. 4.0 ± 2.5 mmol/L; $P = 0.029$), low-density lipoprotein (2.8 ± 1.0 vs. 2.2 ± 0.7 mmol/L; $P = 0.001$), and triglycerides [2.7 (1.5–4.1) vs. 1.1 (0.9–1.9) mmol/L; $P < 0.001$] (**Table 3**).

Of 106 patients with the electrocardiogram records, 20 (18.9%) patients developed ST-T changes. However, the distribution was not significantly different between patients with and without elevated cTnI/T levels.

COVID-19 patients with myocardial injury showed no change in the pH values of arterial blood while having a higher prevalence of hypoxia (SaPO2 < 95%) than those without cardiac injury (**Table 3**), implying increased severity of COVID-19 injury toward the respiratory system in patients with myocardial injury.

Chest CT Scan Assessment of EATV Predicating Myocardial Injury

The chest CT scan performed on admission showed that EATV in patients with myocardial injury was significantly larger than the non-injury patients [139.1 (83.8–195.9) vs. 92.6 (76.2–134.4) cm^2; $P = 0.036$]. **Figure 2** illustrates chest CT images in COVID-19 cases with and without myocardial injury. Using the receiver operating characteristic (ROC) curve analysis, we found that a cut-off value of 137.1 cm^2 in EATV had predicted the occurrence of myocardial injury at 55% sensitivity, 77% specificity, and the area under the curve of 0.642. The positive likelihood ratio is 0.193, while the negative likelihood ratio is 0.046. Patients with EATV over 137.1 cm^2 on admission were more commonly diagnosed with myocardial injury than those not [11/68 (16.2%) vs. 9/204 (4.4%); $P = 0.001$]. In the univariable logistic analysis, odds of myocardial injury were greater in patients with EATV

TABLE 2 | Comparison in demographic and clinical characteristics of COVID-19 patients with and without myocardial injury.

	Total	Myocardial injury	Non-myocardial injury	P-value[a]
	(n = 400)	(n = 46)	(n = 354)	
Age (yrs)	49.0 (37.0–61.0)	52.5 (42.8–68.0)	49.0 (36.0–60.0)	0.046
Female	191 (47.8%)	20 (43.5%)	171 (48.3%)	0.538
Hypertension	62 (15.5%)	12 (26.1%)	51 (14.1%)	0.035
Diabetes	37 (9.3%)	8 (17.4%)	29 (8.2%)	0.056
Hyperlipidemia	11 (2.8%)	4 (8.7%)	7 (2.0%)	0.028
Liver Disease	7 (1.8%)	2 (4.3%)	5 (1.4%)	0.187
Kidney disease	5 (1.3%)	3 (6.5%)	2 (0.6%)	0.012
Signs and symptoms				
Fever	334 (83.5%)	40 (87.0%)	294 (83.1%)	0.502
Cough	295 (73.8%)	33 (71.7%)	262 (74.0%)	0.724
Fatigue	91 (22.8%)	16 (34.8%)	75 (21.2%)	0.039
Abdominal discomfort/ diarrhea/vomiting	43 (10.8%)	6 (13.0%)	37 (10.5%)	0.612
Sore throat	35 (8.8%)	7 (15.2%)	28 (7.9%)	0.102
Weight (Kg)	65.0 (57.0–72.0)	65.0 (57.0–75.0)	65.0 (57.0–71.8)	0.889
Respiratory rate >20 breaths/min	162 (40.5%)	19 (42.2%)	143 (40.5%)	0.826
Pulse rate, median (bpm)	83.6 ± 12.9	86.3 ± 10.6	83.3 ± 13.1	0.171
Peak pulse rate, (bpm)	97.3 ± 11.9	103.2 ± 14.0	96.8 ± 11.6	0.012

[a]Significant difference (p < 0.05) was determined between the myocardial and non-myocardial injury groups.

TABLE 3 | Laboratory and electrocardiographic findings of COVID-19 patients with or without myocardial injury.

	Total	Myocardial injury	Non-myocardial injury	P-value[a]
	(n = 400)	(n = 46)	(n = 354)	
Laboratory findings				
White blood cells, mean, × 10^9/L	5.0 (4.0–5.8)	5.3 (3.8–6.7)	5.0 (4.0–5.8)	0.455
Neutrophils, mean, × 10^9/L	3.2 (2.2–4.2)	3.3 (2.3–5.2)	3.2 (2.2–4.2)	0.567
Lymphocytes, mean, × 10^9/L	1.0 (0.9–1.5)	1.0 (0.8–1.3)	1.0 (0.9–1.5)	0.058
Platelets, median, × 10^9/L (n = 388)	173.5 ± 59.3	166.8 ± 61.4	174.4 ± 59.1	0.420
Alanine aminotransferase, U/L (n = 392)	24.0 (15.0–39.5)	20.0 (14.8–28.3)	24.0 (15.0–41.0)	0.130
Aspartate aminotransferase, U/L (n = 392)	26.0 (19.0–34.0)	27.5 (21.0–34.2)	26.0 (19.0–34.0)	0.259
Creatinine, μmol/L (n = 391)	57.6 (46.9–71.3)	66.4 (51.8–76.4)	56.9(46.1–70.0)	0.007
Creatine kinase, U/L (n = 391)	61.0 (41.0–100.0)	84.0 (54.6–150.8)	60.0 (39.5–92.9)	0.002
Lactate dehydrogenase, U/L (n = 391)	191.0 (154.0–263.0)	227.0 (167.5.0–311.5)	188.0 (152.5–256.0)	0.015
Interleukin-6, pg/mL (n = 103)	5.2 (1.5–7.2)	6.5 (5.2–17.9)	2.3 (1.5–6.3)	<0.001
C-reactive protein, mg/L (n = 393)	18.5 (4.6–38.8)	20.7 (5.8–43.3)	18.4 (4.1–37.8)	0.709
NT-Pro-BNP, pg/mL (n = 80)	68.0 (27.3–330.5)	663.6 (103.8–2450.5)	51 (24.2–179.8)	<0.001
Total cholesterol, mmol/L (n = 211)	4.1 ± 2.4	4.7 ± 1.1	4.0 ± 2.5	0.029
Low-density lipoprotein, mmol/L (n = 210)	2.2 ± 0.8	2.8 ± 1.0	2.2 ± 0.7	0.001
Triglycerides, mmol/L (n = 211)	1.1 (0.9–2.2)	2.7 (1.5–4.1)	1.1 (0.9–1.9)	<0.001
Arterial pH, (n = 80)	7.46 ± 0.05	7.45 ± 0.05	7.46 ± 0.05	0.322
SaPO$_2$ <95%	28/167 (16.8%)	7/18(38.9%)	21/149(14.1%)	0.015
Electrocardiographic findings				
ST-T change	20/106 (18.9%)	1/16(6.3%)	19/90(21.1%)	0.296
Left bundle branch block	3/106 (2.8%)	0/16 (0.0%)	3/90(3.3%)	>0.999

[a]Significant difference (p < 0.05) was determined between the myocardial and non-myocardial injury groups.

on admission over 137.1 cm^2. Age, and pre-existing health conditions, such as diabetes, hyperlipidemia, and coronary heart disease, were also significantly associated with myocardial injury. In a multivariable logistic regression model which included 265 patients with necessary data (20 with myocardial injury and 245 without myocardial injury), we found that EATV

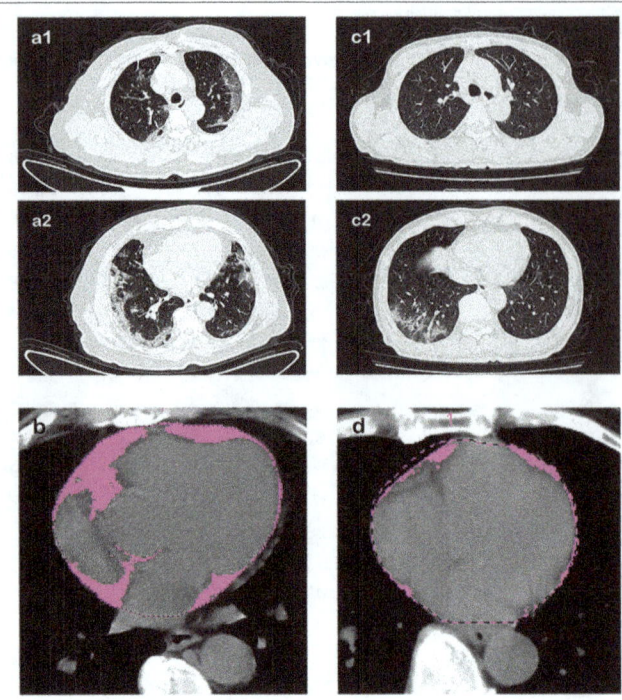

FIGURE 2 | Chest CT scan images and EATV assessment in COVID-19 patients with and without myocardial injury. Transverse chest CT images at two different positions were collected during the first 24 h of hospital admission. Epicardial adipose tissue volume was assessed and calculated in the pink area. Case A, in the age range of 60–70 years, who presented myocardial injury during hospitalization, representative chest CT scan image at two different pulmonary and cardiac positions: **(a1)** Upper position of heart and lung, and **(a2)** middle-lower position of heart and lung), showing subpleural strip-like ground-glass opacities and patchy consolidation scattering in the left upper lobe, right middle lobe, and bilateral lower lobes, the typical imaging findings of lung involvement in COVID-19. **(b)** The epicardial adipose tissue volume was 221 cm^3, presented as the pink area. Case B, also in the age range of 60–70 years but did not present myocardial injury during hospitalization. **(c1,c2)** Representative CT scan images at the lung window showing similar images of lung injury characteristic of COVID-19: subpleural irregular patchy and grid-like hyperdense shallows with blurred edges in the right lower lobe. **(d)** The epicardial adipose tissue volume or EATV was 86.5 cm^3 in this case. The volume of hypodense tissue surrounding the myocardium appearing much smaller than that shown in case A.

on admission over 137.1 cm^2 was associated with the higher incidence of myocardial injury [adjusted odds ratio (OR) 3.058, (95%CI, 1.032–9.063); $P = 0.044$], after adjusting the influence of age, body weight, the history of coronary heart disease and hyperlipidemia. Age and the history of hyperlipidemia also remained significant in this model (**Table 4**).

Therapeutic Approaches and Outcomes in COVID-19 Patients With and Without Myocardial Injury

Almost all the enrolled patients received various antiviral treatments. No differences in therapeutics were found between the myocardial injury and non-myocardial injury groups, except for the usage of corticosteroids [17/46 (37.0%) vs. 83/354

(23.4%); $P = 0.047$] (**Table 5**). In myocardial injury patients, corticosteroid therapies had markedly decreased the blood levels of IL-6 [6.0 (4.9–7.6) vs. 15.4 (5.8–34.9) pg/mL; $P = 0.03$] as well as the incidence of in-hospital adverse events [1/17 (5.9%) vs. 11/29 (37.9%); $P = 0.034$].

In-hospital adverse events (admission to an ICU, invasive mechanical ventilation, or death) occurred in 47 patients (11.8%), including 40 (10.0%) of whom were admitted to ICU, 5 (1.3%) underwent invasive mechanical ventilation, and 8 (2.0%) died (**Table 5**). Compared with those without myocardial injury, myocardial injury patients underwent more in-hospital adverse events [12/46 (26.1%) vs. 35/354 (9.9%); $P = 0.001$], while the incidence of death and ICU admission were higher too.

In the multivariable logistic regression model including all 400 patients (46 patients with myocardial injury and 354 without myocardial injury), the myocardial injury was independently associated with the risk of in-hospital adverse events [adjusted OR 2.607 (95%CI: 1.166–5.830); $P = 0.020$] after adjusting for age, sex, history of hypertension, diabetes and coronary heart disease. Age also remained significant in this model, indicating that it also contributes to in-hospital adverse events (**Supplementary Table 2**). This association remained stable in patients with EATV value ($n = 272$) in subgroup analysis (**Supplementary Table 3**).

DISCUSSION

In the current cohort study we investigated and compared the clinical characteristics between COVID-19 patients with and without myocardial injury, who were admitted to six hospitals and regional medical centers outside of the epicenter of Wuhan. This group of patients demonstrated certain pathophysiological characteristics, to a certain degree, different from those hospitalized and treated in Wuhan or other epicenters of COVID-19 around the world. We observed that many of the patients had pre-existing health conditions and increased values of EATV on admission which might be predisposed to the pathogenesis of myocardial injury. The average age of patients with myocardial injury appears higher than those without myocardial injury, but the age gap only marginable, suggesting that in this cohort, pre-existing health conditions, rather than age, might serve as the major risk factors for the development of myocardial injury. Pre-existing cardiovascular and metabolic comorbidities were more commonly observed in COVID-19 patients with myocardial injury, along with abnormal levels of metabolic indicators, indicating COVID-19 patients with underlying cardiovascular conditions, especially abnormal lipid metabolism, are exposed to an increased risk for myocardial injury. Myocardial injury serves as a contributor to the severity and mortality of COVID-19, with reported hazard ratio ranging from 2.1 to 8.9 (9, 16, 17), and odds ratio from 6.6 to 26.9 (18–20) in different studies. Our logistic regression analysis also suggests that myocardial injury is an independent adverse event, which precipitates poor prognosis. Thus, it is of great importance to timely detect and treat patients with a high risk of myocardial injury and to offer a special care to avoid relevant adverse events.

TABLE 4 | Predictors for the incidence of myocardial injury ($n = 265$).

	Univariable OR (95% CI)	P-value[a]	Multivariable OR (95% CI)	P-value[b]
Age, 10 years	1.225 (1.004–1.495)	0.045	1.602 (1.035–2.477)	0.034
Male sex (vs female)	1.215 (0.654–2.256)	0.538	–	–
Hyperlipidemia (vs not present)	4.721 (1.326–16.803)	0.017	5.247 (1.122–24.551)	0.035
Coronary heart disease (vs not present)	8.000 (1.099–58.224)	0.040	8.273 (0.742–92.187)	0.086
Epicardial adipose tissue volume on admission >137.1 cm² (vs. not present)	4.181 (1.651–10.588)	0.003	3.058 (1.032–9.063)	0.044
Weight	0.997 (0.972–1.023)	0.814	1.021 (0.973–1.072)	0.402

OR, odd ratio; CI, confidence intervals.
[a]Significant difference (p < 0.05) was determined using univariable logistic regression model.
[b]Significant difference (p <0.05) was determined using multivariable logistic regression model.

TABLE 5 | Therapeutics received and outcomes of COVID-19 patients with or without myocardial injury.

	Total ($n = 400$)	Myocardial injury ($n = 46$)	Non-myocardial injury ($n = 354$)	P-value[a]
Treatment				
Oxygen therapy	199 (49.8%)	24 (52.2%)	175 (49.7%)	0.754
Invasive mechanic ventilation	5 (1.3%)	1 (2.2%)	4 (1.1%)	0.459
Non-invasive mechanic ventilation	25 (6.3%)	2/46 (4.3%)	23 (6.5%)	0.459
Lopinavir/ritonavir	236 (59.0%)	29 (63.0%)	207 (58.5%)	0.553
Arbidol	160 (40.0%)	22 (47.8%)	138 (39.0%)	0.266
Oseltamivir	94 (23.5%)	14 (30.4%)	80 (22.6%)	0.238
Antibiotics	282 (70.6%)	31 (67.4%)	251 (71.1%)	0.608
Corticosteroids	100 (25.0%)	17 (37.0%)	83 (23.4%)	0.047
Outcomes				
ICU admission	40 (10.0%)	11 (23.9%)	29 (8.2%)	0.003
Death	8 (2.0%)	5 (10.9%)	3 (0.8%)	0.001

ICU, intensive care unit.
[a]Significant difference (p < 0.05) was determined between the myocardial and non-myocardial injury groups.

Patients with the deadly contagious disease COVID-19 often receive medical attention in ICU or emergency room. Upon admission, less likely, they will have a comprehensive imaging assessment of cardiac complications, including echocardiography and CMR. Moreover, echocardiographic findings in patients with myocardial injury are mostly non-specific (9). Slight injury may not lead to functional or structural changes, and often it is undetectable by echocardiography and cardiac magnetic reasoning imaging. Only 20% of COVID-19 patients with myocardial injury showed abnormality on echocardiogram, left others with normal performance (21). CMR is reportedly helpful in revealing the cardiac involvement of COVID-19 in recovered patients, but its predicting value in COVID-19 patients is doubtful (22).

In the current cohort study, we explored the feasibility of using cardiac images from routine chest CT scan as a potential index of myocardial injury. Our findings demonstrate the correlation between EATV on admission and the occurrence of myocardial injury. First, the mean value of EATV is significantly larger in COVID-19 patients with myocardial injury than those without myocardial injury. Second, 137.1 cm² is the optimal cut-off point of EATV for predicting in-hospital myocardial injury on ROC analysis. Third, EATV over 137.1 cm² is the strong independent

indicator for myocardial injury in general COVID-19 patients, with a valuable negative predictive value.

For the diagnosis and assessment of pneumonia, the predominant manifestation of COVID-19, patients are routinely examined by chest CT scan. Strictly speaking, EATV is a measurement of not mere fat tissue expansion but also peri- or epicardiac soft tissue (perhaps consisting of both fat and inflammatory connective tissues) enlargement with inflammatory responses (10, 23). It is exquisitely sensitive to the adjacent inflammatory states associated with coronary atherosclerotic plaque, atrial fibrillation, and systemic inflammatory disorders (24).

To date, the precise mechanisms that cause myocardial injury in COVID-19 patients are not entirely understood. The cytokine storm (i.e., excessive and uncontrollable cytokine production in response to SARS-CoV-2 infection, may be one of the main contributors to the pathogenic injury of myocardium). There have been plenty of studies indicating that serum levels of cytokines are significantly increased in COVID-19 patients (3, 4). Moreover, cytokine levels were associated with disease mortality and the incidence of myocardial injury (2, 25, 26), indicating the contributing role of cytokine storm in COVID-19 associated myocardial injury. In our population, compared with patients without myocardial injury, IL-6 levels were significantly higher in myocardial injury patients, implying the possible pathogenic role of the cytokine storm in the development of myocardial injury. CRP levels were increased too, but statistically no significance was found between the groups of COVID-19 patients. Myocardial injury patients treated with corticosteroids had markedly decreased levels of IL-6. This observation may partially explain the improved outcome in myocardial injury patients treated with the steroids.

Epicardial fat may represent a transducer that mediates the detrimental impacts of systemic inflammation on the adjacent myocardium (27). We observed the significantly enlarged EATV in COVID-19 patients with myocardial injury, which may be due to inflammatory cell infiltration and temporary edema related to systemic cytokine storm and pericarditis and micro-myocarditis.

Increased EATV has been shown in obese individuals with increased chest and abdominal obesity, a possible risk factor for myocardial injury. Abdominal obesity is proved to be the major risk factor for disease progression and mortality in COVID-19 patients, independent of obesity-related comorbidities (28, 29). So high body mass index (BMI) and waist-hip ratio indicate a high risk of hospitalization (30). As a reflection of total visceral fatness, EATV is associated with BMI and waist circumference (31, 32), so the strong association between high EATV and myocardial injury may reveal the possible contributing role of overall and abdominal obesity to the development of myocardial injury. In this study, we observed hyperlipidemia in COVID-19 patients with myocardial injury. The elevation of EATV values in COVID-19 patients may also reflect this pathological condition.

Taken together, observations from the current study clearly document that EATV enlargement may serve as a potentially important parameter or predictor for the development of myocardial injury. Although the exact mechanism behind the association of high EATV and in-hospital myocardial injury remains unclear, it is recommendable to employ the CT scan measurement of EATV as an early risk evaluation for myocardial injury in COVID-19, in combination with other imaging methods.

Study Limitations

First, given the retrospective nature of this study, some parameters were not available in all the patients enrolled in the study. There were 128 enrolled patients who lacked the mediastinal window images, so the predicting value of EATV was analyzed based on data from the other 272 patients. Systemic bias might be introduced, though the baseline characteristics between patients with and without EATV values were roughly the same. Second, the inconsistency of troponin type between study centers deters us from clarifying the correlation between EATV and the severity of myocardial injury, which may offer a more comprehensive picture for EATV study in COVID-19 patients with cardiovascular complications. Third, myocardial injury was identified by a combination of biomarkers and clinical symptoms, primarily the abnormal levels of TnI/T during hospitalization. However, TnI/T levels could be affected by other determinants, such as the infection status, hypoxia, and renal insufficiency, which might lead to the false-positive diagnosis. On the other hand, false positive diagnosis might exist as some patients approaching to stable conditions might have a decreased likelihood of myocardial injury identification. This could cause a systematic bias when assessing the relationship between myocardial injury and disease severity. Fourth, echocardiographic data were not available in enrolled patients. A comprehensive assessment of the heart function using electrocardiography, imaging, and laboratory testing would help a deeper understanding of clinical profiles of myocardial injury.

Furthermore, we only account for weight in logistic regression, instead of other better indicator for obesity like BMI or waist-hip ratio. So as an early predictor for myocardial injury, EATV may not be independent of obesity. Whether simple anthropometric data is a predictor for myocardial injury will be explored in our further study. The role of abdominal obesity in myocardial injury development is also worthy of being investigated in the future, leveraging specific indicators like adiponectin. And finally, the cohort is relatively smaller and restricted to the Han Chinese COVID-19 patients. Thus, the conclusion should be further confirmed by large-scale prospective cohort studies in ethnically diverse cohorts.

CONCLUSIONS

Myocardial injury is the major in-hospital adverse event that contributes to the mortality of COVID-19 patients. Pre-existing health conditions, inflammatory cytokine production, and augmented EATV on admission may serve as potentially independent risk factors for the development of myocardial injury in COVID-19 patients. EATV at less than the threshold 137.1 cm^2 or so in a chest CT scan on admission may predict a better outcome for COVID-19 patients with increased risks of myocardial injury.

AUTHOR CONTRIBUTIONS

Z-YW, H-YQ, W-XY, and Y-JG designed the study. Z-YW, H-YQ, and Y-JG drafted the manuscript. RQ, JC, W-JW, HY, JX, HW, CW, and C-HG acquired and analyzed the data. Z-YW and YW contributed to the statistical analysis. JH, ML, CL, JY, H-MD, M-JL, K-WL, and H-FS made technical support. All authors contributed to the article and approved the submitted version.

ACKNOWLEDGMENTS

We thank all health-care workers in the six clinical centers for their tireless and bravely supporting patient enrollment, data collection, and processing. We especially thank Drs. Chun Zhou, Gui-Rong Xiong (Yichang Central People's Hospital), Li-Zheng Song, and Ying-Hua Zhong (Fifth Affiliated Hospital of Sun Yat-sen University) for their works on the collection of clinical data. Special thanks are also given to the imaging analyzing team members Drs. Jun-Long Pan and Song Yu (Yichang Central People's Hospital).

REFERENCES

1. World Health Organization. *Coronavirus disease (COVID-19) outbreak.* Available online at: https://www.who.int/emergencies/diseases/novel-coronavirus-2019 (accessed February 8, 2020).

2. Huang C, Wang Y, Li X, Ren L, Zhao J, Hu Y, et al. Clinical features of patients infected with 2019 novel coronavirus in Wuhan, China. *Lancet.* (2020) 395:497–506. doi: 10.1016/S0140-6736(20)30183-5

3. Geng YJ, Wei ZY, Qian HY, Huang J, Lodato R, Castriotta RJ. Pathophysiological characteristics and therapeutic approaches for pulmonary injury and cardiovascular complications of coronavirus disease 2019. *Cardiovasc Pathol.* (2020) 47:107228. doi: 10.1016/j.carpath.2020.107228

4. Wei ZY, Geng YJ, Huang J, Qian HY. Pathogenesis and management of myocardial injury in coronavirus disease 2019. *Eur J Heart Fail.* (2020) 22:1994–2006. doi: 10.1002/ejhf.1967

5. Inciardi RM, Lupi L, Zaccone G, Italia L, Raffo M, Tomasoni D, et al. Cardiac involvement in a patient with coronavirus disease 2019 (COVID-19). *JAMA Cardiol.* (2020) 5:819–24. doi: 10.1001/jamacardio.2020.1096

6. Guo T, Fan Y, Chen M, Wu X, Zhang L, He T, et al. Cardiovascular implications of fatal outcomes of patients with coronavirus disease 2019 (COVID-19). *JAMA Cardiol.* (2020) 5:811–8. doi: 10.1001/jamacardio.2020.1017

7. Zhou F, Yu T, Du R, Fan G, Liu Y, Liu Z, et al. Clinical course and risk factors for mortality of adult inpatients with COVID-19 in Wuhan, China: a retrospective cohort study. *Lancet.* (2020) 395:1054–62. doi: 10.1016/S0140-6736(20)30566-3

8. Du Y, Tu L, Zhu P, Mu M, Wang R, Yang P, et al. Clinical features of 85 fatal cases of COVID-19 from wuhan: a retrospective observational study. *Am J Respir Crit Care Med.* (2020) 201:1372–79. doi: 10.1164/rccm.202003-0543OC

9. Deng Q, Hu B, Zhang Y, Wang H, Zhou X, Hu W, et al. Suspected myocardial injury in patients with COVID-19: evidence from front-line clinical observation in Wuhan, China. *Int J Cardiol.* (2020) 311:116–21. doi: 10.1016/j.ijcard.2020.03.087

10. Braha A, Timar B, Diaconu L, Lupusoru R, Vasiluta L, Sima A, et al. Dynamics of epicardiac fat and heart function in type 2 diabetic patients initiated with SGLT-2 inhibitors. *Diabetes Metab Syndr Obes.* (2019) 12:2559–66. doi: 10.2147/DMSO.S223629

11. World Health Organization. *Clinical Management of Severe Acute Respiratory Infection when Novel Coronavirus (nCoV) Infection is Suspected: Interim Guidance.* Available online at: https://www.who.int/publications-detail/clinical-management-of-severe-acute-respiratory-infection-when-novel-coronavirus-(ncov)-infection-is-suspected (accessed January 28, 2020).

12. National Health Commission. *Notification for the Practice Guideline of the 2019 Novel Coronavirus Diease (version seventh)* Available online at: http://www.gov.cn/zhengce/zhengceku/2020-03/04/content_5486705.htm (accessed March 04, 2020).

13. Thygesen K, Alpert JS, Jaffe AS, Chaitman BR, Bax JJ, Morrow DA, et al. Fourth universal definition of myocardial infarction 2018. *Circulation.* (2019) 138:e618–51. doi: 10.1161/CIR.0000000000000617

14. Guan WJ, Ni ZY, Hu Y, Liang WH, Ou CQ, He JX, et al. Clinical characteristics of coronavirus disease 2019 in China. *N Engl J Med.* (2020) 382:1708–20. doi: 10.1056/NEJMoa2002032

15. Guan WJ, Liang WH, Zhao Y, Liang HR, Chen ZS, Li YM, et al. Comorbidity and its impact on 1590 patients with COVID-19 in China: a nationwide analysis. *Eur Respir J.* (2020) 55:2000547. doi: 10.1183/13993003.01227-2020

16. Shi S, Qin M, Shen B, Cai Y, Liu T, Yang F, et al. Association of cardiac injury with mortality in hospitalized patients with COVID-19 in Wuhan, China. *JAMA Cardiol.* (2020) 5:802–10. doi: 10.1001/jamacardio.2020.0950

17. Shi S, Qin M, Cai Y, Liu T, Shen B, Yang F, et al. Characteristics and clinical significance of myocardial injury in patients with severe coronavirus disease 2019. *Eur Heart J.* (2020) 41:2070–9. doi: 10.1093/eurheartj/ehaa408

18. Chen C, Chen C, Yan JT, Zhou N, Zhao JP, Wang DW. Analysis of myocardial injury in patients with COVID-19 and association between concomitant cardiovascular diseases and severity of COVID-19. *Zhonghua xin xue guan bing za zhi.* (2020) 48:567–71. doi: 10.3760/cma.j.cn112148-20200225-00123

19. Ni W, Yang X, Liu J, Bao J, Li R, Xu Y, et al. Acute myocardial injury at hospital admission is associated with all-cause mortality in COVID-19. *J Am Coll Cardiol.* (2020) 76:124–5. doi: 10.1016/j.jacc.2020.05.007

20. Wei J-F, Huang F-Y, Xiong T-Y, Liu Q, Chen H, Wang H, et al. Acute myocardial injury is common in patients with covid-19 and impairs their prognosis. *Heart.* (2020) 106:1154–9. doi: 10.1136/heartjnl-2020-317007

21. Bangalore S, Sharma A, Slotwiner A, Yatskar L, Harari R, Shah B, et al. ST-segment elevation in patients with covid-19 - a case series. *N Engl J Med.* (2020) 382:2478–80. doi: 10.1056/NEJMc2009020

22. Puntmann VO, Carerj ML, Wieters I, Fahim M, Arendt C, Hoffmann J, et al. Outcomes of cardiovascular magnetic resonance imaging in patients recently recovered from coronavirus disease 2019 (COVID-19). *JAMA Cardiol.* (2020) 5:1265–73. doi: 10.1001/jamacardio.2020.3557

23. Wang J, Chen D, Cheng XM, Zhang QG, Peng YP, Wang LJ, et al. Influence of phenotype conversion of epicardial adipocytes on the coronary atherosclerosis and its potential molecular mechanism. *Am J Transl Res.* (2015) 7:1712–23.

24. Wang J, Chen D, Cheng XM, Zhang QG, Peng YP, Wang LJ, et al. Epicardial adipose tissue may mediate deleterious effects of obesity and inflammation on the myocardium. *J Am Coll Cardiol.* (2018) 71:2360–72. doi: 10.1016/j.jacc.2018.03.509

25. Chen T, Wu D, Chen H, Yan W, Yang D, Chen G, et al. Clinical characteristics of 113 deceased patients with coronavirus disease 2019: retrospective study. *BMJ.* (2020) 368:m1091. doi: 10.1136/bmj.m1091

26. Song Y, Gao P, Ran T, Qian H, Guo F, Chang L, et al. High inflammatory burden: a potential cause of myocardial injury in critically Ill patients with COVID-19. *Front Cardiovasc Med.* (2020) 7:128. doi: 10.3389/fcvm.2020.00128

27. Patel VB, Shah S, Verma S, Oudit GY. Epicardial adipose tissue as a metabolic transducer: role in heart failure and coronary artery disease. *Heart Fail Rev.* (2017) 22:889–902. doi: 10.1007/s10741-017-9644-1

28. Tartof S, Qian L, Hong V, Wei R, Nadjafi R, Fischer H, et al. Obesity and mortality among patients diagnosed with COVID-19: results from an integrated health care organization. *Ann Intern Med.* (2020) 173:773–81. doi: 10.7326/M20-3742

29. Sales-Peres S, de Azevedo-Silva L, Bonato R, Sales-Peres M, Pinto A, Santiago Junior JJOr, et al. Coronavirus (SARS-CoV-2) and the risk of obesity for critically illness and ICU admitted: Meta-analysis of the epidemiological evidence. *Obes Res Clin Pract.* (2020) 14:389–97. doi: 10.2139/ssrn.3612053

30. Hamer M, Gale C, Kivimäki M, Batty G. Overweight, obesity, and risk of hospitalization for COVID-19: a community-based cohort study of adults in the United Kingdom. *Proc Natl Acad Sci USA.* (2020) 117:21011–3. doi: 10.1073/pnas.2011086117

31. Alexopoulos N, McLean DS, Janik M, Arepalli CD, Stillman AE, Raggi P. Epicardial adipose tissue and coronary artery plaque characteristics. *Atherosclerosis.* (2010) 210:150–4. doi: 10.1016/j.atherosclerosis.2009.11.020

32. de Vos AM, Prokop M, Roos CJ, Meijs MFL, van der Schouw YT, Rutten A, et al. Peri-coronary epicardial adipose tissue is related to cardiovascular risk factors and coronary artery calcification in post-menopausal women. *Eur Heart J.* (2008) 29:777–83. doi: 10.1093/eurheartj/ehm564

19

Lung Ultrasound Score as a Predictor of Mortality in Patients with COVID-19

Zhenxing Sun [1,2†], Ziming Zhang [1,2†], Jie Liu [1,2†], Yue Song [1,2], Shi Qiao [1,2], Yilian Duan [1,2], Haiyan Cao [1,2], Yuji Xie [1,2], Rui Wang [1,2], Wen Zhang [1,2], Manjie You [1,2], Cheng Yu [1,2], Li Ji [1,2], Chunyan Cao [1,2], Jing Wang [1,2], Yali Yang [1,2], Qing Lv [1,2], Hongbo Wang [3*‡], Haotian Gu [4*‡] and Mingxing Xie [1,2*‡]

[1] Department of Ultrasound Medicine, Union Hospital, Tongji Medical College, Huazhong University of Science and Technology, Wuhan, China, [2] Hubei Province Key Laboratory of Molecular Imaging, Wuhan, China, [3] Department of Gynecology and Obstetrics, Union Hospital, Tongji Medical College, Huazhong University of Science and Technology, Wuhan, China, [4] British Heart Foundation Centre of Research Excellence, King's College London, London, United Kingdom

*Correspondence:
Haotian Gu
haotian.gu@kcl.ac.uk
Hongbo Wang
drwanghb69@sina.com
Mingxing Xie
xiemx@hust.edu.cn

[†] These authors share first authorship

[‡] These authors share senior authorship

Background: Lung injury is a common condition among hospitalized patients with coronavirus disease 2019 (COVID-19). However, whether lung ultrasound (LUS) score predicts all-cause mortality in patients with COVID-19 is unknown. The aim of the present study was to explore the predictive value of lung ultrasound score for mortality in patients with COVID-19.

Methods: Patients with COVID-19 who underwent lung ultrasound were prospectively enrolled from three hospitals in Wuhan, China between February 2020 and March 2020. Demographic, clinical, and laboratory data were collected from digital patient records. Lung ultrasound scores were analyzed offline by two observers. Primary outcome was in-hospital mortality.

Results: Of the 402 patients, 318 (79.1%) had abnormal lung ultrasound. Compared with survivors ($n = 360$), non-survivors ($n = 42$) presented with more B2 lines, pleural line abnormalities, pulmonary consolidation, and pleural effusion (all $p < 0.05$). Moreover, non-survivors had higher global and anterolateral lung ultrasound score than survivors. In the receiver operating characteristic analysis, areas under the curve were 0.936 and 0.913 for global and anterolateral lung ultrasound score, respectively. A cutoff value of 15 for global lung ultrasound score had a sensitivity of 92.9% and specificity of 85.3%, and 9 for anterolateral score had a sensitivity of 88.1% and specificity of 83.3% for prediction of death. Kaplan–Meier analysis showed that both global and anterolateral scores were strong predictors of death (both $p < 0.001$). Multivariate Cox regression analysis showed that global lung ultrasound score was an independent predictor (hazard ratio, 1.08; 95% confidence interval, 1.01–1.16; $p = 0.03$) of death together with age, male sex, C-reactive protein, and creatine kinase-myocardial band.

Conclusion: Lung ultrasound score as a semiquantitative tool can be easily measured by bedside lung ultrasound. It is a powerful predictor of in-hospital mortality and may play a crucial role in risk stratification of patients with COVID-19.

Keywords: COVID-19, SARS-CoV-2, lung ultrasound score, mortality, prognosis

BACKGROUND

The coronavirus disease 2019 (COVID-19) is a newly recognized infectious disease caused by the severe acute respiratory syndrome coronavirus 2 (SARS-CoV-2). Although chest computed tomography (CT) has been regarded as an important diagnostic tool for COVID-19 diagnosis (1), it is limited by high cost, radiation exposure, infection control challenges, and lack of continuous monitoring, particularly for critically ill patients (2). Lung ultrasound (LUS), with the advantage of being non-invasive, low cost, and radiation free, has been increasingly used as a bed-side tool for evaluation and monitoring of lung diseases, particularly in the intensive care unit (ICU) (2, 3). It was found to have high accuracy in diagnosing viral community-acquired pneumonia with 94% sensitivity and 89% specificity for the detection of viral pneumonia in symptomatic patients (4). Global LUS score, a semiquantitative numerical score of lung aeration across 12 lung regions, has been shown as a useful tool to diagnose acute respiratory distress syndrome (ARDS) (5).

We therefore hypothesized that LUS score may play an important role in detecting lung lesions and optimizing risk stratification in patients with COVID-19. To test this hypothesis, LUS images in patients prospectively recruited from three hospitals in Wuhan, China were analyzed to evaluate the prognostic value of LUS score for in-hospital mortality in patients with COVID-19.

MATERIALS AND METHODS

Patient Population

Patients with confirmed COVID-19 who underwent lung ultrasound were consecutively recruited from the West Branch of Wuhan Union Hospital, Cancer Centre of Union Hospital, and Jianghan Mobile Cabin Hospital Wuhan, China between February 6, 2020 and March 15, 2020. The study was approved by the ethics committee, Union Hospital, Tongji Medical College, Huazhong University of Science and Technology (No. 20200021). Written informed consent was waived because of the unprecedented nature of COVID-19 pandemic.

Inclusion criteria were age $\geq$18 years and confirmed COVID-19. Exclusion criteria were incomplete image acquisition, missing clinical data, and cardiac failure causing cardiogenic pulmonary oedema.

Demographic, clinical history, comorbidities, laboratory data, and outcomes of all patients were obtained from electronic medical records (Dthealth Medical Systems CO, Tianjin, China). Primary outcome was all-cause mortality. All patients were followed up until April 7, 2020 when the last patient in the study was discharged.

Lung Ultrasound

LUS examinations were performed by nine qualified ultrasound doctors using Mindray M9 potable ultrasound machines (Mindray Bio-medical electronics Co, Shenzhen, China) with 1- to 5- MHz convex probes. LUS consisted of 12 different regions (two anterior, two lateral, and two posterior thoracic regions) (**Supplementary Figure 1**) as previously described (6).

All video files were recorded in a hospital local archive and were interpreted and scored offline by two experienced observers within 24 h of LUS examinations who were blinded to the clinical data and outcomes. In case of disagreement between observers, the two observers agreed by consensus on the LUS score.

Examples of ultrasound findings including the patterns of B lines, consolidations, pleural line abnormalities, pleural effusion, and the lesion distribution are shown in **Figure 1**.

Lung Ultrasound Score

LUS score was determined based on four lung patterns (**Supplementary Table 1**): N = 0, B1 = 1, B2 = 2, and C = 3 as described previously (7):

a. N pattern—normal aeration: A lines or <3 isolated B lines;
b. B1 pattern—moderate loss of lung aeration: a clear number of multiple visible B lines with horizontal spacing between adjacent B lines $\leq$7 mm (B1 lines);
c. B2 pattern—severe loss of lung aeration: multiple B lines fused together with horizontal spacing between adjacent B lines $\leq$3 mm, including "white lung" (B2 lines); and
d. C pattern—complete loss of aeration: pulmonary consolidation, presence of tissue pattern accompanied by static or dynamic air bronchograms.

Global LUS score was calculated by summing the scores of all 12 lung regions (ranging from 0 to 36). An adjusted composite score, antero-lateral score, was also derived by summing the anterior and lateral regional scores (range from 0 to 24) (5, 7).

Repeatability and Reproducibility of Lung Ultrasound Score

Intra- and interobserver variability of global LUS score was assessed in 30 randomly selected subjects by repeat measurements on the same images 1 month apart by two observers. Bland–Altman plots were produced.

Statistical Analysis

Demographic, clinical, and outcome variables were presented as percentages for categorical variables and as medians with interquartile ranges (IQRs) for continuous variables. The Mann–Whitney U-test was used to compare LUS scores between survivors and non-survivors.

Receiver operating characteristic (ROC) curves for death were drafted for global and anterolateral score. The area under the receiver operating characteristic curves (AUCs) was calculated to determine the diagnostic accuracy for death. The optimal cutoffs were determined as the highest Youden's index (sensitivity + specificity – 1).

Kaplan–Meier curves were used to examine cumulative death rate, and differences between groups were tested using a log rank test. Univariate and multivariate Cox regression analysis was performed to identify potential predictors of death. Multivariate models were constructed to assess the prognostic utility of global and anterolateral scores, incorporating covariables that were significant ($p < 0.05$) in the univariate analysis. All statistical analyses were performed using SPSS version 25 (SPSS Inc. Chicago, Illinois).

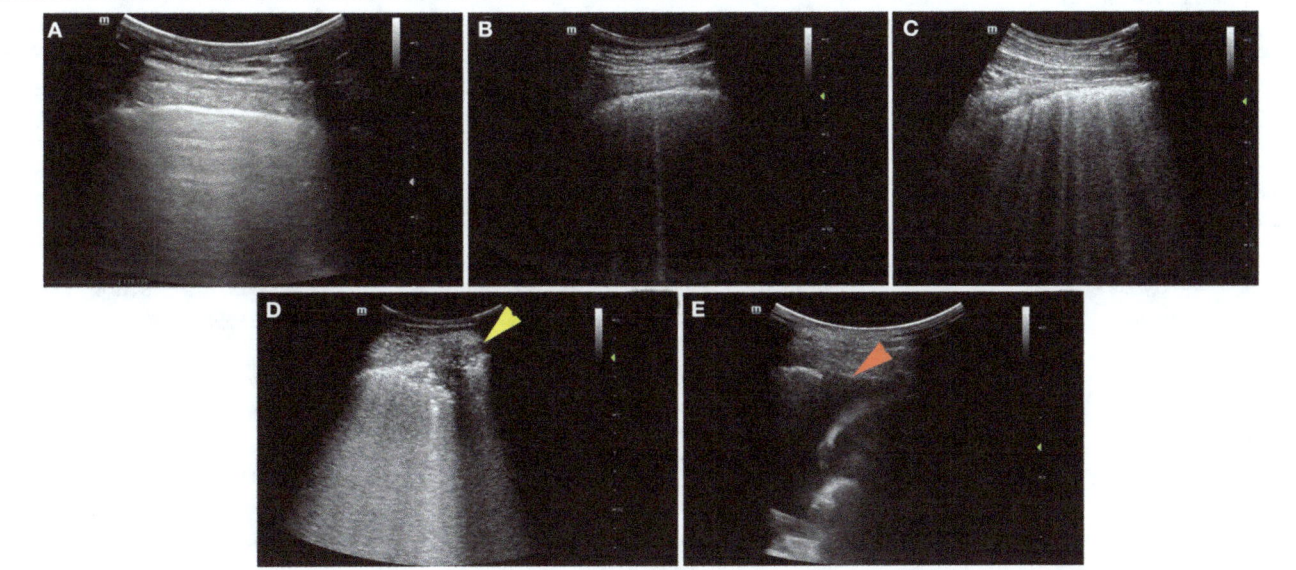

FIGURE 1 | Ultrasonographic features and lung ultrasound (LUS) score in patients with coronavirus disease 2019 (COVID-19). **(A)** Normal: the presence of A lines beyond the pleural line characterizes mornal pulmonay aeration, LUS score: 0. **(B)** B1 line: the presence of multiple vertical B lines (comet tails) with well-defined spacing regularly spaced B lines 7 mm apart, LUS score: 1. **(C)** B2 line: the presence of coalescent B lines <3 mm apart, LUS score: 2. **(D)** Lung consolidation: the presence of a tissue pattern (yellow arrowhead), LUS score: 3. **(E)** Pleural effusion at costophrenic angle (red arrowhead).

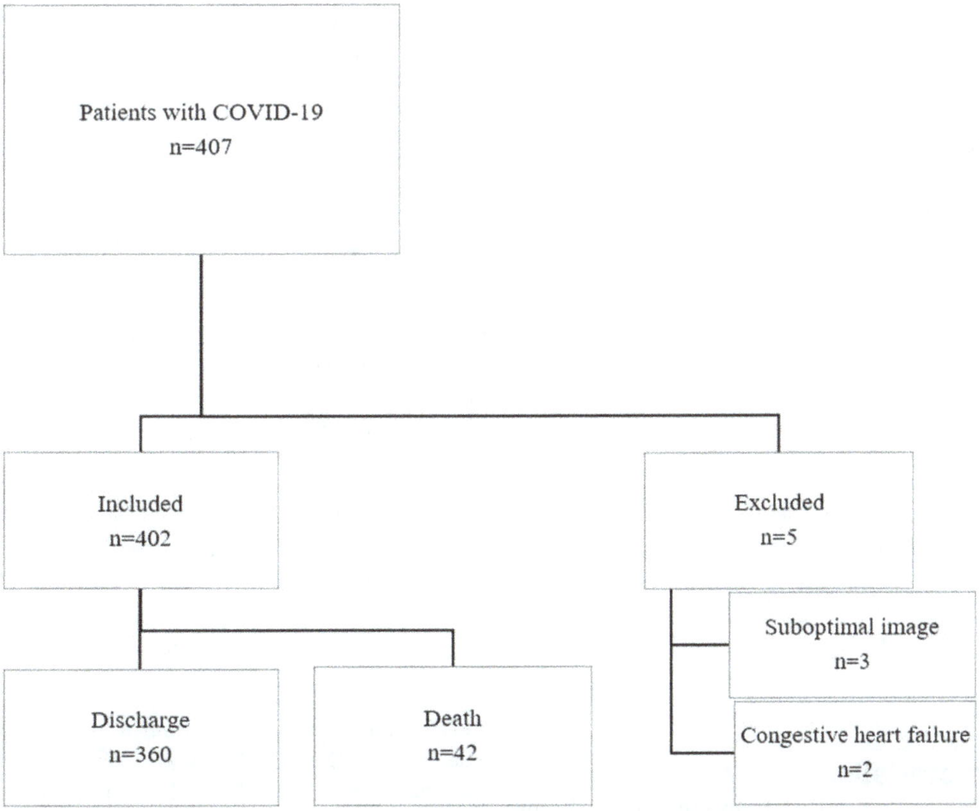

Patients with COVID-19
n=407

Included
n=402

Excluded
n=5

Discharge
n=360

Death
n=42

Suboptimal image
n=3

Congestive heart failure
n=2

FIGURE 2 | Study flow chart.

TABLE 1 | Patient characteristics.

	No. (%)			p-value	No. (%)		p-value
	Total (N = 402)	Survivors (N = 360)	Non-survivors (N = 42)		Global LUS Score <15 (N = 310)	Global LUS Score ≥15 (N = 92)	
Age, median (IQR), years	63 (52–70)	62 (52–69)	69 (61–77)	<0.001	61 (51–68)	69 (61–77)	<0.001
Age distribution	–	–	–	<0.001	–	–	<0.001
20–40 years	39 (9.7)	39 (10.8)	0		36 (11.6)	4 (4.3)	
40–60 years	125 (31.1)	124 (34.5)	1 (2.4)		112 (36.1)	18 (19.6)	
≥60 years	238 (59.2)	197 (54.7)	41 (97.6)		162 (52.3)	70 (76.1)	
Sex	–	–	–	0.002	–	–	0.002
Female	210 (52.2)	199 (55.3)	11 (26.2)		175 (56.5)	35 (38.0)	
Male	192 (47.8)	161 (44.7)	31 (73.8)		135 (43.5)	57 (62.0)	
Clinical presentation							
Fever	395 (98.2)	353 (98.0)	42 (100)	0.36	304 (98.1)	91 (98.9)	0.93
Dry cough	279 (69.4)	246 (68.3)	33 (78.6)	0.17	209 (67.4)	70 (76.1)	0.11
Headache	23 (5.7)	18 (5.0)	5 (11.9)	0.14	14 (4.8)	9 (9.8)	0.06
Sore throat	45 (11.1)	42 (11.7)	3 (7.1)	0.53	31 (10.0)	14 (15.3)	0.16
Myalgia	135 (33.6)	116 (32.2)	19 (45.2)	0.09	97 (31.3)	38 (41.3)	0.07
Fatigue	131 (32.6)	115 (31.9)	16 (38.1)	0.42	100 (32.3)	31 (33.7)	0.80
Dyspnea	124 (30.8)	104 (23.2)	20 (34.8)	0.01	72 (23.2)	32 (34.8)	0.03
Rhinorrhea	43 (10.7)	35 (9.4)	8 (21.4)	0.11	32 (18.6)	11 (16.8)	0.66
Nausea and vomiting	26 (6.5)	24 (6.7)	2 (4.8)	0.89	23 (7.4)	3 (3.3)	0.15
Diarrhea	51 (12.7)	47 (13.1)	4 (9.5)	0.52	37 (11.9)	14 (15.2)	0.41
Comorbidities							
Hypertension	97 (24.1)	80 (22.2)	17 (40.5)	0.009	64 (20.6)	33 (35.9)	0.003
Coronary heart disease	50 (12.4)	35 (9.7)	15 (35.7)	<0.001	30 (9.7)	20 (21.7)	0.002
Arrhythmia	10 (2.5)	9 (2.5)	1 (2.4)	1.00	8 (2.6)	2 (2.2)	1.00
Diabetes	40 (10.0)	36 (10.0)	4 (9.5)	1.00	27 (8.7)	13 (14.1)	0.13
Cerebrovascular disease	12 (3.0)	9 (2.5)	3 (7.1)	0.23	6 (1.9)	6 (6.5)	0.06
Chronic pulmonary Disease	15 (3.7)	11 (3.1)	4 (9.5)	0.01	9 (2.9)	6 (6.5)	0.11
Chronic liver disease	17 (4.2)	15 (4.2)	2 (4.8)	1.00	12 (3.9)	5 (5.4)	0.72
Chronic kidney disease	5 (1.2)	4 (1.1)	1 (2.4)	1.00	3 (1.0)	2 (2.2)	0.70
Malignancy	25 (6.2)	18 (5.0)	7 (16.7)	0.009	14 (4.5)	11 (12.0)	0.01
Clinical outcome	–	–	–	<0.001	–	–	<0.001
Discharged	360 (89.6)	360 (100)	0		305 (98.4)	55 (59.8)	
Died	42 (10.4)	0	42 (100)		5 (1.6)	37 (40.2)	
ARDS	85 (21.1)	43 (11.9)	42 (100)	<0.001	17 (5.5)	68 (73.9)	<0.001
ICU admission	79 (19.7)	38 (10.5)	41 (97.6)	<0.001	15 (4.8)	64 (69.6)	<0.001
Mechanical Ventilation	76 (18.9)	36 (10.0)	40 (95.2)	<0.001	13 (4.2)	63 (68.5)	<0.001
Days from admission to ultrasonic examination, median (IQR), days	3 (2–5)	3 (2–5)	3 (1–4)	0.44	3 (2–5)	3 (2–5)	0.32
Length of hospital stay, median (IQR), days	27 (20–39)	28 (21–40)	23 (15–31)	0.002	27 (20–40)	27 (19–37)	0.88

Global LUS score: summing the scores of all 12 lung regions (two anterior, two lateral, and two posterior thoracic regions) (ranging from 0 to 36).

ARDS, acute respiratory distress syndrome; ICU, intensive care unit.

RESULTS

Patient Characteristics

A total of 407 patients with COVID-19 meeting the inclusion criteria were recruited, of whom 5 were excluded due to suboptimal LUS images ($n = 3$) and congestive heart failure ($n = 2$) (**Figure 2**). Four hundred two patients were included in the final analysis, of whom 42 died with median time to death 21 (IQR, 14–29) days. Cause of death was recorded as multiorgan failure (42.9%), respiratory failure (26.1%), cardiac (9.5%), septic shock (9.5%), unknown (7.1%), and stroke (4.8%). Baseline characteristics are summarized in **Table 1**. Non-survivors were older and more male gender compared to survivors. There was a higher prevalence of

TABLE 2 | Laboratory findings.

	Median (IQR)			p-value	Median (IQR)		p-value
	Total (N =402)	Survivors (N = 360)	Non-survivors (N = 42)		Global LUS Score <15 (N = 310)	Global LUS Score ≥15 (N = 92)	
Blood count							
WBC count, ×109/L	5.94 (4.73–7.56)	5.85 (4.62–6.87)	6.99 (4.98–10.51)	0.045	5.85 (4.62–6.87)	6.99 (4.98–10.51)	<0.001
Lymphocyte count, ×109/L	1.49 (1.11–1.87)	1.45 (1.09–1.85)	0.45 (0.28–0.78)	<0.001	1.60 (1.25–1.96)	0.97 (0.45–1.38)	<0.001
Platelet count, ×109/L	205 (160–250)	210 (167–255)	140 (92–208)	<0.001	211 (168–256)	179 (139–223)	<0.001
Hemoglobin, g/dl	120 (107–132)	121 (109–132)	104 (92–124)	0.001	122 (112–134)	107 (95–124)	<0.001
Coagulation function							
PT, s, (n = 384)	13.0 (12.4–13.8)	12.9 (12.4–13.6)	15.8 (13.9–18.4)	<0.001	12.9 (12.4–13.6)	13.8 (12.8–16.2)	<0.001
APTT, s, (n = 384)	37.1 (34.5–41.7)	36.7 (34.2–40.4)	47.9 (39.3–58.4)	<0.001	36.5 (34.2–40.3)	40.5 (35.1–49.5)	<0.001
D-dimer, mg/L, (n = 384)	0.44 (0.22–1.22)	0.39 (0.21–0.93)	3.08 (1.36–8.00)	<0.001	0.37 (0.20–0.84)	1.10 (0.39–3.01)	<0.001
Blood biochemistry							
TP, g/L	66.3 (62.7–70.2)	66.7 (63.5–70.6)	59.5 (54.8–65.4)	<0.001	66.7 (63.6–70.5)	64.3 (57.7–68.4)	0.003
Albumin, g/L	38.6 (35.0–41.5)	39.2 (36.3–41.8)	26.9 (24.4–30.1)	<0.001	39.6 (365. −41.9)	33.7 (27.0–38.2)	<0.001
ALT, U/L	28 (19–47)	29 (19–46)	37.0 (22–70)	0.06	29.0 (19.5–46.0)	26.0 (18.0–47.0)	0.08
AST, U/L	24 (19–32)	23 (19.0–31)	42 (29–75)	0.01	23.0 (18.0–30.5)	31 (22.0–45.0)	0.02
TB, μmol/L	10.4 (7.8–13.7)	10.0 (7.7–13.1)	14.7 (9.5–28.8)	0.002	10.2 (7.8–13.2)	11.0 (7.5–15.4)	0.05
Sodium, mmol/L	139.8 (138.5–141.6)	139.7 (138.5–141.3)	141.5 (138.6–144.3)	0.05	139.8 (138.7–141.4)	139.8 (137.5–142.5)	0.98
Potassium, mmol/L	4.15 (3.90–4.37)	4.16 (3.93–4.37)	3.96 (3.55–4.39)	0.73	4.17 (3.94–4.37)	4.10 (3.79–4.40)	0.58
BUN, mmol/L, (n = 382)	4.92 (3.90–6.01)	4.75 (3.84–5.69)	10.61 (6.85–18.48)	<0.001	4.70 (3.87–5.70)	5.65 (4.23–10.52)	<0.001
Creatinine, μmol/L	64.3 (53.8–77.0)	63.8 (53.9–75.5)	76.9 (50.7–140.3)	0.024	63.5 (54.3–75.7)	68.7 (50.3–91.0)	0.05
hs-cTnI, pg/mL, (n = 382)	3.3 (1.7–12.1)	2.6 (1.6–6.5)	100.6 (29.3–407.4)	<0.001	2.50 (1.53–5.18)	15.4 (4.12–98.05)	<0.001
LDH, U/L	180 (153–228)	174 (151–206)	393 (278–670)	<0.001	174 (150–206)	216 (166–365)	0.001
CK-MB, U/L (n = 347)	0.9 (0.4–9.0)	0.8 (0.4–7.0)	21.6 (9.0–34.3)	0.008	0.8 (0.4–8.0)	1.9 (0.6–21.1)	0.03
Infection-related biomarkers							
CRP, mg/L, (n = 370)	3.03 (0.72–10.4)	2.43 (0.62–5.92)	90.19 (53.7–125.8)	<0.001	2.37 (0.59–5.8)	24.93 (2.21–105.6)	<0.001
PCT, ng/ml, (n = 370)	0.06 (0.04–0.13)	0.06 (0.04–0.11)	0.38 (0.14–1.51)	<0.001	0.06 (0.04–0.10)	0.07 (0.07–0.43)	0.03

WBC, white blood cell; PT, prothrombin time; APTT, activated partial thromboplastin time; TP, total protein; ALT, alanine transaminase; AST, aspartate aminotransferase; TB, total bilirubin; BUN, blood urea nitrogen; hs-cTnI, hypersensitive troponin I; LDH, lactate dehydrogenase; CK-MB, creatine kinase–MB; CRP, hypersensitive C-reactive protein; PCT, procalcitonin.

preexisting conditions including hypertension, coronary heart disease (CHD), and malignancy in non-survivors compared to survivors.

Laboratory Findings

Laboratory data on hospital admission are summarized in **Table 2**. Overall, non-survivors had significant worse

TABLE 3 | Lung ultrasound findings.

	No. (%)			p-value
	Total (N = 402)	Survivors (N = 360)	Non-survivors (N = 42)	
Normal baseline lung ultrasound	84 (20.9)	84 (23.3)	0	<0.001
Abnormal baseline lung ultrasound	318 (79.1)	276 (76.7)	42 (100)	
Characteristics of lung ultrasound				
B line	318 (79.1)	276 (76.7)	42 (100)	<0.001
B1 line	236 (58.7)	210 (58.3)	26 (61.9)	0.66
B2 line	213 (51.5)	171 (45.8)	42 (100)	<0.001
Pleural line abnormalities	137 (31.8)	103 (26.4)	34 (78.6)	<0.001
Pulmonary consolidation	117 (25.6)	83 (20.6)	34 (69.0)	<0.001
Pleural effusion	36 (8.2)	18 (4.4)	18 (40.5)	<0.001
Distribution at baseline ultrasound				<0.001
Right lung	63 (15.7)	63 (17.5)	0	
Left lung	30 (7.5)	30 (8.3)	0	
Bilateral lungs	223 (55.5)	181 (50.3)	42 (100)	
Abnormalities at lung region				
Left anterior superior	129 (32.1)	93 (25.8)	36 (85.7)	<0.001
Left anterior inferior	112 (28.4)	74 (20.6)	38 (90.5)	<0.001
Left lateral superior	128 (31.8)	100 (27.8)	28 (66.7)	<0.001
Left lateral inferior	153 (38.1)	112 (31.1)	41 (97.6)	<0.001
Left posterior superior	111 (27.6)	81 (22.5)	30 (71.4)	<0.001
Left posterior inferior	156 (38.8)	125 (34.7)	31 (73.8)	<0.001
Right anterior superior	139 (34.5)	108 (30.0)	31 (73.8)	<0.001
Right anterior inferior	138 (34.3)	102 (28.3)	36 (85.7)	<0.001
Right lateral superior	129 (32.1)	103 (28.6)	26 (61.9)	<0.001
Right lateral inferior	160 (39.8)	120 (33.3)	40 (95.2)	<0.001
Right posterior superior	142 (35.3)	107 (29.7)	35 (83.3)	<0.001
Right posterior inferior	150 (37.3)	130 (36.1)	20 (47.6)	0.14
Global LUS score, median (IQR)	4 (1–13)	3 (1–9)	20 (18–23)	<0.001
Anterolateral LUS score, median (IQR)	2 (0–8)	5 (0–9)	14 (11–15)	0.001

laboratory results, including increased white blood cell count, prothrombin time, activated partial thromboplastin time, D-dimer, aspartate aminotransferase, total bilirubin, blood urea nitrogen, creatinine, hypersensitive troponin I (hs-TnI), lactate dehydrogenase (LDH), creatine kinase–myocardial band (CK-MB), hypersensitive C-reactive protein (CRP), and procalcitonin and decreased lymphocyte count, platelet count, hemoglobin, total protein, and albumin (all $p < 0.05$) compared to survivors. Patients with a higher global LUS score (>15) had significant worse laboratory results, in particular, significantly increased D-dimer and CRP compared to those with a global LUS score <15.

Lung Ultrasound Findings and Lung Ultrasound Score

Lung ultrasound was performed within a median of 3 (IQR, 2–5) days from hospital admission. Lung ultrasound findings are shown in **Table 3**. Eighty-four patients (20.9%)

had normal LUS. The presence of B lines was the most common finding (318/402, 79.1%), followed by pleural line abnormalities (137/402, 31.8%) and consolidation (117/402, 25.6%). Pleural effusions were detected in 36 (8.2%) patients. Compared to survivors, non-survivors were more likely to have B2 lines, pleural line abnormalities, pulmonary consolidation, and pleural effusion, but there was no difference in the presence of B1 lines. All non-survivors had bilateral involvement. Survivors had significantly lower global and anterior–lateral LUS scores compared to non-survivors (**Figure 3**). Findings of each of 12 lung regions are shown in **Supplementary Figure 2**. Regional LUS scores including anterior, lateral, and posterior scores are presented in **Supplementary Figure 3**. Bland–Altman plots for intra- and interobserver variability of global LUS score are shown in **Supplementary Figure 4**. All repeated measures were within 1.96 × standard deviation of the mean, which suggested a good reproducibility of global LUS score.

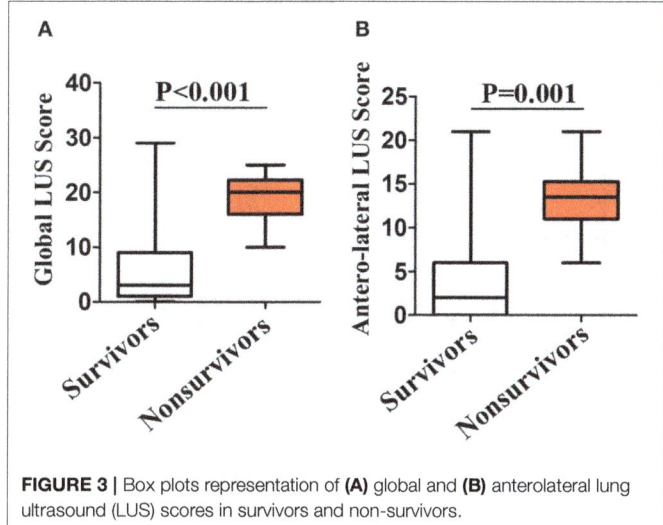

FIGURE 3 | Box plots representation of **(A)** global and **(B)** anterolateral lung ultrasound (LUS) scores in survivors and non-survivors.

Prediction of Mortality by LUS Global and Anterolateral Score

After a median of 27 (IQR, 20–39) days of follow-up, 42 patients died. ROC curve analyses of global and anterolateral LUS score for predicting mortality are shown in **Figure 4**. The area under the curve were 0.936 and 0.913 for global and anterolateral LUS score, respectively. A cutoff value of 15 for global LUS score had a sensitivity of 92.9% and specificity of 85.3% for prediction of death, and a cutoff value of 9 for anterolateral LUS score had a sensitivity of 88.1% and specificity of 83.3%. Clinical characteristics and laboratory findings dichotomized according to global LUS score optimal value of 15 are shown in **Tables 1**, **2**.

Kaplan–Meier analysis showed that both global and anterolateral LUS scores were strong predictors of death (**Figure 5**). When global LUS score was >15, 37/92 (40.2%) patients died compared to only 5/310 (1.6%) death in those with a global LUS score <15. When patients were dichotomized by anterolateral LUS score of 9, there were 36/97 (37.1%) deaths in patients with a high score compared to 6/305 (2.0%) deaths in those with a low anterolateral score.

On univariate Cox regression analysis, age, male gender, malignancy, CHD, CRP, hs-cTnl, CK-MB, D-dimer, global LUS score, and anterolateral LUS score were significantly associated with mortality (**Table 4**). In multivariate model 1, considering global LUS score together with other significant predictors in the univariate model, age, male sex, CRP, CK-MB, and global LUS score [hazard ratio (HR), 1.08; 95%CI, 1.01–1.16, $p = 0.03$) remained as a significant predictor. In multivariate model 2, when anterolateral LUS score was tested with other variables, the predictive power of anterolateral LUS score did not remain significant.

DISCUSSION

Our data suggested that global LUS score was a predictor of in-hospital mortality independent of age, gender, comorbidities, and biochemical markers and was superior to LUS anterolateral

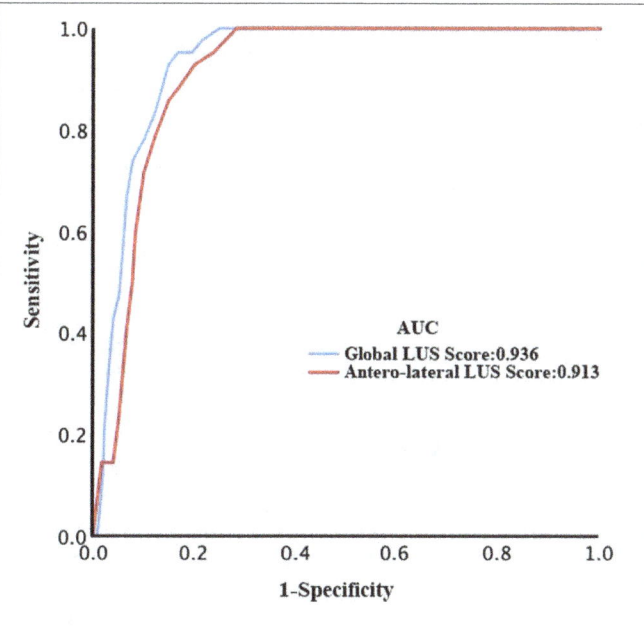

FIGURE 4 | Receiver operating characteristic (ROC) curves of global and anterolateral lung ultrasound (LUS) score for prediction of death.

score. The optimal threshold of 15 for global LUS score and 9 for anterolateral LUS score were in line with those derived from previous investigations (5, 8). These findings supported the clinical utility of LUS in patients with COVID-19 (7, 9) given its ease of use at point of care, low cost, lack of radiation exposure, and ready combination with other components of critical care ultrasonography (10, 11).

LUS features in patients with COVID-19 in our study manifested as multiple lesions, various types of B lines, irregularly pleural lines, and subpleural consolidations. B lines presented in 79.1% patients. B2 lines and consolidations were more common in non-survivors than in survivors. Pleural effusion, pleural thickening, and pneumothorax were less common in COVID-19 patients, which were consistent with the latest autopsy report (12) that COVID-19 patients presented with acute interstitial lung disease.

Bass et al. showed that LUS had high sensitivity for detection of interstitial and alveolar–interstitial lung disease with peripheral distribution (13). Consistent with these features, our findings suggested that global LUS score was highly predictive of death in COVID-19 and independent of other previously identified predictors. Non-survivors in our study were older and more male with higher prevalence of preexisting conditions including hypertension, CHD, and malignancy and higher levels of cardiac injury and systematic inflammation markers than survivors, which were in consistence with previous studies (14).

Another interesting finding of our study was that when the posterior regions were excluded, the predictive power of anterolateral LUS score disappeared in the multivariate cox regression model. This finding was consistent with chest CT findings that the most commonly involved lung segments in patients with COVID-19 were the dorsal segment of the right

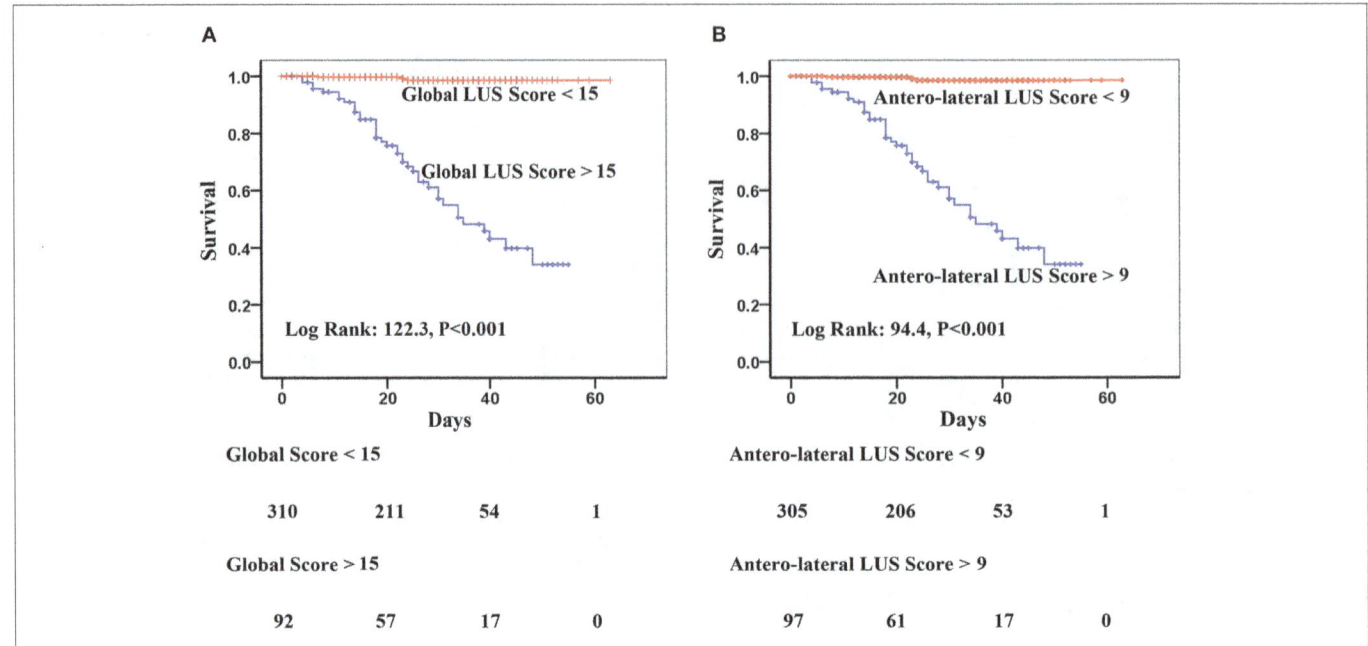

FIGURE 5 | Kaplan–Meier curves of **(A)** global lung ultrasound (LUS) score with optimal cutoff value of 15 and **(B)** anterolateral LUS score with optimal cutoff value of 9 for prediction of in-hospital mortality.

TABLE 4 | Univariate and multivariate Cox regression.

	HR	CI (95%)	p	HR	CI (95%)	p	HR	CI (95%)	p
		Univariate			Model 1			Model 2	
Age	1.04	1.01–1.07	**0.005**	1.05	1.00–1.10	**0.04**	1.05	1.00–1.09	**0.05**
Male sex	0.33	0.17–0.67	**0.002**	0.31	0.11–0.89	**0.03**	0.34	0.12–0.92	**0.03**
Hypertension	0.55	0.30–1.03	0.06						
Malignancy	0.32	0.14–0.72	**0.006**	0.57	0.18–1.81	0.34	0.57	0.18–1.82	0.34
CHD	0.28	0.15–0.52	**<0.001**	0.99	0.45–2.18	0.99	0.93	0.43–2.02	0.85
CRP	2.58	1.99–3.35	**<0.001**	1.60	1.17–2.20	**0.004**	1.69	1.23–2.31	**0.001**
hs-cTnl	1.82	1.61–2.04	**<0.001**	1.11	0.90–1.37	0.34	1.17	0.95–1.44	0.14
CK-MB	2.11	1.75–2.54	**<0.001**	1.47	1.09–1.99	**0.01**	1.54	1.13–2.08	**0.006**
D-Dimer	2.75	2.08–3.65	**<0.001**	1.19	0.83–1.69	0.34	1.17	0.82–1.66	0.38
Global LUS score	1.20	1.15–1.26	**<0.001**	1.08	1.01–1.16	**0.03**			
Anterolateral LUS score	1.23	1.17–1.29	**<0.001**				1.04	0.96–1.13	0.34
C-index					**0.995**			**0.994**	

CHD, coronary heart disease; CRP, C-reactive protein; hs-cTnl, hypersensitive troponin I; CK-MB, creatine kinase–myocardial band.
Global LUS score: summing the scores of all 12 lung regions (two anterior, two lateral, and two posterior thoracic regions) (ranging from 0 to 36). The values in bold represent statistical differences in data.

lower lobe, the posterior basal segment of the right lower lobe, the lateral basal segment of the right lower lobe, and the dorsal segment and the posterior basal segment of the left lower lobe (15). Despite some studies showing that the posterior regions had the lowest diagnostic accuracy (5), scores from these regions could play an important role in risk stratification. In the present study, lung lesions were mainly located in the right lateral inferior area (39.8%), left lateral inferior area (38.1%), left posterior inferior area (38.8%), and right posterior inferior area (37.3%) (the lower posterior and lateral segments of the lungs). This finding also supported that the potential benefit of prone position

in patients affected with COVID-19 acute respiratory distress syndrome (ARDS) due to a more even distribution of the gas–tissue ratios along the dependent–non-dependent axis and a more homogeneous distribution of lung stress and strain (16).

Although anterolateral LUS score had less predive power compared to global LUS score, it may still play an important role particularly in patients on ICU.

Clinical Implications

COVID-19 as a global pandemic imposes a huge burden on medical systems. Early quantification of patients with severe lung involvement may be critical for optimization of treatment and management. LUS as a non-invasive and cost-effective diagnostic tool can be performed rapidly, particularly in ICU. Severe studies have also demonstrated that echocardiography is a crucial tool in detecting cardiovascular complications (in particular on assessment of left and right ventricular function) and predicts poor prognosis in patients COVID-19 (17, 18). Combining LUS with echocardiography may add additional value to identify patients at higher risk of poor outcomes.

Limitations

Our study has several limitations. First, mortality rate was relatively low, which limits the strength of our conclusion. Low mortality rate may be due to the fact that majority of patients in the present study were not in ICU, while this rate was similar to previously published data (19). Second, the follow-up period was relatively short, as majority of patients were discharged within 28 days from admission.

Although our findings suggested that LUS may add additional value in risk stratification, the strength of our conclusion may be limited by the nature of an observational study. There are several other limitations of LUS that cannot be ignored such as the requirement of special training to perform high-quality LUS, lack of evidence-based guidelines, the high risk of infection when performing LUS examination in patients with COVID-19 (20, 21).

Patients included in this study were recruited from three hardest-hit hospitals in Wuhan, and these patients may not represent the population in other areas. Finally, the relationship between LUS and lung CT was not explored, as the majority of patients did not have lung CT due to limited availabilities and the nature of infectious disease.

CONCLUSION

Global LUS score as a semiquantitative measure of lung conditions is a powerful predictor of in-hospital mortality in patients with COVID-19 and may add additional value in patient monitoring and risk stratification.

AUTHOR CONTRIBUTIONS

ZS, HW, HG, and MX conceived and designed the study. ZZ and JL contributed to the literature search. ZS, CC, SQ, YS, YD, WZ, MY, and LJ contributed to data collection. ZZ, CY, and HG contributed to data analysis. JW, YY, QL, and HG contributed to data interpretation. YX and RW contributed to the figures. ZS, HG, ZZ, and JL drafted the article. All authors contributed to the article and approved the submitted version.

ACKNOWLEDGMENTS

We are grateful for all our colleagues, especially Dr. Li Zhang and Hongliang Yuan, for their support to the present study. We are also grateful to the many frontline medical staffs for their dedication in the face of this outbreak despite the potential threat to their own lives and the lives of their families.

REFERENCES

1. Shi H, Han X, Jiang N, Cao Y, Alwalid O, Gu J, et al. Radiological findings from 81 patients with COVID-19 pneumonia in Wuhan, China: a descriptive study. *Lancet Infect Dis.* (2020) 20:425–34. doi: 10.1016/S1473-3099(20)30086-4

2. Lepri G, Orlandi M, Lazzeri C, Bruni C, Hughes M, Bonizzoli M, et al. The emerging role of lung ultrasound in COVID-19 pneumonia. *Eur J Rheumatol.* (2020) 7:129–33. doi: 10.5152/eurjrheum.2020.2063

3. Volpicelli G, Lamorte A, Villen T. What's new in lung ultrasound during the COVID-19 pandemic. *Intensive Care Med.* (2020) 46:1445–48. doi: 10.1007/s00134-020-06048-9

4. Zhang YK, Li J, Yang JP, Zhan Y, Chen J. Lung ultrasonography for the diagnosis of 11 patients with acute respiratory distress syndrome due to bird flu H7N9 infection. *Virol J.* (2015) 12:176. doi: 10.1186/s12985-015-0406-1

5. Pisani L, Vercesi V, van Tongeren PSI, Lagrand WK, Leopold SJ, Huson MAM, et al. The diagnostic accuracy for ARDS of global versus regional lung ultrasound scores - a post hoc analysis of an observational study in invasively ventilated ICU patients. *Intensive Care Med Exp.* (2019) 7:44. doi: 10.1186/s40635-019-0241-6

6. Bouhemad B, Mongodi S, Via G, Rouquette I. Ultrasound for "lung monitoring" of ventilated patients. *Anesthesiology.* (2015) 122:437–47. doi: 10.1097/ALN.0000000000000558

7. Volpicelli G, Elbarbary M, Blaivas M, Lichtenstein DA, Mathis G, Kirkpatrick AW, et al. International evidence-based recommendations for point-of-care lung ultrasound. *Intensive Care Med.* (2012) 38:577–91. doi: 10.1007/s00134-012-2513-4

8. Tierney DM, Boland LL, Overgaard JD, Huelster JS, Jorgenson A, Normington JP, et al. Pulmonary ultrasound scoring system for intubated critically ill patients and its association with clinical metrics and mortality: a prospective cohort study. *J Clin Ultrasound.* (2018) 46:14–22. doi: 10.1002/jcu.22526

9. Nazerian P, Volpicelli G, Vanni S, Gigli C, Betti L, Bartolucci M, et al. Accuracy of lung ultrasound for the diagnosis of consolidations when compared to chest computed tomography. *Am J Emerg Med.* (2015) 33:620–5. doi: 10.1016/j.ajem.2015.01.035

10. Peng QY, Wang XT, Zhang LN. Findings of lung ultrasonography of novel corona virus pneumonia during the 2019-2020 epidemic. *Intensive Care Med.* (2020) 46:849–50. doi: 10.1007/s00134-020-05996-6

11. Vetrugno L, Bove T, Orso D, Barbariol F, Bassi F, Boero E, et al. Our Italian experience using lung ultrasound for identification, grading and serial follow-up of severity of lung involvement for management of patients with COVID-19. *Echocardiography.* (2020) 37:625–27. doi: 10.1111/echo.14664

12. Xu Z, Shi L, Wang Y, Zhang J, Huang L, Zhang C, et al. Pathological findings of COVID-19 associated with acute respiratory distress syndrome. *Lancet Respir Med.* (2020) 8:420–22. doi: 10.1016/S2213-2600(20)30076-X

13. Bass CM, Sajed DR, Adedipe AA, West TE. Pulmonary ultrasound and pulse oximetry versus chest radiography and arterial blood gas analysis for the diagnosis of acute respiratory distress syndrome: a pilot study. *Crit Care.* (2015) 19:282. doi: 10.1186/s13054-015-0995-5

14. Luo X, Zhou W, Yan X, Guo T, Wang B, Xia H, et al. Prognostic value of C-reactive protein in patients with COVID-19. *Clin Infect Dis.* (2020) 71:2174–9. doi: 10.1093/cid/ciaa641

15. Wu J, Wu X, Zeng W, Guo D, Fang Z, Chen L, et al. Chest CT findings in patients with coronavirus disease 2019 and its relationship with clinical features. *Invest Radiol.* (2020) 55:257–61. doi: 10.1097/RLI.0000000000 000670

16. Guérin C, Albert RK, Beitler J, Gattinoni L, Jaber S, Marini JJ, et al. Prone position in ARDS patients: why, when, how and for whom. *Intensive Care Med.* (2020) 46:2385–96. doi: 10.1007/s00134-020-06306-w

17. Moody WE, Mahmoud-Elsayed HM, Senior J, Gul U, Khan-Kheil AM, Horne S, et al. Impact of right ventricular dysfunction on mortality in patients hospitalized with COVID-19, according to race. *CJC Open.* (2021) 3:91–100. doi: 10.1016/j.cjco.2020.09.016

18. Cameli M, Pastore MC, Soliman Aboumarie H, Mandoli GE, D'Ascenzi F, et al. Usefulness of echocardiography to detect cardiac involvement in COVID-19 patients. *Echocardiography.* (2020) 37:1278–86. doi: 10.1111/echo.14779

19. Chen N, Zhou M, Dong X, Qu J, Gong F, Han Y, et al. Epidemiological and clinical characteristics of 99 cases of 2019 novel coronavirus pneumonia in Wuhan, China: a descriptive study. *Lancet.* (2020) 395:507–13. doi: 10.1016/S0140-6736(20)30211-7

20. Gargani L, Soliman-Aboumarie H, Volpicelli G, Corradi F, Pastore MC, Cameli M. Why, when, and how to use lung ultrasound during the COVID-19 pandemic: enthusiasm and caution. *Eur Heart J Cardiovasc Imaging.* (2020) 21:941–8. doi: 10.1093/ehjci/jeaa163

21. Di Serafino M, Notaro M, Rea G, Iacobellis F, Delli Paoli V, Acampora C, et al. The lung ultrasound: facts or artifacts? In the era of COVID-19 outbreak. *Radiol Med.* (2020) 125:738–53. doi: 10.1007/s11547-020-01236-5

20

Renin-Angiotensin System and Coronavirus Disease 2019

Annamaria Mascolo [1,2]*, Cristina Scavone [1,2], Concetta Rafaniello [1,2], Carmen Ferrajolo [1,2], Giorgio Racagni [3], Liberato Berrino [1], Giuseppe Paolisso [4], Francesco Rossi [1,2†] and Annalisa Capuano [1,2†]

[1] Section of Pharmacology "L. Donatelli", Department of Experimental Medicine, University of Campania "Luigi Vanvitelli", Naples, Italy, [2] Campania Regional Centre for Pharmacovigilance and Pharmacoepidemiology, Naples, Italy, [3] Department of Pharmacological and Biomolecular Sciences, Università degli Studi di Milano, Milan, Italy, [4] Department of Advanced Medical and Surgical Sciences, University of Campania "Luigi Vanvitelli", Naples, Italy

*Correspondence:
Annamaria Mascolo
annamaria.mascolo@unicampania.it

[†] *These authors have contributed equally to this work and share lead authorship*

Although clinical manifestations of the 2019 novel coronavirus disease pandemic (COVID-19), caused by the novel severe acute respiratory syndrome coronavirus 2 (SARS-COV-2), are mainly respiratory symptoms, patients can also develop severe cardiovascular damage. Therefore, understanding the damage caused by SARS-COV-2 to the cardiovascular system and the underlying mechanisms is fundamental. The cardiovascular damage may be related to the imbalance of the renin-angiotensin-system (RAS) as this virus binds the Angiotensin-Converting-Enzyme 2 (ACE2), expressed on the lung alveolar epithelial cells, to enter into cells. Virus internalization may cause a downregulation of ACE2 on host cell surface that could lead to a local increased level of angiotensin II (AII) and a reduced level of angiotensin 1-7 (A1-7). An imbalance between these angiotensins may be responsible for the lung and heart damage. Pharmacological strategies that interfere with the viral attachment to ACE2 (umifenovir and hydroxychloroquine/chloroquine) or that modulate the RAS (analogous of A1-7 and ACE2, losartan) are in clinical development for COVID-19. The use of RAS inhibitors has also become a matter of public concern as these drugs may increase the mRNA expression and levels of ACE2 and impact the virulence and transmission of SARS-COV-2. Data on the effect of RAS inhibitors on ACE2 mRNA expression are scarce. Scientific societies expressed their opinion on continuing the therapy with RAS inhibitors in patients with COVID-19 and underlying cardiovascular diseases. In conclusion, RAS may play a role in SARS-COV-2-induced cardiac and pulmonary damage. Further studies are needed to better understand the role of RAS in COVID-19 and to guide decision on the use of RAS inhibitors.

Keywords: COVID-19, renin-angiotensin system, SARS-COV-2, heart damage, pulmonary damage, RAS inhibitors

INTRODUCTION

The renin–angiotensin system (RAS) is a complex hormonal system composed by different mediators that can affect the cardiovascular, renal, immune, and nervous functions (1, 2). Many components of the RAS have been isolated from different tissues (3), including the lung (4). This system is composed by two pathways: the classic RAS and the non-classic RAS, which have opposite activities, especially for renal, and cardiovascular functions (2, 5). A component of the non-classic RAS, the Angiotensin-Converting-Enzyme 2 (ACE2) present on the lung surface, has been discovered to be a functional receptor for coronaviruses, essential for triggering their infection (1). Severe acute respiratory syndrome coronavirus 1 (SARS-COV-1) and SARS-COV-2, which are responsible for the SARS and the more recent coronavirus disease 2019 (COVID-19), respectively, are both able to bind the ACE2 in the lung (6, 7). Patients affected with COVID-19 show respiratory and flu-like symptoms, which can be complicated by lymphopenia and interstitial pneumonia with high levels of pro-inflammatory cytokines that can lead to acute respiratory distress syndrome (ARDS) and organ failure (8). Although the clinical manifestations of COVID-19 are mainly represented by respiratory symptoms, some patients also developed severe cardiovascular damage (9). In addition, an increased risk of death was found in patients with cardiovascular diseases (9).

Understanding the mechanisms by which the RAS interacts with SARS-COV-2 is fundamental for the treatment of patients with cardiac diseases as showed in the context of metabolic diseases (10). Moreover, considering the interaction between these viruses and the ACE2, concerns were also raised about the use of RAS inhibitors in patients with COVID-19 as they may alter ACE2 mRNA expression and levels and, in this way, impact the virulence and transmission of SARS-COV-2 (11). Therefore, in this review, we aim to summarize the physiological role of the RAS, its implication in the SARS-COV-2 infection, the actual evidence and recommendation on the use of RAS inhibitors, and the ongoing researches of drugs with a potential for the treatment of COVID-19 and acting either by influencing the RAS or disrupting the viral attachment to ACE2.

CLINICAL CHARACTERISTICS OF COVID-19

First evidence regarding the clinical characteristics of patients with COVID-19 showed the presence of bilateral lung ground glass opacity on computed tomography (CT) imaging (12). CT abnormalities were observed in both asymptomatic or symptomatic patients with SARS-CoV-2 infection, making it a useful diagnostic tool. Asymptomatic individuals with CT abnormalities rarely developed severe pneumonia (13). Initial symptoms were fever, cough, dyspnea, myalgia or fatigue, sputum production, headache, hemoptysis, and diarrhea. In most severe cases, there was a progression to ARDS, to acute cardiac injury, to acute kidney injury (AKI), or to shock. Other symptoms that were identified pertained to the gastrointestinal system (nausea and diarrhea) (12). However, other studies showed a lower development of gastrointestinal symptoms (14, 15). Moreover, an increase in serum lactate dehydrogenase as marker of lung tissue damage was observed in COVID-19 patients (13), and it was associated with higher odds of severe disease (14). Additionally, older age and lymphopenia were identified as potential risk factors for severe COVID-19 (13).

CLASSIC AND NON-CLASSIC RAS

The classic RAS involves as main effector peptide the angiotensin II (AII), whose synthesis starts with the cleavage of angiotensinogen into angiotensin I (AI) by the renin and then its conversion into AII by the ACE (16) (**Figure 1**). Despite this represent the main pathway for the AII production, also other enzymes can be involved (5). The main effects of AII are explained by its interaction with three receptors (AT1, AT2, and nonAT1nonAT2). AT1 and AT2 are classified as G protein-coupled receptors (16), while nonAT1nonAT2 seems more prone to be an angiotensin clearance receptor or an angiotensinase (17). The stimulation of the AT1 receptor can induce vasoconstriction, increase the release of catecholamines and the synthesis of aldosterone (16). Moreover, AT1 receptors can stimulate fibrosis, inflammatory processes, reduction of collagenase activity, and expression of mitogen-activated protein kinase (MAPK) (2, 5). As pro-inflammatory action, these receptors seem to be involved in several pathways: down-regulation of the NADPH oxidase expression in smooth muscle cells; enhancement of the production of reactive oxygen species (ROS) and the activity of pro-inflammatory transcription nuclear factors like nuclear factor-kappaB (NF-kB) and E26 transformation-specific sequence (Ets) (18); release of different types of cytokines such as TNF-α, IL-6, and MCP-1 (19); shifting of the macrophage phenotype toward the pro-inflammatory M1 polarization state (20). The stimulation of AT2 receptors, instead, has a protective role in the RAS activation inducing anti-inflammatory, anti-oxidative, and anti-fibrotic effects (16).

The non-classic RAS involves, instead, other peptide mediators and enzymes. Specifically, the main mediator is the angiotensin 1-7 (A1-7), whose synthesis can involve two different pathways. One starts with the cleavage of AII into A1-7 by the carboxypeptidase ACE2, while another through the cleavage of AI into angiotensin 1-9 (A1-9) by ACE2 and its subsequent conversion into A1-7 by ACE (5) (**Figure 1**). Today, two forms of ACE2 are recognized, one soluble and another transmembrane, both contributing to the generation of A1-7. The A1-7 stimulates the G protein-coupled receptor MAS1, promoting the nitric oxide release (21), Akt phosphorylation (22), and anti-inflammatory effects (23). Moreover, the activation of MAS1 receptors, expressed on the macrophage surface, inhibits the inflammatory macrophage phenotype and the release of pro-inflammatory cytokines (5). Therefore, A1-7 is a component of a beneficial axis of the RAS that exerts opposite cardiovascular and renal effects compared to the ACE/AII/AT1 axis (24).

Interestingly, it has been found that human monocytes can express ACE and ACE2 and metabolize AI to multiple angiotensin peptides. In particular, classical monocytes (CD14^{++}CD16^{-}) produce both AII and A1–9/A1-7, whereas the non-classical subtype (CD14^{+}CD16^{++}) produces mainly A1-7 (25). This indicates that ACE and ACE2 participate to the inflammation also as components of a local RAS at sites infiltrated by monocytes/macrophages.

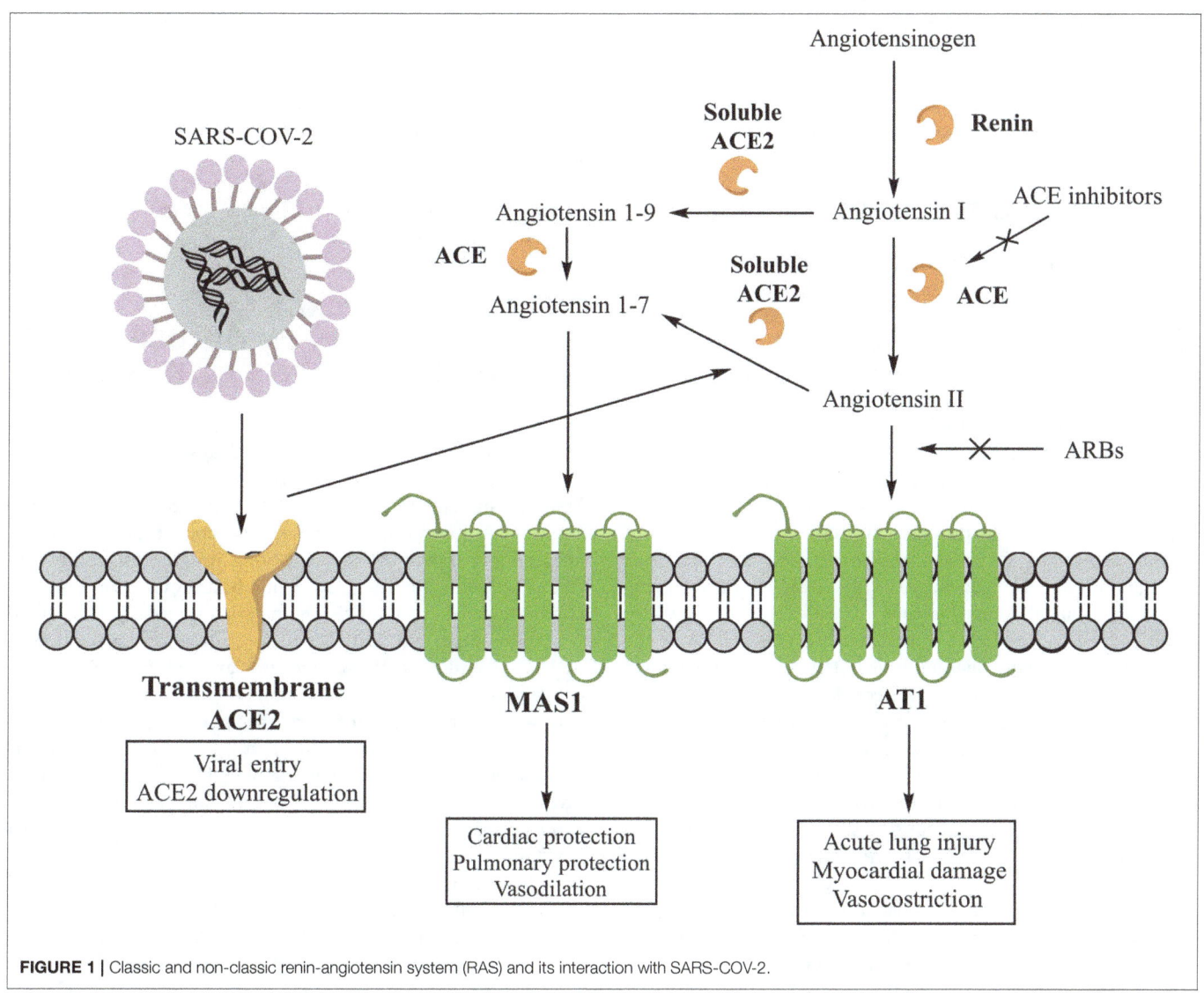

FIGURE 1 | Classic and non-classic renin-angiotensin system (RAS) and its interaction with SARS-COV-2.

SARS-COV-2 AND ACE2 IN THE LUNG

SARS-COV-2 is a betacoronavirus with a single-stranded positive-sense RNA genome encapsulated within a membrane envelope (26). The genome encodes for several structural proteins, including the glycosylated spike (S) protein that is a major inducer of host immune response. The S protein is also important because mediates host cell invasion by SARS-COV-2 via binding to the receptor protein ACE2 present on the surface of lung alveolar epithelial cells (host cells) (6, 27). The affinity of S protein binding region to the extracellular domain of ACE2 has been estimated of 15 nM (27, 28). The invasion process requires the activation of the S protein, which is facilitated by the human androgen-sensitive transmembrane serine protease type 2 (TMPRSS211) (6, 26). Specifically, TMPRSS211 cleaves the S protein and generates the S1 and S2 subunits. This is a critical step as both subunits are essential for viral entry in the host cells (28). S1 is the subunit recognized by ACE2 and the one that facilitates

viral attachment, whereas S2 is the subunit that drives membrane fusion and viral internalization in the pulmonary epithelium (6). The greater virulence of SARS-COV-2 compared to SARS-COV-1 was supposed to be related to the higher affinity of S1 subunit for ACE2 (26, 28). In fact, a Cryo-EM structure analysis revealed that the affinity of the S protein of SARS-COV-2 to ACE2 is about 10–20 times greater than that observed with the S protein of SARS-COV-1 (27).

Another important consideration is that the ACE2 internalization mediated by SARS-COV-2 could potentially result in a reduced presence of ACE2 on cell surface, leading to the absence of a key factor for AII degradation and A1-7 synthesis. An imbalance between AII and A1-7 levels may further exacerbate the damage of lung provoked by SARS-COV-2. Therefore, a decrease in ACE2 may contribute to the reduction of pulmonary function and the increase of tissue fibrosis and inflammation due to COVID-19 (28). This hypothesis was already investigated with SARS-COV-1 infection, which was associated with a reduced presence of ACE2 on cell membranes and an increased severity of lung injury (29). Because SARS-COV-1 and SARS-COV-2 share the same cellular invasion process, they may also share similar pathogenesis and pathological manifestations of lung injury (29).

SARS-COV-2 AND ACE2 IN THE HEART

Potentially, once the SARS-COV-2 enters the circulation, it can infect any tissue expressing the ACE2, including the heart or other cardiovascular tissues (28). Evidence showed that patients with COVID-19 had a high occurrence of cardiovascular symptoms, in addition to respiratory ones, and that these symptoms were also reported in patients without underlying cardiovascular diseases (30). The National Health Commission of China (NHC) reported that cardiovascular symptoms (such as heart palpitations and chest tightness) occurred at the beginning of the SARS-COV-2 infection in some of confirmed cases. Moreover, the 11.8% of patients who died for COVID-19 but without underlying cardiovascular diseases had substantial heart damage (30). These data suggest the necessity of involving cardiologists in the management of patients with COVID-19 (31). However, the real contribute of SARS-COV-2 in the development of myocardial injury is not clear (32). It is known that the infection itself may directly impact cardiovascular diseases and the development of cardiovascular complications (30, 33). Another factor that should be considered is also the expression in the tissue of TMPRSS211 or other proteases able to trigger the viral entry (6). Another hypothesis for the induction of heart damage considers the reduction of ACE2 caused by SARS-COV-2, which might exacerbate symptoms in patients with underlying cardiovascular diseases (28, 34). This could be due to the imbalance between the classic and non-classic RAS in favor of AII that may further compromise cardiac function apart from the viral infection (28). In fact, a preclinical study shows that ACE2 knockout animal models had a worse left ventricular remodeling in response to the AII-induced acute injury, suggesting a protective role of non-classic RAS in myocardial recovery (35). This finding may also explain the heart damage found in patients with COVID-19 but without cardiovascular diseases (30). To corroborate this hypothesis, a study demonstrated that the AII level in the plasma sample of SARS-COV-2 infected patients was markedly high and linearly associated with the viral load and lung injury (32). Moreover, another study found in the 35% of heart samples from patients with SARS the presence of viral RNA associated with a reduced ACE2 protein expression (36). Another proposed mechanism of myocardial injury includes the cytokine storm (32) as the systemic inflammatory response and immune system disorders during disease progression may be responsible for the myocardial damage (30). Also, in this case, other than the viral infection itself, a minor role in potentiating the inflammation might be played by the classic RAS cascade. Moreover, needs to be considered that also some drugs that are being investigated for COVID-19 are potential risk factors for the cardiovascular toxicity (31).

Finally, evidence showed that COVID-19 may produce a form of disseminated intravascular coagulation (DIC) as the presence of microthrombi have been reported from the autopsy of patients with COVID-19 (37). To date, the exact causes of DIC are many and unclear. Potential suggested mechanisms are as follows: inflammation (e.g., IL-6) stimulates the synthesis of fibrinogen (38); or the virus may directly bind to endothelial cells; or a mutual relationship between DIC and cytokine storm (wherein each exacerbates the other) exists.

CONCERNS, EVIDENCE AND RECOMMENDATION ON THE USE OF RAS INHIBITORS IN PATIENTS WITH COVID-19

Concerns were raised on the use of RAS inhibitors in patients with COVID-19 as the use of these drugs may determine an increase of ACE2 and then of SARS-COV-2 virulence (11, 30). Among drugs able to inhibit the RAS, there are renin inhibitors, ACE inhibitors, and the Angiotensin Receptor Blockers (ARBs). ACE inhibitors and ARBs are among drugs most commonly used worldwide for the treatment of cardiovascular diseases. Therefore, concerns on their use in patients with COVID-19 are even more important. Initial evidence showed that patients with COVID-19 and coexisting cardiovascular conditions had a more severe illness, a more frequent admission to the intensive care unit, were more prone to receive mechanical ventilation, or to die (11). The first hypothesis was that the medical management of these conditions, including the use of RAS inhibitors, may have contributed to the adverse health outcomes. So far, there is no rigorous report accounting for key factors as potential confounders in risk prediction; moreover, available evidence on the effect of RAS inhibitors on ACE2 mRNA expression and levels are conflicting and scarce, highlighting also the absence of data on lung-specific mRNA expression of ACE2 (11). Researches have also suggested that this effect of RAS inhibitors may not be uniform among molecules (11, 39). Moreover, even if there was a relationship between the RAS inhibition and the up-regulation of ACE2, there is no evidence demonstrating a causal relationship between the ACE2 activity and the SARS-COV-2 associated mortality (40). Furthermore, the presence of ACE2 on cell surface may not be the only factor participating in the infection process. In fact, additional co-factors might participate in the cell invasion process as SARS-COV-1 infection was not observed in some cells expressing ACE2 on the surface, whereas it was found in cells apparently without ACE2 (41). Moreover, the lethal outcome observed in patients with COVID-19 may also be driven by the severity of the lung damage. In this regard, a preclinical study suggested a beneficial role of RAS blockers in limiting the SARS-COV-1-induced lung injury (42), so that, a protective role is played by RAS inhibitors. This finding could rise a new hypothesis in which the activation of the classic RAS, rather than its inhibition, may predispose patients toward a more deleterious outcome.

Finally, another aspect that should be considered is the potential harm associated with the withdrawal of a RAS inhibitor in a patient with a stable cardiovascular condition. In fact,

RAS inhibitors are known to determine clinical benefits and to protect both myocardium and kidney. Therefore, their sudden withdrawal may expose patients to an unjustified risk related to decompensation and symptoms exacerbation, especially in high cardiovascular risk patients. In this regard, clinical trials have demonstrated a rapid relapse of the dilated cardiomyopathy or a decline of the clinical condition after the discontinuation of the pharmacological treatment with a RAS inhibitor (43).

Moreover, there are solid evidence on the effect of RAS inhibitors in reducing mortality in patients with cardiovascular diseases. These drugs are indeed the cornerstone therapy for a favorable prognosis in patients with heart failure, with the highest level of evidence in reducing mortality (44). Finally, Scientific Societies have expressed their opinion on the use of RAS inhibitors, highlighting the absence of evidence suggesting an eventual discontinuation of ACE-inhibitors, or ARBs in patients with COVID-19. Therefore, they recommend to continue the treatment with the usual anti-hypertensive agent in patients with COVID-19 (45–49). This recommendation has been supported by different observational studies published in the last few months. In this regards, a population-based case–control study carried out in the Lombardy region of Italy did not show any association between the use of ARBs or ACE-inhibitors with COVID-19 among all patients (adjusted odds ratio, 0.95 [95% confidence interval (CI), 0.86 to 1.05] for ARBs and 0.96 [95% CI, 0.87 to 1.07] for ACE inhibitors) or among patients with a severe or fatal course of the disease (adjusted odds ratio, 0.83 [95% CI, 0.63 to 1.10] for ARBs and 0.91 [95% CI, 0.69 to 1.21] for ACE inhibitors) (50).

Accordingly, another Italian nested case-control study showed no increased risk of being infected by SARS-COV-2 in patients treated with RAS inhibitors (51). Moreover, a case-population study showed that RAS inhibitors had an adjusted odds ratio for COVID-19 requiring admission to hospital of 0.94 (95% CI, 0.77 to 1.15) compared with users of other antihypertensive drugs (52). In relation to the mortality outcome, instead, a retrospective observational study showed similar mortality rates between the RAS inhibitor and non-RAS inhibitor cohorts (2.2 vs. 3.6%, adjusted hazard ratio [HR] 0.85; 95% CI, 0.28 to 2.58) (53). Similarly, a Korean nationwide population-based cohort study showed no difference for mortality between RAS inhibitors users and non-users (adjusted odds ratio, 0.88; 95% CI, 0.53 to 1.44) (54). Finally, a retrospective, multi-center study demonstrated a lower risk of COVID-19 mortality in inhospital patients with hypertension and hospitalized due to COVID-19 who received ACE inhibitor/ARB compared to those who did not receive an ACE inhibitor/ARB (adjusted HR, 0.37; 95% CI, 0.15 to 0.89) (55). Different other published studies supported the aforementioned findings (56–58). Moreover, it is ongoing an observational study that will enroll about 2,000 participants to assess if the chronic intake of RAS inhibitors modifies the prevalence and severity of clinical manifestations of COVID-19 (ClinicalTrials.gov identifier, NCT04331574).

Clinical trials are also ongoing to assess instead clinical benefits of continuing or not the treatment with ARBs or ACE inhibitors in patients with COVID-19 (NCT04330300, NCT04351581, NCT04353596, and NCT04329195). In particular, the NCT04330300 is a randomized, open label, parallel assignment clinical trial that will randomize patients with primary essential hypertension who are already taking ACE inhibitor/ARB to either switch to an alternative antihypertensive agent or continue with the ACE inhibitor/ARB treatment. The NCT04351581 is a randomized, single mask (outcome assessor), parallel assignment clinical trial that will randomize hospitalized patients with COVID-19 to continue or discontinue their treatment with the ACE inhibitor or ARB. The NCT04353596 is also a randomized, single mask (outcome assessor), parallel assignment clinical trial that will randomize symptomatic SARS-CoV2-infected patients to stop/replace the chronic treatment with the ACE inhibitor/ARB or to continue this chronic treatment. The NCT04329195 is instead a randomized, open label, parallel assignment clinical trial that will randomize patients with a history of cardiovascular disease treated with RAS blockers, and infected by SARS-CoV-2 to stop or continue the treatment with the RAS blocker. Moreover, the substudy of the Austrian Coronavirus Adaptive Clinical Trial (ACOVACT), which is a randomized, controlled, multicenter, open-label basket trial that aims to compare various antiviral treatments for COVID-19, will also compare the sub-arm with RAS blockade vs. no RAS blockade for patients with blood pressure >120/80 mmHg (NCT04351724). Characteristics of the ongoing clinical trials are showed in **Table 1**.

NEW PHARMACOLOGICAL APPROACHES FOR PREVENTING VIRAL ENTRY OF SARS-COV-2 WITH A FOCUS ON THE DISRUPTION OF S PROTEIN/ACE2 INTERACTION

To prevent viral infection, molecules like camostat mesylate, nafamostat mesylate, gabexate, umifenovir, and hydroxychloroquine/chloroquine are being considered (26). Nafamostat and camostat are inhibitors of the protease TMPRSS211 (26). Gabexate has instead multiple mechanisms of action. It has anticoagulant and anti-platelet activities on one hand, and it is a serine protease inhibitor with antiviral and anti-inflammatory properties on the other (59, 60).

While these drugs act on the protease inhibition, umifenovir and hydroxychloroquine/chloroquine directly influence the S protein/ACE2 interaction (**Table 2**) (26). Hydroxychloroquine and chloroquine, in addition to their use for malaria and autoimmune diseases, may be effective also for the treatment of COVID-19. These drugs are able to elevate endosomal pH and interfere with ACE2 glycosylation (26, 70). The efficacy of chloroquine was already demonstrated with SARS-COV-1 infection, in which the treatment was effective either if administrated prior or after the infection, suggesting that chloroquine may have both a prophylactic and therapeutic use (70). Moreover, preliminary *in vitro* results demonstrated that remdesivir and chloroquine are highly effective in the inhibition of SARS-COV-2 infection (71). Clinical findings also confirmed the efficacy of chloroquine in terms of reduction of exacerbation of pneumonia and duration of symptoms in a cohort of 100

TABLE 1 | Characteristics of ongoing clinical trials on drugs acting either by influencing the RAS or disrupting the viral attachment to ACE2 in patients with COVID-19.

Clinical trial number	Clinical phase; multicenter	Arms	Estimated enrollment	Primary outcome	Estimated study completion date
NCT04330300	4; No	• Experimental arm: switching to an alternative anti-hypertensive medication (specifically a calcium channel blocker or thiazide/thiazide-like diuretic at an equipotent blood pressure lowering dose). The choice of the alternative anti-hypertensive will be at the discretion of the patient's treating physician. • Comparator arm: continuing the treatment with ACE inhibitor/ARB	2,414	1. Number of COVID-19 positive participants who die, require intubation in intensive care unit, or require hospitalization for non-invasive ventilation at 12 months. Time from randomization to the first occurrence of any of the clinical events above.	March 1, 2021
NCT04351581	Not reported; No	• Experimental arm: continuing the treatment with ACE inhibitor/ARB. The clinicians will be encouraged to continue the medication throughout the hospital admission but it will be permissible for the clinician to stop treatment if necessary (e.g., due to hypotension). • Experimental arm: discontinuing the treatment with ACE inhibitor/ARB. If hypertensive treatment is necessary during hospital admission, the clinicians will first be encouraged to start non-ACE inhibitor/non-ARB treatment.	215	1. Days alive and out of hospital within 14 days after recruitment	December 2020
NCT04353596	4; Yes	• Experimental arm: chronic treatment with ACE inhibitor or ARB will be stopped or replaced. • Comparator arm: no intervention, which means to continue the treatment with ACE inhibitor or ARB.	208	1. Combination of maximum Sequential Organ Failure Assessment (SOFA) Score and death at 30 days. 2. Composite of admission to an intensive care unit, the use of mechanical ventilation, or all-cause death at 30 days.	May 15, 2022
NCT04329195	3; No	• Experimental arm: discontinuation of RAS blocker therapy • Comparator arm: continuation of RAS blocker therapy	554	1. Time to clinical improvement from day 0 to day 28 (improvement of two points on a seven-category ordinal scale, or live discharge from the hospital, whichever comes first)	August 9, 2020
NCT04351724 substudy	2/3; Yes	• Experimental arm: candesartan at 4 mg once daily and titrated to normotension • Comparator arm: non-RAS antihypertensive agents titrated to normotension. Those with normal blood pressure may be controlled without further treatment.	500	1. Sustained improvement (>48 h) of one point on the WHO Scale within 29 days (daily evaluation).	December 31, 2020
NCT04260594	4; Not reported	• Experimental arm: umifenovir tablets (2 tablets/time, 3 times/day for 14–20 days) + basic treatment • Comparator arm: basic treatment • The basic treatment is based on the condition of the patient.	380	1. Virus negative conversion rate in the first week	December 30, 2020
NCT04252885	4; No	• Experimental arm: standard treatment + lopinavir/ritonavir. Specifically, 50 participants are given ordinary treatment plus a regimen of lopinavir (200 mg) and ritonavir (50 mg) (oral, q12h, every time 2 tablets of each, taking for 7–14 days).	125	1. The rate of virus inhibition at Day 0, 2, 4, 7, 10, 14, and 21. Novel corona viral nucleic acid is measured in nose/throat swab at each time point.	July 31, 2020

(Continued)

TABLE 1 | Continued

Clinical trial number	Clinical phase; multicenter	Arms	Estimated enrollment	Primary outcome	Estimated study completion date
		• Comparator arm: standard treatment + umifenovir. Specifically, 50 participants are given ordinary treatment plus a regimen of umifenovir (100 mg) (oral, tid, 200 mg each time, taking for 7–14 days). • No intervention arm: standard treatment. Specifically, 25 cases are only given ordinary treatment.			
NCT04255017	4; No	• Experimental arm: addition of umifenovir (0.2 g once, 3 times a day for 2 weeks) • Experimental arm: addition of oseltamivir (75 mg once, twice a day for 2 weeks) • Experimental arm: addition of lopinavir/ritonavir (500 mg once, twice a day for 2 weeks) • No intervention arm: symptomatic supportive treatment	400	1. Rate of disease remission at 2 weeks. Defined for mild patients as fever, cough and other symptoms relieved with improved lung CT, and for severe patients as fever, cough and other symptoms relieved with improved lung CT, SPO2> 93% or PaO2/FiO2 > 300 mmHg (1 mmHg = 0.133 Kpa); 2. Time for lung recovery at 2 weeks. Defined as the comparison of the average time of lung imaging recovery after 2 weeks of treatment in each group.	July 1, 2020
NCT04350684	4; No	• Experimental arm: umifenovir + interferon-β 1a + lopinavir/ritonavir + single dose of hydroxychloroquine + standards of care • Comparator arm: interferon-β 1a + lopinavir/ritonavir + single dose of hydroxychloroquine + standards of care	40	1. Time to clinical improvement from the date of randomization until 14 days later. Improvement of two points on a seven-category ordinal scale (recommended by the World Health Organization: COVID-2019) R&D. Geneva: World Health Organization) or discharge from the hospital, whichever came first.	April 24, 2020
NCT04312009	2; Yes	• Experimental arm: losartan (50 mg daily, oral) • Control arm: placebo (microcrystalline methylcellulose, gelatin capsule, oral)	200	1. Difference in Estimated Positive End-expiratory Pressure (PEEP adjusted) P/F Ratio at 7 days. Outcome calculated from the partial pressure of oxygen or peripheral saturation of oxygen by pulse oximetry divided by the fraction of inspired oxygen (PaO2 or SaO2: FiO2 ratio). PaO2 is preferentially used if available. A correction is applied for endotracheal intubation and/or positive end-expiratory pressure. Patients discharged prior to day 7 will have a home pulse oximeter send home for measurement of the day 7 value, and will be adjusted for home O2 use, if applicable. Patients who died will be applied a penalty with a P/F ratio of 0.	April 1, 2021
NCT04311177	2; Yes	• Experimental arm: losartan (25 mg daily, oral) • Comparator arm: placebo (microcrystalline methylcellulose, gelatin capsule, oral)	580	1. Hospital Admission within 15 days. Outcome reported as the number of participants per arm admitted to inpatient hospital care due to COVID-19-related disease within 15 days of randomization.	April 1, 2021

(Continued)

TABLE 1 | Continued

Clinical trial number	Clinical phase; multicenter	Arms	Estimated enrollment	Primary outcome	Estimated study completion date
NCT04328012	2/3; Yes	• Experimental arm: lopinavir/ritonavir (400 mg/200 mg, oral, BID X 5–14 days depending on availability) • Experimental arm: hydroxychloroquine (400 mg BID on Day 0, and 200 mg BID Days 1–4, days 1–13 if available) • Experimental arm: losartan (25 mg, oral, daily X 5–14 days depending on availability) • Comparator arm: placebo (BID X 14 days)	4,000	1. National Institute of Allergy and Infectious Diseases COVID-19 Ordinal Severity Scale (NCOSS) at 60 days. Difference in NCOSS scores between the different treatment groups	April 1, 2021
NCT04335786	4; Yes	• Experimental arm: valsartan for 14 days at a dosage and frequency titrated to blood pressure with 80 mg or 160 mg tablets up to a maximum dose of 160 mg b.i.d. • Comparator arm: placebo for 14 days (matching 80 or 160 mg placebo tablets at a dosage and frequency titrated to systolic blood pressure)	651	1. First occurrence of intensive care unit admission, mechanical ventilation or death within 14 days. Death is defined as all-cause mortality	December 2021
NCT04360551	2; No	• Experimental arm: telmisartan (40 mg, oral, daily X 21 days) • Comparator arm: placebo (once daily X 21 days)	40	1. Maximum clinical severity of disease over the 21 day period of study. Based on a modified World Health Organization (WHO) COVID-19 7-point ordinal scale	June 30, 2021

subjects (72, 73). This finding led the China Authority to include these medicines in the recommendations for the prevention and treatment of COVID-19 pneumonia (73). Many other clinical studies are ongoing to evaluate the efficacy and safety of hydroxychloroquine for the pre-exposure prophylaxis, post-exposure prophylaxis, and treatment of COVID-19 (www.clinicaltrials.gov) (74). However, it should be noted that current evidence on the effects of chloroquine is conflicting. Authors of a recent systematic review underlined that, even though a rationale to justify clinical research on chloroquine in patients with COVID-19 exists, high-quality clinical trials are urgently needed (75). In addition, a further literature review (76) reported that there is limited *in vitro* evidence on the efficacy of this drug against SARS-COV-2 and that clinical data based on studies with small sample size and affected by methodological limitations (77, 78). Therefore, high quality randomized clinical trials are strongly needed. Umifenovir interferes instead with the attachment of viral envelope protein to host cells (26). Umifenovir is an antiviral agent actually authorized in Russia, but not in Europe, for the treatment of Influenza A and B. This drug is considered safe and it is patented for the SARS treatment (79). The opinion of the Italian Medicine Agency on this drug is that evidence on its efficacy are not sufficient to support its use in patients with COVID-19 (80). Currently, a randomized, open label, parallel assignment clinical study is evaluating the efficacy and safety of umifenovir for the treatment of pneumonia in patients infected with SARS-COV-2 (NCT04260594). In this

study, patients will be randomized to receive umifenovir plus basic treatment or just the basic treatment (**Table 1**). Moreover, two clinical trials are ongoing to assess the efficacy and safety of umifenovir and lopinavir/ritonavir (NCT04252885) or umifenovir, oseltamivir, and lopinavir/ritonavir (NCT04255017). Specifically, the NCT04252885 is a randomized, open label, parallel assignment clinical trial that will randomize patients with SARS-COV-2 infection in three groups (2:2:1). One group will receive the standard treatment plus lopinavir/ritonavir; the second group will receive standard treatment plus umifenovir; finally, the third group will just receive the standard treatment. The NCT04255017 is instead a randomized, single mask (participants), parallel assignment clinical trial that will randomize COVID-19 patients in four arms. One arm will receive the treatment with umifenovir; the second arm will receive the treatment with oseltamivir; the third arm will receive the treatment with lopinavir/ritonavir; the last arm will just receive the symptomatic supportive treatment (**Table 1**). Another small, randomized, triple mask (Participant, Care Provider, Investigator), parallel assignment clinical trial will be conducted on patients who have a positive test confirming COVID-19 to evaluate the combined treatment with umifenovir, interferon-β 1a, lopinavir/ritonavir, single dose of hydroxychloroquine, and the standards of care compared to the same combined treatment without umifenovir (NCT04350684).

In addition, speculations were done on the possible use for COVID-19 of new compounds, never approved before, which

TABLE 2 | Mechanism of action, main adverse events and potential drug-drug interactions of inhibitors of viral invasion interfering with the S protein/ACE2 interaction, RAS inhibitors, and analogous ACE2 and A1-7 under clinical evaluation for the treatment of COVID-19.

Therapeutic class	Drugs	Main mechanism of action	Main adverse events	Drug-drug interactions	References
Inhibitors of S protein/ACE2 interaction	Chloroquine/ Hydroxychloroquine	Increase of endosomal pH and interference with ACE2 glycosylation	Cardiovascular disorders, including prolongation of QT	Digoxin, class IA and III antiarrhythmic, tricyclic antidepressants, antipsychotics	(61, 62)
	Umifenovir	Interference with the attachment of the viral protein to host cells	Gastrointestinal symptoms and increased transaminase	As UDP-glucuronosyltransferase 1A9 and 2B7 inhibitor, umifenovir can increase levels of its substrates (paracetamol, buprenorphine, etc.) Cytochrome 3A4 inducers can reduce umifenovir levels	(63, 64)
ARBs	Losartan	Blocks the AII-induced lung injury	Dizziness, anemia, renal failure, asthenia, hyperkaliemia	Fluconazole and Rifampicine can increase losartan levels, Potassium-sparing diuretics can increase the risk of hyperkaelemia	(65, 66)
Analogous of ACE2 and A1-7	A1-7	Restores the beneficial effect of the non-classic RAS	Headache, fatigue, injection site reaction	Not Available	(29, 67, 68)
	ACE2	Restores the beneficial effect of the non-classic RAS	Hypernatremia, rash, dysphagia, and pneumonia	Not Available	(69)

have shown the ability of interfering with S protein/ACE2 interaction (74). The compound SSAA09E2 showed the ability of blocking the early interaction of SARS-S protein with ACE2 in ACE2-expressing 293T cells (81). Moreover, the agent VE607 also showed a significant inhibition of SARS-pseudovirus entry in the same cellular model (82).

NEW PHARMACOLOGICAL PERSPECTIVE FOR COVID-19 ACTING ON THE RAS

Based on the beneficial role of the non-classic RAS, which seems lacking in patients with COVID-19, hypotheses have been made on the potential therapeutic approach of restoring the ACE2/A1-7 pathway. This hypothesis is based on preclinical evidence showing an improvement of oxygenation, reduction of inflammation, and reduction of tissue fibrosis after infusion of A1-7 in two models of ARDS (65, 83). Evidence also showed that the administration of the soluble human recombinant ACE2 was able to reverse the lung-injury process in preclinical models of other viral infections (84, 85). The rationale to administer soluble ACE2 is to stimulate the RAS protective pathway without increasing the ACE2 transmembrane form that could instead potentiate the viral entry into the cells. Clinical evidence on this aspect is scarce (86). A phase 2 trial conducted in patients with ARDS showed that ACE2 infusion safely reduced the AII level, but this trial was not powered enough to show efficacy in terms of pulmonary function (69). Restoring the ACE2 activity may also be beneficial for the myocardial protection in patients with COVID-19 (87). To date, clinical researches are

ongoing to assess the clinical impact of a restoration of the non-classic RAS (ACE2 and A1-7) in patients with COVID-19. Is underway a controlled trial aimed to assess the efficacy, safety and clinical impact of A1-7 infusion in a cohort of COVID-19 patients requiring mechanical ventilation (NCT04332666). It was, instead, suspended a further clinical trial that aimed to assess preliminary biologic, physiologic, and clinical data with the use of ACE2 recombinant compared to the standard care in patients with COVID-19 (NCT04287686).

In addition, based on the organ protective effects of RAS inhibitors, many studies are being conducted to investigate their efficacy in COVID-19 patients. The beneficial effects of ACE inhibitors and ARB may be related to the prevalence of ACE2/A1-7 effects as demonstrated in experimental studies (88, 89). Moreover, experimental evidence strongly suggests that AII could promote acute lung injury induced by different coronaviruses, including SARS-COV-1 and SARS-COV-2 (42, 65). Therefore, the use of RAS inhibitors may block the deleterious effect associated with AII. Two trials are ongoing to investigate the role of losartan for the treatment of COVID-19 in patients who have not previously received a RAS inhibitor and are either hospitalized (NCT04312009) or not hospitalized (NCT04311177). In particular, both trails (NCT04312009 and NCT04311177) are randomized, quadruple mask (participant, care provider, investigator, outcomes assessor), parallel assignment clinical trials that will compare the treatment with losartan vs. placebo in COVID-19 patients, including those with ARDS. Moreover, a pragmatic adaptive, randomized, quadruple mask (participant, care provider, investigator, outcomes assessor), parallel assignment trial is comparing the treatment with lopinavir/ritonavir, or hydroxychloroquine, or losartan vs. placebo in patients with COVID-19 (NCT04328012). Another randomized, quadruple mask (participant, care provider, investigator, outcomes assessor), parallel assignment clinical trial will evaluate the treatment with valsartan compared to placebo for the prevention of ARDS in hospitalized patients with COVID-19 (NCT04335786). Finally, a pilot, randomized, triple mask (participant, care provider, investigator), parallel assignment clinical trial is ongoing to assess the safety and efficacy of telmisartan compared to placebo for the mitigation of pulmonary and cardiac complications in COVID-19 patients (NCT04360551). Characteristics of the mentioned clinical trials are showed in **Table 1**. The mechanism of action, main adverse events and potential drug-drug interactions of RAS inhibitors and analogous of A1-7 and ACE2 under clinical evaluation for COVID-19 are summarized in **Table 1**.

Finally, other compounds that may be useful for the treatment of COVID-19, but not currently evaluated, are molecules that may adjust the imbalance between AT1 and AT2 receptors such as compound 21 (C-21), CGP-42112A, and L-163491 (26). C-21 and CGP-42112A are two agonists of AT2 receptors, whereas L-163491 has a dual action as a partial agonist of AT2 receptors and a partial antagonist of AT1 receptors (26).

CONCLUSION

The RAS may play a complex role in SARS-COV-2 infection. SARS-COV-2 internalization may cause a reduction of ACE2 on cell surface. A reduction in ACE2 can further contribute to the pulmonary function deterioration and the myocardial damage. However, there is a paucity of clinical evidence on the efficacy of restoring the ACE2 functionality for the treatment of viral-induced lung injury. A clinical trial is ongoing to evaluate the effect of A1-7 in COVID-19 patients. To date, there is no effective drug for the treatment of COVID-19 and few clinical data are available. Some clinical trials are ongoing to evaluate the efficacy of drugs that could interfere with the S protein/ACE2 interaction such as umifenovir and hydroxychloroquine/chloroquine.

Data instead on the increased mRNA expression and levels of ACE2 after treatment with RAS inhibitors are scarce and to date not associated with an increased mortality in patients with COVID-19. Currently, clinical trials are ongoing to investigate the use of a RAS inhibitor for the reduction of the lung damage in patients with COVID-19. Substantial evidence is needed to guide decision-making on the use of ACE inhibitors and ARBs in such patients, until then we need to base on the available data that place RAS inhibitors among the safe choices for cardiovascular diseases.

AUTHOR CONTRIBUTIONS

AM, CS, CR, CF, GR, LB, GP, FR, and AC: drafting the work, revising it for important intellectual content, final approval of the version to be published, and agreement to be accountable for all aspects of the work in ensuring that questions related to the accuracy or integrity of any part of the work are appropriately discussed. FR and AC developed the concept and designed the study. AM wrote the paper. All authors contributed to the article and approved the submitted version.

ACKNOWLEDGMENTS

We are grateful for the help and support of the Italian Society of Pharmacology (SIF) and its Section of Clinical Pharmacology Giampaolo Velo. All authors who contributed significantly to the work are listed.

REFERENCES

1. Turner AJ, Hiscox JA, Hooper NM. ACE2: from vasopeptidase to SARS virus receptor. *Trends Pharmacol Sci.* (2004) 25:291–4. doi: 10.1016/j.tips.2004.04.001

2. Mascolo A, Sessa M, Scavone C, De Angelis A, Vitale C, Berrino L, et al. New and old roles of the peripheral and brain renin–angiotensin–aldosterone system (RAAS): focus on cardiovascular and neurological diseases. *Int J Cardiol.* (2017) 227:734–42. doi: 10.1016/j.ijcard.2016.10.069

3. Skov J, Persson F, Frøkiær J, Christiansen JS. Tissue renin-angiotensin systems: a unifying hypothesis of metabolic disease. *Front Endocrinol.* (2014) 5:23. doi: 10.3389/fendo.2014.00023

4. Marshall R. The pulmonary renin-angiotensin system. *Curr Pharm Des.* (2005) 9:715–22. doi: 10.2174/1381612033455431

5. Mascolo A, Urbanek K, De Angelis A, Sessa M, Scavone C, Berrino L, et al. Angiotensin II and angiotensin 1-7: which is their role in atrial fibrillation? *Heart Fail Rev.* (2020) 25:367–80. doi: 10.1007/s10741-019-09837-7

6. Hoffmann M, Kleine-Weber H, Schroeder S, Krüger N, Herrler T, Erichsen S, et al. SARS-CoV-2 cell entry depends on ACE2 and TMPRSS2 and is blocked by a clinically proven protease inhibitor. *Cell.* (2020) 181:271–80.e8. doi: 10.1016/j.cell.2020.02.052

7. Li W, Moore MJ, Vasllieva N, Sui J, Wong SK, Berne MA, et al. Angiotensin-converting enzyme 2 is a functional receptor for the SARS coronavirus. *Nature.* (2003) 426:450–4. doi: 10.1038/nature02145

8. Guo YR, Cao QD, Hong ZS, Tan YY, Chen SD, Jin HJ, et al. The origin, transmission and clinical therapies on coronavirus disease 2019 (COVID-19) outbreak - an update on the status. *Mil Med Res.* (2020) 7:11. doi: 10.1186/s40779-020-00240-0

9. Huang C, Wang Y, Li X, Ren L, Zhao J, Hu Y, et al. Clinical features of patients infected with 2019 novel coronavirus in Wuhan, China. *Lancet.* (2020) 395:497–506. doi: 10.1016/S0140-6736(20)30183-5

10. Mori J, Oudit GY, Lopaschuk GD. SARS-CoV-2 perturbs the renin-angiotensin system and energy metabolism. *Am J Physiol Metab.* (2020) 319:E43–7. doi: 10.1152/ajpendo.00219.2020

11. Vaduganathan M, Vardeny O, Michel T, McMurray JJ V, Pfeffer MA, Solomon SD. Renin-angiotensin-aldosterone system inhibitors in patients with covid-19. *N Engl J Med.* (2020) 382:1653–9. doi: 10.1056/NEJMsr2005760

12. Jiang F, Deng L, Zhang L, Cai Y, Cheung CW, Xia Z. Review of the clinical characteristics of coronavirus disease 2019 (COVID-19). *J Gen Intern Med.* (2020) 35:1545–9. doi: 10.1007/s11606-020-05762-w

13. Tabata S, Imai K, Kawano S, Ikeda M, Kodama T, Miyoshi K, et al. Clinical characteristics of COVID-19 in 104 people with SARS-CoV-2 infection on the diamond princess cruise ship: a retrospective analysis. *Lancet Infect Dis.* (2020). doi: 10.1016/S1473-3099(20)30482-5. [Epub ahead of print].

14. Colaneri M, Sacchi P, Zuccaro V, Biscarini S, Sachs M, Roda S, et al. Clinical characteristics of coronavirus disease (COVID-19) early findings from a teaching hospital in Pavia, North Italy, 21 to 28 February 2020. *Eurosurveillance.* (2020) 25:2000460. doi: 10.2807/1560-7917.ES.2020.25.16.2000460

15. Guan WJ, Ni ZY, Hu Y, Liang WH, Ou CQ, He JX, et al. Clinical characteristics of coronavirus disease 2019 in China. *N Engl J Med.* (2020) 382:1708–20. doi: 10.1056/NEJMoa2002032

16. Unger T. The role of the renin-angiotensin system in the development of cardiovascular disease. *Am J Cardiol.* (2002) 89:3A–9. doi: 10.1016/S0002-9149(01)02321-9

17. Karamyan VT, Arsenault J, Escher E, Speth RC. Preliminary biochemical characterization of the novel, non-AT1, non-AT2 angiotensin binding site from the rat brain. *Endocrine.* (2010) 37:442–8. doi: 10.1007/s12020-010-9328-2

18. Marchesi C, Paradis P, Schiffrin EL. Role of the renin-angiotensin system in vascular inflammation. *Trends Pharmacol Sci.* (2008) 29:367–74. doi: 10.1016/j.tips.2008.05.003

19. Dandona P, Dhindsa S, Ghanim H, Chaudhuri A. Angiotensin II and inflammation: the effect of angiotensin-converting enzyme inhibition and angiotensin II receptor blockade. *J Hum Hypertens.* (2007) 21:20–7. doi: 10.1038/sj.jhh.1002101

20. Yamamoto S, Yancey PG, Zuo Y, Ma LJ, Kaseda R, Fogo AB, et al. Macrophage polarization by angiotensin II-type 1 receptor aggravates renal injury-acceleration of atherosclerosis. *Arterioscler Thromb Vasc Biol.* (2011) 31:2856–64. doi: 10.1161/ATVBAHA.111.237198

21. Fraga-Silva RA, Pinheiro SVB, Gonçalves ACC, Alenina N, Bader M, Santos RAS, et al. The antithrombotic effect of angiotensin-(1-7) involves mas-mediated NO release from platelets. *Mol Med.* (2008) 14:28–35. doi: 10.2119/2007-00073.Fraga-Silva

22. Dias-Peixoto MF, Santos RAS, Gomes ERM, Alves MNM, Almeida PWM, Greco L, et al. Molecular mechanisms involved in the angiotensin-(1-7)/Mas signaling pathway in cardiomyocytes. *Hypertension.* (2008) 52:542–8. doi: 10.1161/HYPERTENSIONAHA.108.114280

23. da Silveira KD, Coelho FM, Vieira AT, Sachs D, Barroso LC, Costa VV, et al. Anti-inflammatory effects of the activation of the angiotensin-(1-7) receptor, MAS, in experimental models of arthritis. *J Immunol.* (2010) 185:5569–76. doi: 10.4049/jimmunol.1000314

24. Santos RAS, Ferreira AJ, Verano-Braga T, Bader M. Angiotensin-converting enzyme 2, angiotensin-(1-7) and mas: new players of the renin-angiotensin system. *J Endocrinol.* (2013) 216:R1–17. doi: 10.1530/JOE-12-0341

25. Rutkowska-Zapała M, Suski M, Szatanek R, Lenart M, Weglarczyk K, Olszanecki R, et al. Human monocyte subsets exhibit divergent angiotensin I-converting activity. *Clin Exp Immunol.* (2015) 181:126–32. doi: 10.1111/cei.12612

26. Liu C, Zhou Q, Li Y, Garner LV, Watkins SP, Carter LJ, et al. Research and development on therapeutic agents and vaccines for COVID-19 and related human coronavirus diseases. *ACS Cent Sci.* (2020) 6:315. doi: 10.1021/acscentsci.0c00272

27. Wrapp D, Wang N, Corbett KS, Goldsmith JA, Hsieh CL, Abiona O, et al. Cryo-EM structure of the 2019-nCoV spike in the prefusion conformation. *Science.* (2020) 367:1260–3. doi: 10.1126/science.abb2507

28. South AM, Diz D, Chappell MC. COVID-19, ACE2 and the cardiovascular consequences. *Am J Physiol Hear Circ Physiol.* (2020) 318:H1084–90. doi: 10.1152/ajpheart.00217.2020

29. Cheng H, Wang Y, Wang GQ. Organ-protective effect of angiotensin-converting enzyme 2 and its effect on the prognosis of COVID-19. *J Med Virol.* (2020) 96:726–30. doi: 10.1002/jmv.25785

30. Zheng YY, Ma YT, Zhang JY, Xie X. COVID-19 and the cardiovascular system. *Nat Rev Cardiol.* (2020) 17:259–60. doi: 10.1038/s41569-020-0360-5

31. Driggin E, Madhavan MV, Bikdeli B, Chuich T, Laracy J, Bondi-Zoccai G, et al. Cardiovascular considerations for patients, health care workers, and health systems during the coronavirus disease 2019. (COVID-19) Pandemic. *J Am Coll Cardiol.* (2020) 75:2352–71. doi: 10.1016/j.jacc.2020.03.031

32. Liu Y, Yang Y, Zhang C, Huang F, Wang F, Yuan J, et al. Clinical and biochemical indexes from 2019-nCoV infected patients linked to viral loads and lung injury. *Sci China Life Sci.* (2020) 63:364–74. doi: 10.1007/s11427-020-1643-8

33. Du L, He Y, Zhou Y, Liu S, Zheng BJ, Jiang S. The spike protein of SARS-CoV - a target for vaccine and therapeutic development. *Nat Rev Microbiol.* (2009) 7:226–36. doi: 10.1038/nrmicro2090

34. Yousif MHM, Dhaunsi GS, Makki BM, Qabazard BA, Akhtar S, Benter IF. Characterization of angiotensin-(1-7) effects on the cardiovascular system in an experimental model of type-1 diabetes. *Pharmacol Res.* (2012) 66:269–75. doi: 10.1016/j.phrs.2012.05.001

35. Kassiri Z, Zhong J, Guo D, Basu R, Wang X, Liu PP, et al. Loss of angiotensin-converting enzyme 2 accelerates maladaptive left ventricular remodeling in response to myocardial infarction. *Circ Hear Fail.* (2009) 2:446–55. doi: 10.1161/CIRCHEARTFAILURE.108.840124

36. Oudit GY, Kassiri Z, Jiang C, Liu PP, Poutanen SM, Penninger JM, et al. SARS-coronavirus modulation of myocardial ACE2 expression and inflammation in patients with SARS. *Eur J Clin Invest.* (2009) 39:618–25. doi: 10.1111/j.1365-2362.2009.02153.x

37. Luo W, Yu H, Gou J, Li X, Sun Y, Li J, et al. Clinical pathology of critical patient with novel coronavirus pneumonia (COVID-19) List of authors. *Preprints.* (2020). [Epub ahead of print].

38. Carty CL, Heagerty P, Heckbert SR, Jarvik GP, Lange LA, Cushman M, et al. Interaction between fibrinogen and IL-6 genetic variants and associations with cardiovascular disease risk in the cardiovascular health study. *Ann Hum Genet.* (2010) 74:1–10. doi: 10.1111/j.1469-1809.2009.00551.x

39. Mourad JJ, Levy BI. Interaction between RAAS inhibitors and ACE2 in the context of COVID-19. *Nat Rev Cardiol.* (2020) 17:313. doi: 10.1038/s41569-020-0368-x

40. Kuster GM, Pfister O, Burkard T, Zhou Q, Twerenbold R, Haaf P, et al. SARS-CoV2: should inhibitors of the renin-angiotensin system be withdrawn in patients with COVID-19? *Eur Hear J.* (2020) 41:1801–3. doi: 10.1093/eurheartj/ehaa235

41. Gu J, Korteweg C. Pathology and pathogenesis of severe acute respiratory syndrome. *Am J Pathol.* (2007) 170:1136–47. doi: 10.2353/ajpath.2007.061088

42. Kuba K, Imai Y, Rao S, Gao H, Guo F, Guan B, et al. A crucial role of angiotensin converting enzyme 2 (ACE2) in SARS coronavirus-induced lung injury. *Nat Med.* (2005) 11:875–9. doi: 10.1038/nm1267

43. Halliday BP, Wassall R, Lota AS, Khalique Z, Gregson J, Newsome S, et al. Withdrawal of pharmacological treatment for heart failure in patients with recovered dilated cardiomyopathy (TRED-HF): an open-label, pilot, randomised trial. *Lancet.* (2019) 393:61–73. doi: 10.1016/S0140-6736(18)32484-X

44. Ponikowski P, Voors AA, Anker SD, Bueno H, Cleland JGF, Coats AJS, et al. ESC Guidelines for the diagnosis and treatment of acute and chronic heart failure: the task force for the diagnosis and treatment of acute and chronic heart failure of the European Society of Cardiology (ESC). Developed with the special contribution. *Eur J Heart Fail.* (2016) 37:2129–200. doi: 10.1093/eurheartj/ehw128

45. Italian Society of Hypertension. *Farmaci antiipertensivi e rischio di COVID-19. Il comunicato della SIIA | SIIA.* Available online at: https://siia.it/notizie-siia/farmaci-antiipertensivi-e-rischio-di-covid-19-il-comunicato-della-siia/ (accessed April 4, 2020).

46. Italian Society of Cardiology. *GUIDA CLINICA COVID-19 PER CARDIOLOGI.* (2020). Available online at: https://www.sicardiologia.it/public/Documento-SIC-COVID-19.pdf (accessed April 20, 2020).

47. European Society of Cardiology. *Position Statement of the ESC Council on Hypertension on ACE-Inhibitors and Angiotensin Receptor Blockers.* (2020). Available online at: https://www.escardio.org/Councils/Council-on-Hypertension-(CHT)/News/position-statement-of-the-esc-council-on-hypertension-on-ace-inhibitors-and-ang (accessed April 20, 2020).

48. American Heart Association. *HFSA/ACC/AHA statement addresses concerns re: using RAAS antagonists in COVID-19.* (2020). Available online at: https://www.acc.org/latest-in-cardiology/articles/2020/03/17/08/59/hfsa-acc-aha-statement-addresses-concerns-re-using-raas-antagonists-in-covid-19 (accessed April 20, 2020).

49. Italian Society of Pharmacology. *SIF | Documento Informativo della Società Italiana di Farmacologia - Uso di Ace-Inibitori/Sartani ed infezione da COVID-19.* (2020). Available online at: https://www.sifweb.org/documenti/document_2020-03-13_documento-informativo-della-societa-italiana-di-farmacologia-uso-di-ace-inibitori-sartani-ed-infezione-da-covid-19 (accessed April 17, 2020).

50. Mancia G, Rea F, Ludergnani M, Apolone G, Corrao G. Renin–angiotensin–aldosterone system blockers and the risk of Covid-19. *N Engl J Med.* (2020) 382:2431–40. doi: 10.1056/NEJMoa2006923

51. Gnavi R, Demaria M, Picariello Roberta, Dalmasso M, Ricceri F, Costa G. Therapy with agents acting on the renin-angiotensin system and risk of severe acute respiratory syndrome coronavirus 2 infection. *Clin Infect Dis.* (2020) 174:30–3. doi: 10.1093/cid/ciaa634

52. de Abajo FJ, Rodríguez-Martín S, Lerma V, Mejía-Abril G, Aguilar M, García-Luque A, et al. Use of renin–angiotensin–aldosterone system inhibitors and risk of COVID-19 requiring admission to hospital: a case-population study. *Lancet.* (2020) 395:1705–14. doi: 10.1016/S0140-6736(20)31030-8

53. Gao C, Cai Y, Zhang K, Zhou L, Zhang Y, Zhang X, et al. Association of hypertension and antihypertensive treatment with COVID-19 mortality: a retrospective observational study. *Eur Heart J.* (2020) 41:2058–66. doi: 10.1093/eurheartj/ehaa433

54. Jung SY, Choi JC, You SH, Kim WY. Association of renin-angiotensin-aldosterone system inhibitors with COVID-19-related outcomes in korea: a nationwide population-based cohort study. *Clin Infect Dis.* (2020) 22:ciaa624. doi: 10.1093/cid/ciaa624

55. Zhang P, Zhu L, Cai J, Lei F, Qin JJ, Xie J, et al. Association of inpatient use of angiotensin-converting enzyme inhibitors and angiotensin II receptor blockers with mortality among patients with hypertension hospitalized with COVID-19. *Circ Res.* (2020) 126:1671–81. doi: 10.1161/CIRCRESAHA.120.317242

56. Reynolds HR, Adhikari S, Pulgarin C, Troxel AB, Iturrate E, Johnson SB, et al. Renin–angiotensin–aldosterone system inhibitors and risk of covid-19. *N Engl J Med.* (2020) 382:2441–8. doi: 10.1056/NEJMoa2008975

57. Li J, Wang X, Chen J, Zhang H, Deng A. Association of renin-angiotensin system inhibitors with severity or risk of death in patients with hypertension hospitalized for coronavirus disease 2019 (COVID-19) infection in Wuhan, China. *JAMA Cardiol.* (2020) 5:1–6. doi: 10.1001/jamacardio.2020.1624

58. Meng J, Xiao G, Zhang J, He X, Ou M, Bi J, et al. Renin-angiotensin system inhibitors improve the clinical outcomes of COVID-19 patients with hypertension. *Emerg Microbes Infect.* (2020) 9:757–60. doi: 10.1080/22221751.2020.1746200

59. Yuksel M, Okajima K, Uchiba M, Okabe H. Gabexate mesilate, a synthetic protease inhibitor, inhibits lipopolysaccharide-induced tumor necrosis factor-α production by inhibiting activation of both nuclear factor-κB and activator protein-1 in human monocytes. *J Pharmacol Exp Ther.* (2003) 305:298–305. doi: 10.1124/jpet.102.041988

60. Tamura Y, Hirado M, Okamura K, Minato Y, Fujii S. Synthetic inhibitors of trypsin, plasmin, kallikrein, thrombin, C1r, and C1 esterase. *Biochim Biophys Acta.* (1977) 484:417–22. doi: 10.1016/0005-2744(77)90097-3

61. Dong L, Hu S, Gao J. Discovering drugs to treat coronavirus disease 2019 (COVID-19). *Drug Discov Ther.* (2020) 14:58–60. doi: 10.5582/ddt.2020.01012

62. Italian Medicine Agency. *Plaquenil, Summary of Product Characteristics.* Available online at: https://farmaci.agenziafarmaco.gov.it/aifa/servlet/PdfDownloadServlet?pdfFileName=footer_008055_013967_RCP.pdf&retry=0&sys=m0b1l3 (accessed April 8, 2020).

63. Wang M, Cai B, Li L, Lin J, Su N, Yu H, et al. [Efficacy and safety of arbidol in treatment of naturally acquired influenza] - pubmed. *Zhongguo Yi Xue Ke Xue Yuan Xue Bao.* (2004) 26:289–93.

64. Liu X, Huang T, Chen JX, Zeng J, Fan XR, Xu-Zhu, et al. Arbidol exhibits strong inhibition towards UDP-glucuronosyltransferase (UGT) 1A9 and 2B7. *Pharmazie.* (2013) 68:945–50.

65. Wösten-Van Asperen RM, Lutter R, Specht PA, Moll GN, Van Woensel JB, Van Der Loos CM, et al. Acute respiratory distress syndrome leads to reduced ratio of ACE/ACE2 activities and is prevented by angiotensin-(1-7) or an angiotensin II receptor antagonist. *J Pathol.* (2011) 225:618–27. doi: 10.1002/path.2987

66. Italian Medicine Agency. *Losaprex, Summary of Product Cherateristics.* Available online at: https://farmaci.agenziafarmaco.gov.it/aifa/servlet/PdfDownloadServlet?pdfFileName=footer_004375_029393_RCP.pdf&retry=0&sys=m0b1l3 (accessed April 8, 2020).

67. Savage PD, Lovato J, Brosnihan KB, Miller AA, Petty WJ. Phase II trial of angiotensin-(1-7) for the treatment of patients with metastatic sarcoma. *Sarcoma.* (2016) 2016:1–7. doi: 10.1155/2016/4592768

68. Chappell MC. Emerging evidence for a functional angiotensin-converting enzyme 2-angiotensin-(1-7)-Mas receptor axis: more than regulation of blood pressure? *Hypertension.* (2007) 50:596–9. doi: 10.1161/HYPERTENSIONAHA.106.076216

69. Khan A, Benthin C, Zeno B, Albertson TE, Boyd J, Christie JD, et al. A pilot clinical trial of recombinant human angiotensin-converting enzyme 2 in acute respiratory distress syndrome. *Crit Care.* (2017) 21:234. doi: 10.1186/s13054-017-1823-x

70. Vincent MJ, Bergeron E, Benjannet S, Erickson BR, Rollin PE, Ksiazek TG, et al. Chloroquine is a potent inhibitor of SARS coronavirus infection and spread. *Virol J.* (2005) 2:69. doi: 10.1186/1743-422X-2-69

71. Wang M, Cao R, Zhang L, Yang X, Liu J, Xu M, et al. Remdesivir and chloroquine effectively inhibit the recently emerged novel coronavirus (2019-nCoV) *in vitro. Cell Res.* (2020) 30:269–71. doi: 10.1038/s41422-020-0282-0

72. Gao J, Tian Z, Yang X. Breakthrough: chloroquine phosphate has shown apparent efficacy in treatment of COVID-19 associated pneumonia in clinical studies. *Biosci Trends.* (2020) 14:72–3. doi: 10.5582/bst.2020.01047

73. Colson P, Rolain JM, Lagier JC, Brouqui P, Raoult D. Chloroquine and hydroxychloroquine as available weapons to fight COVID-19. *Int J Antimicrob Agents.* (2020) 55:105932. doi: 10.1016/j.ijantimicag.2020.105932

74. U.S. National Library of Medicine. *Search of: hydroxychloroquine | Covid-19 - List Results - ClinicalTrials.gov.* (2020). Available online at: https://clinicaltrials.gov/ct2/results?cond=Covid-19&term=hydroxychloroquine&cntry=&state=&city=&dist= (accessed April 6, 2020).

75. Cortegiani A, Ingoglia G, Ippolito M, Giarratano A, Einav S. A systematic review on the efficacy and safety of chloroquine for the treatment of COVID-19. *J Crit Care.* (2020) 57:279–83. doi: 10.1016/j.jcrc.2020.03.005

76. Gbinigie K, Frie K. Should chloroquine and hydroxychloroquine be used to treat COVID-19? a rapid review. *BJGP Open.* (2020) 4:bjgpopen20X101069. doi: 10.3399/bjgpopen20X101069

77. Chen J, Liu D, Liu L, Liu P, Xu Q, Xia L, et al. A pilot study of hydroxychloroquine in treatment of patients with common coronavirus disease-19 (COVID-19). *J Zhejiang Univ.* (2020) 49:1–10.

78. Gautret P, Lagier J-C, Parola P, Hoang VT, Meddeb L, Mailhe M, et al. Hydroxychloroquine and azithromycin as a treatment of COVID-19: results of an open-label non-randomized clinical trial. *Int J Antimicrob Agents.* (2020) 56:105949. doi: 10.1016/j.ijantimicag.2020.105949

79. Blaising J, Polyak SJ, Pécheur EI. Arbidol as a broad-spectrum antiviral: an update. *Antiviral Res.* (2014) 107:84–94. doi: 10.1016/j.antiviral.2014.04.006

80. Italian Medicine Agency. *AIFA precisa: uso umifenovir su COVID-19 non autorizzato in Europa e USA, scarse evidenze scientifiche sull'efficacia.* (2020). Available online at: https://www.aifa.gov.it/web/guest/-/aifa-precisa-uso-umifenovir-su-covid-19-non-autorizzato-in-europa-e-usa-scarse-evidenze-scientifiche-sull-efficacia (accessed April 5, 2020).

81. Adedeji AO, Severson W, Jonsson C, Singh K, Weiss SR, Sarafianos SG. Novel inhibitors of severe acute respiratory syndrome coronavirus entry that act by three distinct mechanisms. *J Virol.* (2013) 87:8017–28. doi: 10.1128/JVI.00998-13

82. Kao RY, Tsui WHW, Lee TSW, Tanner JA, Watt RM, Huang JD, et al. Identification of novel small-molecule inhibitors of severe acute respiratory syndrome-associated coronavirus by chemical genetics. *Chem Biol.* (2004) 11:1293–9. doi: 10.1016/j.chembiol.2004.07.013

83. Zambelli V, Bellani G, Borsa R, Pozzi F, Grassi A, Scanziani M, et al. Angiotensin-(1-7) improves oxygenation, while reducing cellular infiltrate and fibrosis in experimental acute respiratory distress syndrome. *Intensive Care Med Exp.* (2015) 3:44. doi: 10.1186/s40635-015-0044-3

84. Zou Z, Yan Y, Shu Y, Gao R, Sun Y, Li X, et al. Angiotensin-converting enzyme 2 protects from lethal avian influenza A H5N1 infections. *Nat Commun.* (2014) 5:3594. doi: 10.1038/ncomms4594

85. Gu H, Xie Z, Li T, Zhang S, Lai C, Zhu P, et al. Angiotensin-converting enzyme 2 inhibits lung injury induced by respiratory syncytial virus. *Sci Rep.* (2016) 6:19840. doi: 10.1038/srep19840

86. Patel AB, Verma A. COVID-19 and angiotensin-converting enzyme inhibitors and angiotensin receptor blockers: what is the evidence? *JAMA.* (2020) 323:1769–70. doi: 10.1001/jama.2020. 4812

87. Basu R, Poglitsch M, Yogasundaram H, Thomas J, Rowe BH, Oudit GY. Roles of angiotensin peptides and recombinant human ACE2 in heart failure. *J Am Coll Cardiol.* (2017) 69:805–19. doi: 10.1016/j.jacc.2016. 11.064

88. Chappell MC. Biochemical evaluation of the renin-angiotensin system: the good, bad, and absolute? *Am J Physiol - Hear Circ Physiol.* (2016) 310:H137–52. doi: 10.1152/ajpheart.00618. 2015

89. Santos RAS, Oudit GY, Verano-Braga T, Canta G, Steckelings UM, Bader M. The renin-angiotensin system: going beyond the classical paradigms. *Am J Physiol Hear Circ Physiol.* (2019) 316:H958–70. doi: 10.1152/ajpheart.00723.2018

21

IL-10 and IL-12 (P70) Levels Predict the Risk of Covid-19 Progression in Hypertensive Patients: Insights from the BRACE-CORONA Trial

Renata Moll-Bernardes[1], Andrea Silvestre de Sousa[1,2], Ariane V. S. Macedo[1,3,4],
Renato D. Lopes[1,5,6], Narendra Vera[7], Luciana C. R. Maia[7], André Feldman[1,8],
Guilherme D. A. S. Arruda[9], Mauro J. C. Castro[10], Pedro M. Pimentel-Coelho[7],
Denílson C. de Albuquerque[1,11], Thiago Ceccatto de Paula[3], Thyago A. B. Furquim[12],
Vitor A. Loures[8], Karla G. D. Giusti[13], Nathália M. de Oliveira[13], Fábio A. De Luca[14],
Marisol D. M. Kotsugai[14], Rafael A. M. Domiciano[8], Mayara Fraga Santos[1],
Olga Ferreira de Souza[1,15], Fernando A. Bozza[1,2], Ronir Raggio Luiz[1,16†] and
Emiliano Medei[1,7,17*†]

[1] D'Or Institute for Research and Education, Rio de Janeiro, Brazil, [2] Evandro Chagas National Institute of Infectious Disease, Oswaldo Cruz Foundation, Rio de Janeiro, Brazil, [3] Hospital São Luiz Jabaquara, São Paulo, Brazil, [4] Santa Casa de São Paulo, São Paulo, Brazil, [5] Duke Clinical Research Institute, Duke University Medical Center, Durham, NC, United States, [6] Brazilian Clinical Research Institute, São Paulo, Brazil, [7] Institute of Biophysics Carlos Chagas Filho, Federal University of Rio de Janeiro, Rio de Janeiro, Brazil, [8] Hospital São Luiz Anália Franco, São Paulo, Brazil, [9] Hospital São Luiz São Caetano, São Caetano do Sul, Brazil, [10] Instituto de Microbiologia Paulo de Góes, Federal University of Rio de Janeiro, Rio de Janeiro, Brazil, [11] Cardiology Department, Rio de Janeiro State University, Rio de Janeiro, Brazil, [12] Hospital Sino Brasileiro, Osasco, Brazil, [13] Hospital Villa Lobos, São Paulo, Brazil, [14] Hospital São Luiz Morumbi, São Paulo, Brazil, [15] Hospital Copa Star, Rio de Janeiro, Brazil, [16] Institute for Studies in Public Health—IESC, Federal University of Rio de Janeiro, Rio de Janeiro, Brazil, [17] National Center for Structural Biology and Bioimaging, Federal University of Rio de Janeiro, Rio de Janeiro, Brazil

*Correspondence:
Emiliano Medei
emedei70@biof.ufrj.br

† These authors have contributed equally to this work and share last authorship

Background: Cardiovascular comorbidities such as hypertension and inflammatory response dysregulation are associated with worse COVID-19 prognoses. Different cytokines have been proposed to play vital pathophysiological roles in COVID-19 progression, but appropriate prognostic biomarkers remain lacking. We hypothesized that the combination of immunological and clinical variables at admission could predict the clinical progression of COVID-19 in hypertensive patients.

Methods: The levels of biomarkers, including C-reactive protein, lymphocytes, monocytes, and a panel of 29 cytokines, were measured in blood samples from 167 hypertensive patients included in the BRACE-CORONA trial. The primary outcome was the highest score during hospitalization on the modified WHO Ordinal Scale for Clinical Improvement. The probability of progression to severe disease was estimated using a logistic regression model that included clinical variables and biomarkers associated significantly with the primary outcome.

Results: During hospitalization, 13 (7.8%) patients showed progression to more severe forms of COVID-19, including three deaths. Obesity, diabetes, oxygen saturation, lung involvement on computed tomography examination, the C-reactive protein level, levels of 15 cytokines, and lymphopenia on admission were associated with progression to severe COVID-19. Elevated levels of interleukin-10 and interleukin-12 (p70) combined with two or three of the abovementioned clinical comorbidities were associated strongly with progression to severe COVID-19. The risk of progression to severe disease reached 97.5% in the presence of the five variables included in our model.

Conclusions: This study demonstrated that interleukin-10 and interleukin-12 (p70) levels, in combination with clinical variables, at hospital admission are key biomarkers associated with an increased risk of disease progression in hypertensive patients with COVID-19.

Keywords: hypertension, cytokine, COVID-19, biomarker, inflammation, prognosis

INTRODUCTION

COVID-19 may evolve to severe viral pneumonia and acute respiratory distress syndrome with a high mortality rate. Importantly, patients with cardiac comorbidities have been found in various studies to be at greater risk of severe disease (1–6). In addition, patients with cardiovascular disease are more prone to myocardial injury development after SARS-CoV-2 infection (7–9).

The pathophysiological mechanisms related to these increased risks in patients with cardiac comorbidities are not completely understood. Concern has been raised about the use of angiotensin-converting enzyme inhibitors (ACEIs) and angiotensin receptor blockers (ARBs) in hypertensive patients, as preclinical studies have suggested that renin-angiotensin-aldosterone system inhibitors increase the expression of angiotensin-converting enzyme 2, the functional SARS-CoV-2 receptor (10–12). A recent randomized trial from our group (the BRACE-CORONA trial), in which 659 hypertensive patients were included, demonstrated that the discontinuation of ACEIs and ARBs for 30 days does not impact the number of days over a 30-day follow-up period that patients hospitalized with mild to moderate COVID-19 remain alive and out of the hospital (13, 14).

In addition to cardiac risk factors, several studies have suggested the occurrence of a dysregulated inflammatory response, characterized by the simultaneous release of pro- and anti-inflammatory mediators, known as a cytokine storm and established as a key factor in the physiopathology and clinical progression of COVID-19 in a subset of patients (15, 16). An exacerbated immune response is well-accepted to potentially strongly impair cardiac function (17–20). Several cytokines have been proposed to be potential biomarkers of COVID-19 severity (21–24); interferon gamma–induced protein 10 (IP-10), interleukin (IL)-6, and IL-10 have been associated consistently with greater severity of this disease (25–28).

The uncertainty and variability of the innate immune response, associated with an unpredictable disease course ranging from mild to fatal, highlights the need to identify prognostic factors related to a greater risk of progression to severe disease, particularly in more susceptible patients with comorbidities such as hypertension. To our knowledge, however, no data have been provided about biomarkers that could allow clinicians to identify, in the first 48 h after hospital admission, hypertensive patients at increased risk of disease progression, thereby helping them to choose the best therapeutic option.

This study was conducted to test the hypothesis that the immunological profiles of hypertensive patients upon admission to hospital with COVID-19 provide additional information about disease severity and progression. The analysis of cellular components, such as lymphocytes and monocytes, and the quantification of cytokine concentrations were performed to identify potential biomarkers.

MATERIALS AND METHODS

Population and Design

Patients included in this study were from the BRACE-CORONA trial (14), an academically led, investigator-initiated phase IV multicenter open-label registry-based randomized trial involving 659 patients on ACEIs/ARBs with confirmed COVID-19 diagnoses at 29 centers in Brazil. The present study was conducted with blood samples from 167 hospitalized hypertensive patients enrolled consecutively in the trial at six centers in the state of São Paulo, Brazil. The samples were collected within 24 h of COVID-19 diagnosis confirmation between 21 May and 27 June 2020. The trial protocol (13) was approved by the Brazilian Ministry of Health National Commission for Research Ethics and by institutional review boards or ethics committees at participating sites. All patients provided informed consent before enrollment.

Patients eligible for the BRACE-CORONA trial were aged ≥18 years and chronic ACEI/ARB users. Patients with clinical indications for ACEI/ARB treatment termination, such as hypotension, acute kidney injury, and/or shock, were excluded. Patients on mechanical ventilation and those with hemodynamic instability, acute renal failure, or shock also were excluded (14). The inclusion and exclusion criteria are provided in full in the **Supplementary Data.**

Abbreviations: ACEI, angiotensin-converting enzyme inhibitor; ARB, angiotensin receptor blocker; AUC, area under the receiver operating characteristic curve; CI, confidence interval; CRP, C-reactive protein; CT, computed tomography; G-CSF, granulocyte colony-stimulating factor; GM-CSF, granulocyte-macrophage colony-stimulating factor; ICU, intensive care unit; IFN, interferon; IL, interleukin; IP-10, interferon gamma–induced protein 10; LOS, length of stay; MCP-1, monocyte chemoattractant protein-1; MIP, macrophage inflammatory protein; OR, odds ratio; TNF, tumor necrosis factor; WHO, World Health Organization.

Outcomes

The primary outcome was defined as the highest score during hospitalization on the modified WHO Ordinal Scale for Clinical Improvement [range, 0 (no evidence of infection) to 8 (death)]. COVID-19 was classified as non-severe (mild to moderate, scores of 3–5), ranging from the lack of need for oxygen therapy to conditions requiring noninvasive ventilation, and severe (scores of 6–8), including disease necessitating the use of mechanical ventilation, inotropic support, and/or renal replacement therapy, and that causing death (**Supplementary Table 1**) (29). Secondary outcomes were the lengths of stay (LOSs) in the hospital and intensive care unit (ICU), acute myocardial infarction, new or worsening heart failure, hypertensive crisis, transient ischemic attack, stroke, myocarditis, pericarditis, arrhythmias requiring treatment, and thromboembolic events.

Biomarker Quantification

Blood samples were collected in tubes containing ethylenediaminetetraacetic acid as an anticoagulant and centrifuged immediately for plasma separation. Plasma samples were then frozen and stored at $-20°C$ until analysis. Levels of epidermal growth factor, eotaxin, granulocyte colony-stimulating factor (G-CSF), granulocyte-macrophage colony-stimulating factor (GM-CSF), interferon (IFN)-α2, IFN-γ, IL-1α, IL-1β, IL-1ra, IL-2–8, IL-10, IL-12 (p40), IL-12 (p70), IL-13, IL-15, IL-17A, IP-10, monocyte chemoattractant protein-1 (MCP-1), macrophage inflammatory protein (MIP)-1α, MIP-1β, tumor necrosis factor (TNF)-α, TNF-β, and vascular endothelial growth factor in undiluted samples were measured using the MILLIPLEX MAP human cytokine/chemokine magnetic bead panel (HCYTMAG-60K-PX29; Merck Millipore, Billerica, MA, USA) according to the manufacturer's instructions. The assay plates were read immediately and analyzed in a MAGPIX® system (Merck Millipore). All samples and standards were measured in duplicate. Lymphocyte and monocyte quantification was performed in an automized Horiba ABX Micros 60 system (Horiba Medical, Montpellier, France) using photometry. C-reactive protein (CRP) was measured by latex-enhanced immunoturbidimetric assay. Cytokines not detected in >50% of the patient samples were excluded from further analyses.

TABLE 1 | Baseline patient characteristics by primary outcome*.

Clinical Conditions	Total	Score 3–5 (n = 154/167)	Score 6–8 (n= 13/167)	Fisher's exact test P-value
	n	n (%)	n (%)	
Sex				
Male	110	99 (90.0)	11 (10.0)	0.22
Female	57	55 (96.5)	2 (3.5)	
Age				
<60 years old	114	105 (92.1)	9 (7.9)	1.00
60 and older	53	49 (92.5)	4 (7.5)	
Signs of pulmonary involvement				
O$_2$ sat > 93% and CT ≤ 50%[†]	131	126 (96.2)	5 (3.8)	0.001
O$_2$ sat ≤ 93% or CT > 50%	36	28 (77.8)	8 (22.2)	
Obesity				
No (BMI < 30 kg/m²) [†]	79	78 (98.7)	1 (1.3)	0.003
Yes (BMI ≥ 30 kg/m²)	88	76 (86.4)	12 (13.6)	
Diabetes				
No	126	123 (97.6)	3 (2.4)	< 0.001
Yes	41	31 (75.6)	10 (24.4)	
Asthma/COPD				
No	164	151 (92.1)	13 (7.9)	1.00
Yes	3	3 (100.0)	0 (0.0)	
Dyslipidemia				
No	138	128 (92.8)	10 (7.2)	0.70
Yes	29	26 (89.7)	3 (10.3)	
Coronary disease				
No	163	151 (92.6)	12 (7.4)	0.28
Yes	4	3 (75.0)	1 (25.0)	

*Highest modified World Health Organization WHO Ordinal Scale for Clinical Improvement.
[†]Extent of lung involvement on CT examination.
BMI, body mass index; O$_2$ sat, oxygen saturation; COPD, chronic obstructive pulmonary disease; CT, computed tomography.

Statistical Analysis

Continuous variables were described as medians, means, and standard deviations; categorical variables were characterized by proportions. For the primary outcome, 95% confidence intervals (CIs) were calculated. Fisher's exact test was used to detect statistical associations between the outcome and categorical clinical variables. For continuous variables, receiver operating characteristic (ROC) curves were used to discriminate between severe and non-severe cases, and those associated statistically with the primary outcome were dichotomized using cutoff points of 90% sensitivity. $P \leq 0.05$ was used to define significance and for automatic forward stepwise selection of clinical variables for inclusion in a binary logistic regression model. The significance levels for entry and removal of variables selected by the automatic regression model were defined at 5 and 10%, respectively. The beta coefficients and odd ratios were calculated for all variables in each step of the model to quantify the association with the outcome. The goodness of fit for the final model was evaluated by the Hosmer–Lemeshow test and by ROC curve. Predicted probabilities for the primary outcome were estimated using variables showing significant associations in the final model. All analysis were performed using SPSS software (version 24.0; IBM Corporation, Armonk, NY, USA).

RESULTS

Of the 167 hypertensive patients, 13.8% were using ACEIs and 86.2% were using ARBs. The mean patient age was 54.1 $\pm$ 12.3 years; 57 (34.1%) patients were female, 88 (52.7%) were obese, 41 (24.6%) had diabetes, and 29 (17.4%) had dyslipidemia. Coronary artery disease and chronic pulmonary disease were present in 2.4% of the cases each, and 2.4% of the patients were smokers. Data on all comorbidities are provided in **Supplementary Figure 1**.

Cough (62.3%), fever (57.5%), myalgia (46.7%), shortness of breath (44.9%), and fatigue (44.9%) were the most common symptoms at presentation (**Supplementary Figure 2**). The mean interval from symptom onset to hospital presentation was 5 $\pm$ 3.1 days, and 20.4% of patients had $\leq$93% baseline oxygen saturation. All patients included in this study had non-severe COVID-19 (WHO scores of 3–5) on admission. On chest computed tomography (CT) examinations, 59.9% of patients showed $\leq$25% lung involvement, 35.3% showed 26–50% involvement, and 4.8% showed >50% lung involvement. Thirty-six (21.6%) cases presented criteria for significant pulmonary involvement (oxygen saturation $\leq$ 93% and/or >50% lung involvement on CT) at admission (**Supplementary Table 2**).

Primary Outcome

Worst WHO clinical improvement scores during hospitalization were 3 (mild disease) in 81 (48.5%; 95% CI, 41.0–56.1%) cases, 4 or 5 (moderate disease) in 73 (43.7%; 95% CI, 36.3–51.3%) cases, and 6–8 (severe disease) in 13 (7.8%; 95% CI, 4.4–12.6) cases (**Supplementary Table 3**). Progression to severe disease was associated with obesity ($p = 0.003$), diabetes ($p < 0.001$), and oxygen saturation ($p = 0.001$) and lung involvement ($p = 0.001$) on admission, but not with age or sex (**Table 1**).

Secondary Outcomes

The mean hospital LOS was 9.1 $\pm$ 6.9 days. In total, 119 patients were admitted to the ICU; the mean ICU LOS was 7.6 $\pm$ 6.8 days (**Supplementary Table 4**). According to the report on the

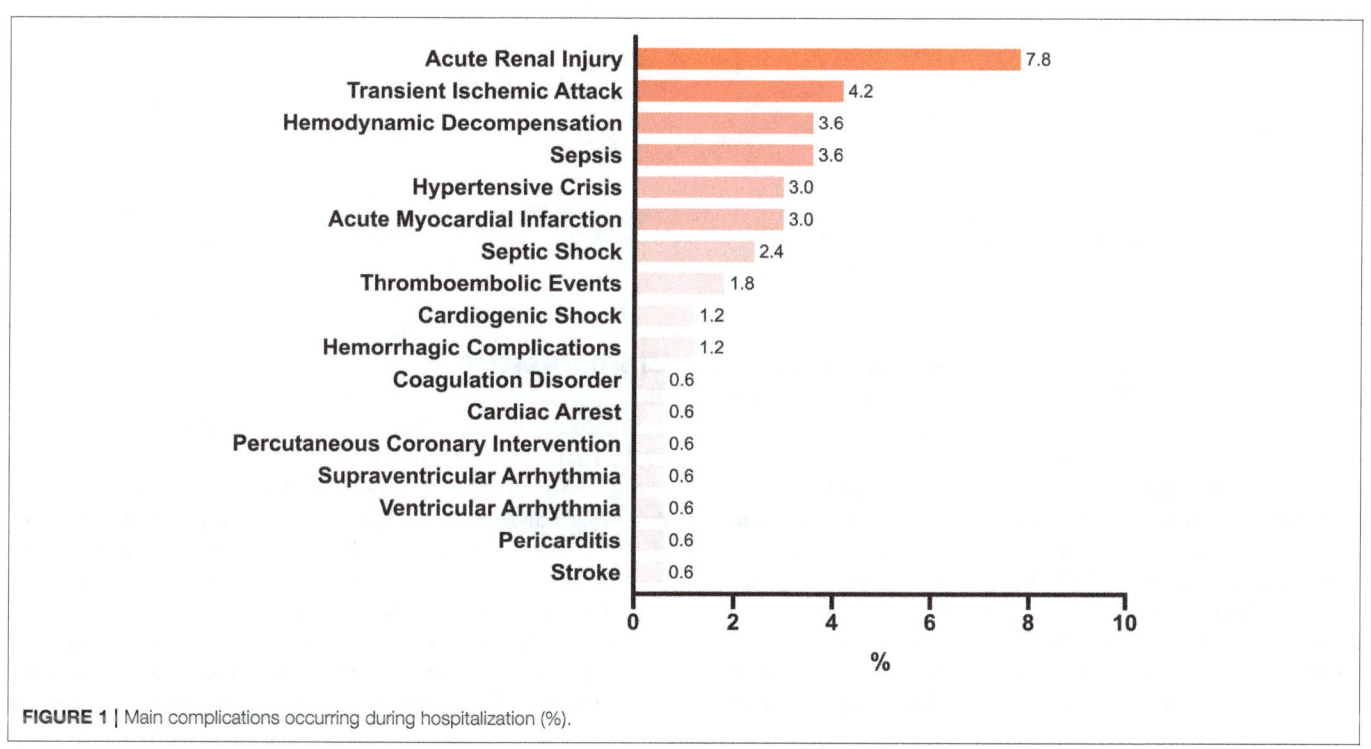

FIGURE 1 | Main complications occurring during hospitalization (%).

TABLE 2 | Biomarker levels according to WHO Ordinal Scale for Clinical Improvement.

	All			Non-severe (score 3–5)			Severe (score 6–8)		
	Median	Mean	SD	Median	Mean	SD	Median	Mean	SD
Lymphocytes*	1.40	1.51	0.74	1.44	1.53	0.65	0.73	1.30	1.45
Monocytes*	0.23	0.36	0.38	0.23	0.35	0.32	0.10	0.53	0.82
CRP†	2.23	4.53	5.28	2.08	4.05	4.95	10.70	10.20	6.01
MIP-1β	21.8	22.5	11.1	22.0	22.9	11.0	13.8	17.6	10.5
VEGF	57.2	80.5	83.9	55.0	81.1	86.8	67.4	72.8	34.6
TNF-β	0.9	27.1	102.1	0.8	28.9	106.1	2.6	6.4	11.1
TNF-α	15.8	16.0	7.4	15.6	15.8	7.4	18.5	18.1	6.6
MIP-1α	5.1	7.3	11.0	5.1	7.3	11.4	7.6	7.4	5.1
MCP-1	466	584	428	435	573	435	792	721	316
IP-10	2,357	2,765	2,482	1,842	2,509	2,155	5,434	5,798	3,904
IL-17A	0.4	2.7	5.9	0.2	2.6	6.0	2.0	4.3	5.2
IL-15	5.1	6.1	4.8	5.1	5.9	4.8	9.2	9.2	3.9
IL-13	1.7	13.1	43.0	1.3	13.8	44.6	1.7	4.7	11.4
IL-12 (p70)	0.8	1.4	2.1	0.6	1.4	2.0	1.6	2.5	2.3
IL-12 (p40)	1.3	4.2	6.6	1.2	4.1	6.6	4.3	6.3	6.2
IL-10	15.5	26.3	29.4	13.4	23.2	25.2	43.8	62.0	49.2
IL-8	8.9	14.2	18.5	8.6	13.8	18.5	13.9	18.8	19.2
IL-7	7.7	10.0	12.7	7.0	10.1	13.2	9.1	9.1	5.0
IL-6	5.5	28.4	76.8	5.1	28.1	78.8	12.6	32.1	49.3
IL-5	1.5	6.4	19.1	1.4	6.6	19.8	2.0	4.3	6.8
IL-4	0.0	239	916	0.0	254	951	10	62	185
IL-3	0.0	0.06	0.11	0.0	0.05	0.11	0.13	0.12	0.08
IL-2	0.48	1.11	2.01	0.29	1.06	2.03	1.15	1.72	1.71
IL-1ra	52	112	196	48	91	138	231	358	464
IL-1β	0.58	1.25	2.08	0.58	1.26	2.15	0.83	1.12	0.93
IL-1α	25.4	59.6	137.8	23.6	59.9	143.1	48.7	55.9	39.0
IFN-γ	5.5	12.6	22.5	5.4	12.5	23.2	11.9	13.4	11.2
IFN-α2	28.2	40.8	54.2	26.4	37.8	54.1	74.1	75.7	43.2
GM-CSF	2.68	4.01	5.00	1.92	3.84	5.09	5.37	5.97	3.37
G-CSF	57.8	65.7	55.4	53.4	61.3	52.7	118.6	118.3	61.2
eotaxin	177	195	96	177	196	99	182	186	51
EGF	208	247	205	204	251	211	214	197	111

CRP, C-reactive protein; EGF, epidermal growth factor; G-CSF, granulocyte colony-stimulating factor; GM-CSF, granulocyte-macrophage colony-stimulating factor; IFN, interferon; IL, interleukin; IP-10, interferon gamma-induced protein 10; MCP-1, monocyte chemoattractant protein 1; MIP, macrophage inflammatory protein; SD, standard deviation; TNF, tumor necrosis factor; VEGF, vascular endothelial growth factor; WHO, World Health Organization.
*10^9 cells/L, †mg/L; all other biomarker units are pg/mL.

BRACE-CORONA trial (13), the mean numbers of days alive and out of hospital did not differ among patients hospitalized with mild to moderate COVID-19 according to ACEI/ARB discontinuation or continuation.

At least one complication occurred during hospitalization in 29 (17.4%) patients. The number of complications per patient ranged from one to nine. The most common complication was acute renal injury [$n = 13$ (7.8%); **Figure 1**]. The criteria used for the identification of these complications have been provided in the BRACE-CORONA trial (13). The most commonly administered treatments were antibiotics (98.2%), anticoagulants (68.3%), and corticosteroids (59.9%; **Supplementary Figure 3**).

Biomarkers

Blood samples were collected a mean of 2.8 days after hospitalization. Levels of IL-10, IP-10, G-CSF, IFN-α2, IL-1ra, IL-15, IL-1α, IL-12 (p70), IL-2, IL-17A, GM-CSF, IL-8, IL-6, MCP-1, and CRP were higher in patients with severe than in those with non-severe disease. In contrast, levels of lymphocytes and MIP-1β were lower in patients with severe than in those with non-severe disease (**Table 2**). IL-3 and IL-4 were not detected in >50% of patients and were excluded from further analyses.

Fifteen cytokines were found to be useful for the prediction of progression to severe COVID-19 [areas under the ROC curve (AUCs), 0.667–0.836]. Increased levels of 14 cytokines

IL-10 and IL-12 (P70) Levels Predict the Risk of Covid-19 Progression in Hypertensive Patients: Insights...

181

TABLE 3 | Distinction of severe (modified WHO score 6–8) and non-severe (modified WHO score 3–5) cases by areas under ROC curves.

Biomarkers	Area under curve	P-value	Cut-off for 90% sensitivity
IL-10	**0.836**	**<0.001**	**26.0**
CRP[†]	**0.825**	**<0.001**	**2.70**
IP-10	**0.812**	**<0.001**	**2400**
G-CSF	**0.788**	**0.001**	**54.0**
IFN-α2	**0.775**	**0.001**	**19.4**
IL-1ra	**0.759**	**0.002**	**29.5**
IL-15	**0.750**	**0.003**	**5.1**
Lymphocytes*[§]	**0.742**	**0.004**	**2.11**
IL-1α	**0.731**	**0.006**	**26.1**
IL-12 (p70)	**0.730**	**0.006**	**0.91**
IL-2	**0.715**	**0.010**	**0.35**
IL-17A	**0.711**	**0.012**	**0.21**
GMCSF	**0.710**	**0.012**	**2.69**
MIP-1β[§]	**0.686**	**0.026**	**32.6**
IL-8	**0.682**	**0.030**	**6.2**
IL-6	**0.678**	**0.033**	**2.6**
MCP-1	**0.667**	**0.045**	**406**
IL-12 (p40)	0.664	0.051	#
TNF-β	0.644	0.085	#
TNF-α	0.607	0.202	#
IFN-γ	0.607	0.200	#
IL-1β	0.601	0.225	#
MIP-1α	0.584	0.313	#
IL-5	0.581	0.330	#
IL-7	0.576	0.366	#
VEGF	0.564	0.441	#
IL-13	0.539	0.637	#
Eotaxin	0.503	0.971	#
EGF	0.473	0.743	#
Monocytes*	0.378	0.143	#

CRP, C-reactive protein; EGF, epidermal growth factor; G-CSF, granulocyte colony-stimulating factor; GM-CSF, granulocyte-macrophage colony-stimulating factor; IFN, interferon; IL, interleukin; IP-10, interferon gamma-induced protein 10; MCP-1, monocyte chemoattractant protein 1; MIP, macrophage inflammatory protein; ROC, receiver operating characteristic; SD, standard deviation; TNF, tumor necrosis factor; VEGF, vascular endothelial growth factor; WHO, World Health Organization.
*10^9 cells/L, [†]mg/L; all other biomarker units are pg/mL; [§]In contrast to other biomarkers, reduced values are predictors of disease progression; Bold values indicate significance at p < 0.05.
[#]Not calculated due to lack of statistical association at established value.

and decreased levels of MIP-1β were associated with COVID-19 severity. AUCs for IL-10, IP-10, G-CSF, IFN- α2, IL-1ra, and IL-15 were ≥0.75 (**Table 3**). Increased CRP levels and reduced lymphocyte counts were also associated with disease severity (AUCs, 0.825 and 0.742, respectively; **Supplementary Figure 4**).

Predictive Model

The initial model for the prediction of the risk of progression of COVID-19 included diabetes, obesity, hypoxemia, lung involvement on CT, the CRP level, the lymphocyte count, and levels of 15 cytokines. Five variables were selected automatically

TABLE 4 | Forward stepwise logistic regression results for COVID-19 severity.

Variables in the equation		β	P-value	Odds ratio
Step 1	IL-10 > 26	3.47	0.001	32.0
Step 2	Diabetes	2.82	< 0,001	16.8
	IL-10 > 26	3.68	0.001	39.6
Step 3	IL-12 (p70) > 0.91	3.30	0.009	27.1
	Diabetes	3.54	0.000	34.3
	IL-10 > 26	3.89	0.002	49.1
Step 4	Obesity	2.86	0.046	17.5
	IL-12 (p70) > 0.91	3.33	0.024	28.0
	Diabetes	3.89	0.001	49.0
	IL-10 > 26	4.35	0.002	77.2
Step 5 (final model)*	Lung involvement[†]	2.16	0.045	8.7
	Obesity	3.81	0.032	45.2
	IL-12p70 > 0.91	3.89	0.026	49.0
	Diabetes	3.58	0.004	35.9
	IL-10 > 26	4.36	0.005	78.3

IL, interleukin.
*Constant = −14.15 and Hosmer–Lemeshow test p = 1.000.
[†]Significant lung involvement on admission (oxygen saturation ≤ 93% or >50% lung involvement on computed tomography examination).
Biomarker values are presented in pg/mL.

in a forward stepwise manner: the IL-10 level (>26.0 pg/mL), diabetes, the IL-12 (p70) level (>0.91 pg/mL), obesity, and significant lung involvement on admission (oxygen saturation ≤ 93% or >50% lung involvement on CT). The IL-10 level was associated strongly with disease severity [odds ratio (OR) = 32]. The ORs for the other four variables also showed associations with progression to severe disease (**Table 4**), and the predictive value of the model increased strongly with the addition of these variables (OR = 78.3). The ROC curve for the predictive model showed a very high discriminatory power between the two groups with an AUC of 0.981 (**Supplementary Figure 5**).

In the presence of two or three clinical comorbidities, the predictive capability of these biomarkers increased markedly (**Figure 2**). In patients with diabetes and obesity, for example, the likelihood of disease progression increased from 0.1% with low IL-10 and IL-12 (p70) levels to >80% with levels of these cytokines exceeding the 90% sensitivity thresholds. Similarly, the risk of progression to severe disease in the presence of three clinical comorbidities was 1.0% with IL-10 and IL-12 (p70) levels below the thresholds and 97.5% with levels exceeding the thresholds (**Table 5**).

DISCUSSION

In this study, we analyzed immune response patterns, including levels of 29 cytokines, CRP, monocytes, and lymphocytes, in a large sample (n = 167) of hospitalized hypertensive patients from the BRACE-CORONA trial (13). In univariate analysis, progression to severe COVID-19 was associated with clinical factors (diabetes, obesity, and lung involvement on admission) and levels of biomarkers, including 15 cytokines, CRP, and lymphocytes. We propose a logistic regression model that includes clinical variables (diabetes, obesity, and significant lung involvement) and critical biomarkers [IL-10 and IL-12 (p70)]. This combined use of clinical risk factors and biomarkers for the prediction of COVID-19 severity at admission is novel.

Clinical comorbidities, particularly diabetes, hypertension, and other cardiovascular diseases, have been associated with COVID-19 severity, as they are more prevalent in non-survivors and patients requiring ICU care (1, 30–32). However, the mechanisms involved in the increased risk of COVID-19 in these patients are not understood completely. Infections are

more prevalent and have more complicated courses in patients with diabetes, possibly due to disturbances in humoral and cellular immunity and exaggerated pro-inflammatory cytokine responses (33, 34). In addition, obesity has been associated with ICU admission and mortality in patients with COVID-19, which may be related to the presence of angiotensin-converting enzyme 2 receptors in adipose tissue, elevated pro-inflammatory cytokine levels, increased susceptibility to infection by various pathogens (35), and pro-coagulant profiles (36). Moreover, the extent of CT lung involvement has been correlated with COVID-19 severity, and severity scores for chest CT findings have been proposed to enable the differentiation of clinical forms and prediction of clinical outcomes (37, 38). The lack of association between age and the outcome in the present study may be related to the relative young mean age of our sample, due to the exclusion of patients with severe disease in the first 24 h after admission.

In this study, admission levels of 17 biomarkers (increased levels of CRP and 14 cytokines and reduced levels of MIP-1β and lymphocytes) were associated significantly with progression to severe disease. Our biomarker findings are similar to previously reported associations of the levels of several cytokines (e.g., IL-1ra, IL-2, IL-6, IL-8, IL-10, and IP-10) with COVID-19 severity and mortality (25, 27, 39–41). The association of the IL-10 level with COVID-19 progression to severity has been reported in a considerable number of publications (40–42). IL-10 is an immunoregulatory cytokine with the main functions of limiting inflammatory responses and regulating immune cell differentiation and proliferation (43). Information about the role of IL-12 (p70) in COVID-19 is more limited. Consistent with our findings, higher levels of IL-12 (p70) have been associated with severe COVID-19 (44, 45). IL-12 is a heterodimeric cytokine composed of p35 and p40 subunits that enhances connections between the innate and adaptive immune responses; its expression is induced via a pathogen-associated molecular response when a virus enters a cell (46).

Although the ability of clinical and laboratory variables to independently predict COVID-19 severity has been assessed

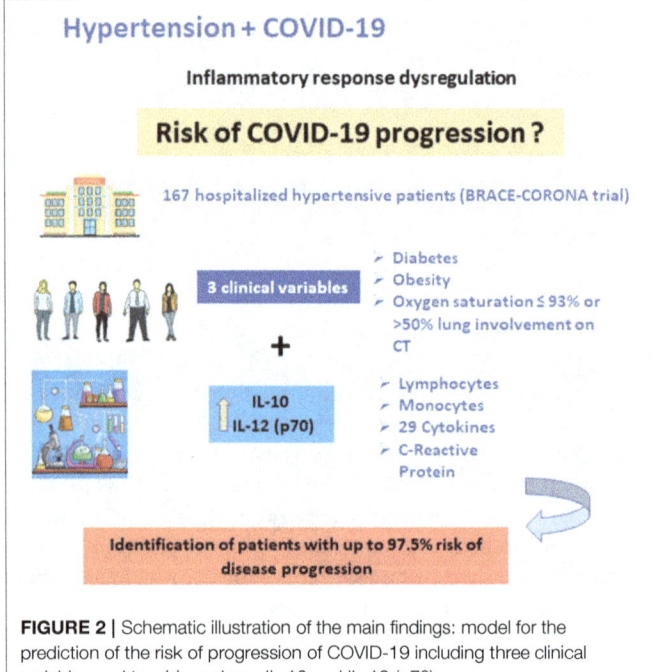

FIGURE 2 | Schematic illustration of the main findings: model for the prediction of the risk of progression of COVID-19 including three clinical variables and two biomarkers: IL-10 and IL-12 (p70).

TABLE 5 | Probability of COVID-19 progression according to the final logistic model.

	IL-10 ≤ 26 and IL12p70 ≤ 0.91	IL10 ≤ 26 and IL12p70 > 0.91	IL10 > 26 and IL12p70 ≤ 0.91	IL10 > 26 and IL12p70 > 0.91
No clinical risk factors[†]	<0.1%	<0.1%	<0.1%	0.3%
Only diabetes	<0.1%	0.1%	0.2%	8.9%
Only obesity	<0.1%	0.2%	0.3%	10.9%
Only significant lung involvement[‡]	<0.1%	<0.1%	<0.1%	2.3%
Diabetes + obesity	0.1%	5.3%	8.3%	81.5%
Diabetes + significant lung involvement	< 0.1%	1.1%	1.7%	45.9%
Obesity + significant lung involvement	< 0.1%	1.3%	2.1%	51.6%
Diabetes + obesity + significant lung involvement	1.0%	32.8%	43.9%	97.5%

IL, interleukin.
Biomarker values are presented in pg/mL.
[†]Clinical risk factors in the model are diabetes, obesity, and significant lung involvement on admission.
[‡]Oxygen saturation ≤ 93% or >50% lung involvement on computed tomography examination.

extensively and predictive models have been proposed, no definitive prognostic biomarker or effective predictive model for the identification, at the time of hospital admission, of patients who will require ICU care, mechanical ventilation, or inotropic support has emerged (47, 48). According to the model we propose, the probability of progression to severe disease in hypertensive patients with obesity and diabetes is 0.1% in the absence of increased IL-10 and IL-12 (p70) levels, but 81.5% with levels of these two cytokines exceeding the 90% sensitivity thresholds. Similarly, in the presence of the three clinical comorbidities (obesity, diabetes, and oxygen saturation ≤93% or >50% lung involvement on CT), the probability of progression is 1% with lower IL-10 and IL-12 (p70) levels, but 97.5% with elevated levels of these biomarkers. A practical approach to model application for the estimation of the risk of progression to severe COVID-19 would be to measure IL-10 and IL-12 (p70) levels on admission in hypertensive patients with two or three of the relevant clinical comorbidities.

Limitations

This study has some limitations. Blood samples were collected a mean of 2.8 days after hospitalization (usually within 24 h after confirmation of SARS-CoV-2 infection); with a median 6-day interval between symptom onset and hospital admission, and our population included only hypertensive patients who were taking ACEi or ARBs, which might limit the generalizability of our results. Nevertheless, we believe that the widespread use of these drugs in the hypertensive population associated with the multicentric nature of the study might help to ensure a good external validity. Besides, we were not able to validate our model with a different patient sample. Additional studies are needed to validate the results obtained here in more heterogeneous populations of hypertensive patients and also to evaluate the applicability of the proposed model in non-hypertensive COVID-19 populations.

CONCLUSION

The measurement of IL-10 and IL-12 (p70) levels on admission may be useful for the identification of hypertensive patients at greater risk of COVID-19 progression, particularly in the presence of classical clinical comorbidities (obesity, diabetes, and extensive lung involvement). We propose a new biomarker-based approach to improve the prediction of COVID-19 progression in hypertensive patients, which may help physicians identify patients at high risk who would benefit from more intensive surveillance and treatment.

AUTHOR CONTRIBUTIONS

RM-B, EM, AS, FB, and RRL: study design. OS, AM, RDL, AF, GA, DA, and MS: patient recruitment, data, and sample collection organization. RM-B and EM: application for the funding and writing-original draft preparation. AM, AF, GA, TP, TF, VL, KG, NO, FD, MK, and RD: patient recruitment and sample collection. NV, LM, MC, and PP-C: biomarker processing and analyses. RDL, RM-B, AM, and RRL: data curation. RRL: statistical analyses. AS, FB, and RDL writing-review and editing. All authors contributed to the article and approved the submitted version.

ACKNOWLEDGMENTS

We thank all staff and research assistants from: D'Or Institute of Research and Education (IDOR), Brazilian Clinical Research Institute (BCRI) and Rede D'Or Hospitals which took part in this study. In addition, the authors thank all patients for accepting participating in this project.

REFERENCES

1. Clerkin KJ, Fried JA, Raikhelkar J, Sayer G, Griffin JM, Masoumi A, et al. COVID-19 and cardiovascular disease. *Circulation.* (2020) 141:1648–55. doi: 10.1161/CIRCULATIONAHA.120.046941

2. Mehra MR, Desai SS, Kuy S, Henry TD, Patel AN. Cardiovascular disease, drug therapy, and mortality in Covid-19. *N Engl J Med.* (2020) 382:e102. doi: 10.1056/NEJMoa2007621

3. Wang D, Hu B, Hu C, Zhu F, Liu X, Zhang J, et al. Clinical characteristics of 138 hospitalized patients with 2019 novel coronavirus-infected pneumonia in Wuhan, China. *JAMA.* (2020) 323:1061–69. doi: 10.1001/jama.2020.1585

4. Zheng YY, Ma YT, Zhang JY, Xie X. COVID-19 and the cardiovascular system. *Nat Rev Cardiol.* (2020) 17:259–60. doi: 10.1038/s41569-020-0360-5

5. Zhou F, Yu T, Du R, Fan G, Liu Y, Liu Z, et al. Clinical course and risk factors for mortality of adult inpatients with COVID-19 in Wuhan, China: a retrospective cohort study. *Lancet.* (2020) 395:1054–62. doi: 10.1016/S0140-6736(20)30566-3

6. Wu C, Chen X, Cai Y, Xia J, Zhou X, Xu S, et al. Risk factors associated with acute respiratory distress syndrome and death in patients with coronavirus disease 2019 pneumonia in Wuhan, China. *JAMA Intern Med.* (2020) 180:934–43. doi: 10.1001/jamainternmed.2020.0994

7. Guo T, Fan Y, Chen M, Wu X, Zhang L, He T, et al. Cardiovascular implications of fatal outcomes of patients with coronavirus disease 2019 (COVID-19). *JAMA Cardiol.* (2020) 5:811–8. doi: 10.1001/jamacardio.2020.1017

8. Liu PP, Blet A, Smyth D, Li H. The science underlying COVID-19: implications for the cardiovascular system. *Circulation.* (2020) 142:68–78. doi: 10.1161/CIRCULATIONAHA.120.047549

9. Nguyen LS, Dolladille C, Drici M-D, Fenioux C, Alexandre J, Mira J-P, et al. Cardiovascular toxicities associated with hydroxychloroquine and azithromycin: an analysis of the World Health Organization Pharmacovigilance Database. *Circulation.* (2020) 142:303–5. doi: 10.1161/CIRCULATIONAHA.120.048238

10. Vaduganathan M, Vardeny O, Michel T, McMurray JJ, Pfeffer MA, Solomon SD. Renin-angiotensin-aldosterone system inhibitors in patients with Covid-19. *N Engl J Med.* (2020) 382:1653–9. doi: 10.1056/NEJMsr2005760

11. Gheblawi M, Wang K, Viveiros A, Nguyen Q, Zhong J-C, Turner AJ, et al. Angiotensin-converting enzyme 2: SARS-CoV-2 receptor and regulator of the renin-angiotensin system: celebrating the 20th anniversary of the discovery of ACE2. *Circ Res.* (2020) 126:1456–74. doi: 10.1161/CIRCRESAHA.120.317015

12. Reynolds HR, Adhikari S, Pulgarin C, Troxel AB, Iturrate E, Johnson SB, et al. Renin-angiotensin-aldosterone system inhibitors and risk of Covid-19. *N Engl J Med.* (2020) 382:2441–8. doi: 10.1056/NEJMoa2008975

13. Lopes RD, Macedo AVS, de Barros ESPGM, Moll-Bernardes RJ, Dos Santos TM, Mazza L, et al. Effect of discontinuing vs continuing angiotensin-converting enzyme inhibitors and angiotensin II receptor blockers on days alive and out of the hospital in patients admitted with COVID-19: a randomized clinical trial. *JAMA*. (2021) 325:254–64. doi: 10.1001/jama.2020.25864

14. Lopes RD, Macedo AVS, de Barros ESPGM, Moll-Bernardes RJ, Feldman A, D'Andrea Saba Arruda G, et al. Continuing versus suspending angiotensin-converting enzyme inhibitors and angiotensin receptor blockers: Impact on adverse outcomes in hospitalized patients with severe acute respiratory syndrome coronavirus 2 (SARS-CoV-2)–The BRACE CORONA Trial. *Am Heart J*. (2020) 226:49–59. doi: 10.1016/j.ahj.2020.05.002

15. Mehta P, McAuley DF, Brown M, Sanchez E, Tattersall RS, Manson JJ. COVID-19: consider cytokine storm syndromes and immunosuppression. *Lancet*. (2020) 395:1033–4. doi: 10.1016/S0140-6736(20)30628-0

16. Lowenstein CJ, Solomon SD. Severe COVID-19 is a microvascular disease. *Circulation*. (2020) 142:1609–11. doi: 10.1161/CIRCULATIONAHA.120.050354

17. Monnerat G, Alarcón ML, Vasconcellos LR, Hochman-Mendez C, Brasil G, Bassani RA, et al. Macrophage-dependent IL-1β production induces cardiac arrhythmias in diabetic mice. *Nat Commun*. (2016) 7:1–15. doi: 10.1038/ncomms13344

18. Alarcon MML, Trentin-Sonoda M, Panico K, Schleier Y, Duque T, Moreno-Loaiza O, et al. Cardiac arrhythmias after renal I/R depend on IL-1β. *J Mol Cell Cardiol*. (2019) 131:101–11. doi: 10.1016/j.yjmcc.2019.04.025

19. Belhadjer Z, Méot M, Bajolle F, Khraiche D, Legendre A, Abakka S, et al. Acute heart failure in multisystem inflammatory syndrome in children in the context of global SARS-CoV-2 pandemic. *Circulation*. (2020) 142:429–36. doi: 10.1161/CIRCULATIONAHA.120.048360

20. Lazzerini PE, Boutjdir M, Capecchi PL. COVID-19, arrhythmic risk, and inflammation: mind the gap! *Circulation*. (2020) 142:7–9. doi: 10.1161/CIRCULATIONAHA.120.047293

21. Wan S, Yi Q, Fan S, Lv J, Zhang X, Guo L, et al. Relationships among lymphocyte subsets, cytokines, and the pulmonary inflammation index in coronavirus (COVID-19) infected patients. *Br J Haematol*. (2020) 189:428–37. doi: 10.1111/bjh.16659

22. Costela-Ruiz VJ, Illescas-Montes R, Puerta-Puerta JM, Ruiz C, Melguizo-Rodriguez L. SARS-CoV-2 infection: the role of cytokines in COVID-19 disease. *Cytokine Growth Factor Rev*. (2020) 54:62–75. doi: 10.1016/j.cytogfr.2020.06.001

23. Conti P, Ronconi G, Caraffa A, Gallenga CE, Ross R, Frydas I, Kritas SK. Induction of pro-inflammatory cytokines (IL-1 and IL-6) and lung inflammation by Coronavirus-19 (COVI-19 or SARS-CoV-2): anti-inflammatory strategies. *J Biol Regul Homeost Agents*. (2020) 34:327–31. doi: 10.23812/CONTI-E

24. Han H, Ma Q, Li C, Liu R, Zhao L, Wang W, et al. Profiling serum cytokines in COVID-19 patients reveals IL-6 and IL-10 are disease severity predictors. *Emerg Microbes Infect*. (2020) 9:1123–30. doi: 10.1080/22221751.2020.1770129

25. Yang Y, Shen C, Li J, Yuan J, Wei J, Huang F, et al. Plasma IP-10 and MCP-3 levels are highly associated with disease severity and predict the progression of COVID-19. *J Allergy Clin Immunol*. (2020) 146:119–27.e114. doi: 10.1016/j.jaci.2020.04.027

26. Chen G, Wu D, Guo W, Cao Y, Huang D, Wang H, et al. Clinical and immunological features of severe and moderate coronavirus disease 2019. *J Clin Invest*. (2020) 130:2620–9. doi: 10.1172/JCI137244

27. Sun HB, Zhang YM, Huang LG, Lai QN, Mo Q, Ye XZ, et al. The changes of the peripheral CD4+ lymphocytes and inflammatory cytokines in Patients with COVID-19. *PLoS One*. (2020) 15:e0239532. doi: 10.1371/journal.pone.0239532

28. Dhar SK, K V, Damodar S, Gujar S, Das M. IL-6 and IL-10 as predictors of disease severity in COVID-19 patients: results from meta-analysis and regression. *Heliyon*. (2021) 7:e06155. doi: 10.1016/j.heliyon.2021.e06155

29. World Health Organization. *WHO R&D Blueprint: COVID-19 Therapeutic Trial Synopsis*. (2020). Available online at: https://www.who.int/publications/i/item/covid-19-therapeutic-trial-synopsis (accessed October 20, 2020).

30. Iaccarino G, Grassi G, Borghi C, Ferri C, Salvetti M, Volpe M. Age and multimorbidity predict death among COVID-19 patients: results of the SARS-RAS study of the Italian Society of Hypertension. *Hypertension*. (2020) 76:366–72. doi: 10.1161/HYPERTENSIONAHA.120.15324

31. Semenzato L, Botton J, Drouin J, Baricault B, Vabre C, Cuenot F, et al. Antihypertensive drugs and COVID-19 risk: a cohort study of 2 million hypertensive patients. *Hypertension*. (2021) 77:833–42. doi: 10.1161/HYPERTENSIONAHA.120.16314

32. Silverio A, Di Maio M, Citro R, Esposito L, Iuliano G, Bellino M, et al. Cardiovascular risk factors and mortality in hospitalized patients with COVID-19: systematic review and meta-analysis of 45 studies and 18,300 patients. *BMC Cardiovasc Disord*. (2021) 21:23. doi: 10.1186/s12872-020-01816-3

33. Geerlings SE, Hoepelman AI. Immune dysfunction in patients with diabetes mellitus (DM). *FEMS Immunol Med Microbiol*. (1999) 26:259–65. doi: 10.1111/j.1574-695X.1999.tb01397.x

34. Pal R, Bhansali A. COVID-19, diabetes mellitus and ACE2: the conundrum. *Diabetes Res Clin Pract*. (2020) 162:108132. doi: 10.1016/j.diabres.2020.108132

35. Dicker D, Bettini S, Farpour-Lambert N, Frühbeck G, Golan R, Goossens G, et al. Obesity and COVID-19: the two sides of the coin. *Obes Facts*. (2020) 13:430–8. doi: 10.1159/000510005

36. Sattar N, McInnes IB, McMurray JJ. Obesity is a risk factor for severe COVID-19 infection: multiple potential mechanisms. *Circulation*. (2020) 142:4–6. doi: 10.1161/CIRCULATIONAHA.120.047659

37. Yang R, Li X, Liu H, Zhen Y, Zhang X, Xiong Q, et al. Chest CT severity score: an imaging tool for assessing severe COVID-19. *Radiology*. (2020) 2:e200047. doi: 10.1148/ryct.2020200047

38. Francone M, Iafrate F, Masci GM, Coco S, Cilia F, Manganaro L, et al. Chest CT score in COVID-19 patients: correlation with disease severity and short-term prognosis. *Eur Radiol*. (2020) 30:6808–17. doi: 10.1007/s00330-020-07033-y

39. Jin M, Shi N, Wang M, Shi C, Lu S, Chang Q, et al. CD45: a critical regulator in immune cells to predict severe and non-severe COVID-19 patients. *Aging (Albany NY)*. (2020) 12:19867. doi: 10.18632/aging.103941

40. Varchetta S, Mele D, Oliviero B, Mantovani S, Ludovisi S, Cerino A, et al. Unique immunological profile in patients with COVID-19. *Cell Mol Immunol*. (2020) 18:1–11. doi: 10.21203/rs.3.rs-23953/v1

41. Li Q, Xu W, Li W, Huang C, Chen L. Dynamics of cytokines and lymphocyte subsets associated with the poor prognosis of severe COVID-19. *Eur Rev Med Pharmacol Sci*. (2020) 24:12536–44. doi: 10.26355/eurrev_202012_24051

42. Liu QQ, Cheng A, Wang Y, Li H, Hu L, Zhao X, et al. Cytokines and their relationship with the severity and prognosis of coronavirus disease 2019 (COVID-19): a retrospective cohort study. *BMJ Open*. (2020) 10:e041471. doi: 10.1136/bmjopen-2020-041471

43. Asadullah K, Sterry W, Volk H. Interleukin-10 therapy-review of a new approach. *Pharmacol Rev*. (2003) 55:241–69. doi: 10.1124/pr.55.2.4

44. Young BE, Ong SWX, Ng LFP, Anderson DE, Chia WN, Chia PY, et al. Viral dynamics and immune correlates of COVID-19 disease severity. *Clin Infect Dis*. (2020). doi: 10.1093/cid/ciaa1280. [Epub ahead of print].

45. Liu Y, Chen D, Hou J, Li H, Cao D, Guo M, et al. An inter-correlated cytokine network identified at the center of cytokine storm predicted COVID-19 prognosis. *Cytokine*. (2021) 138:155365. doi: 10.1016/j.cyto.2020.155365

46. Guo Y, Cao W, Zhu Y. Immunoregulatory functions of the IL-12 family of cytokines in antiviral systems. *Viruses*. (2019) 11:772. doi: 10.3390/v11090772

47. Wynants L, Van Calster B, Collins GS, Riley RD, Heinze G, Schuit E, et al. Prediction models for diagnosis and prognosis of covid-19: systematic review and critical appraisal. *BMJ*. (2020) 369:m1328. doi: 10.1136/bmj.m1328

48. Collins GS, van Smeden M Riley RD. COVID-19 prediction models should adhere to methodological and reporting standards. *Eur Respir J*. (2020) 56:2002643. doi: 10.1183/13993003.02643-2020

Higher Incidence of Stroke in Severe COVID-19 is not Associated with a Higher Burden of Arrhythmias: Comparison with Other Types of Severe Pneumonia

Peter Jirak [1*†], Zornitsa Shomanova [2†], Robert Larbig [3,4], Daniel Dankl [5], Nino Frank [5], Clemens Seelmaier [1], Dominyka Butkiene [4], Michael Lichtenauer [1], Moritz Mirna [1], Bernhard Strohmer [1], Jan Sackarnd [2], Uta C. Hoppe [1], Jürgen Sindermann [2], Holger Reinecke [2], Gerrit Frommeyer [3], Lukas J. Motloch [1‡] and Rudin Pistulli [2‡]

[1] Clinic II for Internal Medicine, University Hospital Salzburg, Paracelsus Medical University, Salzburg, Austria, [2] Department of Cardiology I—Coronary and Peripheral Vascular Disease, Heart Failure, University Hospital Münster, Münster, Germany, [3] Department of Cardiology II—Electrophysiology, University Hospital Münster, Münster, Germany, [4] Division of Cardiology, Hospital Maria Hilf Mönchengladbach, Mönchengladbach, Germany, [5] Department of Anesthesiology, Perioperative Care, and Intensive Care Medicine, University Hospital Salzburg, Paracelsurs Medical University, Salzburg, Austria

*Correspondence:
Peter Jirak
p.jirak@salk.at

[†] These authors have contributed equally to this work and share first authorship

[‡] These authors have contributed equally to this work and share senior authorship

Aims: Thromboembolic events, including stroke, are typical complications of COVID-19. Whether arrhythmias, frequently described in severe COVID-19, are disease-specific and thus promote strokes is unclear. We investigated the occurrence of arrhythmias and stroke during rhythm monitoring in critically ill patients with COVID-19, compared with severe pneumonia of other origins.

Methods and Results: This retrospective study included 120 critically ill patients requiring mechanical ventilation in three European tertiary hospitals, including $n = 60$ COVID-19, matched according to risk factors for the occurrence of arrhythmias in $n = 60$ patients from a retrospective consecutive cohort of severe pneumonia of other origins. Arrhythmias, mainly atrial fibrillation (AF), were frequent in COVID-19. However, when compared with non-COVID-19, no difference was observed with respect to ventricular tachycardias (VT) and relevant bradyarrhythmias (VT 10.0 vs. 8.4 %, $p = ns$ and asystole 5.0 vs. 3.3%, $p = ns$) with consequent similar rates of cardiopulmonary resuscitation (6.7 vs. 10.0%, $p = ns$). AF was even more common in non-COVID-19 (AF 18.3 vs. 43.3%, $p = 0.003$; newly onset AF 10.0 vs. 30.0%, $p = 0.006$), which resulted in a higher need for electrical cardioversion (6.7 vs. 20.0%, $p = 0.029$). Despite these findings and comparable rates of therapeutic anticoagulation (TAC), the incidence of stroke was higher in COVID-19 (6.7.% vs. 0.0, $p = 0.042$). These events also happened in the absence of AF (50%) and with TAC (50%).

Conclusions: Arrhythmias were common in severe COVID-19, consisting mainly of AF, yet less frequent than in matched pneumonia of other origins. A contrasting higher incidence of stroke independent of arrhythmias also observed with TAC, seems to be an arrhythmia-unrelated disease-specific feature of COVID-19.

Keywords: COVID-19, arrhythmias, atrial fibrillation, stroke, pneumonia, ventricular tachycardia, anticoagulation

INTRODUCTION

The novel coronavirus disease COVID-19 caused by severe acute respiratory syndrome coronavirus 2 (SARS-CoV-2) has caused a worldwide healthcare crisis with an overstrain of hospital resources (1, 2). Given its diverse cardiovascular involvement, further investigation of potential disease-specific processes is crucial to optimize its medical management (3–5). Although previous studies observed a high rate of cardiac injury in COVID-19 infections (3), two recent publications reported rates of cardiac injury to be similar to non-COVID-19 pneumonia, pointing against a COVID-19 specific cardiac involvement (6, 7). Similarly, the impact of COVID-19 on cardiac arrhythmias and thromboembolic events is also yet to be covered to the full extent. The arrhythmic burden is high in COVID-19 patients. The first investigation from Wang et al. reported cardiac arrhythmias in 17% of all their included patients and in 44.4% of those admitted to ICU (8). However, the missing definition of arrhythmias in that study should be taken into account when interpreting results (8). A recent work of Bertini et al. analyzed ECGs in critically ill COVID-19 patients and reported a high rate of ECG abnormalities (93%) with atrial fibrillation/flutter being the most common arrhythmia (22%) (9). In this context, the high incidence of stroke in COVID-19, as the most frequent thromboembolic complication of atrial fibrillation, attracts special attention (10–12). Similar investigations on thromboembolic events including stroke, deep vein thrombosis (DVT), and pulmonary embolism reported overall rates of up to 43% in critically ill COVID-19 patients (13–15). Of note, the majority of patients in those studies received at least a prophylactic anticoagulation (13–15). These findings suggest a potential correlation between cardiac arrhythmias and high rates of stroke and other thromboembolic events. Moreover, it remains unclear, whether the high arrhythmic burden in COVID 19 is the effect of unspecific proarrhythmogenic states promoted by cardiac injury as well as the systemic inflammatory burden, or whether a COVID-19 specific mechanism exists, which promotes cardiac arrhythmias. Given its considerable clinical impact, further investigation on COVID-19 associated arrhythmias and their potential link to thromboembolic events is urgently needed. Accordingly, in our multicentre study, we aimed for a comparative analysis of cardiac arrhythmias as well as stroke and other thromboembolic events in critically ill patients requiring ventilator therapy due to SARS-CoV-2 induced pneumonia matched to a historical cohort requiring respiratory support due to severe pneumonia of non-COVID-19 origin (non-COVID-19).

METHODS

The present retrospective study was conducted in three European tertiary centers in Germany and Austria (University Hospital Münster, Maria Hilf Hospital Mönchengladbach and the University Hospital Salzburg). The study was conducted in accordance with the Declaration of Helsinki and the standards of good clinical practice. All three local ethic committees approved the present study (University Hospital Münster Nr. 2020-306-f-S, Maria Hilf Hospital Mönchengladbach: Nr. 143/2020, and University Hospital Salzburg: Nr. 1071/2020).

Study Cohorts

A total of 120 patients were involved in this study (60 COVID-19 vs. 60 non-COVID-19). The COVID-19 cohort consisted of 60 consecutive patients with available ICU rhythm monitoring who suffered severe pneumonia. Severe pneumonia was defined as pneumonia-associated respiratory failure requiring mechanical ventilation [noninvasive ventilation (NIV) or invasive ventilation]; the term NIV in this study refers to mechanical ventilation involving end-expiratory and inspiratory positive air pressure support *via* a tightly fitted face mask or helmet, as opposed to invasive ventilation necessitating endotracheal intubation. All patients included in the study had some form of mechanical ventilation (patients who merely needed oxygen insufflations were not included) between March and May 2020. Patients were treated according to recent recommendations (1). All patients received anticoagulation during their ICU stay. A detailed description with regards to anticoagulation is given in the **Supplementary Methods** section. Patients with a history of hyperthyroid disease, of inherited arrhythmic disorders, and a history of persistent or permanent atrial fibrillation (AF) were excluded from the analyses. The diagnosis of COVID-19 was established in the presence of a positive result in real-time reverse transcription–polymerase chain reaction assay (performed according to the manufacturer) for COVID-19 and a chest radiography and/or computer tomography of the thorax indicative for COVID-19 related pneumonia according to current recommendations (2).

The control group was recruited from a consecutive collective of 1,222 patients suffering severe pneumonia of non-COVID-19 origin. All patients in the control group were treated between January 2014 and Mach 2020 at the ICU according to current intensive care guidelines (3). Patients from the control group requiring mechanical ventilation (non-invasive/invasive ventilation) were primarily matched to the COVID-19 population according to the medical history of paroxysmal AF. To account for potential confounders as proarrhythmic comorbidities, patients were further matched for known risk factors associated with cardiac arrhythmias. Matching was conducted stepwise and manually according to age, gender, heart failure, coronary artery disease, atrial flutter, diabetes mellitus, arterial hypertension, valvular heart disease, and previous stroke/TIA. If more than one candidate in the retrospective non-COVID-19 cohort fully fulfilled the matching criteria, the patient with the closest admission time point as compared with the time point of the beginning of the recruitment of the COVID-19 cohort (March 2020) was chosen for matching. To further validate the matching process, covariate imbalance was assessed. Standardized differences and omnibus test revealed no statistically significant covariate imbalance between the two investigated groups (**Supplementary Table 6**).

Higher Incidence of Stroke in Severe COVID-19 is not Associated with a Higher Burden...

187

TABLE 1 | Baseline characteristics.

	COVID-19 (n = 60)		Non-COVID-19 (n=60)		p
	n	Mean ± SD, median (Q3–Q1) or %	n	Mean ± SD, median (Q3–Q1) or %	
Gender (female)	14/60	23.3%	14/60	23.3%	>0.999
Age (years)	60	66.5 ± 12.6	60	65.9 ± 11.61	0.813
BMI (kg/m^2)	51	27.7 (5.1)	50	25.6 (6.7)	0.493
Medical history					
Arterial hypertension	31/60	51.7%	33/60	55%	0.714
Coronary artery disease	9/60	15.0%	9/60	15.0%	>0.999
Peripheral vascular disease	4/60	6.7%	2/60	3.3%	0.679
Diabetes mellitus	13/60	21.7%	14/60	23.3%	0.827
Current smoking	10/60	16.7%	16/60	26.7%	0.184
Heart failure	7/60	11.7%	7/60	11.7%	>0.999
Valvular heart disease	3/60	5.0%	5/60	8.3%	0.717
Paroxysmal AF	9/60	15.0%	9/60	15.0%	>0.999
Atrial flutter	1/60	1.7%	0/60	0%	>0.999
Pulmonary arterial hypertension	2/60	3.3%	1/60	1.7%	>0.999
Obstructive lung disease	8/60	13.3%	12/60	20.0%	0.327
Structural lung disease	0/60	0%	1/60	1.7%	>0.999
Stroke/TIA	6/60	10.0%	3/60	5.0%	0.491
Medication					
Beta-blockers	18/60	30.0%	22/60	36.7%	0.439
NOAK/AOK	7/60	11.7%	8/60	13.3%	0.783
Amiodarone	0/60	0%	2/60	3.3%	0.496

AF, atrial fibrillation; BMI, body mass index; SD, standard deviation.
*p<0.05.

Data Collection and Analyses

In all eligible patients, data were retrospectively collected from electronic medical records. Data obtained comprises demographics, medical history, laboratory examinations, comorbidities, complications, specific treatment measures, and outcomes, and also 12-lead ECGs at ICU admission and complete rhythm monitoring during ICU stay (continuous standard three-lead ECG during complete ICU stay). Laboratory samples were collected within the first hours after ICU admittance, and follow-up was conducted on a daily routine according to the need for clinical assessment. With regards to rhythm monitoring, baseline rhythm was evaluated and documented every hour during the entire ICU stay. Analyses of ECGs, classification of arrhythmias, and quantification of the duration of arrhythmias in the rhythm monitoring were analyzed and documented by a trained team of ICU nurses and physicians in one of the recruiting centers. Cardiac arrhythmias during ICU rhythm monitoring were classified according to current guidelines (4–6). AF was defined as the presence of an irregular rhythm with fibrillatory waves and no defined P-waves for at least 30 s during rhythm monitoring. Other SVTs were defined as regular rhythm when atrial and/or ventricular rates exceeded 100 bpm for at least 30 s during monitoring, consistent with atrial flutter, focal atrial tachycardia, atrioventricular nodal tachycardia, or atrioventricular tachycardia. Non-sustained ventricular tachycardia was defined as three or more consecutive ventricular beats occurring at a rate of ≥100 bpm and sustained

ventricular tachycardia lasting ≥30 s. High grade atrioventricular block was defined as the presence of second- or third-degree heart block. Bradyarrhythmia absoluta was defined as the presence of an irregular rhythm with fibrillatory waves and no defined P-waves as well as heart rate <40/min for at least 30 s. Asystole was defined as the absence of electrical activity during rhythm monitoring lasting >6 s. New-onset AF was defined as AF during ICU monitoring in the absence of AF history, as indicated by the medical record of the patient.

Diagnosis of thromboembolic/thrombotic events including pulmonary embolism, thromboembolic stroke, and transient ischemic attack was established in agreement with current guidelines (7, 8). The diagnosis of thromboembolic stroke and transient ischemic attack of thromboembolic origin was verified by an experienced neurologist. Acquired data were independently reviewed and entered into the computer database by two blinded analysts. During ICU stay all recruited patients received standard prophylactic anticoagulation or therapeutic anticoagulation (TAC), if indicated, using low molecular weight heparin.

Statistical Analysis

Statistical analysis was conducted using R (version 4.0.2., R Core Team (2013), R Foundation for Statistical Computing, Vienna, Austria; http://www.R-project.org/) using the packages "MatchIt," "optmatch" and "RItools," "stddiff," and also SPSS (Version 23.0, IBM, Armonk, New York, USA), and was carried out blindly by our statistical analytic team. Descriptive

TABLE 2 | Continuous rhythm monitoring during ICU stay.

	COVID-19 ($n = 60$)		Non-COVID-19 ($n = 60$)		p
	n	Median (Q3–Q1) or %	n	Median (Q3–Q1) or %	
Supraventricular tachyarrhythmias					
AF during ICU stay	11/60	18.3%	26/60	43.3%	0.003*
New-onset of AF	6/60	10.0%	18/60	30.0%	0.006*
Duration of total AF burden (minutes)	60	780.0 (1,680.0)	60	960.0 (4,035.0)	0.855
Other SVTs$	5/60	8.3%	8/60	13.3%	0.378
Ventricular tachyarrhythmias					
nsVT	4/60	6.7%	4/60	6.7%	>0.999
Sustained VT or VF	2/60	3.3%	1/60	1.7%	>0.999
Bradyarrhythmias					
High grade AVB§	0/60	0%	0/60	0%	>0.999
Asystole	3/60	5.0%	2/60	3.3%	>0.999
Bradyarrhytmia absoluta	0/60	0%	1/60	1.7%	>0.999
eCV	4/60	6.7%	12/60	20.0%	0.029*
Reason for eCV					
AF	3/60	5.0%	10/60	16.6%	0.040*
Other SVTs$	0/60	0%	1/60	1.7%	>0.999
Sustained VT or VF	1/60	1.7%	1/60	1.7%	>0.999

*AF, atrial fibrillation; AVB, atrioventricular block; ICU, intensive care unit; eCV, electrical cardioversion; nsVT, non-sustained ventricular tachycardia; SVT, supraventricular tachycardia; VF, ventricular fibrillation; VT, ventricular tachycardia; $definition other SVT see method section; § For definition of high grade AVB see Method section;*p < 0.05.*

statistics were obtained for all study variables. All categorical variables were compared by using the Fisher exact test. Ordinal data are presented as median (interquartile range [IQR]). Median values were compared using the Mann–Whitney-U test. Normal distribution of continuous variables was tested using the Kolmogorov–Smirnov test. According to results, continuous variables were compared using the independent student t-test or the Mann-Whitney U test, as appropriate. Continuous data are expressed as mean and standard deviation (SD) or median (interquartile range [IQR]) values. A $p < 0.05$ was regarded as statistically significant. Covariate imbalance was assessed by calculating standardized differences for the covariates age, gender, coronary artery disease, valvular heart disease, arterial hypertension, diabetes mellitus, atrial fibrillation, atrial flutter, stroke, and heart failure, and also by calculating an omnibus test and significant differences between the two investigated groups using Wilcoxon rank-sum test and χ^2 test."

Patient and Public Involvement

Patients or the public were not involved in the design, or conduct, or reporting, or dissemination of our research.

RESULTS

With regards to the assessment of covariate imbalance, standardized differences and omnibus test ($p = 0.556$) revealed no statistically significant differences between the two investigated groups (standardized differences >0.25 were considered significant covariate imbalance) (**Supplementary Table 6**).

The baseline characteristics of both patient cohorts are presented in **Table 1**. According to matching criteria, the same rates of heart failure, coronary artery disease, and paroxysmal AF were present in both groups at inclusion. Similarly, no significant differences were observed with regards to other comorbidities and predisposing risk factors for cardiac arrhythmias including arterial hypertension, diabetes mellitus and relevant valvular heart disease as well as sex and gender. No significant differences with regards to antiarrhythmics were observed (**Table 1**). Origin of pneumonia in the control group is depicted in **Supplementary Table 4**.

The analyses of the continuous rhythm monitoring during the ICU stay are presented in **Table 2** and **Figure 1**. Additionally, a separate analysis of patients displaying a QTc-time over 500 ms in the admission ECG is depicted in **Supplementary Table 5**. Expectedly, COVID-19 presented a high rate of cardiac arrhythmias. Nevertheless, when matched to non-COVID-19, rates of relevant ventricular tachyarrhythmias were similar (**Table 1**; **Figure 1D**). With regards to bradyarrhythmias, there was no significant difference in the incidence of high grade AVBs or asystole (**Table 1**; **Figure 1E**). Although the rates of AF diagnosed by 12-lead ECG at admission were similar in both groups (**Supplementary Table 1**), the incidence of AF during rhythm-monitoring was significantly higher in the non-COVID-19 population despite comparable risk factors for the development of arrhythmias. This was reflected by higher rates of AF during ICU stay, but similar AF duration during the monitoring period in affected patients was observed. The higher rates of AF also corresponded to a significantly

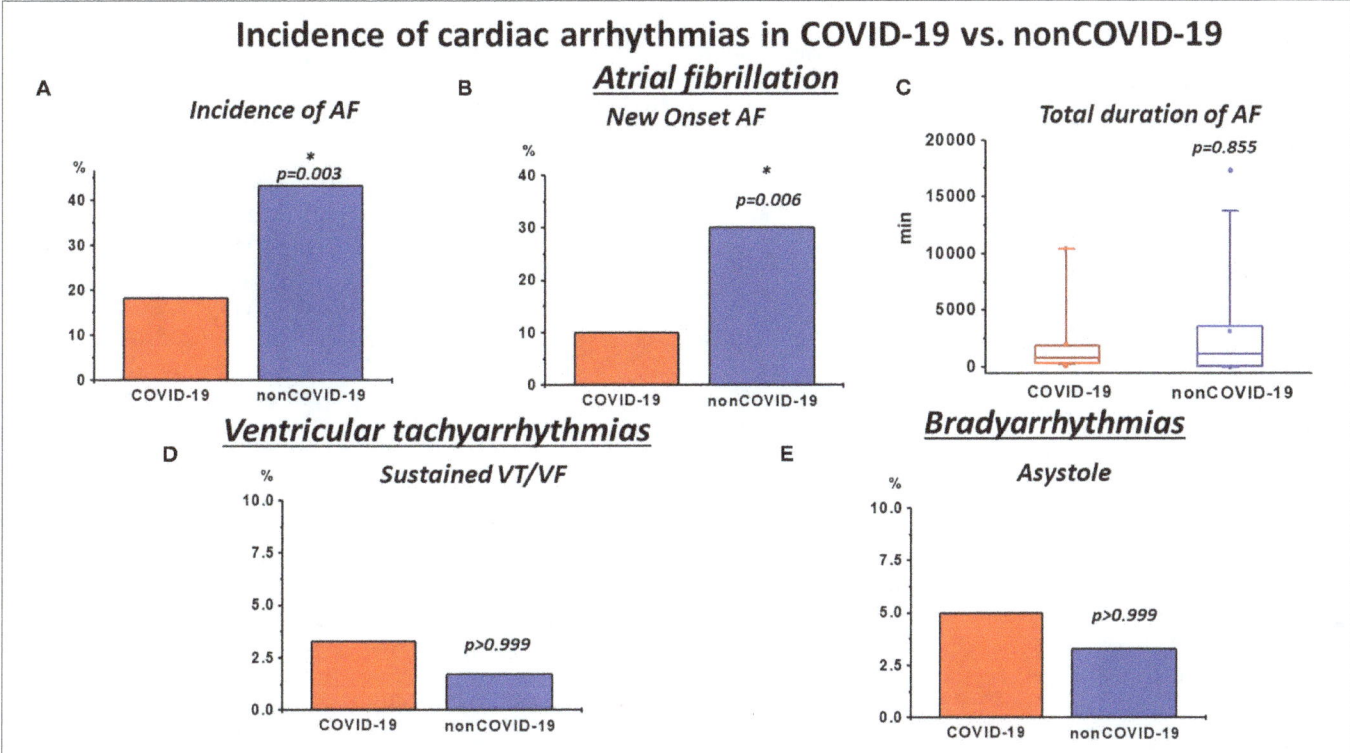

FIGURE 1 | Incidence of relevant cardiac arrhythmias during intensive care (ICU) rhythm monitoring in COVID-19 vs. non-COVID-19: **(A)** incidence of atrial fibrillation (AF) and **(B)** newly diagnosed AF was high in both groups. However, non-COVID-19 patients presented a higher burden of AF and newly diagnosed AF, **(C)** while the total duration of AF was not different in affected patients. **(D)** The incidence of sustained VTs/ventricular fibrillation (VF) was similar in both groups **(E)** and the frequency of asystole was also not significantly different. $*p < 0.050$.

higher necessity for electrical cardioversion in the non-COVID-19 group (**Table 2**). Furthermore, the incidence of newly diagnosed AF was significantly higher in non-COVID-19 indicating a more pronounced arrhythmic substrate in this population.

With regards to inflammatory activity and disease severity, non-COVID-19 revealed higher leucocytes and procalcitonin (PCT) levels. This was further accompanied by increased lactate levels and decreased pH (**Table 4**) in non-COVID-19. Consequently, while mortality was high in both groups, a significantly higher rate in the non-COVID-19 group was observed (**Table 3**), indicating a more pronounced critical patient status.

In contrast to these observations and in line with previous reports (9), we observed a higher rate of pulmonary embolisms in COVID-19 (**Table 3**). This observation was consistent with high stroke rates in COVID-19. Of note, despite a lower burden of AF as well as similarly high rates of anticoagulation and comparable CHA_2DS_2-Vasc scores, a significantly higher incidence of thrombotic strokes/TIA was revealed (**Table 3**; **Figure 2**). Of note, these events were also observed in patients receiving TAC and with continuous sinus rhythm (**Figure 2**; **Supplementary Table 2**), indicating disease-specific events that occur independently of cardiac arrhythmias.

DISCUSSION

The typical finding in severe COVID-19 disease is pneumonia accompanied by acute lung injury (10). In this context, many recent studies covered the topic of COVID-19-related cardiac injury (11, 12). Nevertheless, despite described cases of COVID-19 specific myocarditis, recent publications in critically ill patients, indicated that in this population cardiac injury is rather explained by the high inflammatory burden, similar to cardiac injury in other severe inflammatory processes such as in acute respiratory distress syndrome and severe pneumonia (11, 12). A further point of interest is the burden of arrhythmias in COVID-19 patients. Only a few studies on this topic have been published, pointing toward a high arrhythmic burden in this patient collective (13, 14). Nevertheless, comparable with findings on myocardial injury, arrhythmias and especially AF are a frequent finding in patients with severe pneumonia and sepsis (15). Accordingly, the present study aimed to further evaluate this issue.

To account for underlying medical conditions predisposing to cardiac arrhythmias, the study cohorts were matched for preexisting AF as well as age, gender, coronary artery disease, valvular heart disease, arterial hypertension, diabetes mellitus, atrial fibrillation, atrial flutter, stroke, and heart failure. Reliability of the matching process was further confirmed by analyzing

TABLE 3 | Patients' outcome and relevant therapies during ICU stay.

	COVID-19 (*n* = 60)		Non-COVID-19 (*n* = 60)		*p*
	n	Median (Q3–Q1) or %	*n*	Median (Q3–Q1) or %	
Outcome ICU					
Death	21/60	35.0%	34/60	56.7%	0.017*
Discharged from ICU	39/60	65.0%	26/60	43.3%	0.017*
Duration of ICU stay (days)	60	13.0 (18.0)	60	11.5 (17.0)	0.308
Required ICU therapy					
ECMO	9/60	15.0%	14/60	23.3%	0.246
Hemofiltration	17/60	28.3%	25/60	41.7%	0.126
Catecholamines	45/60	75.0%	53/60	88.3%	0.059
Required catecholamines	60	1.0 (1.0)	60	1.0 (1.0)	0.640
Ventilation therapy					
NIV	9/60	15.0%	7/60	11.7%	0.591
Intubation	51/60	85.0%	53/60	88.3%	0.591
Duration of intubation	60/60	9.0 (20.0)	60/60	5.0 (10.0)	0.711
Relevant bleedings	4/60	6.7%	4/60	6.7%	>0.999
CPR	4/60	6.7%	6/60	10.0%	0.509
Reason for CPR					
Asystole	1/60	1.7%	3/60	5.0%	0.619
VF/VT	1/60	1.7%	1/60	1.7%	>0.999
Pulseless electrical activity	2/60	3.3%	2/60	3.3%	>0.999
Therapeutic anticoagulation	24/60	40.0%	30/60	50.0%	0.271
Thrombosis/thromboembolic events					
Pulmonary embolism	10/60	16.7%	2/60	3.3%	0.015*
Peripheral thrombosis/thromboembolism	3/60	5.0%	5/60	8.3%	0.717
Stroke/TIA	4/60	6.7%	0/60	0%	0.042*

CPR, cardiopulmonary resuscitation; ECMO, extracorporal membrane oxygenation; ICU, intensive care unit; NIV, non-invasive ventilation; TIA, transient ischemic attack; VF, ventricular fibrillation; VT, ventricular tachycardia.
*$p < 0.05$.

covariate imbalance between the two investigated, showing no significant differences.

In contrast to former studies conducted on arrhythmias in COVID-19, the present project included monitoring data on arrhythmias for the entire ICU-stay in addition to standard 12-lead ECGs, thus allowing for a more precise analysis of the arrhythmic burden. To avoid potential interference of novel treatment options, such as dexamethasone, with our findings, patients were recruited during the first wave of the pandemic before publication of the "RECOVERY Trial in July 2020." The impact of COVID-19 disease on myocardial arrhythmias might be better reflected through this approach, since outcomes are not influenced by this treatment regime, which is now routinely applied in the involved study centers. Accordingly, COVID-19 specific therapy is low in the present patient collective as it was mostly experimental during this investigated period.

In the COVID-19 group, AF was the most frequent arrhythmia and was observed in 18.3% of all patients (**Table 2**; **Figure 1A**). It is in line with a recent publication by Bertini et al. (14), which reported an AF rate of about 22% in a similar patient collective, documented by ECG at hospital admission. Of note, the mean patient age in that study tended to be higher compared

with our collectives, which might explain the slightly higher AF rate (14). Interestingly, the AF burden in the non-COVID-19 group in our study was even higher, ranging at around 43% and requiring a higher need for electrical cardioversion (**Table 2**; **Figure 1A**). This was also reflected by an increased incidence of new-onset of AF (**Table 2**; **Figure 1B**), indicating a more pronounced proarrhythmic substrate in this population. Of note, the rates of AF in our control group are in line with former studies conducted on AF in sepsis and septic shock, with rates of new onset of AF ranging between 7% and 46%, depending on disease severity (16, 17). Apart from AF, rates of other supraventricular and also ventricular tachyarrhythmias and relevant bradyarrhythmias with consequent need for cardiopulmonary resuscitation were similar in both COVID-19 and non-COVID-19 patients (**Tables 2**, **3**; **Figures 1D,E**). With respect to ventricular arrhythmias, one has to keep in mind the comparably low amount of heart failure (11.7%) and coronary artery disease (15%) in our patient collective resulting in a low percentage of patients with a predisposing myocardial substrate, which could facilitate ventricular tachycardias (VT).

Since inflammatory processes are known to increase the vulnerability for arrhythmias (15, 18), the higher inflammatory

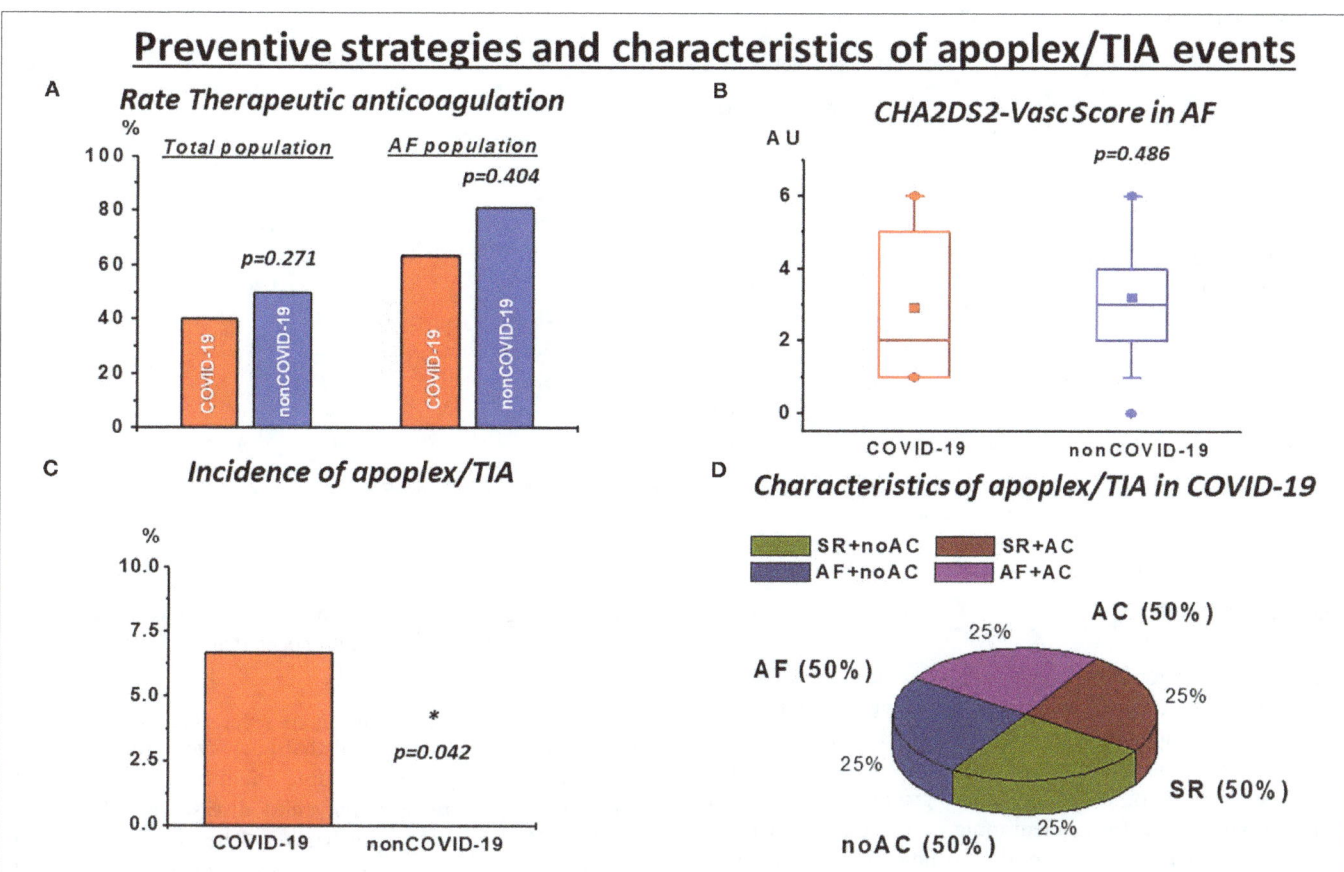

FIGURE 2 | Preventive strategies and characteristics of stroke/TIA events: **(A)** despite high but not different rates of therapeutic anticoagulation (TAC) in the total population and in patients with atrial fibrillation (AF) during rhythm monitoring as well as **(B)** similar CHA2DS2-Vasc Scores in this subgroup, **(C)** incidence of stroke/TIA events was significantly higher in COVID-19. **(D)** These events were also observed with AC (50%) and with continuous sinus rhythm (SR; 50%) during rhythm monitoring. noAC, no application of TAC. *$p < 0.05$.

burden and disease severity in the non-COVID-19 group, reflected by higher levels of leucocytes, PCT, lactate, and also lower pH levels with consequent higher mortality rates in non-COVID-19 (**Tables 3, 4**), represents an important factor in this regard (15). Consequently, one might speculate that similar to other critically ill patients, in COVID-19, cardiac arrhythmias are primarily driven by inflammatory processes and disease burden, rather than by disease-specific effects of COVID-19.

While no significant increase of arrhythmias in the COVID-19 cohort was evident, thromboembolic events showed a significant increase compared with non-COVID-19 patients. This is reflected by a higher incidence of pulmonary embolism and stroke/TIA in our COVID-19 cohort (**Table 3**). Accordingly, this finding suggests a COVID-19 specific thromboembolic effect independent of arrhythmic burden. In AF, the most common observed arrhythmia in our study, TAC, is recommended according to preexisting risk factors with a high risk of thromboembolic strokes (6). This therapy is known to be efficient as indicated in our non-COVID-19 cohort with no stroke stoke/TIA events despite a higher incidence of AF (**Table 2**) but also with a high rate of TAC (**Figure 2A**). Whether in COVID-19, AF and the associated preexisting risk factors

might further drive thromboembolic events, is still a matter of debate. Concerning our results, this seems questionable since the rate of neurologic events was higher in COVID-19 despite a lower incidence of AF, comparable CHA2DS2-Vasc scores (**Figures 2B,C**) and also the appearance of these events in patients with continuous sinus rhythm during monitoring (**Figure 2D**). This emphasizes the need for effective prevention strategies in critically ill COVID-19. However, in our study, the rate of TAC in critically COVID-19 was comparable with non-COVID-19, despite the lower rate of AF (**Figure 2A**). It could be argued, that, given the high incidence of thromboembolic events, more, if not all critical COVID-19 patients should receive effective anticoagulation. While a mortality benefit seems to be associated with anticoagulatory treatment in COVID-19, the clinical evidence for efficacy and safety of such an approach is a topic for ongoing investigations (19, 20). Importantly, we observed thrombotic/thromboembolic neurological events despite sufficient TAC (**Figure 2D**; **Supplementary Table 2**), indicating TAC to be probably less effective in this population. Thus, taken together our data emphasize that thromboembolic events seem to be a disease-specific in severe COVID-19 patients unrelated to the presence of arrhythmias.

TABLE 4 | Relevant laboratory markers during ICU stay.

	COVID-19 ($n = 60$)		Non-COVID-19 ($n = 60$)		p
	n	Median (Q3–Q1)	n	Median (Q3–Q1)	
Lactate (U/L)	60	2.6 (2.1)	60	3.5 (4.8)	0.017*
Min. pH	60	7.19 (0.1)	60	7.13 (0.1)	0.045*
Creatinine (mg/dl)	60	1.7 (2.1)	60	2.3 (2.6)	0.404
Min potassium (mmol/L)	60	3.4 (0.4)	60	3.3 (0.5)	0.720
Leukocytes (10^9/L)	60	14.8 (11.5)	60	20.2 (11.8)	0.002*
Min. lymphocytes (10^9/L)	60	4.4 (6.6)	45	4.9 (6.5)	0.712
CRP (ng/ml)	59	25.5 (17.7)	60	28.2 (15.4)	0.493
PCT (ng/ml)	60	1.9 (5.1)	57	3.0 (17.9)	0.013*
Interleukin 6 (pg/ml)	53	513.8 (2,395.2)	23	394.8 (1,080.6)	0.923
Fibrinogen (mg/dl)	34	672.5 (298)	54	602.5 (270.0)	0.175

CRP, C-reactive protein; Min., lowest level of laboratory biomarker obtained during the total period of ICU stay; PCT, procalcitonin. Relevant laboratory findings obtained during intensive care unit (ICU) stay. If not other indicated, the highest obtained value during the whole period of ICU stay is presented.
*$p < 0.05$.

LIMITATIONS

The present study has by design its limitations, while contributing novel clinical findings. Our sample size may be too small to detect differences in arrhythmias with low incidence, such as ventricular tachyarrhythmias and bradyarrhythmias. The heterogeneity of our comparison group, which consists of patients suffering from pneumonia of diverse origin might in part differ with regards to the pathogenetic mechanisms compared with COVID-19 pneumonia. Thus, the findings of the present study have to be considered as hypothesis generating. The passionate use of untested treatments in a number of COVID-19 patients (such as tocilizumab or hydroxychloroquine, **Supplementary Table 3**) might have affected the results, especially concerning arrhythmia burden due to effects on QT interval. However, while QT prolongation is suspected to promote this issue, QTc in our COVID-19 cohort was in the normal range with shorter QTc compared with non-COVID-19 (**Supplementary Table 1**). Instead of screening, diagnostic workups for thromboembolic events were only performed when clinically suspected and therefore, they are probably underestimated.

In summary, AF is common in severe COVID-19, but we found it to be less frequent than in severe pneumonia of non-COVID-19 origin. Arrhythmia might be mainly attributed to a high inflammatory activity and disease severity, instead of a COVID-19 specific mechanism. The contrasting higher incidence of stroke, despite the lower rate of AF, seems to be a disease-specific feature of critical COVID-19, consistent with high rates of pulmonary embolisms. Further research will hopefully clarify the potential role of TAC to prevent thromboembolic events, which are independent of AF.

AUTHOR CONTRIBUTIONS

All authors listed have made a substantial, direct, and intellectual contribution to the work and approved it for publication.

REFERENCES

1. Alhazzani W, Møller MH, Arabi YM, Loeb M, Gong MN, Fan E, et al. Surviving sepsis campaign: guidelines on the management of critically ill adults with coronavirus disease 2019 (COVID-19). *Intensive Care Med.* (2020) 46:854–87. doi: 10.1007/s00134-020-06022-5
2. Rubin GD, Ryerson CJ, Haramati LB, Sverzellati N, Kanne JP, Raoof S, et al. The role of chest imaging in patient management during the COVID-19 pandemic: a multinational consensus statement from the Fleischner Society. *Radiology.* (2020) 7:2020201365. doi: 10.1148/radiol.2020201365
3. Papazian L, Aubron C, Brochard L, Chiche JD, Combes A, Dreyfuss D, et al. Formal guidelines: management of acute respiratory distress syndrome. *Ann Intensive Care.* (2019) 9:019–0540. doi: 10.1186/s13613-019-0540-9
4. Boriani G, Fauchier L, Aguinaga L, Beattie JM, Blomstrom Lundqvist C, Cohen A, et al. European Heart Rhythm Association (EHRA) consensus

document on management of arrhythmias and cardiac electronic devices in the critically ill and post-surgery patient, endorsed by Heart Rhythm Society (HRS), Asia Pacific Heart Rhythm Society (APHRS), Cardiac Arrhythmia Society of Southern Africa (CASSA), and Latin American Heart Rhythm Society (LAHRS). *Europace.* (2019) 21:7–8. doi: 10.1093/europace/euy110
5. Cronin EM, Bogun FM, Maury P, Peichl P, Chen M, Namboodiri N, et al. 2019 HRS/EHRA/APHRS/LAHRS expert consensus statement on catheter ablation of ventricular arrhythmias. *Europace.* (2019) 21:1143–4. doi: 10.1093/europace/euz132
6. Katritsis DG, Boriani G, Cosio FG, Hindricks G, Jaïs P, Josephson ME, et al. European Heart Rhythm Association (EHRA) consensus document on the management of supraventricular arrhythmias, endorsed by Heart Rhythm Society (HRS), Asia-Pacific Heart Rhythm Society (APHRS), and Sociedad Latinoamericana de Estimulación Cardiaca y Electrofisiologia (SOLAECE). *Europace.* (2017) 19:465–511. doi: 10.1093/europace/euw301

7. Konstantinides SV, Meyer G, Becattini C, Bueno H, Geersing GJ, Harjola VP, et al. 2019 ESC Guidelines for the diagnosis and management of acute pulmonary embolism developed in collaboration with the European Respiratory Society (ERS). *Eur Heart J.* (2020) 41:543–603. doi: 10.1093/eurheartj/ehz405

8. Powers WJ, Rabinstein AA, Ackerson T, Adeoye OM, Bambakidis NC, Becker K, et al. 2018 guidelines for the early management of patients with acute ischemic stroke: a guideline for healthcare professionals from the American Heart Association/American Stroke Association. *Stroke.* (2018) 49:e46–110. doi: 10.1161/STR.0000000000000158

9. Klok FA, Kruip M, van der Meer NJM, Arbous MS, Gommers D, Kant KM, et al. Incidence of thrombotic complications in critically ill ICU patients with COVID-19. *Thromb Res.* (2020) 191:145–7. doi: 10.1016/j.thromres.2020.04.013

10. Guan WJ, Ni ZY, Hu Y, Liang WH, Ou CQ, He JX, et al. Clinical characteristics of coronavirus disease 2019 in China. *N Engl J Med.* (2020) 382:1708–20. doi: 10.1056/NEJMoa2002032

11. Jirak P, Larbig R, Shomanova Z, Fröb EJ, Dankl D, Torgersen C, et al. Myocardial injury in severe COVID-19 is similar to pneumonias of other origin: results from a multicentre study. *ESC Heart Fail.* (2020) 17:13136. doi: 10.1002/ehf2.13136

12. Metkus TS, Sokoll LJ, Barth AS, Czarny MJ, Hays AG, Lowenstein CJ, et al. Myocardial injury in severe COVID-19 compared to non-COVID acute respiratory distress syndrome. *Circulation.* (2020) 13:050543. doi: 10.1161/CIRCULATIONAHA.120.050543

13. Wang D, Hu B, Hu C, Zhu F, Liu X, Zhang J, et al. Clinical characteristics of 138 hospitalized patients with 2019 novel coronavirus-infected pneumonia in Wuhan, China. *JAMA.* (2020) 7:1585. doi: 10.1001/jama.2020.1585

14. Bertini M, Ferrari R, Guardigli G, Malagù M, Vitali F, Zucchetti O, et al. Electrocardiographic features of 431 consecutive, critically ill COVID-19 patients: an insight into the mechanisms of cardiac involvement. *EP Europace.* (2020) 22:1848–54. doi: 10.1093/europace/euaa258

15. Shahreyar M, Fahhoum R, Akinseye O, Bhandari S, Dang G, Khouzam RN. Severe sepsis and cardiac arrhythmias. *Ann Transl Med.* (2018) 6:26. doi: 10.21037/atm.2017.12.26

16. Meierhenrich R, Steinhilber E, Eggermann C, Weiss M, Voglic S, Bögelein D, et al. Incidence and prognostic impact of new-onset atrial fibrillation in patients with septic shock: a prospective observational study. *Crit Care.* (2010) 14:10. doi: 10.1186/cc9057

17. Walkey AJ, Hammill BG, Curtis LH, Benjamin EJ. Long-term outcomes following development of new-onset atrial fibrillation during sepsis. *Chest.* (2014) 146:1187–95. doi: 10.1378/chest.14-0003

18. Boos CJ. Infection and atrial fibrillation: inflammation begets AF. *Eur Heart J.* (2020) 41:1120–22. doi: 10.1093/eurheartj/ehz953

19. Hadid T, Kafri Z, Al-Katib A. Coagulation and anticoagulation in COVID-19. *Blood Rev.* (2021) 47:8. doi: 10.1016/j.blre.2020.100761

20. McBane RD. 2nd, Torres Roldan VD, Niven AS, Pruthi RK, Franco PM, Linderbaum JA, et al. Anticoagulation in COVID-19: a systematic review, meta-analysis, and rapid guidance from Mayo clinic. *Mayo Clin Proc.* (2020) 95:2467–86. doi: 10.1016/j.mayocp.2020.08.030

23

Reduction of Emergency Calls and Hospitalizations for Cardiac Causes: Effects of Covid-19 Pandemic and Lockdown in Tuscany Region

Flavio D'Ascenzi[1]*, Matteo Cameli[1], Silvia Forni[2], Fabrizio Gemmi[2], Claudia Szasz[2], Valeria Di Fabrizio[2], Maria Teresa Mechi[3], Matteo Nocci[3], Sergio Mondillo[1] and Serafina Valente[1]

[1] Division of Cardiology, Department of Medical Biotechnologies, University of Siena, Siena, Italy, [2] Regional Health Agency of Tuscany, Florence, Italy, [3] Quality of Care and Clinical Networks, Regional Health Department of Tuscany, Florence, Italy

Correspondence:
Flavio D'Ascenzi
flavio.dascenzi@unisi.it

Introduction: Containment measures were established to flatten the curve of COVID-19 contagion in order to avoid a crash of the healthcare system. However, these measures influenced the rate of hospitalization of cardiac patients. In this study, we aimed to analyse the impact of COVID-19 and the effects of lockdown measures on hospital admissions and alerts of emergency medical system (EMS) for cardiac causes in the Tuscany region.

Methods: An observational, retrospective analysis from Italian Tuscany region was conducted. We evaluated consecutive patients contacting EMS or admitted to the 39 Emergency Departments (EDs) in Tuscany for cardiac causes in the first trimester of 2020. Data were compared with the same period in 2018/19.

Results: The alerts of EMS for cardiac causes significantly decrease in 2020 and the highest difference between 2018/19 and 2020 was found immediately after national lockdown ($\Delta = -47.4\%$, $p < 0.001$). The number of admissions for chest pain in the EDs also decreased, with a maximum difference of -67.6% ($p < 0.001$) vs. 2018/19. The number of hospital accesses for acute coronary syndromes, atrial fibrillation, and heart failure in the EDs significantly decreased in 2020 as compared to 2018/19 (maximum $\Delta = -58.9\%$, $p < 0.001$; maximum $\Delta = -63.0\%$, $p < 0.001$; maximum $\Delta = -72.7\%$, $p < 0.001$, respectively).

Conclusions: A significant decrease in the contacts to EMS for cardiac causes and in cardiac diagnoses was observed during the first trimester of 2020. Fear of contagion has likely played a relevant role. The lesson learnt from first wave of COVID-19 pandemic suggests that appropriate public information strategies and re-education of people are essential.

Keywords: lockdown, coronavirus, cardiovascular disorders, acute coronary syndrome, atrial fibrillation, heart failure

INTRODUCTION

The pandemic caused by COVID-19 has been associated with thousands of deaths worldwide and multiple cardiovascular risk factors and cardiac disorders have been recognized as high-risk conditions (1). The rapidly increasing number of patients affected by COVID-19 requiring hospitalization has imposed a relevant problem of sustainability for the healthcare system. Accordingly, during the first wave of COVID-19 pandemic, the Italian government has imposed measures promoting social distancing and a stepwise strategy starting from the quarantine for some Italy regions with subsequent lockdown measures adopted for the entire nation as of 11 March (https://www.gazzettaufficiale.it/eli/id/2020/03/08/20A01522/sg, https://www.gazzettaufficiale.it/eli/id/2020/03/11/20A01605/sg). Although these strategies were aimed to flatten the curve of the contagion in order to avoid a crash of the health care system, these measures have significantly influenced the rate of hospitalization of cardiac patients and changes in the pattern of hospital admissions have been noted, particularly in the Northern regions of Italy (2–4).

In this study, we aimed to analyse the epidemiologic impact of COVID-19 and the effects of lockdown measures on the contacts to emergency medical system (EMS) and hospital visits to the emergency department for cardiac causes for the entire Tuscany region. The number of final diagnoses of acute coronary syndrome (ACS), heart failure (HF), and atrial fibrillation (AF) was also considered. These data were compared with the trends observed in the same time frame of the previous 2 years.

METHODS

We conducted an observational, retrospective analysis from the Tuscany region aimed at evaluating the number of patients contacting the EMS for cardiac problems and symptoms, not occurring during COVID-19 infection (i.e., angina, arrhythmias, syncope, chest pain, etc.), with high dispatch priority, established by nurse triage, and the number of consecutive patients admitted to the Emergency Departments for cardiac causes, analyzing the final number of diagnoses of ACS, HF, and AF. In Tuscany there were 3.73 million inhabitants and 39 Emergency Departments that performed 1,537,031 visits (data for the year 2019). The period of observation lasted 3 months, i.e., the first trimester of 2020, from the 1st of January 2020 to the 31th of March 2020. This period was selected taking into account that the first cluster of cases of COVID-19 was identified in Italy the 20th of February and that lockdown measures were adopted for the entire nation as of 11th March. Weekly data observed during this period were compared to the trends observed in the same time frame of 2018 and 2019. Although the first cluster of cases of COVID-19 was identified in Italy the 20th of February 2020, the entire first trimester of 2020 was included in this analysis to show also pre-COVID 19 data and to demonstrate that differences in the rate of hospitalization in March were not due to physiologic fluctuations due to epidemiologic factors. A sub-analysis was also performed dividing the first trimester 2020 into three different periods, according to the events occurred

during this trimester: 1st January-20th February; 21th February-10th March; 11th March-31th March. Number of accesses to Emergency Departments for stroke and sepsis were also analyzed.

The regional information systems of pre-hospital and hospital EMSs and hospital admission abstracts were used as data sources. These databases include calls to EMS, visits to emergency departments and hospital admissions in Tuscany region. In these data each individual has a unique and anonymous identifier that enables complete record linkage at individual level.

Although the comparison of the rate of mortality between the first trimester 2020 and 2018/2019 was beyond the primary scope of this study, the in-hospital mortality for patients admitted for ACS and HF was also analyzed. The rate of hospitalizations for patients admitted to the Emergency Departments and the number of patients with ACS and HF admitted to the intensive care units of the Tuscany Region during the hospitalization was also analyzed for the entire period. Data were analyzed and were checked for missing or contradictory entries and for values out of normal range by Regional Health Agency of Tuscany.

This study was conducted in accordance with the Helsinki Declaration. According to the Italian legislation (legislative decree 211/2003) and the regional procedures, the study does not need ethic approval as it is a purely observational study on routine collected anonymous data. Furthermore, because this was an observational retrospective study, patients had already been treated when the study protocol was written; therefore, it could not have modified their life-trajectories or care pathways in any way.

Statistical Analysis

Mean values of data obtained in the first trimester of 2018 and 2019 were calculated and compared with data collected in the same period of 2020. Ninety-five percentage confidence intervals of values observed in 2018-19 were calculated using Poisson model for each week and for the three periods considered in the study. Differences between periods of observation for 2018/2019 and 2020 were expressed as Δ and statistical significance was tested using Poisson models. The statistical significance was set for a two-tailed p-value < 0.05. Data were collected using Excel software (version 16.35 2019, Microsoft Corporation, Redmond, USA). The statistical software Stata 14 SE (StataCorp LP, College Station, Texas) was used for the data analyses.

RESULTS

A significant decrease in contacts of EMS by the patients for cardiac causes was found between 2019 and 2020, see **Figure 1**. The highest difference was found 1 week after the national lockdown was imposed ($\Delta = -47.4\%$ as compared to the same week of the previous years, $p < 0.001$).

The numbers of hospital visits for chest pain in the Emergency departments in Tuscany significantly decreased in 2020 as compared to 2018 and to 2019, reaching a Δ at the end of the week between 24 February-01 March of -24.0% ($p < 0.01$ vs. the same period of the previous years), see **Figure 2**. The week after the national lockdown, the number of visits for chest pain significantly dropped to -67.6% as compared to the same time

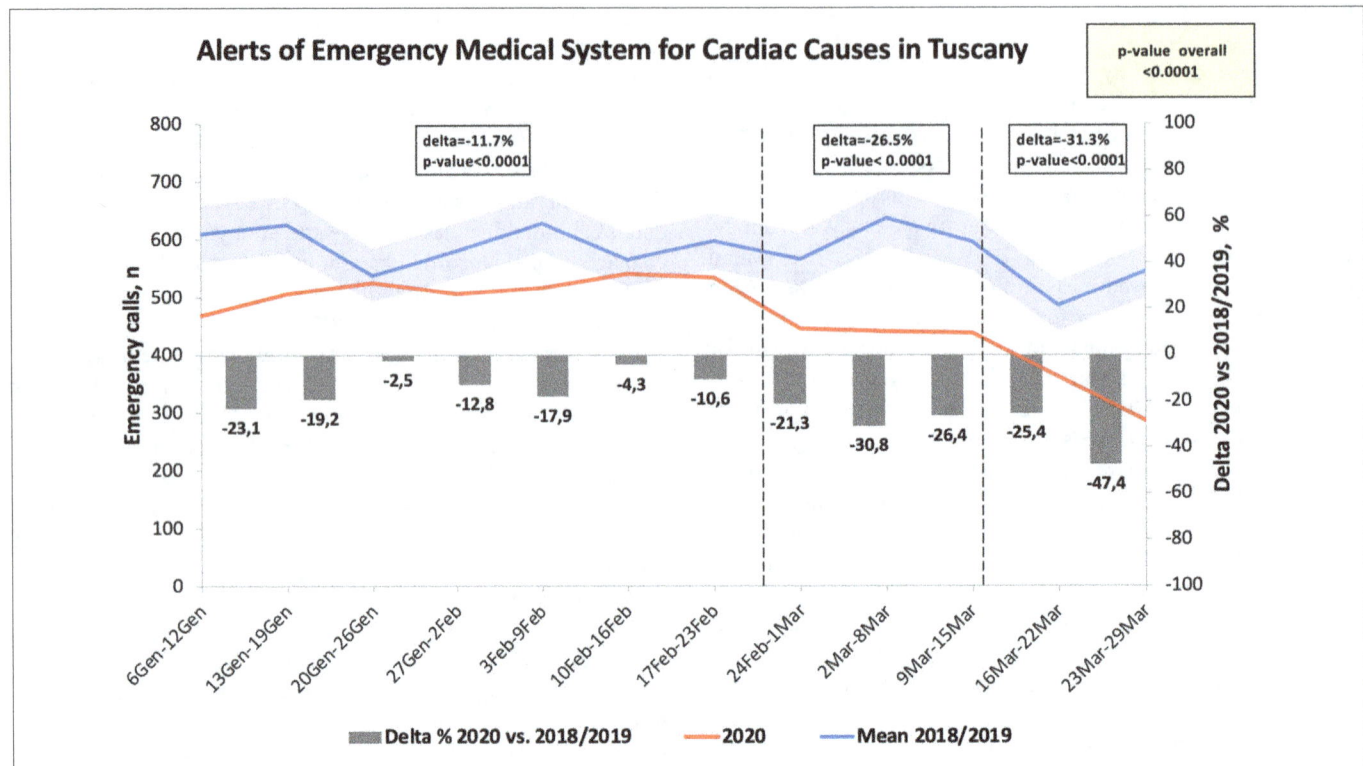

FIGURE 1 | Number of calls to the emergency medical system for cardiac causes in Tuscany. Data obtained in the first trimester were compared to data observed in 2018 and 2019 (an average value of this data was observed). For all the figures data were reported for each week separately (from the 6th of January to the 30th of March) and the delta between 2020 and 2018/2019 was reported and expressed by gray columns as percentage as well as delta and p-values for the three different periods.

frame of 2018 and 2019 ($p < 0.001$) and it represented the highest difference found between 2020 and the previous years. While no significant differences were found before the 24th of February for the visits to the Emergency departments for cardiac causes of chest pain ($p = 0.354$), they significantly decrease after this first period (see **Figure 3**).

The number of hospital visits for ACS in the Emergency departments significantly decreased at the end of February as compared to 2018 and 2019 ($\Delta = -18.3\%$, $p < 0.05$) and the greatest difference was identified at the end of March 2020 ($\Delta = -58.9\%$, $p < 0.001$) (**Figure 4**). Similarly, the diagnosis of AF in the Emergency departments significantly decreased at the end of February 2020 as compared to the same period in 2018 and 2019 ($p < 0.05$), reaching the greatest difference in the week after the national lockdown ($\Delta = -63\%$, $p < 0.001$) (**Figure 5**). The diagnosis of HF significantly decreased during COVID-19 pandemic, reaching the greatest difference in comparison with 2018/2019 data 1 week after the declaration of national lockdown ($\Delta = -72.7\%$, $p < 0.001$, **Figure 6**). The number of accesses to Emergency Departments due to stroke or sepsis were also decreased during the first wave of COVID-19 pandemic as compared to 2018 and 2019 (see **Supplementary Figures 1, 2**).

The rate of hospitalizations for patients admitted to the Emergency Departments did not differ between 2020 and 2018/2019 (overall p-value = 0.68) for ACS and for HF (overall p-value = 0.49). The in-hospital mortality for patients suffering

from an ACS did not differ between the first trimester 2020 and the first trimester of 2018 and 2019 (overall p-value = 0.166). During the three different periods no significant differences were observed ($p = 0.71$, $p = 0.0.92$, and $p = 0.364$, respectively). Among the patients admitted for ACS to the hospitals of the Tuscany Region, the number of patients requiring hospitalization in an intensive care unit did not differ between the first trimester 2020 and 2018/2019 (overall p-value = 0.11).

The in-hospital mortality for HF did not differ between 2020 and 2018/2019 (overall p-value = 0.102), with no differences among the three different periods ($p = 0.053$, $p = 0.269$, and $p = 0.208$, respectively). Among the patients admitted for HF to the hospitals of the Tuscany Region, the number of patients requiring hospitalization in an intensive care unit did not differ between the first trimester 2020 and 2018/2019 (overall p-value = 0.29).

DISCUSSION

The main finding of the present study is that a marked decrease in the number of patients alerting the EMS and visiting the Emergency departments for cardiac causes were observed in Tuscany after the diagnosis of the first cluster of COVID-19 cases in Italy and particularly after the national lockdown, as compared to the same time frame of the previous years (i.e., 2018 and 2019). As a consequence, the number of ACS and

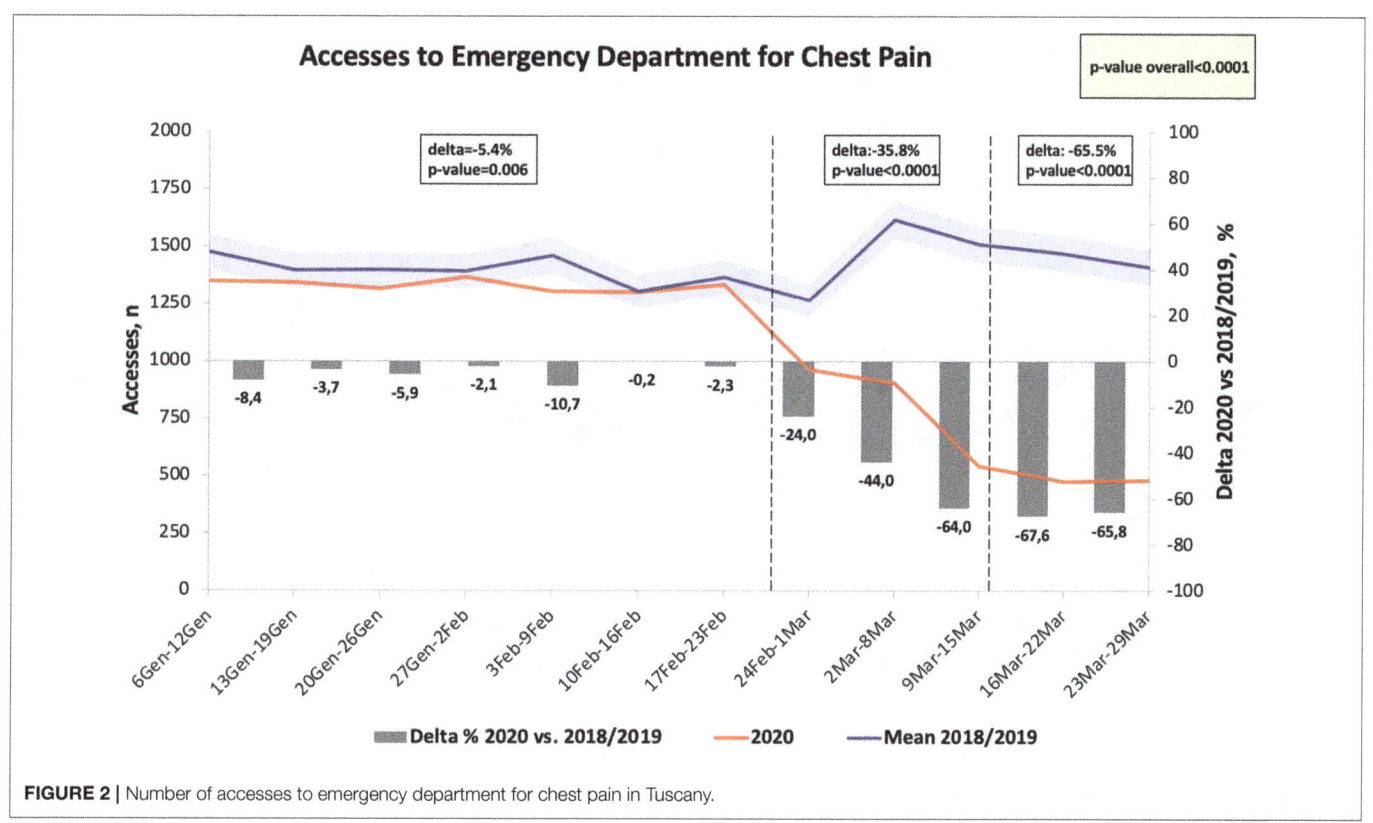

FIGURE 2 | Number of accesses to emergency department for chest pain in Tuscany.

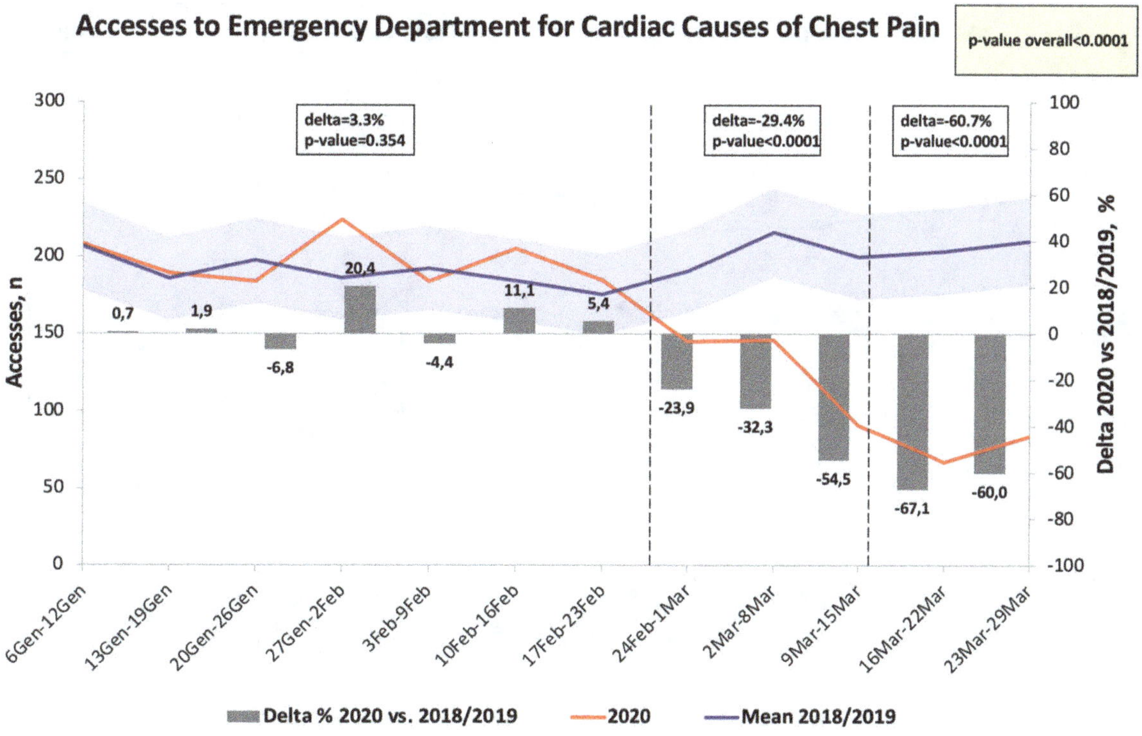

FIGURE 3 | Number of accesses to emergency department for cardiac causes of chest pain in Tuscany.

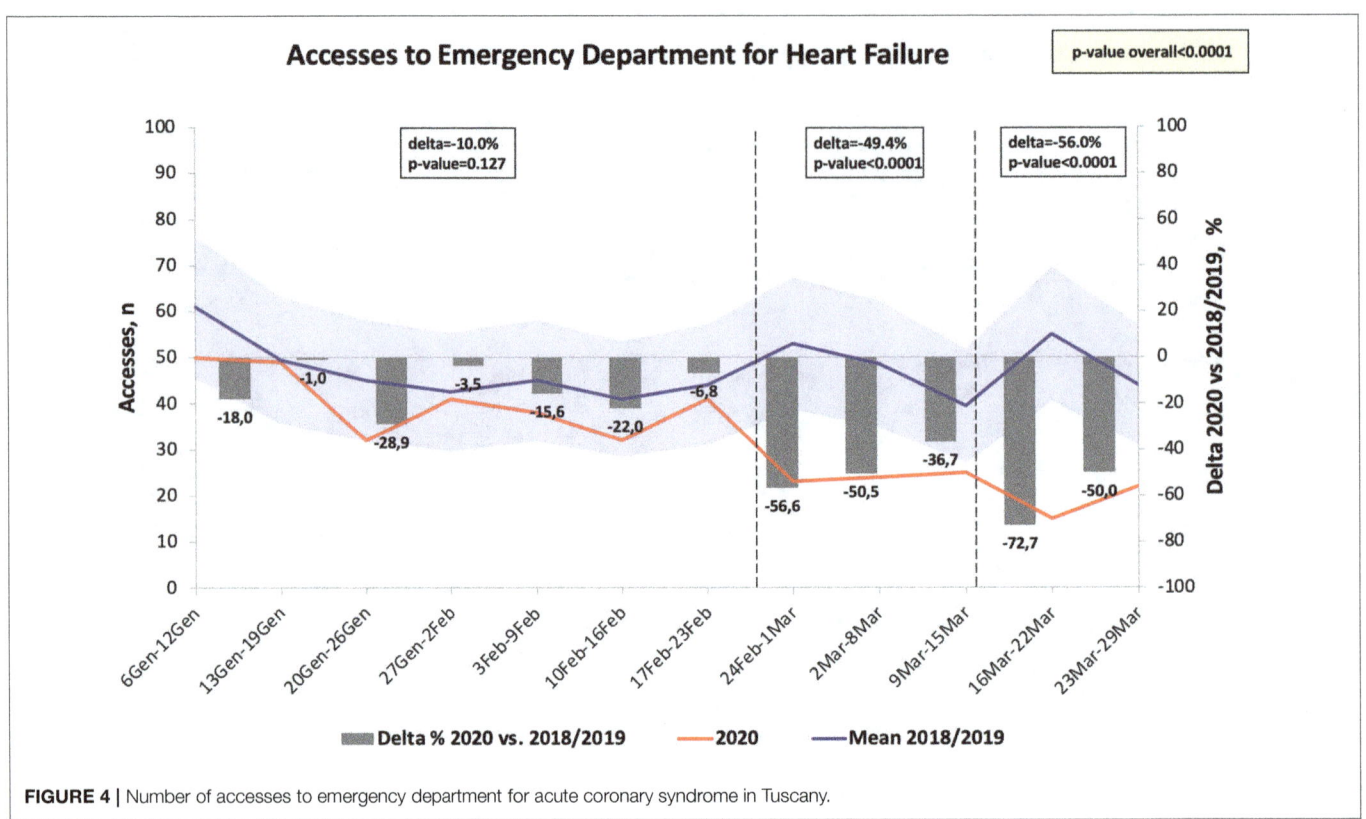

FIGURE 4 | Number of accesses to emergency department for acute coronary syndrome in Tuscany.

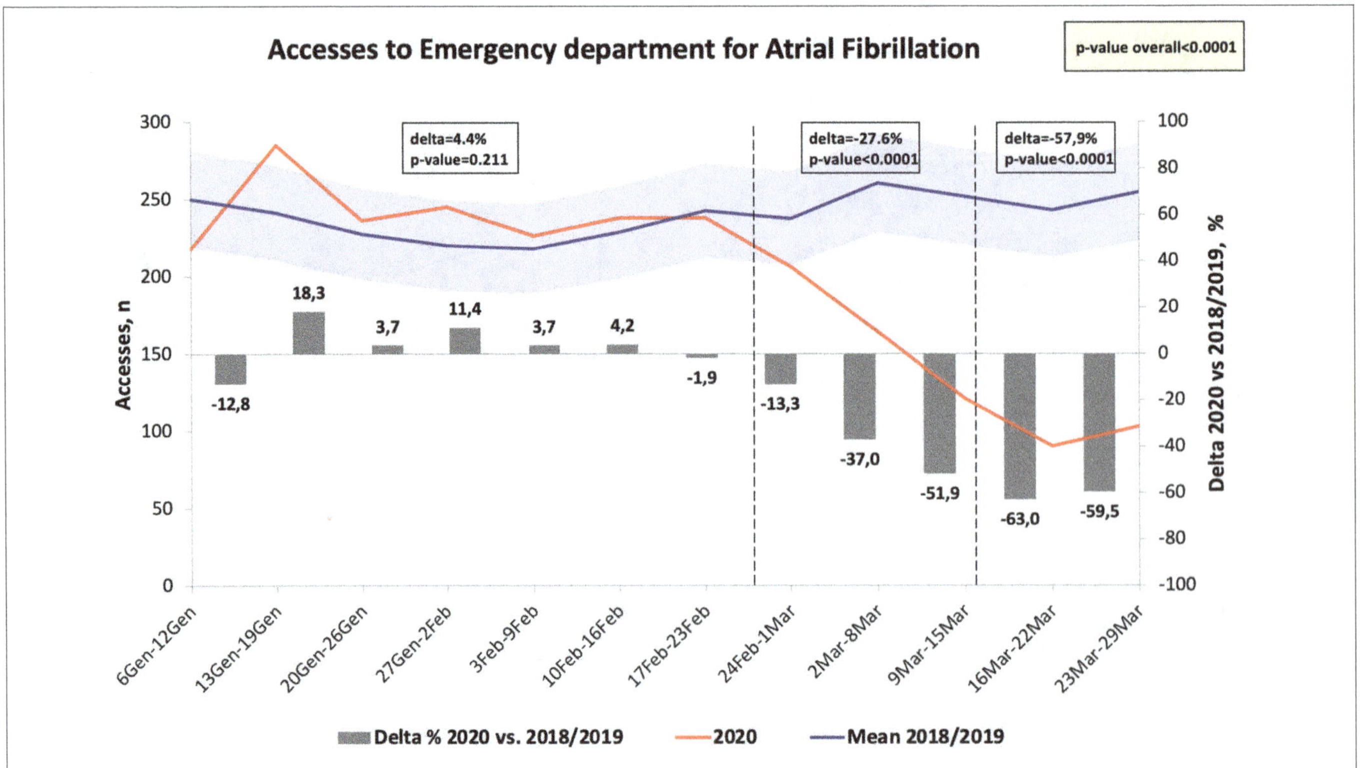

Accesses to Emergency department for Atrial Fibrillation

p-value overall<0.0001

delta=4.4%
p-value=0.211

delta=-27.6%
p-value<0.0001

delta=-57,9%
p-value<0.0001

Delta % 2020 vs. 2018/2019 ▪ 2020 Mean 2018/2019

FIGURE 5 | Number of accesses to emergency department for atrial fibrillation in Tuscany.

Reduction of Emergency Calls and Hospitalizations for Cardiac Causes: Effects of Covid-19 Pandemic...

199

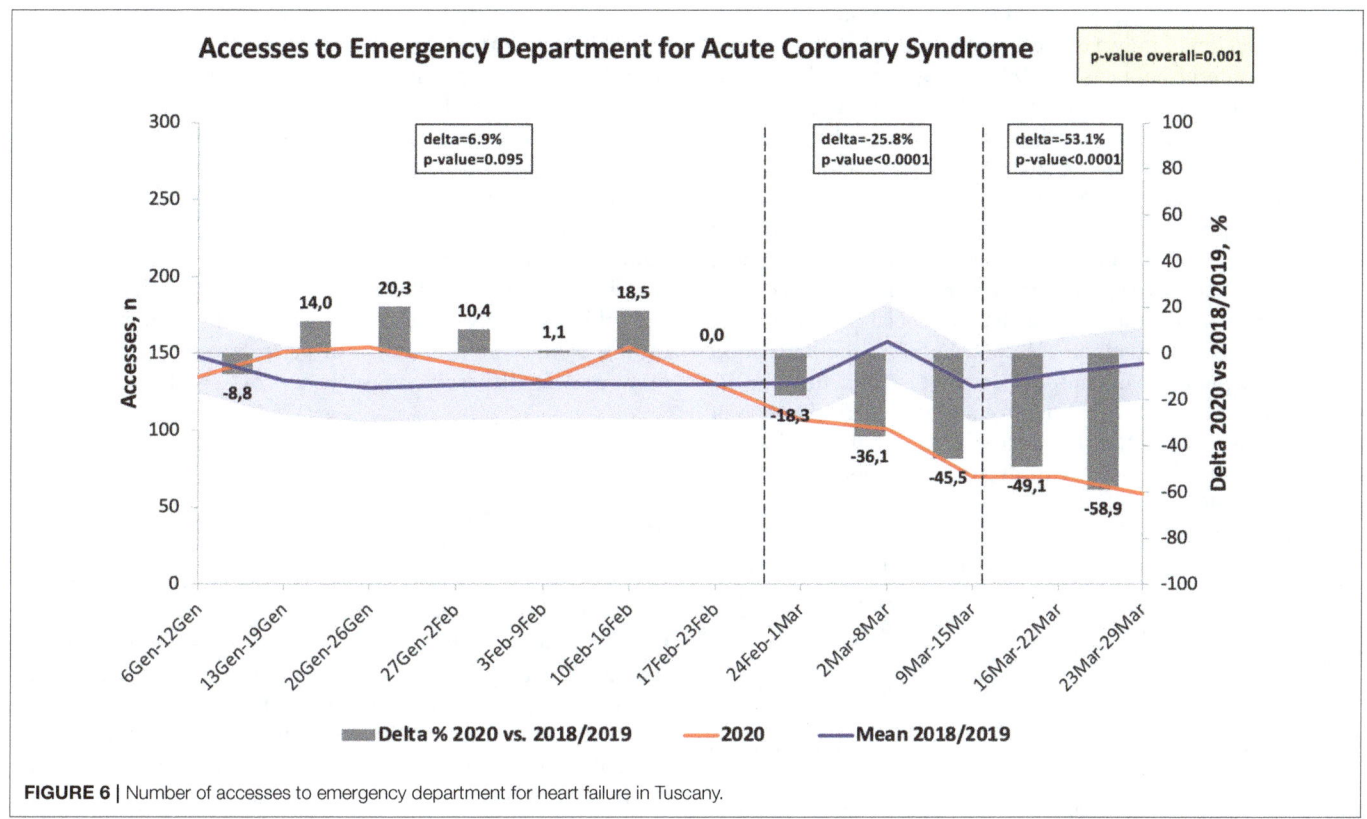

FIGURE 6 | Number of accesses to emergency department for heart failure in Tuscany.

AF diagnosed significantly decreased as compared to the same period of the previous years. Notably, the trend demonstrates a significant drop after the 20th of February and after the 11th of March 2020, i.e., after the first case diagnosed and after the national lockdown. Multiple factors may have affected the rate of visits and hospitalization for cardiac causes during the most dramatic periods of COVID-19 pandemic, as demonstrated also by the unpredictable reduction in hospitalizations for other causes, such stroke and sepsis. However, these findings indirectly suggest that the fear of contagion at the hospital probably have discouraged the patients to alert the EMS during the first wave of COVID-9 pandemic, particularly after the media diffused the news that infection was spread across hospitalized patients and healthcare personnel. The concerns raised by the mass media on the high mortality rate of COVID-19 pneumonia further discouraged patients with cardiac conditions to contact the EMS. As reported by De Rosa et al. (2), a second hypothesis can be that the emergency medical system was focused on COVID-19. However, our study demonstrates that the number of calls to the EMS significantly decrease during this dramatic period; while variations in the rate of ACS and cardiac disease have been demonstrated (5, 6) and cannot be definitely excluded, the marked difference between the same periods of 2018/2019 and 2020, reaching even more than −65% reduction in the visits, suggest that patients intentionally decided not to alert the EMS or to go to the hospital, irrespective of their cardiac conditions and their symptoms. Unfortunately, this phenomenon was

not confined to Italy, but sharp drops in the numbers of persons seeking emergency medical care was observed also in United States, with the total number of US ED visits being 42% lower during the early pandemic period than during the same period a year earlier (7), and in Thailand (−36%) (8). Notably, also in US the decrease in ED visits for acute life-threatening health conditions was observed immediately before and after declaration of the COVID-19 pandemic as a national emergency (9). In agreement with our findings, also Wongtanasarasin et al. observed that the national lockdown in Thailand was associated with a significant reduction in average daily ED visits (8).

A reduction in ACS activations was reported also by US cardiac catheterization laboratories and was noticed also in Spain (10, 11) and in a recent survey conducted by the European Society of Cardiology the respondents declared a reduction in the admission of patients with ACS >40% (12). In Italy, a reduction in the rate of hospital admissions for ACS was reported by De Rosa et al. for the week 12–19 March (2), by Toniolo et al. (3), and by De Filippo et al. (4). Notably, the study by De Rosa was a national registry with analysis confined to 1 week while the other two articles included centers in the Northern part of Italy, i.e., the most affected by COVID-19 pandemic. Indeed, Lombardy and Piedmont regions had 89,526 and 30,758 confirmed cases of COVID-19, respectively, while in Tuscany 10,122 cases were diagnosed (http://opendatadpc.maps.arcgis.com/apps/opsdashboard/index.html#/b0c68bce2cce478eaac82fe38d4138b1 last access, 06/05/2020). In this study we extended the time frame of observation reporting the data of the first trimester 2020 from a different region of Italy, i.e., the Tuscany, and we demonstrated that a low rate of contacts to EMS during this pandemic was observed also in regions of Italy less affected by the pandemic. We found that the reduction in admission was observed also for patients with heart failure, with a delta of -56% for the last period of observation in comparison with 2018 and 2019 ($p <$ 0.0001), in agreement with data reported by Severino et al. and demonstrating a reduction of admission during the lockdown (13). These findings suggest that the ubiquitous presence of COVID-19 news on the mass media and social media and the lack of verified information have contributed to the perception of unsafe hospitals, even if hospital were not overwhelmed by the COVID-19 emergency, as in Tuscany, and an underestimation of mortality and morbidity risks due to cardiac conditions. Indeed, as demonstrated by Barbieri et al., the reduction in hospital admissions observed in 2020 ad compared to the same period of 2019 was associated with increased mortality (14).

Finally, we found in this study that, for the first trimester 2020, the in-hospital mortality did not differ for patients admitted for ACS and for HF, in comparison with the first trimester of 2018 and 2019. Furthermore, the number of patients with ACS and HF requiring hospitalization in an intensive care unit did not differ. Although the impact of the decrease in the number of hospitalizations and visits to the Emergency Departments on the cardiovascular mortality was not the primary scope of this study, these findings suggest that patients were treated with similar standards before and during the first wave of COVID-19 pandemic and with similar outcomes. However, the low rate of hospitalizations for ACS and AF may represent a warning alert for the future development of cardiac and cerebrovascular complications, such as end-stage heart failure, sudden death, or transient ischemic attack and stroke and the negative effects of this marked impact on the pattern of hospitalizations will likely be seen in the next future. Further studies extending the period of observation are needed to report a comprehensive analysis of this phenomenon. Furthermore, the negative impact of the reduction in hospitalization for cardiac causes may have cause an increase in out-of-hospital mortality. Unfortunately, these data were not available.

The present data further strengthen the need of adequate public information policies to reinforce the importance of timely care for medical emergencies. Furthermore, the lesson learnt from the first wave of COVID-19 pandemic suggests that the community of healthcare professionals should continue re-educating the general population to recognize early cardiac symptoms (2) and to be confident with the national healthcare system in case of hospitalization.

Limitations

In this study we observed a dramatic decrease of hospital admissions and emergency contacts, primarily due to the fear of contagion. Although the fear of contagion likely was the primary

mechanisms leading to the reduction of hospital admissions, a multiplicity of factors, rather than a unique mechanism, contributed to this phenomenon. As reported by De Rosa et al. (2), we cannot completely exclude that a true reduction in the incidence of acute cardiovascular disease as the potential result of low physical stress and widespread prevalence of the resting state during the quarantine, especially in the initial phase of the social containment, might have partly contributed to the lower number of admissions.

Although patients affected by SARS-CoV-2 were excluded from the final analysis, we cannot definitively exclude that some cardiac symptoms suffered from patients contacting the EMS may be related to cardiac consequences of COVID-19 infection.

CONCLUSIONS

In Tuscany a significant decrease in the contacts to EMS for symptoms and disease related to cardiac causes and in the hospitalization rate for ACS, AF, and HF was observed during the COVID-19 pandemic. In the comparison with the same period of the previous years, the greatest difference was identified after the first case of COVID-19 in Italy and after the national lockdown. Fear of contagion among the patients has likely played the most relevant role. Therefore, the lesson learnt from the first wave of COVID-19 pandemic suggests that appropriate public information strategies are essential for a proper management of cardiac patients and a re-education of general population to recognize cardiac symptoms and life-threatening cardiovascular disorders and the consequent need of hospitalization should be guaranteed.

AUTHOR CONTRIBUTIONS

FD'A, SM, and SV contributed to the conception of the study while FD'A, SF, FG, and MN contributed to the design of the study. FD'A wrote the manuscript. MC, SF, FG, CS, VD, MM, SM, and SV critically revised the manuscript. All the authors gave the final approval and agrees to be accountable for all aspects of work ensuring integrity and accuracy.

SUPPLEMENTARY MATERIAL

Supplementary Figure 1 | Number of accesses to emergency department for stroke in Tuscany.

Supplementary Figure 2 | Number of accesses to emergency department for sepsis in Tuscany.

REFERENCES

1. Clerkin KJ, Fried JA, Raikhelkar J, Sayer G, Griffin JM, Masoumi A, et al. COVID-19 and cardiovascular disease. *Circulation.* (2020) 141:1648–55. doi: 10.1161/CIRCULATIONAHA.120.046941

2. De Rosa S, Spaccarotella C, Basso C, Calabrò MP, Curcio A, Filardi PP, et al. Reduction of hospitalizations for myocardial infarction in Italy in the COVID-19 era. *Eur Heart J.* (2020) 41:2083–8. doi: 10.1093/eurheartj/ehaa409

3. Toniolo M, Negri F, Antonutti M, Mase M, Facchin D. Unpredictable fall of severe emergent cardiovascular diseases hospital admissions during the COVID-19 pandemic: experience of a single large center in Northern Italy. *J Am Heart Assoc.* (2020) 9:e017122. doi: 10.1161/JAHA.120.017122

4. De Filippo O, D'Ascenzo F, Angelini F, Bocchino PP, Conrotto F, Saglietto A, et al. Reduced rate of hospital admissions for ACS during Covid-19 outbreak in Northern Italy. *N Engl J Med.* (2020) 383:88–9. doi: 10.1056/NEJMc2009166

5. Nagarajan V, Fonarow GC, Ju C, Pencina M, Laskey WK, Maddox TM, et al. Seasonal and circadian variations of acute myocardial infarction: Findings from the Get With The Guidelines-Coronary Artery Disease (GWTG-CAD) program. *Am Heart J.* (2017) 189:85–93. doi: 10.1016/j.ahj.2017.04.002

6. Stewart S, Keates AK, Redfern A, McMurray JJV. Seasonal variations in cardiovascular disease. *Nat Rev Cardiol.* (2017) 14:654–64. doi: 10.1038/nrcardio.2017.76

7. Hartnett KP, Kite-Powell A, DeVies J, Coletta MA, Boehmer TK, Boehmer TK, et al. Impact of the COVID-19 pandemic on emergency department visits—United States, January 1, 2019-May 30, 2020. *MMWR Morb Mortal Wkly Rep.* (2020) 69:699–704. doi: 10.15585/mmwr.mm6923e1

8. Wongtanasarasin W, Srisawang T, Yothiya W, Phinyo P. Impact of national lockdown towards emergency department visits and admission rates during the COVID-19 pandemic in Thailand: a hospital-based study. *Emerg Med Australas.* (2020). doi: 10.1111/1742-6723.13666. [Epub ahead of print].

9. Lange SJ, Ritchey MD, Goodman AB, Dias T, Twentyman E, Fuld J, et al. Potential indirect effects of the COVID-19 pandemic on use of emergency departments for acute life-threatening conditions—United States, January-May 2020. *Am J Transplant.* (2020) 20:2612–7. doi: 10.1111/ajt.16239

10. Garcia S, Albaghdadi MS, Meraj PM, Schmidt C, Garberich R, Jaffer FA, et al. Reduction in ST-segment elevation cardiac catheterization laboratory activations in the United States during COVID-19 pandemic. *J Am Coll Cardiol.* (2020) 75:2871–2. doi: 10.1016/j.jacc.2020.04.011

11. Aldama G, Rebollal F, Flores X, Pinon P, Rodriguez-Leor O, Vazquez JM. Decrease in the number of primary angioplasty procedures during the pandemic and its relationship with mortality from COVID-19. The role of competing risks. *Rev Esp Cardiol (Engl Ed).* (2020). doi: 10.1016/j.rec.2020.11.008

12. Pessoa-Amorim G, Camm CF, Gajendragadkar P, De Maria GL, Arsac C, Laroche C, et al. Admission of patients with STEMI since the outbreak of the COVID-19 pandemic: a survey by the European Society of Cardiology. *Eur Heart J Qual Care Clin Outcomes.* (2020) 6:210–6. doi: 10.1093/ehjqcco/qcaa046

13. Severino P, D'Amato A, Saglietto A, D'Ascenzo F, Marini C, Schiavone M, et al. Reduction in heart failure hospitalization rate during coronavirus disease 19 pandemic outbreak. *ESC Heart Fail.* (2020) 7:4182–8. doi: 10.1002/ehf2.13043

14. Barbieri G, Spinelli S, Filippi M, Foltran F, Giraldi M, Martino MC, et al. COVID-19 pandemic management at the Emergency Department: the changing scenario at the University Hospital of Pisa. *Emerg Care J.* (2020) 16:9146.

24

Interdisciplinary Model for Scheduling Post-Discharge Cardiopulmonary Care of Patients Following Severe and Critical SARS-CoV-2 (Coronavirus) Infection

Kristen Kopp [1†], Michael Lichtenauer [1*†], Lukas Jaroslaw Motloch [1], Uta C. Hoppe [1], Alexander Egle [2], Helmut J. F. Salzer [3,4], Bernd Lamprecht [3,4], Josef Tomasits [5], Hannes M. Müller [6] and Anna Dieplinger [7]

[1] Department of Internal Medicine II, Cardiology, Paracelsus Medical University, Salzburg, Austria, [2] Department of Internal Medicine III, Hematology, Medical Oncology, Hemostaseology, Rheumatology and Infectious Diseases, Paracelsus Medical University, Salzburg, Austria, [3] Department of Pulmonology, Kepler University Hospital, Linz, Austria, [4] Medical Faculty, Johannes Kepler University, Linz, Austria, [5] Institute for Medical and Chemical Laboratory Diagnostics, Kepler University Hospital, Linz, Austria, [6] Department of Cardiac, Vascular, and Thoracic Surgery, Kepler University Hospital, Linz, Austria, [7] Institute for Nursing and Practice, Paracelsus Medical University, Salzburg, Austria

*Correspondence:
Michael Lichtenauer
michael.lichtenauer@chello.at

† These authors have contributed equally to this work

Keywords: Covid-19, severe SARS-CoV-2 infection, post-discharge management, follow-up care, coronavirus

INTRODUCTION

As Covid-19 can severely implicate the respiratory and cardiovascular systems, potential pulmonary, and/or cardiovascular sequelae may be anticipated in patients following severe and critical SARS-CoV-2 infection meriting coordinated post-discharge management to identify residual effects and to mitigate potential worsening of pre-existing conditions. According to current literature, 14% of patients with SARS-CoV-2 infection require hospitalization, of these, 5–14% have severe and 2–5% have critical manifestations of infection (1–4). While Covid-19 is known to primarily cause substantial respiratory pathology in hospitalized patients, such as pneumonia (75%) and acute respiratory distress syndrome (ARDS) (15%), it can also result in systemic complications affecting multiple organ systems including the cardiovascular system such as venous and arterial thromboembolic events (10–25%; 31–59% of ICU patients), myocardial injury (20–30%, >25% of critically ill; >55% in those with pre-existing CVD), cardiomyopathy (7–33% of critically ill), arrhythmias (17%, 44% of ICU patients), and cerebrovascular disease (up to 8%). Additionally, acute kidney injury (9%), hepatocellular injury (19%), hyperglycaemia and ketosis, ocular symptoms, and dermatologic complications have been reported (2, 4–7).

Although long-term outcomes of patients surviving severe SARS-CoV-2 infection are unknown, these patients have the potential to suffer substantial sequelae comparable to those in patients surviving ARDS, sepsis, and other acute illnesses. Survival from sepsis, for example, is associated with increased risks for mortality up to 2 years, new cognitive impairment, new physical disability, recurrent infections, and continued health deterioration (4). Long-term sequelae observed in survivors of severe ARDS during H1N1 influenza include significant exertion dyspnea, decreased diffusion capacity across the blood-gas barrier, as well as reduced quality of life including reduced exercise capacity, anxiety, depression, and/ or development of post-traumatic stress disorder (8).

Follow-up CT imaging at 4 weeks in patients with Severe Acute Respiratory syndrome (SARS) showed that one third of patients with persistent respiratory symptoms had findings of fibrosis, including interlobular and intralobular reticulation, traction bronchiectasis and, more seldomly, honeycombing (9). In another CT study of convalescing SARS patients 51 days after symptom

Interdisciplinary Model for Scheduling Post-Discharge Cardiopulmonary Care of Patients Following Severe...

203

start, follow-up CT showed air trapping (92%) ground-glass opacities GGO (90%) and reticulation (70%). While GGO and reticulation resolved by 5 months, air trapping caused by damage to ciliated respiratory epithelium persisted in 80% of patients (10). In Middle-East Respiratory Syndrome (MERS), 33% of patients showed evidence of lung fibrosis, affecting primarily the elderly, patients with prolonged ICU stays and those with greater lung involvement during the acute phase of infection (9).

With respect to cardiac sequelae following severe respiratory disease in recovered SARS patients, cardiac impairment was observed by echocardiography studies in short-term 30-days follow-up, especially in more critically ill patients (10). In the majority of patients with community-acquired pneumonia (CAP), cardiac injury was seen in 30-days follow-up, likely caused by myocardial oxygen supply and demand mismatch as well as an activated inflammation/coagulation system (11).

The European Society of Cardiology recognizes that SARS-CoV-2 infection has major implications on the cardiovascular system and that patients within the context of Covid-19 have increased risk of morbidity and mortality, especially those with established cardiovascular disease, common in patients with severe infection (12). Severe and critical SARS-CoV-2 infection is associated with acute myocardial injury, cardiac arrhythmias, likely caused by infection-induced myocarditis or ischemia, all with potential for new disease development. Following pneumonia, hypercoagulability, and systemic inflammatory activity can persist thus exposing patients to elevated long-term CV risk, justifying surveillance (12). An interdisciplinary model for scheduling follow-up care may serve as a practical tool for healthcare professionals to ensure that any infection-related sequelae following hospitalization for severe SARS-CoV-2 infection are identified and appropriately managed.

METHODOLOGY

European Center for Disease Prevention and Control reports (ECDC), Center for Disease Control (CDC USA) and National Institutes of Health (NIH USA) reports, WHO Interim Guidance Reports, and current 2020 PubMed articles evaluating SARS-CoV-2 virus manifestations, diagnosis, severity, and discharge criteria of patients with confirmed Covid-19 were reviewed. PubMed Articles describing short and long-term outcomes in SARS, MERS, pneumonia, acute respiratory syndrome ARDS, and sepsis were evaluated.

RATIONALE

The ECDC published a technical report in March 2020 comparing diverging international discharge and de-isolation criteria of patients hospitalized with Covid-19 found in national guidelines of Italy, China, Singapore, and the

USA, and offered its own recommendations for discharge based on:

- Clinical criteria (e.g., no fever >3 days), improved respiratory symptoms, pulmonary imaging evidencing obvious absorption of inflammation, clinical assessment
- Laboratory evidence of SARS-CoV-2 clearance in respiratory samples, 2–4 negative RT- PCR tests for respiratory tract samples (nasopharynx and throat swabs with sampling interval ≥24 h) and if possible, serology with appearance of specific IgG (13).

With respect to post-discharge follow-up care, however, guidance is scant. The CDC China recommends that patients have follow-up visits 2 and 4 weeks after discharge, the National Centre for Infectious Diseases Singapore recommends clinic follow-up if indicated and daily wellness calls until day 14 after exposure, and the ECDC recommends 14 days of further isolation following discharge with regular health monitoring such as follow-up visits and phone calls, although specific guidance with respect to follow-up scope and content is not yet given (13).

The WHO report *Interim Guidance: Clinical Management of Covid 19,* released 27 May 2020 however anticipates potential sequelae in patients with severe and critical SARS-CoV-2 infection following treatment with mechanical ventilation, sedation, and/or prolonged bed rest based on evidence from general critical care populations. Post-intensive care syndrome (PICS) and severe respiratory illness may result in "a range of impairments including (but not limited to) physical deconditioning, reduced exercise tolerance, persisting fatigue, difficulties with activities of daily living, respiratory, swallow, cognitive, and mental health impairments" (14). According to WHO data, older people and patients of all ages with chronic diseases may be most susceptible to its impacts, including some patients recovering from severe COVID-19 who did not require admission to an ICU. The WHO recommends that patients must be referred for tailored inpatient, outpatient or community-based follow-up from post-acute to long term as indicated according to patient needs, with involvement of primary health care providers, relevant specialists, rehabilitation professionals, mental health, and psychosocial providers and social care services for coordinated care (14). A coordinated post-discharge care concept for patients surviving Covid-19 is therefore warranted to identify any cardiopulmonary sequelae and to mitigate possible worsening of preexisting disease following severe and critical SARS-Cov-2 infection. The literature has shown benefit of a well-structured transition phase to improve treatment outcomes and reduce readmission rates in management of other diseases such as heart failure, which may also develop in some patients following the infection (15–17).

While data examining residual effects after recovery from Covid-19 are still sparse, a number of sequelae especially affecting lung and heart function can be extrapolated from current literature. Initially defined by its pulmonary pathology and likely mediated via binding of SARS-CoV2 to ACE2 on

TABLE 1 | Interdisciplinary model for scheduling post-discharge cardiopulmonary care following severe and critical SARS-CoV-2 infection.

Discharge	❖ **Scheduling for patients following severe or critical SARS-CoV-2 infection** ❖ **Scheduling for patients following moderate SARS-CoV-2 infection with exacerbation/worsening of preexisting comorbidities**
Medical professionals at discharge	• Schedule lab work (see parameters below) • Schedule chest CT scan for 1–2 months post discharge (unenhanced low dose CT), at index hospital if possible; chest x-ray (CXR) if CT not available • Schedule follow-up with **General Practitioner** at 1–2 months post-discharge • Evaluate, prescribe, discuss dischargemedications, any O_2 use, care plan / appointments **with patient**, provide written instructions • If transfer to inpatient rehabilitation or long-term care facility, provide written instructions and care plan to managing physician • Involve **social worker/psychologist/nurse** where needed to address short, intermediate, long-term care/support (e.g., PTSD, psychological disorders, care provision) • Discuss potential participation and consent patient for any national/international registries or clinical trials and schedule appointments per protocol
1–2 months post-discharge	❖ **Diagnostic Testing, Care Coordination by GP/Internist,** ❖ **Referral and continued Follow-up when indicated**
Laboratory	• Complete Blood Count, C-Reactive Protein, LDH, AST/ALT, Urea, Glucose, Thrombin Time, Fibrinogen, Ferritin • Cardiac Biomarkers: CK, CK-MB, Troponin, NT-pBNP • For diabetes patients, also: Hemoglobin A1c • For Cancer patients, additional testing as instructed by managing oncologist
Radiologist	• Chest CT, or if not available, chest x-ray (CXR)
General practitioner/internist	• Clinical evaluation of symptoms (dyspnea, fatigue, psychological disorders) • Auscultation (determine signs of pulmonary fibrosis), • Oxygen saturation • ECG • Evaluation of laboratory, radiology and clinical findings, discussion with patient • Referral for further specialist examinations (e.g., **pulmonologist, cardiologist**) if indicated • Referral to **neurologist, nephrologist, endocrinologist** by suspicion of sequelae • Evaluate, prescribe, discuss discharge medications, any O_2 use, and care plan with patient, provide written instructions • Involve social worker/psychologist if further support needed
Pulmonologist (if indicated)	• CT evaluation and discussion with patient • Physical exam: signs and symptoms • Lung function test • 6 min walk test • Blood-gas test • Reevaluation of medications, O_2 use • Determine need for rehabilitation or intermediate/long-term care • Address primary/secondary prevention measures where applicable • Plan 6 and 12 month follow-up by any evidence of reduced functional capacity • Communicate findings and treatment plan to patient and general practitioner
Cardiologist (if indicated)	• Physical exam: signs and symptoms • ECG • Transthoracic echocardiography • Reevaluation/adjustments of medications • For patients with signs of heart failure: enrollment in heart failure program; for all HF patients: evaluate need for visiting heart failure nurse/rehabilitation program • For patients with arrhythmias, plan further evaluation (i.e., Holter monitoring, event recorder) • Address primary/secondary prevention measures where applicable • Schedule follow-up if appropriate • Communicate findings and treatment plan to patient and general practitioner
After 2 months	**Follow-up as needed and at the discretion of managing specialists**

CT, computed tomography; CXR, chest X-ray; LDH, lactate acid dehydrogenase; AST, aspartate aminotransferase; ALT, alanine aminotransferase; CK, Creatinkinase; CK-MB, Creatinkinase-MB; NT-pBNP, N-terminal pro b-type Natriuretic Peptide; O_2, oxygen; QoL, Quality of Life.

lung epithelia, Covid-19 may have significant effects on long term-outcome with respect to pulmonary function. According to Shi et al., lung abnormalities such as bilateral ground-glass opacities progressing to or coexisting with consolidations were observable in CT imaging within 1–3 weeks of SARS-Cov-2 infection (18). Pulmonary fibrosis may occur due to scarring of the lung tissue, as was observed in SARS and MERS, potentially causing significant reduction in lung function and exercise capacity (19, 20), thus warranting follow-up in surviving Covid-19 target populations. Thoracic imaging with chest radiography (CRX) and computed tomography (CT) are key tools for pulmonary disease diagnosis and management (21). CT, however, is more sensitive for detecting parenchymal lung disease, disease progression, and alternate diagnoses. Therefore, in patients with reduced lung capacity and radiological signs of fibrosis at 1–2 months, continued follow-up according to ATS/ACCP guidelines will be required.

Recent publications have also shown direct endothelial cell involvement of vascular beds of different organs by the SARS-CoV-2 virus (22). This should be considered as a reason for cardiovascular events, endotheliitis of lung, heart, kidney, and liver, as well as liver cell necrosis. Covid-19 is characterized by coagulation activation with a high rate of venous and arterial thromboembolic events, including venous thromboembolism, pulmonary embolism, disseminated intravascular coagulation, or cardiovascular events (23). Coagulation testing is therefore warranted and subsequent therapy may be indicated.

Covid-19 may induce new cardiac pathologies and/or exacerbate underlying cardiovascular disease (24). Thus, cardiologists will aim to evaluate residual cardiovascular effects and myocardial injury following SARS-Cov-2 infection. Systemic inflammatory response coupled with localized vascular inflammation may lead to plaque rupture and activation of coagulation cascades, endangering patients for acute coronary syndromes (25). Heart failure may develop following myocarditis, sepsis, or multi-organ failure during infection, or may be caused by treatment side effects. Inflammation and ACE2 downregulation with ensuing endothelial dysfunction can translate into diastolic dysfunction, while hypoxemia may lead to right ventricular dysfunction indicative of myocardial injury. Thus, transthoracic echocardiography may be considered to evaluate left and right ventricular global function, any regional dysfunction, end-diastolic cavity dimensions as well as pericardial thickening or effusion (26). Additionally, cardiac MRI may better reflect structural pathologies of inflammatory myocardial damage. Cardiac arrhythmias, possibly caused by metabolic disarray, hypoxia, neuro-hormonal, or inflammatory stress, have also been associated with the infection (27) and if present will need follow-up evaluation. Cardiologists should be aware of the risk for development of chronic thromboembolic pulmonary hypertension in patients who experienced pulmonary embolism during infection (28). Follow-up is also an opportunity to address primary and secondary prevention strategies for cardiovascular risk control in all patients.

As the short, intermediate and long-term effects of Covid-19 are unknown, patients should be encouraged to participate in national and international registries or clinical studies to facilitate study of this disease. The monitoring of immune effects is also of particular importance.

POST-DISCHARGE CARE MODEL

The proposed interdisciplinary model for scheduling post-discharge cardiopulmonary care of patients following SARS-Cov-2 infection (see **Table 1**) may serve as a practical guide for healthcare professionals to ensure that patients surviving severe and critical infection receive adequate cardiopulmonary follow-up care as we learn more about the residual and potentially chronic effects of the SARS-Cov-2 infection.

Target patient populations for post-discharge Covid-19 follow-up care include:

- Patients who experienced **severe illness*** defined as individuals who had respiratory frequency >30 breaths per minute, SpO_2 < 94% on room air at sea level, a ratio of arterial partial pressure of oxygen to fraction of inspired oxygen (PaO_2/FiO_2) <300 mmHg, or lung infiltrates 50% (e.g., patients treated at an ICU requiring invasive ventilation or CPAP during SARS-CoV-2 infection)
- Patients who experienced **critical illness***, defined as individuals who had respiratory failure, septic shock, and/or multiple organ dysfunction (e.g., patients treated at an ICU requiring ECMO during SARS-CoV-2 infection)
- Patients with chronic conditions (e.g., COPD, cardiomyopathy, coronary artery disease, cancer, chronic kidney disease, hepatic disease, and uncontrolled diabetes) in the presence of disease exacerbation or progression during/following moderate*, severe and critical SARS-CoV-2 infection, where moderate infection is defined as individuals with evidence of lower respiratory disease by clinical assessment, imaging and a saturation of oxygen (SpO_2) > 94% on room air at sea level.

* denotes NIH definitions of moderate, severe and critical illness (5).

As no guidelines on the timing of follow-up care for Covid-19 patients yet exist, this model schedules follow-up to occur at 1–2 months post-discharge based on several considerations. According to the previously cited radiological studies evaluating sequelae in patients following SARS and MERS infection, radiological follow-up was performed 1–2 months after start of infection (9, 10). In patients with confirmed pulmonary fibrosis, the American Thoracic Society recommends mid- to long-term follow up in 4–6-months intervals (29). With respect to cardiac involvement and the timing of follow-ups, the ACCF/AHA Guideline for the Management of Heart Failure was consulted with respect to recommendations for transition of care following hospitalization for acute cardiac decompensation. A follow-up visit within 7–14 days and/or a telephone follow-up within 3 days of discharge for acute cardiac decompensation is deemed a Class IIa recommendation (17). The 2016 *European Society of Cardiology Guidelines for the diagnosis and treatment of acute and chronic heart failure* detail the benefits of regular monitoring of heart failure patients, especially during periods of instability or for optimization of medications, noting benefits especially in older patients. Although timing of follow-up is not detailed, the ESC recommends provision of written action plans and prescheduling follow-up appointments shortly after discharge of patients with acute heart failure to reduce readmission rates (16). Therefore, scheduling transition care for Covid-19 patients potentially suffering from residual cardiopulmonary effects of the infection shortly after discharge is merited. The planning of post-discharge evaluations in the dynamic context of a pandemic, however, must be adapted with respect to post-discharge isolation recommendations, logistics, resource utilization, and health care system overburden. Thus, evaluation within 1–4 weeks post discharge at the height of a pandemic may not feasible for many patients. The model below suggests scheduling follow-up at 1–2 months, if not sooner, according to need and availability.

CARE PATHWAY

Hospital discharge personnel coordinate follow-up laboratory and radiological examinations, schedule a subsequent appointment with the patient's general practitioner or internist, and provide patient with written instructions. The patient's primary care physician or internist will serve as follow-up care coordinator. The interdisciplinary model provides guidance for specialist referral and testing dependent upon the patient's signs and symptoms, as well as radiological and laboratory findings. Due to the association of a more severe course of Covid-19 in those patients with underlying comorbidities, especially those with concomitant cardiovascular and pulmonary diseases, timely follow-up is imperative to identify any worsening of conditions and to initiate or adapt guideline-recommended therapies.

COST ANALYSIS

We estimate that the costs per patient of the basic follow-up (Radiology, Lab, GP) to be € 1,026 according to the Austrian tariff system. In patients requiring specialist evaluation, an additional € 249 for pulmonary consultation and € 527 for cardiological consultation are estimated. However, cost-effectiveness cannot yet be determined until intermediate and long-term data become available for analysis.

CONCLUSION

Short, intermediate and long-term effects following severe and critical SARS-CoV-2 infection are unknown, and significant sequelae may be expected, especially in patient populations experiencing ARDS, sepsis, and/or multiple organ dysfunction, as well as patients with exacerbation or progression of preexisting pulmonary or cardiovascular disease. Coordinated post-discharge management of Covid-19 patients is essential to identify and manage potential pulmonary or cardiovascular sequelae and mitigate worsening of pre-existing conditions following infection. This interdisciplinary model for scheduling follow-up care may serve as a practical tool for healthcare professionals to ensure that patients receive adequate treatment and post-discharge care following hospitalization for severe and critical SARS-CoV-2 infection.

AUTHOR CONTRIBUTIONS

KK wrote the manuscript. ML, LM, AE, HS, JT, and HM revised the manuscript. UH provided supervision. BL and AD provided supervision and revised the manuscript. All authors contributed to the article and approved the submitted version.

REFERENCES

1. Stokes EK, Zambrano LD, Anderson KN, Marder EP, Raz KM, El Burai Felix S, et al. Coronavirus disease 2019 case surveillance—United States, January 22–May 30, 2020. *MMWR*. (2020) 69:759–65. doi: 10.15585/mmwr.mm6924e2

2. Wiersinga WJ, Rhodes A, Cheng AC, Peacock SJ, Prescott HC. Pathophysiology, transmission, diagnosis, and treatment of coronavirus disease 2019 (COVID-19): a review. *JAMA*. (2020). doi: 10.1001/jama.2020.12839. [Epub ahead of print].

3. Wu Z, McGoogan JM. Characteristics of and important lessons from the coronavirus disease 2019 (COVID-19) outbreak in China: summary of a report of 72,314 cases from the Chinese Center for Disease Control and Prevention. *JAMA*. (2020) 323:1239–42. doi: 10.1001/jama.2020.2648

4. Gupta A, Madhavan MV, Sehgal K, Nair N, Mahajan S, Sehrawat TS, et al. Extrapulmonary manifestations of COVID-19. *Nat Med*. (2020) 26:1017–32. doi: 10.1038/s41591-020-0968-3

5. COVID-19 Treatment Guidelines Panel. *Coronavirus Disease 2019 (COVID-19) Treatment Guidelines*. National Institutes of Health. (2020). Available online at: https://www.covid19treatmentguidelines.nih.gov/ (accessed July 20, 2020).

6. Center for Disease Control. *Interim Clinical Guidance for Management of Patients with Confirmed Coronavirus Disease (COVID-19) National Center for Immunization and Respiratory Diseases (NCIRD), Division of Viral Diseases*. Available online at: https://www.cdc.gov/coronavirus/2019-ncov/

hcp/clinical-guidance-management-patients.html#clinical-course (accessed July 20, 2020).

7. Clerkin K, Fried J, Raikhelkar J, Sayer G, Griffin J, Masoumi A, et al. Covid-19 and cardiovascular disease. *Circulation*. (2020). 141:1648–55. doi: 10.1161/CIRCULATIONAHA.120.046941

8. Luyt C, Combes A, Becquemin MH, Beigelman-Aubry C, Hatem S, Brun A-L, et al. Long-term outcomes of pandemic 2009 influenza A(H1N1)-associated severe ARDS. *Chest*. (2012) 142:583–92. doi: 10.1378/chest.11-2196

9. Hosseiny M, Kooraki S, Gholamrezanezhad A, Reddy S, Myers L. Radiology perspective of coronavirus disease 2019 (COVID-19): lessons from severe acute respiratory syndrome and middle east respiratory syndrome. *Am J Roentgenol*. (2020) 214:1078–82. doi: 10.2214/AJR.20.22969

10. Li SS, Cheng C-w, Fu C-l, Chan Y-h, Lee M-p, Chan JW-m, et al. Left ventricular performance in patients with severe acute respiratory syndrome: a 30-days echocardiographic follow-up study. *Circulation*. (2003) 108:1798–803. doi: 10.1161/01.CIR.0000094737.21775.32

11. Frencken JF, van Baal L, Kappen TH, Donker DW, Horn J, van der Poll T, et al. Myocardial injury in critically ill patients with community-acquired pneumonia. A cohort study. *Ann Am Thorac Soc*. (2019) 16:606–12. doi: 10.1513/AnnalsATS.201804-286OC

12. The European Society for Cardiology. *ESC Guidance for the Diagnosis and Management of CV Disease during the COVID-19 Pandemic*. (2020). Available online at: https://www.escardio.org/Education/COVID-19-and-Cardiology/ESC-COVID-19-Guidance (accessed June 10, 2020).

13. European Centre for Disease and Control. *Technical Report: Novel Coronavirus (SARS-CoV-2) Discharge Criteria for Confirmed Covid-19 Cases-When Is it Safe to Discharge Cases Form the Hospital or End Home Isolation?* Available online at: https://www.ecdc.europa.eu/en/publications-data/covid-19-guidance-discharge-and-ending-isolation (accessed July 20, 2020).

14. World Health Organization. *Guidance Document: Clinical Management of Covid-19.* (2020). Available online at: https://www.who.int/publications/i/item/clinical-management-of-covid-19 (accessed July 20, 2020).

15. Mueller C, Bally K, Buser M, Flammer AJ, Gaspoz J-M, Mach F, et al. Roadmap for the treatment of heart failure patients after hospital discharge: an interdisciplinary consensus paper. *Swiss Med Wkly.* (2020) 150:w20159. doi: 10.4414/smw.2020.20159

16. Ponikowski P, Voors A, Anker S. Bueno H, Cleland JGF, Coats AJS, et al. 2016 ESC Guidelines for the diagnosis and treatment of acute and chronic heart failure: The Task Force for the diagnosis and treatment of acute and chronic heart failure of the European Society of Cardiology (ESC) developed with a special contribution of the Heart failure Association (HFA) of the ESC. *Eur Heart J.* (2016) 37:2129–200. doi: 10.1093/eurheartj/ehw128

17. Yancy C, Jessup M, Bozkurt B, Butler J, Casey DE Jr, Colvin MM, et al. 2013 ACCF/AHA guideline for the management of heart of heart failure. A report from the American College of Cardiology Foundation/Amarican Heart Association Task Force on Practical Guidelines. *Circulation.* (2013) 136:e137–161. doi: 10.1161/CIR.0000000000000509

18. Shi H, Han, X, Jiang, N, Cao Y, Alwalid O, Gu J, et al. Radiological Findings from 81 patients with COVID-19 pneumonia in Wuhan, China: a descriptive Study. *Lancet.* (2020) 20:425–34. doi: 10.1016/S1473-3099(20)30086-4

19. Venkataraman T, Frieman MB. The role of epidermal growth factor receptor (EGFR) signaling in SARS. *Antiviral Res.* (2017) 143:142–50. doi: 10.1016/j.antiviral.2017.03.022

20. Hui D, Ko F, Chan D, et al. The long-term impact of severe acute respiratory syndrome (SARS) on pulmonary function, exercise capacity and quality of life in a cohort of survivors. *CHEST J.* (2005) 128 doi: 10.1378/chest.128.4_MeetingAbstracts.148S-b

21. Rubin GD, Ryerson CJ, Haramati LB, Sverzellati N, Kanne JP, Raoof S, et al. The role of chest imaging in patient management during the COVID-19 pandemic: a Multinational Consensus Statement from the Fleischner Society. *Radiology.* (2020) 296:172–80. doi: 10.1148/radiol.2020201365

22. Varga Z, Flammer A., Steiger P, Haberecker M, Andermatt R, Zinkernagel AS, et al. Endothelial cell infection and endotheliitis in Covid-19. *Lancet.* (2020) 395:1417–8. doi: 10.1016/S0140-6736(20)30937-5

23. Lodigiani C, Iapichino G, Carenzo L, Cecconi M, Ferrazzi P, Sebastian T, et al. Venous and arterial thromboembolic complications in COVID-19 patients admitted to an academic hospital in Milan, Italy. *Thromb Res.* (2020) 191:9–14. doi: 10.1016/j.thromres.2020.04.024

24. Madjid M, Safavi-Naeini P, Solomon SD, Vardeny O. Potential effects of coronaviruses on the cardiovascular system: a review. *JAMA Cardiol.* (2020). doi: 10.1001/jamacardio.2020.1286

25. Hansson GK, Libby P, Tabas I. Inflammation and plaque vulnerability. *J Intern Med.* (2015) 278:483–93. doi: 10.1111/joim.12406

26. Moreo A, Pontone G, Gimelli A. *European Association of Cardiovascular Imaging, EACVI Webinar on COVID-19.* (2020). Available online at: https://www.escardio.org/Education/E-Learning/Webinars/EACVI-Webinar-on-COVID-19 (accessed April 30, 2020).

27. Driggin, E, Madhavan, M, Bikdeli, B, Chuich T, Laracy J, Biondi-Zoccai G, et al. Cardiovascular considerations for patients, health care workers and health systems during the coronavirus disease 2019 /Covid-19 pandemic. *JACC.* (2020) 75:31. doi: 10.1016/j.jacc.2020.03.031

28. Poissy J, Goutay J, Caplan M, Parmentier E, Duburcq T, Lassalle F, et al. Pulmonary embolism in COVID-19 patients: awareness of an increased prevalence. *Circulation.* (2020) 142:182–6. doi: 10.1161/CIRCULATIONAHA.120.047430

29. Raghu G, Collard HR, Egan JJ, Martinez FJ, Behr J, Brown KK, et al. An official ATS/ERS/JRS/ALAT statement: idiopathic pulmonary fibrosis: evidence-based guidelines for diagnosis and management an official ATS/ERS/JRS/ALAT statement: idiopathic pulmonary fibrosis: evidence-based guidelines for diagnosis and management. *Am J Respiratory Crit Care Med.* 183:788–824. doi: 10.1164/rccm.2009-040GL

25

Implementation and Evaluation of Virtual Anticoagulation Clinic Care to Provide Incessant Care during COVID-19 Times in an Indian Tertiary Care Teaching Hospital

Sunil Kumar Shambu[1]*, Shyam Prasad Shetty B[2], Oliver Joel Gona[3], Nagaraj Desai[1], Madhu B[4], Ramesh Madhan[3] and Revanth V[3]

[1] Department of Cardiology, Jagadguru Sri Shivarathreeshwara Medical College and Hospital, Jagadguru Sri Shivarathreeshwara Academy of Higher Education and Research (JSS AHER), Mysore, India, [2] Department of Cardiothoracic and Vascular Surgery, Jagadguru Sri Shivarathreeshwara Medical College and Hospital, Jagadguru Sri Shivarathreeshwara Academy of Higher Education and Research (JSS AHER), Mysore, India, [3] Department of Pharmacy Practice, Jagadguru Sri Shivarathreeshwara College of Pharmacy (JSS CPM), Jagadguru Sri Shivarathreeshwara Academy of Higher Education and Research (JSS AHER), Mysore, India, [4] Department of Community Medicine, Jagadguru Sri Shivarathreeshwara Medical College and Hospital, Jagadguru Sri Shivarathreeshwara Academy of Higher Education and Research (JSS AHER), Mysore, India

*Correspondence:
Sunil Kumar Shambu
sunil_cardio@yahoo.co.in;
sunilkumars@jssuni.edu.in

Background: COVID-19 caused by severe acute respiratory syndrome coronavirus 2 (SARS-CoV-II) has become a global pandemic disrupting public health services. Telemedicine has emerged as an important tool to deliver care during these situations. Patients receiving Vitamin K antagonists (VKA) require structured monitoring which has posed a challenge during this pandemic. We aimed to evaluate the impact of Virtual anticoagulation clinic (VAC), a Telehealth model on the quality of anticoagulation, adverse events, and patient satisfaction vis-a-vis standard Anticoagulation clinic (ACC) care.

Materials and methods: A bidirectional cohort study was conducted in the Department of Cardiology, JSS Hospital, Mysore. Two hundred and twenty-eight patients in the VAC and 274 patients in the ACC fulfilling inclusion criteria were the subjects of the study. Telehealth tools like WhatsApp and telephone were used. Time in therapeutic range (TTR), Percentage of International normalized ratio in range (PINRR), and adverse events were analyzed and compared between the VAC group and the ACC group, between pre-COVID and COVID ACC groups, and between the VAC group and the same pre-COVID cohort. Patient satisfaction was assessed by a questionnaire at the end of 8 months. Descriptive statistics were used for the patient characteristics and inferential statistics for the comparisons between pre-VAC and VAC care.

Results: The mean TTR was $75.4 \pm 8.9\%$ and $71.2 \pm 13.4\%$ in the VAC group and ACC group, respectively ($p < 0.001$). The mean PINRR was $66.7 \pm 9.4\%$ and $62.4 \pm 10.9\%$ in the VAC group and ACC group respectively, ($p < 0.001$). There was no significant difference in TTR between the VAC group and the same pre-COVID cohort. The TTR differential between the pre-COVID and COVID ACC groups was significant. In either group, no major adverse events were seen. The most common tools used for data exchange were WhatsApp (83%) and SMS (17%). Seventy-four percent of patients were extremely satisfied with the overall VAC care.

Conclusions: Virtual anticoagulation clinic, a telehealth model can be used as an alternative option to deliver uninterrupted anticoagulation care during pandemic times.

Keywords: anticoagulation clinic, vitamin K antagonist, time in therapeutic range, percentage of international normalized ratio in range, telehealth

INTRODUCTION

COVID-19 caused by severe acute respiratory syndrome coronavirus 2 (SARS-CoV-II) has become a global pandemic disrupting public health services (1). In these time frames, effective clinical care for patients with various chronic cardiovascular and other disorders has gained considerable attention from various stakeholders (2). In this predicament, Telehealth a virtual platform for the care provider and seeker has great potential in providing cardiovascular care which is evidently quite ideal (3). Its utility for patients on oral anticoagulants is one domain that needs to be addressed. Of the anticoagulants, vitamin K antagonists (VKAs) have a narrow therapeutic index with variable dose-response and diet/drug interactions (4). Patients taking VKAs require International normalized ratio (INR) monitoring and dose titration to achieve therapeutic INR for optimal outcomes (5). Patients taking VKAs may have multiple comorbidities like advanced age, hypertension, diabetes mellitus, and others. Studies have shown that patients with these risk factors are susceptible to severe COVID-19 infection necessitating a strategy to mitigate exposure of such patients (6, 7).

Telehealth services help to provide patients with the necessary care while minimizing the risk of transmitting SARS-CoV-II to healthcare workers and patients (8). The notion of telemedicine was incorporated in the Anticoagulation clinic to provide uninterrupted virtual care to patients taking VKAs. This study was conducted to evaluate the impact of Virtual anticoagulation clinic care (VAC) on the quality of anticoagulation, adverse events, and patient satisfaction vis-a-vis standard ACC care.

MATERIALS AND METHODS

Study Design and Participants

A bidirectional observational cohort study was conducted on patients enrolled in the VAC and ACC at the Department of Cardiology, JSS Hospital, Mysore from March to November 2020. Institutional ethical committee approval was taken. A total of 521 patients were registered in ACC till March 2020. Among these, 234 patients opted for VAC care and 287 patients opted for ACC care. For calculation of TTR, patients who had more than 3 months of ACC care before March 2020 with at least 3 INR values in both groups were included in the study. Newly enrolled patients in the ACC and those patients who had less than 3 months of ACC care before March 2020 were excluded from the study. A total of 228 patients in the VAC care group and 274 patients in the standard ACC care group were eligible for analysis. The patient enrolment process is depicted in **Figure 1**.

Anticoagulation Quality Assessment Tools

The anticoagulation related quality measures like Percentage Time in Therapeutic Range (%TTR) (9), Percentage of INR within Range (PINRR) (10), extreme INRs, and adverse events were analyzed. Patient satisfaction toward VAC care was assessed by administering five items self-developed questionnaire with scores 0 to 4 from extremely satisfied to not at all satisfied at the end of 8 months.

Anticoagulation Clinic (ACC)

JSS Hospital, Mysore has an established ACC since February 2017 comprising a multidisciplinary team comprising a Senior cardiologist, Junior cardiologist, Clinical Pharmacist, Clinical Pharmacy interns, and trained nursing staff. Key issues such as patient education (VKA risks/benefits, potential diet/drug interactions), ordering relevant laboratory tests (once a month INR testing), titrating the dose of VKAs to meet the INR target, facilitating procedures requiring interruption of VKAs, and adverse effects associated with VKAs were addressed.

Virtual Anticoagulation Clinic (VAC)

VAC was initiated in March 2020 to provide sustained care to patients taking VKAs registered in ACC during the COVID-19 pandemic. Telehealth tools like WhatsApp and telephone were used as per Telemedicine practice guidelines (11). WhatsApp and SMS were used for the asynchronous exchange of the data. Patients were supposed to undergo INR testing once a month and communicate the INR report and if any symptoms related to bleeding, Transient Ischemic Attack (TIA), or stroke by any of the tools quoting their ACC identification number. Based on the INR value, dose titration was done and advice regarding the next INR testing was given. Patients with INR <1.5 and INR >5.0, major bleeding, and systemic embolic events were advised for the hospital visit. TTR and PINRR were calculated by Rosendaal linear interpolation technique for each patient. Calculations were performed with the assistance of a template made available by INR Pro (12). Major bleeding was defined by the International Society on Thrombosis and Haemostasis criteria (13). Stroke/Systemic embolic events were defined as the combined endpoints of ischaemic stroke, TIA, and systemic embolic events.

Statistical Analysis

Data was entered in MS Office Excel 2019 and analyzed by using IBM SPSS Statistics Version 25. Continuous variables were expressed as mean ± standard deviation (SD). Categorical variables were expressed as absolute numbers and percentages. Descriptive statistics were

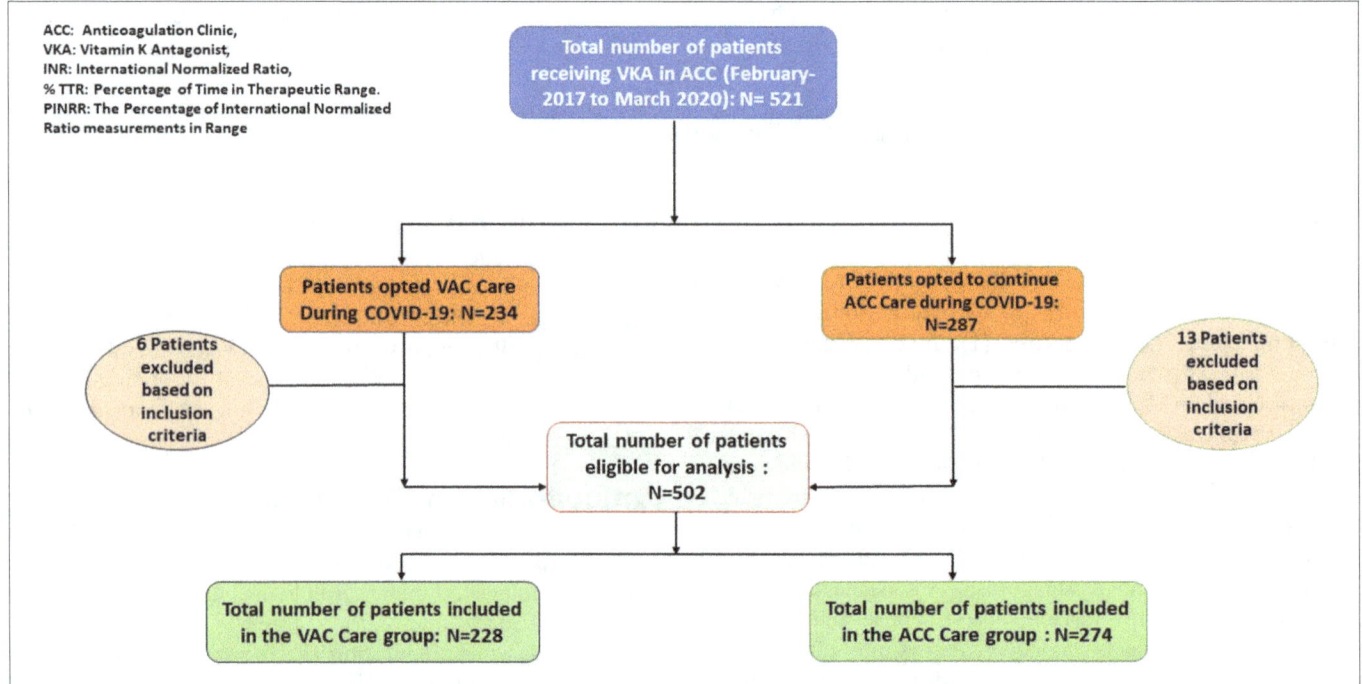

FIGURE 1 | Participant enrolment process. ACC, Anticoagulation clinic; VKA, Vitamin K Antagonist; INR, International Normalized Ratio; % TTR, Percentage of Time in Therapeutic Range; PINRR, The percentage of International Normalized Ratio measurements in Range. * EXCLUSION CRITERIA: Patients having less than 3 months of ACC exposure pre COVID-19 phase and less than 3 INR values were excluded from the study.

used for patient characteristics. *T*-test and chi-square tests (χ^2) were used for comparisons between groups. All tests were two-tailed, $p < 0.05$ was considered to be statistically significant.

RESULTS

The mean age of the patients in the VAC group and ACC group was 55.62 ± 13.77 years and 53.72 ± 11.8 years, respectively. The majority of the patients in the VAC group were from rural areas (57%). On the contrary, only 30% of the patients were from rural areas in the ACC group. Patients characteristics are depicted in **Table 1**. Atrial fibrillation was the most common indication for VKA therapy in both groups. Acenocoumarol was the most common VKA prescribed. Mean TTR in VAC group and ACC group was 75.4 ± 8.9% and 71.2 ± 13.4%, respectively (*p*-value = 0.001). Mean PINRR in the VAC group and ACC group was 66.7 ± 9.4% and 62.4 ± 10.9%, respectively (*p*-value = 0.0002). Patients in the VAC group underwent more frequent INR testing when compared to those in the ACC group. Two patients had a minor lower gastrointestinal bleed in the VAC group. None of the patients had major adverse events in either group. Three patients were scheduled for an in-person visit in the VAC group. Anticoagulation related parameters in the VAC group and ACC group are depicted in **Table 2**. There was no significant difference

in TTR between the VAC group and the same group during pre-COVID ACC care. There was a significant difference in TTR and PINRR between the pre-COVID and COVID-ACC groups (*p* <0.0001). The number of INR tests performed per patient was less in the ACC group during the COVID pandemic. Anticoagulation related parameters between the groups are depicted in **Table 3**.

WhatsApp 189 (83%), followed by SMS 39 (17%) were the most common tools used for the exchange of data. One hundred and sixty-nine (74%) of patients were extremely satisfied with overall VAC care and 187 (82%) of patients were extremely satisfied to continue virtual care as assessed by a 5-item questionnaire. The patient satisfaction score and questionnaire are depicted in **Figure 2** and **Table 4**.

DISCUSSION

In our study, the principal findings were (1) Patients in the VAC group had greater control of anticoagulation in the form of more time spent in the therapeutic range compared to ACC during the COVID pandemic (75.4 and 71.2%, respectively). (2) There was no significant difference in TTR between the VAC group and the same patients in the Pre-COVID ACC care 3). There was a significant difference in TTR between the pre-COVID and COVID ACC groups.

TABLE 1 | Patient characteristics and anticoagulation related parameters.

Variables	VAC (N = 228)	ACC (N = 274)	p-value
Age (years)			
<60	118 (51.6)	156 (57.07)	0.9077
>61	110 (48.4)	118 (42.93)	0.2208
Gender			
Men	129 (57)	167 (60.84)	0.3841
Women	99 (43)	107 (39.16)	
Comorbidities			
Type 2 Diabetes Mellitus	53 (23.4)	89 (32.54)	0.0239
Hypertension	73 (32)	90 (33.01)	0.8102
Congestive heart failure	18 (7.8)	36.1 (13.20)	0.0520
Vascular disease[#]	29 (12.5)	31 (11.32)	0.6842
Educational status			
Literate	162 (71.1)	247 (90.09)	<0.0001[††]
Illiterate	66 (28.9)	27 (9.9)	<0.0001[††]
Location of residence			
Urban	98 (43)	194 (70.82)	<0.0001[††]
Rural	130 (57)	80 (29.18)	<0.0001[††]
HASBLED score			
≥3	69 (30.4)	57 (20.75)	0.0132[††]
<3	158 (69.5)	217 (79.25)	0.0123[††]
Vitamin K Antagonist			
Warfarin	16 (7)	6 (2.36)	0.0121[††]
Acenocoumarol	212 (93)	268 (97.64)	0.0123[††]
Indications for VKA*			
Atrial fibrillation	137 (60)	192 (70.28)	0.0159[††]
Mechanical Valve replacement	8 (3.4)	44 (16.03)	<0.0001[††]
Deep vein thrombosis / Pulmonary embolism	80 (35.1)	38 (13.69)	<0.0001[††]
Cortical venous thrombosis	3 (1.5)	0	–

[#]Vascular disease: Coronary artery disease, Peripheral arterial disease; *VKA: Vitamin K antagonist.
[††] statistically significant p-value has been obtained by performing chi-squared test.

TABLE 2 | Anticoagulation related Quality Parameters.

Variables	VAC (N = 228)	ACC (N = 274)	p-value
Number of INR[†] draws (1,544)	1,324	1,019	-
Average number of INR[†] draws/ Patient	5.8	3.72	-
Mean TTR%[††]	75.4 ± 8.91	71.2 ± 13.4	0.0018[†]
Mean PINRR %**	66.7 ± 9.4 %	62.4 ± 10.9%	0.0002[†]
Tests Over Range	129 (9.7%)	113 (11.11%)	0.2660
Tests Below range	151 (11.7%)	142 (13.9%)	0.1124
Extreme INRs			
INR >5.0	14 (1.06)	15 (1.51)	0.3323
INR < 1.5	30 (2.26)	75 (7.32)	<0.0001
Adverse events			
Major	0 (0%)	0	-
Minor bleeding	2 (0.8%)	0	

[†]INR: International Normalized Ratio; **PINRR: Percentage of International Normalized Ratio in the Therapeutic Range; [††]TTR: Time in Therapeutic Range.
[††] statistically significant p-value has been obtained by performing chi-squared test.
[†] statistically significant p-value has been obtained by performing t-test.

AF on VKA therapy (20). In our study, achieved TTRs in both groups were above the proposed benchmark of >65–70%. One of the main reasons to achieve mean TTR > 70% in our study was because our cohort of patients were those registered in the ACC managed by a multidisciplinary team. Even randomized controlled trials and studies related to Anticoagulation clinics have documented better control of INR compared to community settings that were possible due to frequent monitoring, organized care, and improvement in adherence to VKAs (10, 17).

Other important and desirable points to note were that these patients had multiple comorbidities and could be treated with the reduced risk of exposure to COVID-19 infection during transit to the hospital, cost savings for travel, and no major adverse events. The majority of the patients were satisfied with overall virtual care and opted for virtual care even in the post-COVID state.

The tenable reasons for the patients to continue to benefit from following up in VAC are several. Patients were educated during their initial visits to the regular anticoagulation clinic about the importance of regular follow-up with PT/INR testing, risks of discontinuation, clinical benefits of continuous and uninterrupted use of VKAs. Also, the ease of contacting the care provider through dedicated service like a 24/7 contactable phone number could have helped the patients. Prior consultation on a one-to-one basis with the care provider may also have increased the confidence as it is reflected in the data on the satisfactory questionnaire. In our study, the majority of the patients (74%) were satisfied with overall virtual care. Eighty-two percent of the patients were extremely satisfied in continuing virtual care even in the post-COVID scenario.

In our study, 57% of the patients who availed virtual care were from rural areas. WhatsApp was the most common chat platform used. A recent study by the Internet & Mobile Association of India (IAMAI) and

Due to the COVID pandemic, healthcare was inaccessible to the majority of the patients. Telehealth-based VAC initiated during that period could deliver uninterrupted care to the patients on chronic VKA therapy. Patients in the virtual care group could maintain their mean TTR similar to that of ACC care during the pre-COVID state. Wherein patients in the ACC care group were unable to maintain the mean TTR because of less frequent INR testing and in-person visits. Similar telehealth-based studies conducted on patients with chronic warfarin therapy have reported mean TTRs ranging from 66 to 74% (14–16).

Several meta-analyses of randomized and real-world trials have found that TTRs and PINRRs are generally equal to or below 60% (10, 17, 18). The European consensus document recommends a TTR of >70% for optimal outcomes (19). NICE guidelines recommend a TTR of > 65% for patients with research by Neilsen, reported that there are 227 million active internet users in rural areas in India as of November 2019 (21). This digital penetration can transform the delivery of virtual care to patients with chronic diseases in remote locations.

Preferably, patients who require VKAs, must visit in person initially and ideally should achieve at least two consecutive INRs in the therapeutic range before they could be transitioned to virtual anticoagulation clinic care for optimal patient-centered outcomes.

This pilot study has paved a path of utilizing telehealth to manage patients on chronic VKA therapy during the COVID pandemic. Though short-term results are promising, more extensive and larger multi-centric studies with a longer duration of follow-up are required to assess the feasibility and efficacy of the virtual anticoagulation clinic.

TABLE 3 | Assessment of Anticoagulation parameters among Pre-VAC (pre COVID) and VAC care.

Anticoagulation parameters	VAC care (n = 228)	Pre-COVID care (n = 228)	p-value	ACC COVID-19 care (n = 274)	ACC pre-COVID care (n = 274)	p-value
Number of INR[†] draws	1,324	1,467		1,019	1,551	
Average number of INR[†] draws/ Patient	5.8	6.43	-	3.72	5.66	-
Mean TTR%[*]	75.4 ± 8.91	77.58 ± 8.85	0.0506[#]	71.2 ± 13.4	79.12 ± 9.3	<0.0001[#]
Mean PINRR %[**]	66.7 ± 9.4 %	69.68 ± 11.50	0.0241[#]	62.4 ± 10.9%	67.8 ± 10.4	<0.0001[#]
Tests Over Range	129 (9.7)	118 (8.1)	0.1375	113 (11.11)	96 (6.2)	<0.0001[††]
Tests Below range	151 (11.7)	106 (7.26)	0.0001[††]	142 (13.9)	129 (8.3)	<0.0001[††]
Extreme INRs						
INR >5.0	14 (1.06)	0	-	15 (1.51)	10 (0.66)	0.0339[††]
INR < 1.5	30 (2.26)	11 (0.75)	0.0009[††]	75 (7.32)	8 (0.5)	< 0.0001[††]
Adverse events						
Major	0 (0%)	0	-	0	0	-
Minor bleeding	2 (0.8%)	0		0	0	

[†] INR: International Normalized Ratio; [**]PINRR: Percentage of International Normalized Ratio in the Therapeutic Range [*]TTR: Time in Therapeutic Range.

[††] statistically significant p-value has been obtained by performing chi-squared test.

[#] statistically significant p-value has been obtained by performing t-test.

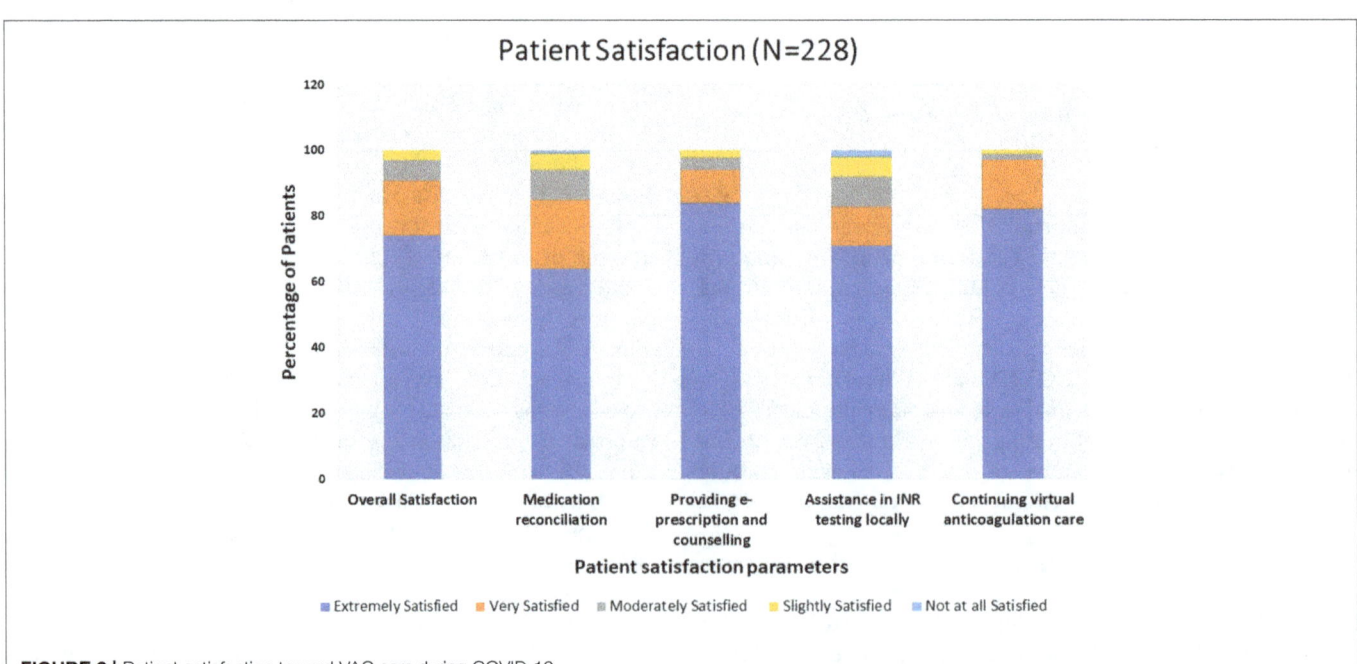

FIGURE 2 | Patient satisfaction toward VAC care during COVID-19.

Implementation and Evaluation of Virtual Anticoagulation Clinic Care to Provide Incessant Care during...

213

TABLE 4 | Patient satisfaction toward virtual anticoagulation care (VAC) during COVID-19 pandemic (N = 228).

S. No	Parameter*		Response** n (%)
1.	Overall satisfaction of patients on VAC care during COVID 19	Extremely satisfied (4)	168 (74)
		Very satisfied (3)	39 (17)
		Moderately satisfied (2)	14 (6)
		Slightly satisfied (1)	7 (3)
		Not at all satisfied (0)	(0)
2.	Medication reconciliation	Extremely satisfied (4)	146 (64)
		Very satisfied (3)	48 (21)
		Moderately satisfied (2)	20 (9)
		Slightly satisfied (1)	12 (5)
		Not at all satisfied (0)	2 (1)
3.	Providing e-prescription and education reinforcement (counseling)	Extremely satisfied (4)	192 (84)
		Very satisfied (3)	23 (10)
		Moderately satisfied (2)	8 (4)
		Slightly satisfied (1)	5 (2)
		Not at all satisfied (0)	(0)
4.	Assistance in INR monitoring locally despite lockdown during COVID 19	Extremely satisfied (4)	162 (71)
		Very satisfied (3)	27 (12)
		Moderately satisfied (2)	20 (9)
		Slightly satisfied (1)	14 (6)
		Not at all satisfied (0)	5 (2)
5.	Continuing virtual anticoagulation care	Extremely satisfied (4)	187 (82)
		Very satisfied (3)	34 (15)
		Moderately satisfied (2)	5 (2)
		Slightly satisfied (1)	2 (1)
		Not at all satisfied (0)	0

*Feedbacks for Q1 – Q7 were obtained through a 5-point Likert scale with scoring 0 – 4, 0 = Not at all Satisfied, 1 = Slightly Satisfied, 2 = Moderately Satisfied, 3 = Very Satisfied, 4 = Extremely Satisfied. **Data represented as frequency and proportion.*

STRENGTHS AND LIMITATIONS

The virtual anticoagulation clinic, a telehealth model that was developed during the onset of the COVID-19 pandemic to facilitate uninterrupted anticoagulation care, which could help maintain the quality of anticoagulation and minimize the risk of exposure to COVID-19. Our study has limitations such as single-center, lack of randomization, small patient population, and shorter duration of follow-up.

CONCLUSIONS

This preliminary study showed that a virtual anticoagulation clinic can serve as a feasible alternate care model to provide uninterrupted anticoagulation care for patients on chronic Vitamin K antagonist therapy during the COVID-19 pandemic.

AUTHOR CONTRIBUTIONS

All authors listed have made a substantial, direct and intellectual contribution to the work. SKS, SPSB, and OJG designed and formulated the hypothesis. RV and OJG performed data collection. SKS and OJG prepared manuscript. ND and RM reviewed the manuscript. MB, OJG, and SKS performed statistical planning and analysis. All the authors approved the manuscript for publication.

ACKNOWLEDGMENTS

We would like to thank JSS Hospital, Mysuru for facilitating the setup of the Virtual Anticoagulation clinic. We immensely thank Prof. Gurunarayana for his contribution to manuscript proofreading.

REFERENCES

1. Castagnoli R, Votto M, Licari A, Brambilla I, Bruno R, Perlini S, et al. Severe acute respiratory syndrome coronavirus 2 (SARS-CoV-II) infection in children and adolescents: a systematic review. *JAMA Pediatr.* (2020) 174:882–9. doi: 10.1001/jamapediatrics.2020.1467
2. Guo T, Fan Y, Chen M, Wu X, Zhang L, He T, et al. Cardiovascular implications of fatal outcomes of patients with coronavirus disease 2019 (COVID-19). *JAMA Cardiol.* (2020) 5:811–8. doi: 10.1001/jamacardio.2020.1017
3. Cutler DM, Nikpay S, Huckman RS. The business of medicine in the era of COVID-19. *JAMA.* (2020) 323:2003–4. doi: 10.1001/jama.2020.7242
4. Vranckx P, Valgimigli M, Heidbuchel H. The Significance of drug—Drug and drug—Food interactions of oral anticoagulation. *Arrhythmia Electrophysiol Rev.* (2018) 7:55. doi: 10.15420/aer.2017.50.1

5. Witt DM, Clark NP, Kaatz S, Schnurr T, Ansell JE. Guidance for the practical management of warfarin therapy in the treatment of venous thromboembolism. *J Thrombosis Thrombolysis.* (2016) 41:187–205. doi: 10.1007/s11239-015-1319-y
6. Shoeb M, Fang MC. Assessing bleeding risk in patients taking anticoagulants. *J Thrombosis Thrombolysis.* (2013) 35:312–9. doi: 10.1007/s11239-013-0899-7
7. Guan WJ, Liang WH, Zhao Y, Liang HR, Chen ZS, Li YM, et al. Comorbidity and its impact on 1590 patients with Covid-19 in China: a nationwide analysis. *Eur Respiratory J.* (2020) 55:2000547. doi: 10.1183/13993003.00547-2020
8. Bhaskar S, Bradley S, Chattu VK, Adisesh A, Nurtazina A, Kyrykbayeva S, et al. Telemedicine as the new outpatient clinic gone digital: position paper from the pandemic health system REsilience PROGRAM (REPROGRAM) international consortium (Part 2). *Front Public Health.* (2020) 8:410. doi: 10.3389/fpubh.2020.00410

9. Schmitt L, Speckman J, Ansell J. Quality assessment of anticoagulation dose management: comparative evaluation of measures of time-in-therapeutic range. *J Thrombosis Thrombolysis*. (2003) 15:213–6. doi: 10.1023/B:THRO.0000011377.78585.63

10. Mearns ES, White CM, Kohn CG, Hawthorne J, Song JS, Meng J, et al. Quality of vitamin K antagonist control and outcomes in atrial fibrillation patients: a meta-analysis and meta-regression. *Thrombosis J*. (2014) 12:1–20. doi: 10.1186/1477-9560-12-14

11. Telemedicine Practice Guidelines. *Enabling Registered Medical Practitioners to Provide Healthcare Using Telemedicine*. Available online at: https://www.mohfw.gov.in/pdf/Telemedicine.pdf (accessed July 1, 2020).

12. INR Pro. *Rosendaal method for % INR in range*. INR Pro. Available online at: www.inrpro.com/rosendaal.asp (accessed July 8, 2020).

13. Schulman S, Kearon C, Subcommittee on Control of Anticoagulation of the Scientific and Standardization Committee of the International Society on Thrombosis and Haemostasis. Definition of major bleeding in clinical investigations of antihemostatic medicinal products in non-surgical patients. *J Thrombosis Haemostasis*. (2005) 3:692–4. doi: 10.1111/j.1538-7836.2005.01204.x

14. Kelly JJ, Sweigard KW, Shields K, Schneider D. Safety, effectiveness, and efficiency: a Web-based virtual anticoagulation clinic. *Joint Commission J Quality Safety*. (2003) 29:646–51. doi: 10.1016/S1549-3741(03)29076-6

15. Chan FW, Wong RS, Lau WH, Chan TY, Cheng G, You JH. Management of Chinese patients on warfarin therapy in two models of anticoagulation service–a prospective randomized trial. *Br J Clin Pharmacol*. (2006) 62:601–9. doi: 10.1111/j.1365-2125.2006.02693.x

16. Ryan F, Byrne S, O'shea S. Randomized controlled trial of supervised patient self-testing of warfarin therapy using an internet-based expert system. *J Thrombosis Haemostasis*. (2009) 7:1284–90. doi: 10.1111/j.1538-7836.2009.03497.x

17. Haas S, Ten Cate H, Accetta G, Angchaisuksiri P, Bassand JP, Camm AJ, et al. Quality of vitamin K antagonist control and 1-year outcomes in patients with atrial fibrillation: a global perspective from the GARFIELD-AF registry. *PLoS ONE*. (2016) 11:e0164076. doi: 10.1371/journal.pone.0164076

18. Erkens PM, ten Cate H, Büller HR, Prins MH. Benchmark for time in therapeutic range in venous thromboembolism: a systematic review and meta-analysis. *PLoS ONE*. (2012) 7:e42269. doi: 10.1371/journal.pone.0042269

19. Camm AJ, Lip GY, De Caterina R, Savelieva I, Atar D, Hohnloser SH, et al. 2012 focused update of the ESC Guidelines for the management of atrial fibrillation: an update of the 2010 ESC Guidelines for the management of atrial fibrillation Developed with the special contribution of the European Heart Rhythm Association. *Eur Heart J*. (2012) 33:2719–47. doi: 10.1093/eurheartj/ehs253

20. National Clinical Guideline Centre (UK). *Atrial Fibrillation: The Management of Atrial Fibrillation*. London: National Institute for Health and Care Excellence (UK) (2014).

21. The Logical Indian. *Internet Usage In Rural India Surpasses Urban Areas For The First Time: Report*. Avaialble online at: https://thelogicalindian.com/news/internet-usage-rural-urban-india-20946 (accessed July 17, 2020).

26

The Notch Pathway: A Link between COVID-19 Pathophysiology and its Cardiovascular Complications

Randa M. Breikaa [1,2] and Brenda Lilly [1,3*]

[1] Center for Cardiovascular Research and The Heart Center, Nationwide Children's Hospital, Columbus, OH, United States,
[2] Molecular, Cellular and Developmental Biology Program, The Ohio State University, Columbus, OH, United States,
[3] Department of Pediatrics, The Ohio State University, Columbus, OH, United States

*Correspondence:
Brenda Lilly
brenda.lilly@nationwidechildrens.org

COVID-19 is associated with a large number of cardiovascular sequelae, including dysrhythmias, myocardial injury, myocarditis and thrombosis. The Notch pathway is one likely culprit leading to these complications due to its direct role in viral entry, inflammation and coagulation processes, all shown to be key parts of COVID-19 pathogenesis. This review highlights links between the pathophysiology of SARS-CoV2 and the Notch signaling pathway that serve as primary drivers of the cardiovascular complications seen in COVID-19 patients.

Keywords: notch signaling pathway, COVID-19, cardiovascular, vascular biology, cardiovascular disease

INTRODUCTION

Beginning in December 2019, the world faced a challenging nemesis presented by a member of the coronaviruses family, SARS-CoV2, later known as Coronavirus Disease 2019 or COVID-19 (1–3). First feared for its aggressive attack on the respiratory system (4, 5), it is now recognized for its severe cardiovascular complications (6–8). These range from hemodynamic instabilities, dysrhythmias, and thromboembolic events, to myocarditis, acute heart failure and cardiac arrest (9, 10). Analyzing patient data from several countries, cardiovascular disease appears in two contexts associated with COVID-19. First, studies have shown that pre-existing cardiovascular disease increases the risk of COVID-19 infection and is indeed present in a high number of cases (11–13). Second, COVID-19 patients develop cardiovascular complications during the course of the disease (14, 15). Despite a clear connection with COVID-19 and the cardiovascular system, we understand little about this relationship.

Notch signaling is a master regulator of cardiovascular function in both health and disease, and has been linked to several biological processes mediating viral infections (16, 17). A recent study by Rosa et al., characterized transcriptional signatures induced in a rhesus macaque model of SARS-CoV2 and showed an increase in Notch signaling in the lungs of the macaques (18). Another group studying human protein interactions with SARS-CoV2 using computational models, showed that proteins interacting with the 5'-region of SARS-CoV2 RNA were associated with Notch2 receptor signaling (19). The Notch pathway is also implicated in the hypoxic response and in coagulopathic processes, both of which are present in COVID-19 patients. These known roles of the Notch pathway make this signaling pathway a likely player in the COVID-19-driven cardiovascular complications.

THE BEGINNING (VIRAL ENTRY)

The angiotensin converting enzyme 2 (ACE2) has been established to play a significant role in SARS-CoV viruses infectivity, including COVID-19, by binding to the viral spike protein and facilitating entry into the host cell (20, 21). ACE2 has distinct roles in the body, ranging from amino acid transportation and catalytic activities, to serving as functional receptors for viruses like the coronaviruses. In the heart, it is localized to cardiomyocytes, cardiac fibroblasts, epicardial adipose tissue, and the coronary vascular endothelium. In the lungs, it is expressed on the cell surface of the inner respiratory tract, protecting against lung injury. This protective effect stems from its negative regulation of the renin-angiotensin system which leads to the inhibition of the vasoconstrictive, pro-inflammatory angiotensin II (ANGII)—ANGII type 1 receptor (AT1) axis (22–24). Its unique location in both organs combined with its function make it a pivotal player in the pulmonary pathogenicity of the virus and its associated cardiovascular complications. Thus, ACE2 on one hand offers protection against injury, while on the other hand facilitates viral entry. Furthermore, upon binding of ACE2 to the viral particle, the receptor itself becomes endocytosed by the cells causing depletion of cell surface ACE2 and its mediated tissue protection (25, 26). This dilemma and the realization of the importance of ACE2 in maintaining cardiovascular homeostasis drove attempts to manipulate the ACE2/ANGII axis to mitigate virus-induced injury, while minimizing the negative effects on the protective functions of ACE2 (20, 23). One solution for this problem and an attractive target for vaccine development are the viral S-proteins, which when targeted make the enzyme unable to bind, preventing viral entry (21, 27).

Notch signaling has been known to interact with many viral particles facilitating their infectivity (**Table 1**). Given that Notch regulates various proliferative and differentiation events in cells, it is no surprise that the pathway is an attractive target for viruses, which are dependent on the cell cycle machinery of the cell. Those viruses tap into the Notch pathway to ensure their own survival (60–62). The first evidence that demonstrated Notch pathway-viral interactions was reported for the Epstein-Barr virus, which targets RBPJ (mouse)/CBF1 (human), the nuclear effector of Notch (28, 63). Other examples include the human papilloma virus (HPV), hepatitis B virus (HBV), and hepatitis C virus (HCV). In the case of HCV, the Notch1 receptor has been shown to facilitate nuclear localization of p65 in response to tumor necrosis factor-alpha (TNF-α) in human hepatocytes, leading to increased pathogenicity of the virus (64). Additionally, the influenza virus has been shown to block the Notch ligand Delta-like 1 (DLL1) causing a heightened inflammatory response and decreased interferon-c levels, which leads to compromised immunity against the virus. In contrast, macrophages were found to enhance their DLL1 production during the course of infection to protect against the same virus (32, 33, 65). In the case of COVID-19, an interesting enzyme that could be linking Notch and COVID-19 activation is FURIN. FURIN is a member of the protein convertases family and is both an activator and a direct target of Notch activity (66, 67). Its enzymatic activity has

been proven to be exploited by a variety of bacteria and viruses, including measles, yellow fever, ebola, and avian influenza, thereby facilitating their virulence and spread (68, 69). To discern the potential role of FURIN in COVID-19, understanding the structure of the viral S-glycoprotein is important. The S-protein has two functional domains: one for receptor binding and the other for mediating fusion of the viral particle with the cell membrane. The S-protein must be cleaved by the protease to expose these fusion sequences and allow cell entry. FURIN takes on this role in coronaviruses including COVID-19 (70–72). Since Notch1 has been shown to transcriptionally induce FURIN, Notch signaling may indirectly lead to enhanced viral entry via enhanced FURIN expression (73, 74).

In addition to having effects on viral infectivity, interestingly both the Notch receptors and ACE2 receptor share a common mechanism of activation through cleavage by the A disintegrin and metalloproteinase (ADAM) family of enzymes, specifically ADAM17 (75, 76). ADAM17 mediates ectodomain shedding of ACE2 which can facilitate viral entry (77, 78). ADAM17 also activates the Notch signaling pathway via receptor cleavage leading to increased viral infectivity through regulation of FURIN. Therefore, Notch activity is indirectly involved in COVID-19 infectivity through FURIN induction and shared activation axis of ACE2, both of which aid in viral entry.

THE CYTOKINE STORM

A balanced innate and adaptive host immunity is key for an effective antiviral response, including activation of T cells, macrophages, and production of various pro-inflammatory cytokines. However, in case of COVID-19, this response becomes heightened, causing a hyperinflammatory reaction known as "The Cytokine Storm Syndrome" (14, 27). The cytokine storm is one of the key factors causing cardiovascular complications in COVID-19 patients. This is attributed to the resulting inflammation-induced vascular injury, myocarditis, arrhythmia, and destabilization of coronary artery plaques leading to myocardial infarcts (79, 80). The common profile of a COVID-19 patient with cytokine storm syndrome includes elevated interleukin-6 (IL-6), IL-2 receptor, TNF-α, granulocyte-colony stimulating factor, among others. IL-6 is secreted by activated leukocytes, promotes differentiation of B lymphocytes and production of acute phase proteins, and is important for thermoregulation (14, 81).

The role of the Notch pathway in inflammation is well-documented, where it has been shown to promote the pro-inflammatory microenvironment (82–84). It is implicated in macrophage polarization and contributes to amplification of the inflammatory loop by promoting the M1 phenotype of macrophages over the M2 phenotype (17, 85). Furthermore, in macrophages, Notch1 directly binds the IL-6 promoter and activates IL-6 transcription in response to interferon-γ (81, 86). Additionally, IL-6 in turn increases the expression of the Notch ligand DLL1, amplifying the Notch signal. This works as a positive feedback loop that further drives the production of

TABLE 1 | Reported link of the Notch signaling pathway to common viral infections.

Viral infection	Link to notch	References
Epstein-barr virus	The Epstein-Barr virus nuclear antigen 2 (EBNA2) is tethered to promoters by targeting RBPJ, the nuclear effector of Notch. Since EBNA2 has been proven to be partly interchangeable with Notch intracellular domain in activation of target genes modulating differentiation processes, it is seen as a biological equivalent of an activated Notch receptor. The Epstein-Barr virus-encoded latent membrane protein 2A (LMP2A) promotes cellular migration mediated by Notch signaling by altering mitochondrial dynamics.	(28–31)
Influenza virus	Macrophages are reported to enhance their Notch ligand DLL1 production in response to the viral infection to protect against the virus. Blocking DLL1 caused heightened inflammatory response and decreased interferon-c levels, leading to a compromised immunity against the virus.	(32–34)
Respiratory syncytial virus (RSV)	Notch signaling has been reported to contribute to the production of inflammatory cytokines induced by the virus in alveolar macrophages. Notch signaling communicates with the Toll-like receptor (TLR) pathway to fine-tune the innate inflammatory responses. In studies where TLR pathway was activated, while Notch signaling was inhibited, RSV-enhanced respiratory disease (ERD) was prevented.	(35, 36)
Human papilloma virus (HPV)	Notch inhibition impairs epithelial differentiation, which is suggested to contribute to HPV replication and viral oncogenesis. HPV8E6 protein inhibits Notch transcriptional activator complexes involving RBPJ and MAML at the Notch target genes, decreasing Notch activity during keratinocyte differentiation. HPV16E6 protein increases Notch levels in keratinocytes. HPV16E6 potentiates Notch activation and differentiation without activating cellular arrest, entirely uncoupling cellular arrest from increased differentiation.	(37–42)
Human T-cell leukemia virus type 1 (HTLV-I)	Notch signaling promotes proliferation and tumor formation of HTLV-I-associated adult T-cell leukemia.	(43, 44)
Hepatitis C virus (HCV)	Notch signaling regulates T Helper 22 Cells in chronic HCV patients. Notch1 receptor has been shown to facilitate nuclear localization of p65 in human hepatocytes in response to TNF-α, leading to increased pathogenicity of the virus. HCV NS3 protein leads to Notch activation by binding to SRCAP transcription factor. HCV causes Notch-dependent modulation in miRNA-449a levels, leading to differential expression of the inflammatory biomarker YKL40.	(45–48)
Hepatitis B virus (HBV)	HBV increases Notch1 and TGF-β levels on intrahepatic T cells in cirrhosis, promoting fibrogenesis and disease progression. HBV X protein activates Notch signaling by increasing DLL4 and Notch1, promoting the growth of hepatocellular carcinoma, in addition to increasing CREB-mediated activation of miR-3188. HBV X protein causes Notch-dependent decrease in nuclear factor-kappa B (NF-κB) signaling. Notch signaling contributes to hepatic inflammation in HBV infection by regulating IL-22-producing cells. Notch signaling aids in transcription of HBV covalently closed circular DNA by a mechanism involving cAMP response element-binding protein and E3 ubiquitin ligase-modulation. In acute hepatitis B (AVH-B) infection, a complementary association between Notch1 and Hes1 in CD8$^+$T cells was reported. In chronic hepatitis B (CHB) infection, repression of the Notch receptors mediates the immune response regulation in patients who progress to cirrhosis and hepatocellular carcinoma.	(49–55)
Human immunodeficiency virus (HIV)	Notch signaling is activated in HIV-associated nephropathy, where Notch ligands (Jagged-1, Jagged-2, DLL1, and DLL4) are all up in kidney tubules, while glomeruli show minimal ligand expression. Notch1 and 4 receptors are up in glomeruli, and only Notch4 is expressed in tubules. Notch inhibition results in improvement of kidney injury scores and renal functions, and blocks podocyte proliferation induced by HIV proteins Nef and Tat.	(56–59)

more IL-6 (87, 88). Nitric Oxide Synthase (iNOS) expression is linked to manifestation of the cytokine storm (89, 90). Direct interaction between the Notch Intracellular Domain (NICD) and TNF-α on the iNOS promoter has also been documented, indicating multiple avenues by which Notch signaling drives hyper-inflammation (91). Further, TNF-α itself has been shown to induce expression of Notch1 and Notch4, in addition to regulating NICD nuclear translocation, which leads to the activation of Notch downstream mediators (92, 93).

This interplay between Notch and pro-inflammatory processes makes the Notch pathway an attractive target for reversing inflammatory events. Indeed, genetic and pharmacological inhibition of Notch signaling was reported to ameliorate disease progression in many inflammatory disease models. These include rheumatoid arthritis, autoimmune encephalomyelitis, and several models of infectious disease (94, 95). In the case of COVID-19, the recommendation to use corticosteroids was discouraged due to controversial efficacy and reports showing exacerbation of patient symptoms. Potentially targeting the Notch pathway to specifically block the inflammatory loop re-enforced by IL-6 and TNF-α may present a viable therapy for these cases (96–98).

THE HYPOXIC RESPONSE

The hypoxic events in COVID-19 patients have been a mystery to medical caretakers and physicians. This is due to the fact that the patients display minimal visible distress, although clinical oxygen levels are remarkably low (99). Its presentation defies its pathophysiology, which initially led to its description of "Happy Hypoxia" (100). Hypoxia is also linked to the thrombotic events seen in these patients, which spirals quickly into more severe cardiovascular complications such as myocarditis and myocardial infarction (101–103).

The Notch pathway plays a significant role in hypoxic events (104). Notch3 is induced under hypoxic conditions in the lungs and vasculature. Notch3 deletion has been shown to protect against the development of pulmonary arterial hypertension in response to hypoxic stimulation (105, 106). Further, Notch3 was found to cooperate with the hypoxia-inducible factor-1 alpha (HIF-1α) (105, 107), a transcription factor upregulated in hypoxia and inflammatory microenvironments and a master regulator of oxygen homeostasis (108). HIF-1α also induces the expression of two of the Notch ligands, DLL4 and Jagged-1 (109–111). Another link between Notch signaling and HIF-1α is through Notch1 receptor. As mentioned previously, Notch1 receptor has been shown to promote M1 macrophage polarization and switching of macrophage metabolism to glycolysis. This is followed by induction of M1 gene transcription, coupled with an increase in mitochondrial oxidative phosphorylation and generation of reactive oxygen species (112). This in turn activates HIF-1α to induce M1 macrophage activation, in a type of positive feedback loop (111).

Additionally, enhanced Notch signaling has been linked to structural changes in air sacs in the lungs that include decreased septation of terminal alveoli, emphysematous patterns and progressive fibrotic changes (113). Furthermore, Notch3 plays a critical role in regulating alveolar epithelium and increased levels of Notch3 are associated with disruption of differentiation processes and altered lung morphology (114). Interestingly in COVID-19-associated hypoxia, the air sacs do not fill up with fluid like in pneumonia, but also show structural changes in the sacs that lead them to collapse (115, 116). Hence, Notch activation in COVID-19 patients is likely directly exacerbating the hypoxic events by cooperating with HIF-1α in addition to promoting structural defects in the air sacs.

THE COAGULOPATHIC RESPONSE

The realization that COVID-19 causes hypercoagulopathy poses more questions than answers, with studies showing severe thrombotic manifestations, while others show postmortem lung sections with extensive bleeding (117, 118). In a recent study by Boonyawa et al. a 28% incidence of venous thromboembolism was reported in COVID-19 patients in the intensive care unit (119). Another study by Klok et al. found a 31% incidence of combined deep vein thrombosis, pulmonary embolism, and arterial thrombosis in critically ill patients (120). Thus, there is an urgent need to understand the rate of bleeding and thrombotic events associated with COVID-19 coagulopathy.

Hypercoagulopathy is an important hallmark of inflammation. In fact, pro-inflammatory cytokines are directly involved in accelerating platelet hyperactivation and driving thrombotic events, while impairing crucial physiological anticoagulation pathways including antithrombin III, tissue factor pathway, and the protein C system (121, 122). The mechanisms involved in COVID-19 coagulopathy have not been fully elucidated yet, but crosstalk between the coagulation and the inflammatory systems is evident, with at least four factors seeming to contribute to this condition (123). First, the pro-inflammatory mediators such as IL-6 and IL-1β produced during the cytokine storm stimulate the production of tissue factor on immune cells. This in turn initiates the activation of the extrinsic coagulation cascade (81, 124). Secondly, those pro-inflammatory mediators directly activate the platelets themselves (125). Thirdly, a decrease in plasminogen activator coupled with an increase in plasminogen activator inhibitor suppresses the fibrinolytic system (126, 127). Lastly, the damage caused to the endothelial cells by the inflammatory reaction results in vascular homeostatic imbalances, causing accelerated local thrombotic events in addition to systemic coagulation defects. Of note is that this damaged endothelium also binds platelets more readily due to enhanced platelet-vessel wall interaction caused by the large von Willebrand factor multimers released by damaged endothelial cells (128).

Despite efforts by the scientific community to understand COVID-19-associated coagulopathy, there is still a lot to clarify regarding mechanisms involved and how to reverse the resulting homeostatic imbalances. Previous studies by Duarte et al. and Gough beautifully demonstrated a link between the Notch pathway and the coagulation pathway through fibroblast growth factor 1 (FGF1) (129, 130). These studies utilized a soluble form of the Notch ligand Jagged-1 to show the effect of Notch inhibition on FGF1 and the coagulation cascade. This link between Notch signaling and coagulation is supported by several previous findings. First, the activation of the coagulation cascade by damaged tissue generates thrombin, which activates the protease-activated receptor 1 (PAR1) and PAR1-dependent FGF1 expression and release. Released FGF1 subsequently promotes angiogenesis and induces Jagged-1 expression in the damaged tissue (131). Second, Alagille syndrome patients, who primarily have mutations in Jagged-1, show bleeding disorders (132). Consistent with this, Jagged-1 null mice show hemorrhage during their embryonic development (133, 134). Lastly, Jagged-1 was found to be the FGF1 response gene responsible for FGF1-dependent endothelial cell differentiation on fibrin matrices (131, 135). Taken together, these studies indicate that there is a Notch-dependent mechanism by which thrombin can regulate FGF1 secretion, which in turn contributes to thrombin's activity, the key protease of the coagulation cascade. Thus, through its established role in both inflammation and coagulation, Notch signaling seems likely responsible for exacerbating COVID-19-associated coagulopathy.

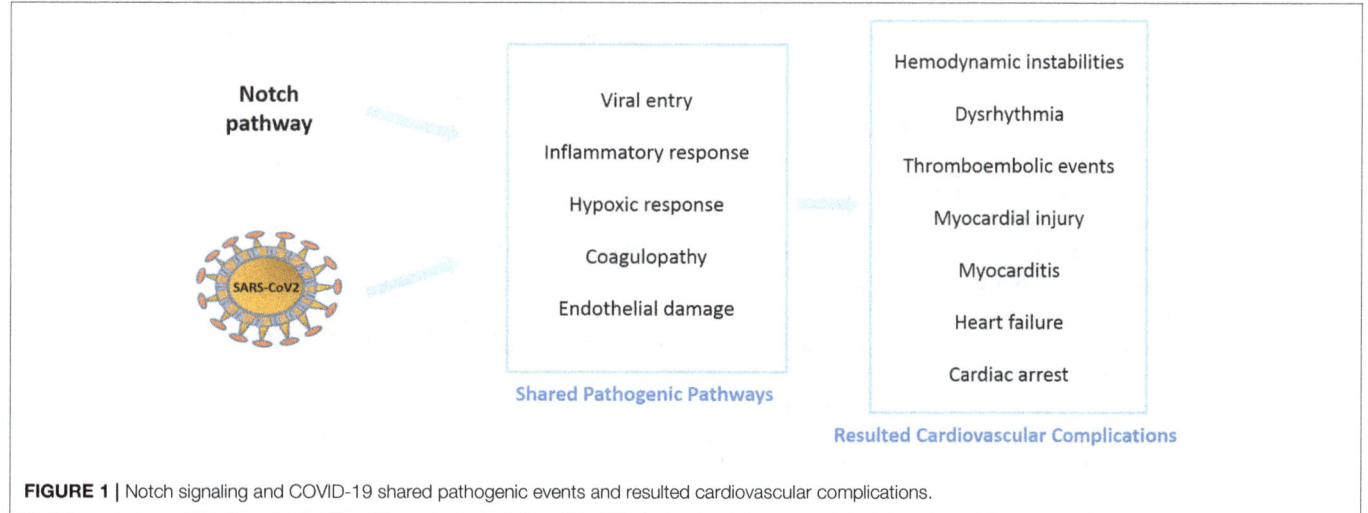

FIGURE 1 | Notch signaling and COVID-19 shared pathogenic events and resulted cardiovascular complications.

ENDOTHELIAL CELL INVOLVEMENT

The endothelium is a single layer of cells lining blood vessels, constituting a barrier between the circulation and the rest of the blood vessel wall. In addition, it is the source for several vasoreactive substances responsible for blood vessel contraction and relaxation such as endothelin and nitric oxide (136). Thus, it is a key regulator of vascular homeostasis, and damage to this layer can lead to loss of the homeostatic state and exacerbation of disease conditions. Indeed, endothelial dysfunction shifts the vascular equilibrium toward an inflammatory, pro-coagulant state (137, 138). Coordination of leukocyte trafficking in particular is critical for the inflammatory response. Under physiological conditions, the endothelial cells prevent binding and extravasation of leukocytes from the blood. However, under disease conditions such as the case in COVID-19 patients, the endothelial junctions are weakened and leaky, resulting in facilitated exit of the leukocytes from the circulation into the tissues (82, 93, 139). Interestingly, immunostaining studies have shown the confinement of Notch4 receptors on endothelial cells at the apical membrane. This localization makes Notch4 ideal for receptor/ligand communication between the endothelial and the inflammatory cells in the blood stream (140). In addition, the Notch ligand DLL4 on the endothelium has been shown to trigger a bidirectional Notch signaling between endothelial cells and monocytes (93, 141).

Several reports have linked endothelial cells to SARS-CoV2 pathology, where histological sections through hearts, kidneys and lungs showed accumulation of both inflammatory cells and viral particles within the endothelium (81, 142, 143). This COVID-19-associated endotheliitis could explain the impaired circulatory function in the various vascular beds and the clinical complications in COVID-19 patients (144–146). Furthermore, endothelial cells express the ACE2 receptor, the entry portal for the virus (147–150). This, coupled with previous reports of development of autoantibodies against endothelial cells after SARS-CoV1 infection, suggests that CoV2 infection of endothelial cells and their subsequent damage is a prominent step in the pathogenesis of COVID-19 (151, 152). Important to consider here is the discrepancy that exists between current studies, where some advocate for the endothelial cell hypothesis of COVID-19 pathology, which reinforces the idea that endothelial cells are the origin for COVID-19-associated cardiovascular impairments. In contrast, others promote a pericyte-COVID-19 hypothesis, where pericytes are the main contributors to disease progression. The studies that propose the pericyte hypothesis are based on the fact that ACE2 expression in the heart is highest in pericytes, and in the brain vasculature ACE2 is on vascular smooth muscle cells and pericytes and not on the endothelium (121, 153). Although the endothelial cell hypothesis seems to be more plausible according to consequences of endotheliitis in COVID-19 patients, these discrepancies highlight the importance of considering tissue type in disease pathology.

CONCLUSIONS

COVID-19 is associated with a large number of cardiovascular sequelae, including dysrhythmias, myocardial injury, myocarditis and thrombosis. Many of these complications seem to be linked to compromised signaling pathways in the patients, including the Notch pathway (**Figure 1**). Notch signaling can indirectly enhance viral entry through inducing FURIN, the protease responsible for exposing the fusion sequences of the viral S-protein. The established role of Notch signaling in both inflammation and coagulation suggests its involvement in COVID-19 cytokine storm and hypercoagulopathy, both of which are main contributors to the cardiovascular complications. Furthermore, Notch activation is known to exacerbate hypoxic events by cooperating with HIF-1α in addition to enhancing structural defects in the air sacs in the lungs, which together may contribute to enhanced lung pathology in COVID-19 patients. Lastly, the suggested role of the endothelium in COVID-19 cardiovascular impairments coupled with the specific localization of Notch4 receptors on the apical membrane of the endothelium reinforces the idea that the Notch pathway serves as a communication channel between endothelial and inflammatory cells.

In summary, several scenarios can be considered regarding the link between the Notch pathway and COVID-19-associated cardiovascular events. COVID-19 may act upstream to increase Notch signaling, leading to enhanced viral entry and associated pathogenic processes. Alternatively, maladaptive responses of Notch signaling due to COVID-19 infection may contribute to the enhanced inflammatory, coagulopathic, and hypoxic events. Both scenarios eventually lead to exacerbation of cardiovascular impairments in COVID-19 patients that are Notch-associated. Gamma-secretase inhibitors, which inhibit Notch receptor cleavage have been used to attenuate Notch signaling in cancer and Alzheimer disease (154, 155). These compounds, however, are associated with significant toxicity. Alternatives include Notch-specific antibodies and decoys. Antibodies allow blockade of individual Notch components, thus are not associated with complications seen with the pan inhibitors (156–158). Notch decoys also selectively block Notch receptors by a unique mechanism that involves mimicking the Notch extracellular domain of a specific Notch ligand or receptor (159, 160). Finally, uncovering new aspects of a Notch-COVID-19 relationship might help mitigate cardiac and pulmonary complications caused by the SARS-CoV family of viruses.

AUTHOR CONTRIBUTIONS

RB wrote, edited, and conceived of topic. BL edited, wrote, and provided topic guidance. All authors contributed to the article and approved the submitted version.

REFERENCES

1. Masters PS. The molecular biology of coronaviruses. *Adv Virus Res.* (2006) 66:193–292. doi: 10.1016/S0065-3527(06)66005-3
2. Chen Y, Liu Q, Guo D. Emerging coronaviruses: genome structure, replication, and pathogenesis. *J Med Virol.* (2020) 92:418–23. doi: 10.1002/jmv.25681
3. Cucinotta D, Vanelli M. WHO declares COVID-19 a pandemic. *Acta biomed.* (2020) 91:157–60. doi: 10.23750/abm.v91i1.9397
4. Menter T, Haslbauer JD, Nienhold R, Savic S, Hopfer H, Deigendesch N, et al. Postmortem examination of COVID-19 patients reveals diffuse alveolar damage with severe capillary congestion and variegated findings in lungs and other organs suggesting vascular dysfunction. *Histopathology.* (2020) 77:198–209. doi: 10.1111/his.14134
5. Wu J, Li X, Huang B, Su H, Li Y, Luo D, et al. Pathological changes of fatal coronavirus disease 2019 (COVID-19) in the lungs: report of 10 cases by postmortem needle autopsy. *Zhonghua Bing Li Xue Za Zhi.* (2020) 49: 568–75. doi: 10.3760/cma.j.cn112151-20200405-00291
6. Lang JP, Wang X, Moura FA, Siddiqi HK, Morrow DA, Bohula EA. A current review of COVID-19 for the cardiovascular specialist. *Am Heart J.* (2020) 226:29–44. doi: 10.1016/j.ahj.2020.04.025
7. Long B, Brady WJ, Koyfman A, Gottlieb M. Cardiovascular complications in COVID-19. *Am J Emerg Med.* (2020) 3:1504–7. doi: 10.1016/j.ajem.2020.04.048
8. Matsushita K, Marchandot B, Jesel L, Ohlmann P, Morel O. Impact of COVID-19 on the cardiovascular system: a review. *J Clin Med.* (2020) 9:1407. doi: 10.3390/jcm9051407
9. Liu PP, Blet A, Smyth D, Li H. The science underlying COVID-19: implications for the cardiovascular system. *Circulation.* (2020) 142:68–78. doi: 10.1161/CIRCULATIONAHA.120.047549
10. Zheng YY, Ma YT. COVID-19 and the cardiovascular system. *Nat Rev Cardiol.* (2020) 17:259–60. doi: 10.1038/s41569-020-0360-5
11. Boureau AS, De Decker L, Berrut G, Hanon O. COVID-19 and cardiovascular diseases: viewpoint for older patients. *Geriatr Psychol Neuropsychiatr Vieil.* (2020) 18:141–9. doi: 10.1684/pnv.2020.0864
12. Chen N, Zhou M, Dong X, Qu J, Gong F, Han Y, et al. Epidemiological and clinical characteristics of 99 cases of 2019 novel coronavirus pneumonia in Wuhan, China: a descriptive study. *Lancet.* (2020) 395:507–13. doi: 10.1016/S0140-6736(20)30211-7
13. Ganatra S, Dani SS, Shah S, Asnani A, Neilan TG, Lenihan D, et al. Management of cardiovascular disease during coronavirus disease (COVID-19) pandemic. *Trends Cardiovasc Med.* (2020) 30:315–25. doi: 10.1016/j.tcm.2020.05.004
14. Ashraf O, Young M, Malik KJ, Cheema T. Systemic complications of COVID-19. *Crit Care Nurs Q.* (2020) 43:390–9. doi: 10.1097/CNQ.0000000000000324
15. Li G, Saguner AM, An J, Ning Y. Cardiovascular disease during the COVID-19 pandemic: think ahead, protect hearts, reduce mortality. *Cardiol J.* (2020) 27:616–24. doi: 10.5603/CJ.a2020.0101
16. Aster JC. In brief: notch signalling in health and disease. *J Pathol.* (2014) 232:1–3. doi: 10.1002/path.4291
17. Shang Y, Smith S, Hu X. Role of Notch signaling in regulating innate immunity and inflammation in health and disease. *Protein Cell.* (2016) 7:159–74. doi: 10.1007/s13238-016-0250-0
18. Rosa BA, Ahmed M, Singh DK, Choreño-Parra JA, Cole J, Jiménez-Álvarez LA, et al. IFN signaling and neutrophil degranulation transcriptional signatures are induced during SARS-CoV-2 infection. *Commun Biol.* (2021) 4:1–14. doi: 10.1038/s42003-021-01829-4
19. Vandelli A, Monti M, Milanetti E, Armaos A, Rupert J, Zacco E, et al. Structural analysis of SARS-CoV-2 genome and predictions of the human interactome. *Nucleic Acids Res.* (2020) 48:11270–83. doi: 10.1093/nar/gkaa864
20. Bourgonje AR, Abdulle AE, Timens W, Hillebrands JL, Navis GJ, Gordijn SJ, et al. Angiotensin-converting enzyme-2 (ACE2), SARS-CoV-2 and pathophysiology of coronavirus disease 2019 (COVID-19). *J Pathol.* (2020) 251:228–48. doi: 10.1002/path.5471
21. Wu J, Deng W, Li S, Yang X. Advances in research on ACE2 as a receptor for 2019-nCoV. *Cell Mol Life Sci.* (2021). 78:531–44. doi: 10.1007/s00018-020-03611-x
22. Eguchi S, Kawai T, Scalia R, Rizzo V. Understanding angiotensin II type 1 receptor signaling in vascular pathophysiology. *Hypertension.* (2018) 71:804–10. doi: 10.1161/HYPERTENSIONAHA.118.10266
23. Gheblawi M, Wang K, Viveiros A, Nguyen Q, Zhong, J-C, et al. Angiotensin-converting enzyme 2: SARS-CoV-2 receptor and regulator of the renin-angiotensin system: celebrating the 20th anniversary of the discovery of ACE2. *Circ Res.* (2020) 126:1456–74. doi: 10.1161/CIRCRESAHA.120.317015
24. Murray E, Tomaszewski M, Guzik TJ. Binding of SARS-CoV-2 and angiotensin-converting enzyme 2: clinical implications. *Cardiovasc Res.* (2020) 116:e87–9. doi: 10.1093/cvr/cvaa096
25. Alsibai KD. Expression of angiotensin-converting enzyme 2 and proteases in COVID-19 patients: a potential role of cellular FURIN in the pathogenesis of SARS-CoV-2. *Med Hypotheses.* (2020) 143:109893. doi: 10.1016/j.mehy.2020.109893
26. Wang Q, Qiu Y. Receptor utilization of angiotensin converting enzyme 2 (ACE2) indicates a narrower host range of SARS-CoV-2 than that

of SARS-CoV. *Transbound Emerg Dis.* (2020) 1–8. doi: 10.1111/tbed. 13792

27. Barillà F, Bassareo PP, Calcaterra G, Romeo F, Mehta JL. Focus on clinical practice: angiotensin-converting enzyme 2 and corona virus disease 2019: pathophysiology and clinical implications. *J Cardiovasc Med (Hagerstown).* (2020) 21:630–3. doi: 10.2459/JCM.0000000000001071

28. Robertson ES, Lin J, Kieff E. The amino-terminal domains of Epstein-Barr virus nuclear proteins 3A, 3B, and 3C interact with RBPJ (kappa). *J Virol.* (1996) 70:3068–74. doi: 10.1128/JVI.70.5.3068-3074.1996

29. Hsieh J, Hayward SD. Masking of the CBF1/RBPJ kappa transcriptional repression domain by Epstein-Barr virus EBNA2. *Science.* (1995) 268:560–3. doi: 10.1126/science.7725102

30. Zimber-Strobl U, Strobl LJ. EBNA2 and Notch signalling in Epstein-Barr virus mediated immortalization of B lymphocytes. *Semin Cancer Biol.* (2001) 11:423–34. doi: 10.1006/scbi.2001.0409

31. Pal AD, Basak NP, Banerjee AS, Banerjee S. Epstein–Barr virus latent membrane protein-2A alters mitochondrial dynamics promoting cellular migration mediated by Notch signaling pathway. *Carcinogenesis.* (2014) 35:1592–601. doi: 10.1093/carcin/bgu069

32. Ito T, Allen RM, Carson Iv WF, Schaller M, Cavassani KA, Hogaboam CM, et al. The critical role of Notch ligand Delta-like 1 in the pathogenesis of influenza A virus (H1N1) infection. *PLoS Pathog.* (2011) 7:e1002341. doi: 10.1371/journal.ppat.1002341

33. Ito T, Matsukawa A. Notch system in influenza A/H1N1 virus infection. *Inflammation and Regeneration.* (2012) 32:132–136. doi: 10.2492/inflammregen.32.132

34. Yang J, Huang X, Liu Y, Zhao D, Han K, Zhang L, et al. Analysis of the microRNA expression profiles of chicken dendritic cells in response to H9N2 avian influenza virus infection. *Vet Res.* (2020) 51:132. doi: 10.1186/s13567-020-00856-z

35. Zhang L, Li H, Hai Y, Yin W, Li W, Zheng B, et al. CpG in combination with an inhibitor of Notch signaling suppresses formalin-inactivated respiratory syncytial virus-enhanced airway hyperresponsiveness and inflammation by inhibiting Th17 memory responses and promoting tissue-resident memory cells in lungs. *J Virol.* (2017) 91:e02111–16. doi: 10.1128/JVI.02111-16

36. Buonvino S, Melino S. New Consensus pattern in Spike CoV-2: potential implications in coagulation process and cell–cell fusion. *Cell Death Discovery.* (2020) 6:134. doi: 10.1038/s41420-020-00372-1

37. Chakrabarti O, Veeraraghavalu K, Tergaonkar V, Liu Y, Androphy EJ, Stanley MA, et al. Human papillomavirus type 16 E6 amino acid 83 variants enhance E6-mediated MAPK signaling and differentially regulate tumorigenesis by notch signaling and oncogenic Ras. *J Virol.* (2004) 78:5934–45. doi: 10.1128/JVI.78.11.5934-5945.2004

38. Tan MJA, White EA, Sowa ME, Harper JW, Aster JC, Howley PM. Cutaneous β-human papillomavirus E6 proteins bind Mastermind-like coactivators and repress Notch signaling. *Proc Natl Acad Sci USA.* (2012) 109:E1473–80. doi: 10.1073/pnas.1205991109

39. Meyers JM, Spangle JM, Munger K. The human papillomavirus type 8 E6 protein interferes with NOTCH activation during keratinocyte differentiation. *J Virol.* (2013) 87:4762–7. doi: 10.1128/JVI.02527-12

40. Vliet-Gregg PA, Hamilton JR, Katzenellenbogen RA. NFX1-123 and human papillomavirus 16E6 increase Notch expression in keratinocytes. *J Virol.* (2013) 87:13741–50. doi: 10.1128/JVI.02582-13

41. Das T, Zhong R, Spiotto MT. Notch signaling and human papillomavirus–associated oral tumorigenesis. *Adv Exp Med Biol.* (2020) 1287:105–22. doi: 10.1007/978-3-030-55031-8_8

42. Vliet-Gregg PA, Hamilton JR, Katzenellenbogen RA. Human papillomavirus 16E6 and NFX1-123 potentiate Notch signaling and differentiation without activating cellular arrest. *Virology.* (2015) 478:50–60. doi: 10.1016/j.virol.2015.02.002

43. Pancewicz J, Taylor JM, Datta A, Baydoun HH, Waldmann TA, Hermine O, et al. Notch signaling contributes to proliferation and tumor formation of human T-cell leukemia virus type 1–associated adult T-cell leukemia. *Proc Natl Acad Sci USA.* (2010) 107:16619–24. doi: 10.1073/pnas.10107 22107

44. Kamdje AHN, Krampera M. Notch signaling in acute lymphoblastic leukemia: any role for stromal microenvironment? *Blood.* (2011) 118:6506–14. doi: 10.1182/blood-2011-08-376061

45. Wurmbach E, Chen YB, Khitrov G, Zhang W, Roayaie S, Schwartz M, et al. Genome-wide molecular profiles of HCV-induced dysplasia and hepatocellular carcinoma. *Hepatology.* (2007) 45:938–47. doi: 10.1002/hep.21622

46. Iwai A, Takegami T, Shiozaki T, Miyazaki T. Hepatitis C virus NS3 protein can activate the notch-signaling pathway through binding to a transcription factor, SRCAP. *PLoS ONE.* (2011) 6:e20718. doi: 10.1371/journal.pone.0020718

47. Jiang BC, Liu X, Liu XH, Li ZS, Zhu GZ. Notch signaling regulates circulating T helper 22 cells in patients with chronic hepatitis C. *Viral Immunol.* (2017) 30:522–32. doi: 10.1089/vim.2017.0007

48. Qin L, Zhou YC, Wu HJ, Zhuo Y, Wang YP, Si CY, et al. Notch signaling modulates the balance of regulatory T cells and T helper 17 cells in patients with chronic hepatitis C. *DNA Cell Biol.* (2017) 36:311–20. doi: 10.1089/dna.2016.3609

49. Wang F, Zhou H, Xia X, Sun Q, Wang Y, Cheng B. Activated Notch signaling is required for hepatitis B virus X protein to promote proliferation and survival of human hepatic cells. *Cancer Lett.* (2010) 298:64–73. doi: 10.1016/j.canlet.2010.06.003

50. Trehanpati N, Shrivastav S, Shivakumar B, Khosla R, Bhardwaj S, Chaturvedi J. Analysis of Notch and TGF-β signaling expression in different stages of disease progression during hepatitis B virus infection. *Clin Transl Gastroenterol.* (2012) 3:e23. doi: 10.1038/ctg.2012.17

51. Luo J, Zhou H, Wang F, Xia X, Sun Q, Wang R, et al. The hepatitis B virus X protein downregulates NF-κB signaling pathways through decreasing the Notch signaling pathway in HBx-transformed L02 cells. *Int J Oncol.* (2013) 42:1636–43. doi: 10.3892/ijo.2013.1842

52. Kongkavitoon P, Tangkijvanich P, Hirankarn N, Palaga T. Hepatitis B virus HBx activates Notch signaling via delta-like 4/Notch1 in hepatocellular carcinoma. *PLoS ONE.* (2016) 11:e0146696. doi: 10.1371/journal.pone.0146696

53. Wei X, Wang JP, Hao CQ, Yang F, Wang LX, Huang CX, et al. Notch Signaling contributes to liver inflammation by regulation of interleukin-22-producing cells in hepatitis B virus infection. *Front Cell Infect Microbiol.* (2016) 6:132. doi: 10.3389/fcimb.2016.00132

54. Zhou SJ, Deng YL, Liang HF, Jaoude JC, Liu FY. Hepatitis B virus X protein promotes CREB-mediated activation of miR-3188 and Notch signaling in hepatocellular carcinoma. *Cell Death Differ.* (2017) 24:1577–87. doi: 10.1038/cdd.2017.87

55. Wang Z, Kawaguchi K, Honda M, Hashimoto S, Shirasaki T, Okada H, et al. Notch signaling facilitates hepatitis B virus covalently closed circular DNA transcription via cAMP response element-binding protein with E3 ubiquitin ligase-modulation. *Sci Rep..* (2019) 9:1–12. doi: 10.1038/s41598-018-38139-5

56. Shoham N, Cohen L, Yaniv A, Gazit A. The Tat protein of the human immunodeficiency virus type 1 (HIV-1) interacts with the EGF-like repeats of the Notch proteins and the EGF precursor. *Virus Res.* (2003) 98:57–61. doi: 10.1016/j.virusres.2003.08.016

57. Sharma M, Callen S, Zhang D, Singhal PC, Vanden Heuvel GB, Buch S. Activation of Notch signaling pathway in HIV-associated nephropathy. *AIDS.* (2010) 24:2161–70. doi: 10.1097/QAD.0b013e32833dbc31

58. Fan Y, Gao X, Chen J, Liu Y, He JJ. HIV tat impairs neurogenesis through functioning as a notch ligand and activation of notch signaling pathway. *J Neurosci.* (2016) 36:11362–73. doi: 10.1523/JNEUROSCI.1208-16.2016

59. Yan Q, Zhao R, Shen C, Wang F, Li W, Gao J, et al. Upregulation of MicroRNA 711 mediates HIV-1 Vpr promotion of kaposi's sarcoma-associated herpesvirus latency and induction of pro-proliferation and pro-survival cytokines by targeting the Notch/NF-κB-signaling axis. *J Virol.* (2018) 92:e00580–18. doi: 10.1128/JVI.00580-18

60. Schaller MA, Neupane R, Rudd BD, Kunkel SL, Kallal LE, Lincoln P, et al. Notch ligand Delta-like 4 regulates disease pathogenesis during respiratory viral infections by modulating Th2 cytokines. *J Exp Med.* (2007) 204:2925–34. doi: 10.1084/jem.20070661

61. Penton AL, Leonard LD, Spinner NB. Notch signaling in human development and disease. *Semin Cell Dev Biol.* (2012) 23:450–7. doi: 10.1016/j.semcdb.2012.01.010

62. Hayward SD. Viral interactions with the Notch pathway. *Semin Cancer Biol.* (2004) 14:387–96. doi: 10.1016/j.semcancer.2004.04.018

63. Kovall RA, Hendrickson WA. Crystal structure of the nuclear effector of Notch signaling, CSL bound to DNA. *EMBO J.* (2004) 23:3441–51. doi: 10.1038/sj.emboj.7600349

64. Sarma NJ, Tiriveedhi V, Subramanian V, Shenoy S, Crippin JS, Chapman WC, et al. Hepatitis C virus mediated changes in miRNA-449a modulates inflammatory biomarker YKL40 through components of the NOTCH signaling pathway. *PLoS ONE.* (2012) 7:e50826. doi: 10.1371/journal.pone.0050826

65. Duval F, Mathieu M, Labrecque N. Notch controls effector CD8+ T cell differentiation. *Oncotarget.* (2015) 6:21787. doi: 10.18632/oncotarget.4886

66. Ma YC, Shi C, Zhang YN, Wang G, Liu H, Jia HT, et al. The tyrosine kinase c-Src directly mediates growth factor-induced Notch-1 and Furin interaction and Notch-1 activation in pancreatic cancer cells. *PLoS ONE.* (2012) 7:e33414. doi: 10.1371/journal.pone.0033414

67. Qiu H, Tang X, Ma J, Shaverdashvili K, Zhang K, Bedogni B. Notch1 autoactivation via transcriptional regulation of furin, which sustains Notch1 signaling by processing Notch1-activating proteases ADAM10 and membrane type 1 matrix metalloproteinase. *Mol Cell Biol.* (2015) 35:3622–32. doi: 10.1128/MCB.00116-15

68. Thomas G. Furin at the cutting edge: from protein traffic to embryogenesis and disease. *Nat Rev Mol Cell Biol.* (2002) 3:753–66. doi: 10.1038/nrm934

69. Braun E, Sauter D. Furin-mediated protein processing in infectious diseases and cancer. *Clin Translational Immunol.* (2019) 8:e1073–e1073. doi: 10.1002/cti2.1073

70. Bradding P, Richardson M, Hinks TS, Howarth PH, Choy DF, Arron JR, et al. ACE2, TMPRSS2, and furin gene expression in the airways of people with asthma—implications for COVID-19. *J Allergy Clin Immunol.* (2020) 146:208–11. doi: 10.1016/j.jaci.2020.05.013

71. Li X, Duan G, Zhang W, Shi J, Chen J, Chen S, et al. A furin cleavage site was discovered in the S protein of the 2019 novel coronavirus. *Chinese J Bioinformatics.* (2020) 18. doi: 10.12113/202002001

72. Wu C, Zheng M, Yang Y, Gu X, Yang K, Li M, et al. Furin: a potential therapeutic target for COVID-19. *Iscience.* (2020) 23:101642. doi: 10.1016/j.isci.2020.101642

73. Bestle D, Heindl MR, Limburg H, Van Lam Van T. TMPRSS2 and furin are both essential for proteolytic activation of SARS-CoV-2 in human airway cells. *bioRxiv [Preprint].* (2020) 3. doi: 10.1101/2020.04.15.042085

74. Xi J, Xu K, Jiang P, Lian J, Hao S, Jia H, et al. Virus strain of a mild COVID-19 patient in Hangzhou representing a new trend in SARS-CoV-2 evolution related to Furin cleavage site. *medRxiv.* (2020). doi: 10.1101/2020.03.10.20033944

75. Bozkulak EC, Weinmaster G. Selective use of ADAM10 and ADAM17 in activation of Notch1 signaling. *Mol Cell Biol.* (2009) 29:5679–95. doi: 10.1128/MCB.00406-09

76. Parr-Sturgess CA, Rushton DJ, Parkin ET. Ectodomain shedding of the Notch ligand Jagged1 is mediated by ADAM17, but is not a lipid-raft-associated event. *Biochem J.* (2010) 432:283–94. doi: 10.1042/BJ20100321

77. Lambert DW, Yarski M, Warner FJ, Thornhill P, Parkin ET, Smith AI, et al. Tumor necrosis factor-α convertase (ADAM17) mediates regulated ectodomain shedding of the severe-acute respiratory syndrome-coronavirus (SARS-CoV) receptor, angiotensin-converting enzyme-2 (ACE2). *J Biol Chem.* (2005) 280:30113–9. doi: 10.1074/jbc.M505111200

78. Rizzo P, Dalla Sega FV, Fortini F, Marracino L, Rapezzi C, Ferrari R. COVID-19 in the heart and the lungs: could we "Notch" the inflammatory storm? *Basic Res Cardiol.* (2020) 115:31. doi: 10.1007/s00395-020-0791-5

79. Collins SD. Excess mortality from causes other than influenza and pneumonia during influenza epidemics. *Public Health Reports.* (1932) 47:2159–79. doi: 10.2307/4580606

80. Corrales-Medina VF, Madjid M, Musher DM. Role of acute infection in triggering acute coronary syndromes. *Lancet Infect Dis.* (2010) 10:83–92. doi: 10.1016/S1473-3099(09)70331-7

81. Zhang C, Wu Z, Li, J-W, Zhao H, Wang Q. The cytokine release syndrome (CRS) of severe COVID-19 and Interleukin-6 receptor (IL-6R) antagonist Tocilizumab may be the key to reduce the mortality. *Int J Antimicrob Agents.* (2020) 55:105954. doi: 10.1016/j.ijantimicag.2020.105954

82. Pabois A, Devallière J, Quillard T, Coulon F, Gérard N, Laboisse C, et al. The disintegrin and metalloproteinase ADAM10 mediates a canonical

83. Fazio C, Ricciardiello L. Inflammation and Notch signaling: a crosstalk with opposite effects on tumorigenesis. *Cell Death Dis.* (2016) 7:e2515. doi: 10.1038/cddis.2016.408

84. Lu Y, Zhang Y, Xiang X, Sharma M, Liu K, Wei J, et al. Notch signaling contributes to the expression of inflammatory cytokines induced by highly pathogenic porcine reproductive and respiratory syndrome virus (HP-PRRSV) infection in porcine alveolar macrophages. *Dev Comp Immunol.* (2020) 108:103690. doi: 10.1016/j.dci.2020.103690

85. Keewan E, Naser SA. The role of Notch signaling in macrophages during inflammation and infection: implication in rheumatoid arthritis? *Cells.* (2020) 9:111. doi: 10.3390/cells9010111

86. Wongchana W, Palaga T. Direct regulation of interleukin-6 expression by Notch signaling in macrophages. *Cell Mol Immunol.* (2012) 9:155–62. doi: 10.1038/cmi.2011.36

87. Guo Y, Xu F, Lu T, Duan Z, Zhang Z. Interleukin-6 signaling pathway in targeted therapy for cancer. *Cancer Treat Rev.* (2012) 38:904–10. doi: 10.1016/j.ctrv.2012.04.007

88. Yang Z, Guo L, Liu D, Sun L, Chen H, Deng Q, et al. Acquisition of resistance to trastuzumab in gastric cancer cells is associated with activation of IL-6/STAT3/Jagged-1/Notch positive feedback loop. *Oncotarget.* (2015) 6:5072. doi: 10.18632/oncotarget.3241

89. Adusumilli NC, Zhang D, Friedman JM, Friedman AJ. Harnessing nitric oxide for preventing, limiting and treating the severe pulmonary consequences of COVID-19. *Nitric Oxide.* (2020) 103:4–8. doi: 10.1016/j.niox.2020.07.003

90. Cespuglio R, Strekalova T, Spencer PS, Román GC, Reis J, Bouteille B, et al. SARS-CoV-2 infection and sleep disturbances: nitric oxide involvement and therapeutic opportunity. *Sleep.* (2021) 44:zsab009. doi: 10.1093/sleep/zsab009

91. Wang R, Li Y, Tsung A, Huang H, Du Q, Yang M, et al. iNOS promotes CD24+ CD133+ liver cancer stem cell phenotype through a TACE/ADAM17-dependent Notch signaling pathway. *Proc Natl Acad Sci USA.* (2018) 115:E10127–36. doi: 10.1073/pnas.1722100115

92. Bell JH, Herrera AH, Li Y, Walcheck B. Role of ADAM17 in the ectodomain shedding of TNF-α and its receptors by neutrophils and macrophages. *J Leukoc Biol.* (2007) 82:173–6. doi: 10.1189/jlb.0307193

93. Quillard T, Devallière J, Coupel S, Charreau B. Inflammation dysregulates Notch signaling in endothelial cells: implication of Notch2 and Notch4 to endothelial dysfunction. *Biochem Pharmacol.* (2010) 80:2032–41. doi: 10.1016/j.bcp.2010.07.010

94. Dees C, Tomcik M, Zerr P, Akhmetshina A, Horn A, Palumbo K, et al. Notch signalling regulates fibroblast activation and collagen release in systemic sclerosis. *Ann Rheum Dis.* (2011) 70:1304–10. doi: 10.1136/ard.2010.134742

95. Liu S, Liu D, Chen C, Hamamura K, Moshaverinia A, Yang R, et al. MSC transplantation improves osteopenia via epigenetic regulation of notch signaling in lupus. *Cell Metab.* (2015) 22:606–18. doi: 10.1016/j.cmet.2015.08.018

96. Russell B, Moss C, Rigg A, Van Hemelrijck M. COVID-19 and treatment with NSAIDs and corticosteroids: should we be limiting their use in the clinical setting? *Ecancermedicalscience.* (2020) 14:1023. doi: 10.3332/ecancer.2020.1023

97. Theoharides T, Conti P. Dexamethasone for COVID-19? Not so fast. *J Biol Regul Homeost Agents.* (2020) 34:1241–3. doi: 10.23812/20-EDITORIAL_1-5

98. Zha L, Li S, Pan L, Tefsen B, Li Y, French N, et al. Corticosteroid treatment of patients with coronavirus disease 2019 (COVID-19). *Med J Australia.* (2020) 212:416–20. doi: 10.5694/mja2.50577

99. Herrmann J, Mori V, Bates JH, Suki B. Can hyperperfusion of nonaerated lung explain COVID-19 hypoxia? *Res Sq. [Preprint].* (2020). doi: 10.21203/rs.3.rs-32949/v1

100. Couzin-Frankel J. The mystery of the pandemic's 'happy hypoxia'. *Science.* (2020) 368:455–6. doi: 10.1126/science.368.6490.455

101. Savla JJ, Levine BD, Sadek HA. The effect of hypoxia on cardiovascular disease: friend or foe? *High Alt Med Biol.* (2018) 19:124–30. doi: 10.1089/ham.2018.0044

102. Kashani KB. Hypoxia in COVID-19: sign of severity or cause for poor outcomes. *Mayo Clin Proc.* (2020) 95:1094–6. doi: 10.1016/j.mayocp.2020.04.021

103. Thachil J. Hypoxia-an overlooked trigger for thrombosis in COVID-19 and other critically ill patients. *J Thromb Haemost.* (2020) 18:3109–10. doi: 10.1111/jth.15029

104. Gustafsson MV, Zheng X, Pereira T, Gradin K, Jin S, Lundkvist J, et al. Hypoxia requires notch signaling to maintain the undifferentiated cell state. *Dev Cell.* (2005) 9:617–28. doi: 10.1016/j.devcel.2005.09.010

105. Li X, Zhang X, Leathers R, Makino A, Huang C, Parsa P, et al. Notch3 signaling promotes the development of pulmonary arterial hypertension. *Nat Med.* (2009) 15:1289–97. doi: 10.1038/nm.2021

106. Thistlethwaite PA, Li X, Zhang X. Notch signaling in pulmonary hypertension. *Adv Exp Med Biol.* (2010) 661:279–98. doi: 10.1007/978-1-60761-500-2_18

107. Liu H, Zhang W, Kennard S, Caldwell RB, Lilly B. Notch3 is critical for proper angiogenesis and mural cell investment. *Circ Res.* (2010) 107:860–70. doi: 10.1161/CIRCRESAHA.110.218271

108. Chun YS, Kim MS, Park JW. Oxygen-dependent and-independent regulation of HIF-1alpha. *J Korean Med Sci.* (2002) 17:581. doi: 10.3346/jkms.2002.17.5.581

109. Sainson RC, Harris AL. Hypoxia-regulated differentiation: let's step it up a Notch. *Trends Mol Med.* (2006) 12:141–3. doi: 10.1016/j.molmed.2006.02.001

110. Fung E, Tang, S-MT, Canner JP, Morishige K, Arboleda-Velasquez JF, et al. Delta-like 4 induces notch signaling in macrophages. *Circulation.* (2007) 115:2948–56. doi: 10.1161/CIRCULATIONAHA.106.675462

111. Zheng X, Linke S, Dias JM, Zheng X, Gradin K, Wallis TP, et al. Interaction with factor inhibiting HIF-1 defines an additional mode of cross-coupling between the Notch and hypoxia signaling pathways. *Proc Natl Acad Sci USA.* (2008) 105:3368–73. doi: 10.1073/pnas.0711591105

112. Xu J, Chi F, Guo T, Punj V, Lee WP, French SW, et al. NOTCH reprograms mitochondrial metabolism for proinflammatory macrophage activation. *J Clin Invest.* (2015) 125:1579–90. doi: 10.1172/JCI76468

113. Jespersen K, Liu Z, Li C, Harding P, Sestak K, Batra R, et al. Enhanced Notch3 signaling contributes to pulmonary emphysema in a Murine Model of Marfan syndrome. *Sci Rep.* (2020) 10:1–11. doi: 10.1038/s41598-020-67941-3

114. Guseh JS, Bores SA, Stanger BZ, Zhou Q, Anderson WJ, Melton DA, et al. Notch signaling promotes airway mucous metaplasia and inhibits alveolar development. *Development.* (2009) 136:1751–9. doi: 10.1242/dev.029249

115. Teo J. Early detection of silent hypoxia in COVID-19 pneumonia using Smartphone pulse oximetry. *J Med Syst.* (2020) 44:1–2. doi: 10.1007/s10916-020-01587-6

116. Wilkerson RG, Adler JD, Shah NG, Brown R. Silent hypoxia: a harbinger of clinical deterioration in patients with COVID-19. *Am J Emerg Med.* (2020) 38:2243.e5–2243.e6. doi: 10.1016/j.ajem.2020.05.044

117. Al-Samkari H, Karp Leaf RS, Dzik WH, Carlson JCT, Fogerty AE, Waheed A, et al. COVID-19 and coagulation: bleeding and thrombotic manifestations of SARS-CoV-2 infection. *Blood.* (2020) 136:489–500. doi: 10.1182/blood.2020006520

118. Chan NC, Weitz JI. COVID-19 coagulopathy, thrombosis, and bleeding. *Blood.* (2020) 136:381–383. doi: 10.1182/blood.2020007335

119. Boonyawat K, Chantrathammachart P, Numthavaj P, Nanthatanti N, Phusanti S, Phuphuakrat A, et al. Incidence of thromboembolism in patients with COVID-19: a systematic review and meta-analysis. *Thromb J.* (2020) 18:34. doi: 10.1186/s12959-020-00248-5

120. Klok FA, Kruip M, Van Der Meer NJM, Arbous MS, Gommers D, Kant KM, et al. Incidence of thrombotic complications in critically ill ICU patients with COVID-19. *Thromb Res.* (2020) 191:145–7. doi: 10.1016/j.thromres.2020.04.013

121. He L, Mae MA, Sun Y, Muhl L, Nahar K, Liebanas EV, et al. Pericyte-specific vascular expression of SARS-CoV-2 receptor ACE2-implications for microvascular inflammation and hypercoagulopathy in COVID-19 patients. *bioRxiv.* (2020). doi: 10.1101/2020.05.11.088500

122. McGonagle D, O'donnell JS, Sharif K, Emery P, Bridgewood C. Immune mechanisms of pulmonary intravascular coagulopathy in COVID-19 pneumonia. *Lancet Rheumatol.* (2020) 2:e437–45. doi: 10.1016/S2665-9913(20)30121-1

123. Colling ME, Kanthi Y. COVID-19-associated coagulopathy: an exploration of mechanisms. *Vasc Med.* (2020) 25:471–8. doi: 10.1177/1358863X20932640

124. Gemmati D, Bramanti B, Serino ML, Secchiero P, Zauli G, Tisato V. COVID-19 and individual genetic susceptibility/receptivity: role of ACE1/ACE2 genes, immunity, inflammation and coagulation. Might the double X-chromosome in females be protective against SARS-CoV-2 compared to the single X-chromosome in males? *Int J Mol Sci.* (2020) 21:3474. doi: 10.3390/ijms21103474

125. Martín-Rojas RM, Pérez-Rus G, Delgado-Pinos VE, Domingo-González A, Regalado-Artamendi I, Alba-Urdiales N, et al. COVID-19 coagulopathy: an in-depth analysis of the coagulation system. *Eur J Haematol.* (2020) 105:741–50. doi: 10.1111/ejh.13501

126. Cesari M, Pahor M, Incalzi RA. Plasminogen activator inhibitor-1 (PAI-1): a key factor linking fibrinolysis and age-related subclinical and clinical conditions. *Cardiovasc Ther.* (2010) 28:e72–e91. doi: 10.1111/j.1755-5922.2010.00171.x

127. Medcalf RL, Keragala CB, Myles PS. Fibrinolysis and COVID-19: a plasmin paradox. *J Thromb Haemost.* (2020) 18:2118–22. doi: 10.1111/jth.14960

128. O'sullivan JM, Mc Gonagle D, Ward SE, Preston RJ, O'donnell JS. Endothelial cells orchestrate COVID-19 coagulopathy. *Lancet Haematol.* (2020) 7:e553–5. doi: 10.1016/S2352-3026(20)30215-5

129. Duarte M, Kolev V, Kacer D, Mouta-Bellum C, Soldi R, Graziani I, et al. Novel cross-talk between three cardiovascular regulators: thrombin cleavage fragment of Jagged1 induces fibroblast growth factor 1 expression and release. *Mol Biol Cell.* (2008) 19:4863–74. doi: 10.1091/mbc.e07-12-1237

130. Gough NR. Thrombin targets notch signaling. *Sci Signal.* (2008) 1:ec375. doi: 10.1126/scisignal.144ec375

131. Zimrin AB, Pepper MS, Mcmahon GA, Nguyen F, Montesano R, Maciag T. An antisense oligonucleotide to the notch ligand jagged enhances fibroblast growth factor-induced angiogenesis *in vitro.* *J Biol Chem.* (1996) 271:32499–502. doi: 10.1074/jbc.271.51.32499

132. Joutel A, Tournier-Lasserve E. Notch signalling pathway and human diseases. In: *Seminars in Cell and Developmental Biology.* Elsevier (1998). p. 619–25. doi: 10.1006/scdb.1998.0261

133. Xue Y, Gao X, Lindsell CE, Norton CR, Chang B, Hicks C, et al. Embryonic lethality and vascular defects in mice lacking the Notch ligand Jagged1. *Hum Mol Genet.* (1999) 8:723–30. doi: 10.1093/hmg/8.5.723

134. Crosnier C, Attié-Bitach T, Encha-Razavi F, Audollent S, Soudy F, Hadchouel M, et al. JAGGED1 gene expression during human embryogenesis elucidates the wide phenotypic spectrum of Alagille syndrome. *Hepatology.* (2000) 32:574–81. doi: 10.1053/jhep.2000.16600

135. Zimrin AB, Villeponteau B, Maciag T. Models of *in vitro* angiogenesis: endothelial cell differentiation on fibrin but not matrigel is transcriptionally dependent. *Biochem Biophys Res Commun.* (1995) 213:630–8. doi: 10.1006/bbrc.1995.2178

136. Sumpio BE, Riley JT, Dardik A. Cells in focus: endothelial cell. *Int J Biochem Cell Biol.* (2002) 34:1508–12. doi: 10.1016/S1357-2725(02)00075-4

137. Rubanyi GM. The role of endothelium in cardiovascular homeostasis and diseases. *J Cardiovasc Pharmacol.* (1993) 22:S1–14. doi: 10.1097/00005344-199322004-00002

138. Kazmi RS, Boyce S, Lwaleed BA. Homeostasis of hemostasis: the role of endothelium. *Semin Thromb Hemost.* (2015) 41:549–55. doi: 10.1055/s-0035-1556586

139. Quillard T, Devalliere J, Chatelais M, Coulon F, Séveno C, Romagnoli M, et al. Notch2 signaling sensitizes endothelial cells to apoptosis by negatively regulating the key protective molecule survivin. *PLoS ONE.* (2009) 4:e8244. doi: 10.1371/journal.pone.0008244

140. Lizama CO, Zovein AC. Polarizing pathways: balancing endothelial polarity, permeability, lumen formation. *Exp Cell Res.* (2013) 319:1247–54. doi: 10.1016/j.yexcr.2013.03.028

141. Pabois A, Pagie S, Gérard N, Laboisse C, Pattier S, Hulin P, et al. Notch signaling mediates crosstalk between endothelial cells and macrophages via Dll4 and IL6 in cardiac microvascular inflammation. *Biochem Pharmacol.* (2016) 104:95–107. doi: 10.1016/j.bcp.2016.01.016

142. Yang X, Chang Y, Wei W. Endothelial dysfunction and inflammation: immunity in rheumatoid arthritis. *Mediators Inflamm.* (2016) 2016:6813016. doi: 10.1155/2016/6813016

143. Ackermann M, Verleden SE, Kuehnel M, Haverich A, Welte T, Laenger F, et al. Pulmonary vascular endothelialitis, thrombosis, and angiogenesis in Covid-19. *N Engl J Med.* (2020) 383:120–8. doi: 10.1056/NEJMoa 2015432

144. Fox SE, Lameira FS, Rinker EB, Vander Heide RS Cardiac Endotheliitis and multisystem inflammatory syndrome after COVID-19. *Ann Intern Med.* (2020) 173:1025–7. doi: 10.7326/L20-0882

145. Endotheliitis and Endothelial Dysfunction in Patients with COVID-19: Its Role in Thrombosis and Adverse Outcomes. *J Clin Med.* (2020) 9:1862. doi: 10.3390/jcm9061862

146. Varga Z, Flammer AJ, Steiger P, Haberecker M, Andermatt R, Zinkernagel AS, et al. Endothelial cell infection and endotheliitis in COVID-19. *Lancet.* (2020) 395:1417–8. doi: 10.1016/S0140-6736(20)30937-5

147. Hamming I, Timens W, Bulthuis M, Lely A, Navis GV, Van Goor. H. Tissue distribution of ACE2 protein, the functional receptor for SARS coronavirus. A first step in understanding SARS pathogenesis. *J Pathol.* (2004) 203:631–7. doi: 10.1002/path.1570

148. Sluimer J, Gasc J, Hamming I, Van Goor H, Michaud A, Van Den Akker L, et al. Angiotensin-converting enzyme 2 (ACE2) expression and activity in human carotid atherosclerotic lesions. *J Pathol.* (2008) 215:273–79. doi: 10.1002/path.2357

149. Muus C, Luecken MD, Eraslan G, Waghray A, Heimberg G, Sikkema L, et al. Integrated analyses of single-cell atlases reveal age, gender, and smoking status associations with cell type-specific expression of mediators of SARS-CoV-2 viral entry and highlights inflammatory programs in putative target cells. *BioRxiv.* (2020). doi: 10.1101/2020.04.19.049254

150. Ratajczak MZ, Bujko K, Ciechanowicz A, Sielatycka K, Cymer M, Marlicz W, et al. SARS-CoV-2 entry receptor ACE2 is expressed on very small CD45– precursors of hematopoietic and endothelial cells and in response to virus spike protein activates the Nlrp3 inflammasome. *Stem Cell Rev Reports.* (2020) 16:1–2. doi: 10.1007/s12015-019-09951-x

151. Rahimi FS, Afaghi S, Tarki FE, Goudarzi K, Alamdari NM. Viral outbreaks of SARS-CoV1, SARS-CoV2, MERS-CoV, influenza H1N1, and ebola in 21st Century; a comparative review of the pathogenesis and clinical characteristics. *School Med Stud J.* 151. (2020). doi: 10.22037/smsj.v2i3. 30455

152. Iba T, Levy JH, Levi M, Thachil J. Coagulopathy in COVID-19. *J Thromb Haemost.* (2020) 18:2103–9. doi: 10.1111/jth.14975

153. Chen L, Li X, Chen M, Feng Y, Xiong C. The ACE2 expression in human heart indicates new potential mechanism of heart injury among patients infected with SARS-CoV-2. *Cardiovasc Res.* (2020) 116:1097–100. doi: 10.1093/cvr/cvaa078

154. Miele L, Miao H, Nickoloff B. NOTCH signaling as a novel cancer therapeutic target. *Curr Cancer Drug Targets.* (2006) 6:313–23. doi: 10.2174/156800906777441771

155. Woo HN, Park JS, Gwon AR, Arumugam TV, Jo DG. Alzheimer's disease and Notch signaling. *Biochem Biophys Res Commun.* (2009) 390:1093–7. doi: 10.1016/j.bbrc.2009.10.093

156. Li K, Li Y, Wu W, Gordon WR, Chang DW, Lu M, et al. Modulation of Notch signaling by antibodies specific for the extracellular negative regulatory region of NOTCH3. *J Biol Chem.* (2008) 283:8046–54. doi: 10.1074/jbc.M800170200

157. Falk R, Falk A, Dyson MR, Melidoni AN, Parthiban K, Young JL, et al. Generation of anti-Notch antibodies and their application in blocking Notch signalling in neural stem cells. *Methods.* (2012) 58:69–78. doi: 10.1016/j.ymeth.2012.07.008

158. Valcourt DM, Dang MN, Scully MA, Day ES. Nanoparticle-mediated co-delivery of Notch-1 antibodies and ABT-737 as a potent treatment strategy for triple-negative breast cancer. *ACS Nano.* (2020) 14:3378–88. doi: 10.1021/acsnano.9b09263

159. Kangsamaksin T, Murtomaki A, Kofler NM, Cuervo H, Chaudhri RA, Tattersall IW, et al. NOTCH decoys that selectively block DLL/NOTCH or JAG/NOTCH disrupt angiogenesis by unique mechanisms to inhibit tumor growth. *Cancer Discovery.* (2015) 5:182–97. doi: 10.1158/2159-8290.CD-14-0650

160. Mitra A, Shanthalingam S, Sherman HL, Singh K, Canakci M, Torres JA, et al. CD28 signaling drives notch ligand expression on CD4 T cells. *Front Immunol.* (2020) 11:735. doi: 10.3389/fimmu.2020. 00735

27

Association between Cardiovascular Risk Factors and the Severity of Coronavirus Disease 2019: Nationwide Epidemiological Study

Kyoung Ae Kong[1†], Sodam Jung[2†], Mina Yu[3], Junbeom Park[2] and In Sook Kang[2]*

[1] Department of Preventive Medicine, College of Medicine, Ewha Womans University, Seoul, South Korea, [2] Division of Cardiology, Department of Internal Medicine, Ewha Womans University Mokdong Hospital, College of Medicine, Ewha Womans University, Seoul, South Korea, [3] Division of Nephrology, Department of Internal Medicine, Ewha Womans University Seoul Hospital, College of Medicine, Ewha Womans University, Seoul, South Korea

Correspondence:
In Sook Kang
pinkvision@ewha.ac.kr

[†] *These authors have contributed equally to this work and share first authorship*

Background: Acute respiratory viral infections can result in cardiovascular involvement, with such patients having a significantly higher mortality rate than those without cardiovascular involvement. Due to the ongoing coronavirus disease 2019 (COVID-19) pandemic, it is important to determine whether cardiovascular risk factors are associated with the severity of COVID-19.

Methods: These nationwide data were provided by the Korea Disease Control and Prevention Agency. We defined a patient as having a "critical illness" if they required more than invasive mechanical ventilation and "fatal illness" if they died.

Results: Among the total 5,307 patients, 2,136 (40.8%) were male. The critical illness rate was 5.1% (males: 6.7, females: 4.0%) and the fatality rate was 4.54%. The multivariable analysis showed that age $\geq$60 years, male sex, diabetes mellitus, hypertension, heart failure, chronic kidney disease, cancer, and dementia were independent risk factors for critical illness. The risk scoring model showed the significance of multiple risk factors. Patients with four risk factors; old age ($\geq$60 years), male sex, hypertension, and diabetes mellitus had a more than a 100 times higher risk for severe COVID-19 than those without these risk factors (OR; 95% confidence interval, 104; 45.6–240.6 for critical, 136.2; 52.3–3547.9 for fatal illness).

Conclusions: This study demonstrated that cardiovascular risk factors are also significant risk factors for severe COVID-19. In particular, patients who have multiple cardiovascular risk factors are more likely to progress to severe COVID-19. Therefore, early and appropriate treatment of these patients is crucial.

Keywords: COVID-19, SARS-CoV-2, cardiovascular disease, risk factor, mortality

INTRODUCTION

The risk of myocardial infarction is known to be proportional to the severity of an acute respiratory infection (1). Acute viral pneumonia can result in cardiovascular diseases, such as heart failure, acute myocardial infarction, arrhythmia, and myocarditis. Patients with cardiovascular involvement have a significantly higher mortality rate than those without cardiovascular involvement (1–4).

Since the end of 2019, coronavirus disease 2019 (COVID-19) caused by a novel coronavirus, severe acute respiratory syndrome coronavirus 2 (SARS-CoV-2), has spread to more than 200 countries around the world. It has displayed high transmission power, severity, and mortality. The clinical manifestation of COVID-19 is broad, ranging from no symptoms to fever, acute respiratory distress syndrome, multiple organ failure, and death (5). Many countries around the world have been struggling to contain COVID-19, and so far, no definite treatment has been developed. Therefore, it is important to assess the risk factors that affect the severity and fatality of COVID-19.

Excess mortality was reported in the United States during the influenza pandemic. Although the association with secondary infections was not identified, cardiovascular event may have been a contributing factor (1, 6). A recent observational study showed that underlying cardiovascular diseases, such as coronary artery disease, congestive heart failure, and arrhythmia were associated with an increased risk of in-hospital death by COVID-19 (7). Early on in the pandemic, studies in China showed that people with underlying conditions such as hypertension, diabetes mellitus, cerebrovascular disease, or cardiovascular disease were more likely to be admitted to the intensive care unit (5).

Hence, in this study, we focused and analyzed the clinical implications of cardiovascular risk factors and the presence or absence of cardiovascular disease on the outcome and severity of COVID-19. Research on cardiovascular risk factors, including hypertension and diabetes mellitus, which are prevalent in the entire population, and the effect of sex and age on the severity of COVID-19 are not only important to cardiologists, but are significant public health topics. Further, this study can provide important prognostic information for patients.

The previous studies are mostly conducted early on in the pandemic and have limited study populations. The Republic of Korea reduced the spread of COVID-19 by proactively and systematically identifying patients with COVID-19 based on the national health insurance system, which is a single-payer, compulsory subscription system. Accordingly, we have a good basis for analyzing the characteristics of the clinical features of COVID-19 using data from across Korea. Here, we analyzed whether cardiovascular disease and/or the associated risk factors affect the severity of COVID-19 using data provided by the Korea Disease Control and Prevention Agency (KDCA).

MATERIALS AND METHODS

Data Source and Study Population

This is a retrospective cohort study, using nationwide data from the Republic of Korea. Study candidates are the patients with COVID-19 who had been hospitalized, among the patients released from isolation or died as of April 30, 2020. Since the first confirmed case of COVID-19 in Korea on January 19, 2020, the KDCA has actively tracked almost all patients and their contacts in an attempt to control the spread of COVID-19. Further, cumulative statistics are released daily on a public web site (http://ncov.mohw.go.kr/en/) and through the media. The KDCA developed a registry of confirmed COVID-19 cases and provided the anonymized data to select researchers. The data includes only COVID-19 patients that had been released from isolation or died until 30 April 2020. We analyzed the data received from the KDCA via encrypted, remote access.

A brief summary of the COVID-19 related quarantine issues in Korea from January 19 to April 30, 2020 is as follows. The approximate total population of the Republic of Korea was 51,780,579 in April 2020 (8). The total number of COVID-19 tests conducted was 623,069 and the number of confirmed cases was 10,774 as of April 30, 2020 (**Figure 1A**). Among the 10,774 confirmed cases, 1,073 (9.96%) were foreign patients. In total, 9,072 patients had been released from isolation, and 248 had died (fatality rate: 2.73%). Of the 9,072 patients who had been released from isolation, 8,976 had accessible medical records. Of these, 5,350 were hospitalized, 3,450 were admitted to community treatment centers, and 176 were isolated at home. Most of the patients who were isolated at home or community treatment center had asymptomatic or mild disease (9). If disease progressed to moderate or severe condition, they were transferred to hospitals. Of the people who initially entered a community treatment center, approximately 270–280 patients were eventually hospitalized (**Figure 1B**) (10). The KDCA allowed select researchers temporary access to the anonymized data of 5,628 patients (under granted permission).

A total of 5,628 raw data points corresponding to inpatients from the KDCA were initially reviewed (**Figure 1B** in the pink box). Finally, 5,307 patients were analyzed after excluding 272 patients under the age of 20 years, 19 pregnant women, 26 without clinical severity information, and four without comorbidity information.

The data included the presence of diabetes mellitus, hypertension, heart failure, chronic heart disease, asthma, chronic obstructive pulmonary disease, chronic kidney disease, malignancy, chronic liver disease, rheumatic/autoimmune disease, and dementia, but did not show the duration of disease and medication history. The co-morbid condition was collected through history taking by medical personnel with questionnaire. There was no available detailed information, disease status and treatment regimens for COVID-19 in the given data.

Study Definitions

A confirmed case was defined as a patient who had tested positive for SARS-CoV-2 after a real-time reverse transcription-polymerase chain reaction (RT-PCR) test with respiratory specimens: upper respiratory specimens (nasopharyngeal and oropharyngeal swabs), with or without a lower respiratory specimen (sputum), regardless of their clinical manifestations (2). To be released from isolation or discharged, patients had to be:

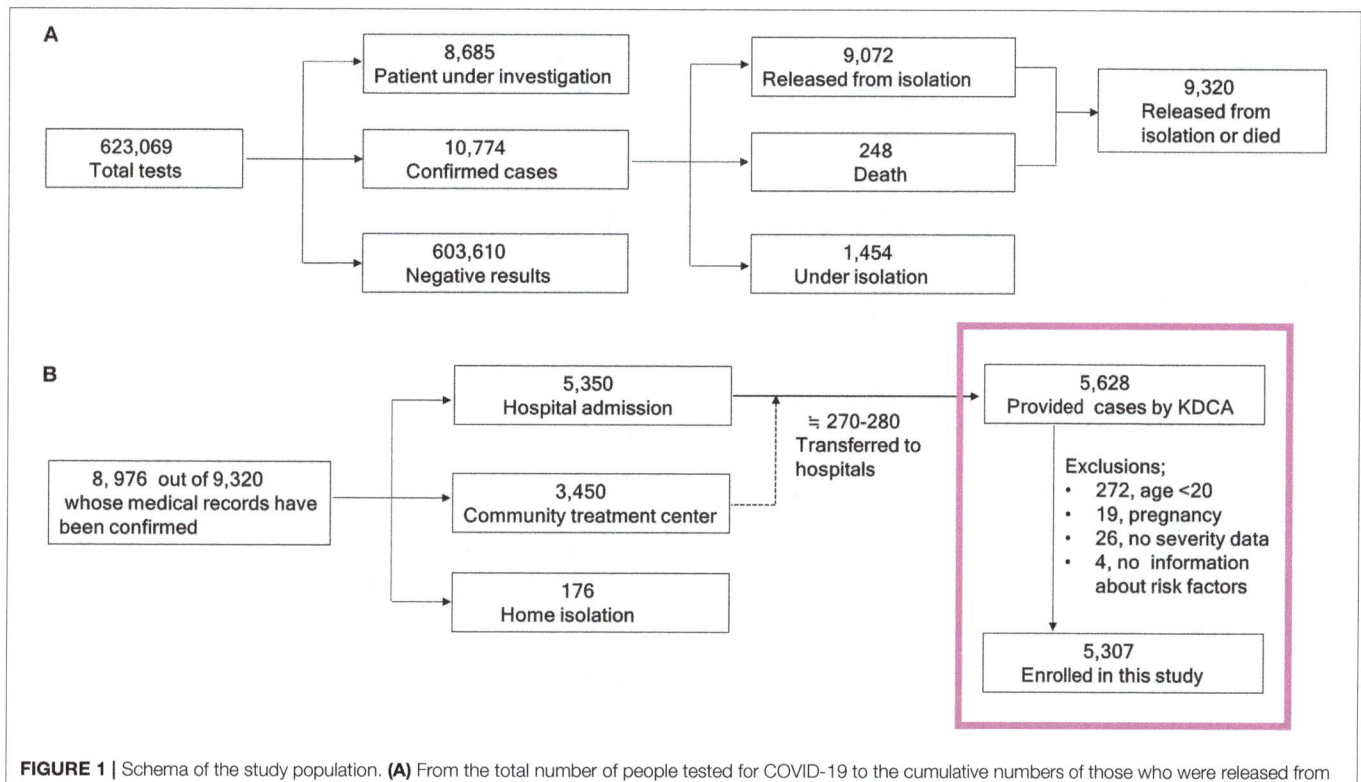

FIGURE 1 | Schema of the study population. **(A)** From the total number of people tested for COVID-19 to the cumulative numbers of those who were released from isolation or died. **(B)** Flow chart of the current study candidates. KDCA, Korea Disease Control and Prevention Agency.

(1) afebrile without symptoms for 10 days and/or (2) have two negative RT-PCR results at least a 24-h interval (11).

Disease severity was defined according to the KDCA and World Health Organization guidelines (11, 12) as follows: level 1, no limitation of daily activities; level 2, limitation of daily activities but no need for oxygen therapy; level 3, oxygen therapy via a nasal cannula; level 4, oxygen therapy via a facial mask; level 5, high-flow supplemental oxygen therapy or non-invasive mechanical ventilation; level 6, needs invasive mechanical ventilation; level 7, multi-organ failure or needs extracorporeal membrane oxygenation (ECMO) therapy; level 8, death. Levels 6–8 were defined as critical illness, whereas 8 was defined as fatal illness. In this study, critical illness is a broader concept that includes fatal illness, and fatal illness refers to a mortality case. The severity evaluation was based on patients with the most severe condition during their hospital stay. For example, fatal illness refers to death of patients regardless of whether they received level 1 or 7 treatment. All fatality cases were made to correspond to level 8. Both critical and fatal illness were considered to be severe COVID-19.

Information on comorbidities was reviewed to determine whether patients had previously been diagnosed with specific comorbidities. Body temperature and body mass index were the initial findings on hospital admission.

Statistical Analysis

The baseline characteristics of the subjects were described as a frequency and proportion for categorical data. The chi-square test was used to compare the categorical variables. The values of continuous variables were expressed as the median and interquartile range (IQR; Q1, Q3). The Mann-Whitney U, or Wilcoxon rank-sum tests were performed for body temperature. Univariate and multivariable logistic regression models were applied to evaluate the risk factors of critical and fatal illness. Age was given as a categorical variable in units of 10 years. There were no critical or death cases reported in the 20–29-year age (20s) group. So, age group was categorized as <40 (20s + 30s) years, 40s, 50s, 60s, 70s, and ≥80 years for logistic regression, and the 60s used as the reference.

Multivariable logistic regression was used to analyze the independent risk of critical and fatal illness after adjusting for several comorbid diseases: diabetes mellitus, hypertension, heart failure, chronic heart disease (other than hypertension and heart failure), bronchial asthma, chronic obstructive lung disease (COPD), chronic kidney disease (CKD), chronic liver disease, rheumatic disease, cancer (excluding cured cases), and dementia.

Utilizing the cardiovascular risk factors, a model for criticality and fatality prediction was made with age ≥60, male sex, medical history of diabetes mellitus, and hypertension as one point each. Theses ranged from a minimum of zero to a maximum of four points.

Next, the criticality and fatality prediction models were analyzed by logistic regression model, odds ratios (ORs) and c-statistics were obtained. The c-statistics were equivalent to the area under the receiver operating characteristic (ROC) curve, based on the predicted probability of the outcomes (the critical or

TABLE 1 | Baseline characteristics of the study population.

Characteristics	Overall (n = 5,307)	Critical illness (n = 271)	Fatal illness (n = 241)	Incidence (%)	
	N (column %)	N (column %)	N (column %)	Critical	Fatal
Age (years)					
20–29	1,104 (20.8)	0 (0)	0 (0)	0	0
30–39	549 (10.3)	3 (1.1)	2 (0.8)	0.5	0.4
40–49	738 (13.9)	2 (0.7)	2 (0.8)	0.3	0.3
50–59	1,141 (21.5)	21 (7.7)	15 (6.2)	1.8	1.3
60-69	906 (17.1)	45 (16.6)	34 (14.1)	5.0	3.8
70–79	545 (10.3)	82 (30.3)	73 (30.3)	15	13.4
≥80	324 (6.1)	118 (43.5)	115 (47.7)	36.4	35.5
Female	3,144 (59.2)	127 (46.9)	114 (47.3)	4	3.6
Male	2,163 (40.8)	144 (53.1)	127 (52.7)	6.7	5.9
Body temperature (°C)	36.9	37.0	37.0		
Median (Q1,Q3)	(36.5, 37.3)	(36.6, 37.9)	(36.5, 37.9)		
Cough*					
Yes	2,231 (42.0)	92 (33.9)	81 (33.6)	4.1	3.6
No	3,075 (57.9)	179 (66.1)	169 (66.4)	5.8	5.2
Sputum*					
Yes	1,549 (29.2)	79 (29.2)	72 (29.9)	5.1	4.6
No	3,757 (70.8)	192 (70.8)	169 (70.1)	5.1	4.5
Sore throat*					
Yes	839 (15.8)	14 (5.2)	13 (5.4)	1.7	1.5
No	4,467 (84.2)	257 (94.8)	228 (94.6)	5.8	5.1
Shortness of breath*					
Yes	658 (12.4)	134 (49.4)	113 (46.9)	20.4	17.2
No	4,648 (87.6)	137 (50.6)	128 (53.1)	2.9	2.8
Diarrhea*					
Yes	504 (9.5)	20 (7.4)	18 (7.5)	4	3.6
No	4,802 (90.5)	251 (92.6)	223 (92.5)	5.2	4.6
Systolic BP†					
<120	1,201 (22.6)	66 (24.4)	58 (24.1)	5.5	4.8
120–129	1,076 (20.3)	33 (12.2)	28 (11.6)	3.1	2.6
130–139	1,039 (19.6)	36 (13.3)	32 (13.3)	3.5	3.1
140–159	1,381 (26.0)	77 (28.4)	68 (28.2)	5.6	4.9
≥160	507 (9.6)	41 (15.1)	37 (15.4)	8.1	7.3
BMI (kg/m²)‡					
<18.5	191 (3.6)	16 (5.9)	16 (6.6)	8.4	8.4
18.5–22.9	1,741 (32.8)	55 (20.3)	46 (19.1)	3.2	2.6
23.0–24.9	1,005 (18.9)	25 (9.2)	20 (8.3)	2.5	2
24.9–29.9	1,011 (19.1)	49 (18.2)	39 (16.2)	4.8	3.9
≥30	193 (3.6)	7 (2.6)	5 (2.1)	3.6	2.6
Diabetes mellitus					
Yes	684 (12.9)	106 (39.1)	98 (40.7)	15.5	14.3
No	4,623 (87.1)	165 (60.9)	143 (59.3)	3.6	3.1
Hypertension					
Yes	1,197 (22.6)	164 (60.5)	144 (59.8)	13.7	12.0
No	4,110 (77.4)	107 (39.5)	97 (40.2)	2.6	2.4
Heart failure					
Yes	59 (1.1)	20 (7.4)	18 (7.5)	33.9	30.5
No	5,248 (98.9)	251 (92.6)	223 (92.5)	4.8	4.2

(Continued)

TABLE 1 | Continued

Characteristics	Overall (n = 5,307)	Critical illness (n = 271)	Fatal illness (n = 241)	Incidence (%)	
	N (column %)	N (column %)	N (column %)	Critical	Fatal
Chronic heart disease					
Yes	179 (3.4)	29 (10.7)	26 (10.8)	16.2	14.5
No	5,112 (96.3)	242 (89.3)	215 (89.2)	4.7	4.2
Missing	16 (0.3)	0	0	0	0
Asthma					
Yes	126 (2.4)	13 (4.8)	13 (5.4)	10.3	10.3
No	5,181 (97.6)	258 (95.2)	228 (94.6)	5	4.4
COPD					
Yes	38 (0.7)	9 (3.3)	8 (3.3)	23.7	21.1
No	5,269 (99.3)	262 (96.7)	233 (96.7)	5	4.4
Chronic kidney disease					
Yes	55 (1.0)	18 (6.6)	16 (6.6)	32.7	29.1
No	5,252 (99.0)	253 (93.4)	225 (93.4)	4.8	4.3
Cancer					
Yes	145 (2.7)	22 (8.1)	22 (9.1)	15.2	15.2
No	5,162 (97.3)	249 (91.9)	219 (90.9)	4.8	4.2
Chronic liver disease[§]					
Yes	83 (1.6)	7 (2.6)	7 (2.9)	8.4	8.4
No	4,912 (92.6)	264 (91.9)	234 (97.1)	5.4	4.8
Rheumatic disease[‖]					
Yes	38 (0.7)	3 (1.1)	3 (1.2)	7.9	7.9
No	4,951 (89.8)	268 (98.9)	238 (98.8)	5.4	4.8
Dementia[¶]					
Yes	224 (4.2)	76 (28.0)	75 (31.1)	33.9	33.5
No	4,768 (89.8)	195 (72.0)	166 (68.9)	4.1	3.5
Severity**					
Level 1	4,179 (78.7)	0 (0)	0 (0)	0	0
Level 2	314 (5.9)	0 (0)	0 (0)	0	0
Level 3	468 (8.8)	0 (0)	0 (0)	0	0
Level 4	43 (0.8)	0 (0)	0 (0)	0	0
Level 5	32 (0.6)	0 (0)	0 (0)	0	0
Level 6	19 (0.4)	19 (7.0)	0 (0)	100	0
Level 7	11 (0.2)	11 (4.1)	0 (0)	100	0
Level 8	241 (4.5)	241 (88.9)	241 (100)	100	100

COPD, chronic obstructive lung disease. *missing n = 1, [†]missing n = 103, [‡]missing n = 1,166, [§]missing n = 312, [‖]missing n = 318, [¶]missing n = 315, **Severity level 1, no limitation of daily activities; level 2, limitation of daily activities but no need oxygen therapy; level 3, oxygen therapy via nasal cannula; level 4, oxygen therapy via facial mask; level 5, high-flow supplemental oxygen therapy or non-invasive mechanical ventilation; level 6, the need for invasive mechanical ventilation; level 7, multi-organ failure or the need for extracorporeal membrane oxygenation therapy; level 8, death.

fatal disease) in the logistic regression models with the risk score as independent variable. In this model, each score was treated as binary category of 0 or 1.

For risk score validation, we performed internal validation using bootstrap resampling. To evaluate the performance of compensating overfitting of logistic regression and the risk score model, a total of 1,000 random bootstrap samples were generated for replacement of the original data, and each bootstrap sample size was the same scale as the original data. Then the means and 95% confidence intervals of bootstrap samples were calculated. The c-statistic difference between original data and bootstrap

samples was defined as optimism. Optimism-corrected c-statistic can be obtained by subtracting the estimated mean of the optimism estimate value from the c-index in the original sample.

A P-value of <0.05 was considered statistically significance. The statistical analysis was performed using the SAS software (version 9.4, SAS Institute, Cary, NC, USA).

Ethics Statement

This study was deemed exempt from ethical review and the requirement for informed consent was waived by the Ewha Womans University Mokdong hospital Institutional

Review Board (EUMC2020-07-002) because all of the data were fully anonymized and did not include personally identifiable information.

RESULTS

The baseline demographic and clinical characteristics are presented in **Table 1**. Among the 5,307 patents, 2,136 (40.8%) were male, the rate of critical illness was 5.1% (male: 6.7, female: 4.0%; $P < 0.001$), and the fatality of the study group was 4.54%. Number of cases is highest in the 20s and 50s, but no critical illness or fatal illness was in the 20s. Meanwhile, critical illness started to rise steeply from the age of 50s, reaching 43.5% in the 80s.

Clinical symptoms including cough, sputum, sore throat and diarrhea did not differ according to severity, but shortness of breath was more frequently reported in the critical illness than in the non-critical illness (20.4 vs. 2.9%) patients. Patients with systolic blood pressures of <120 or ≥140 mmHg were more likely to be critically ill than those with a systolic blood pressure between 120 and 140 mmHg. Underweight patients with a body mass index of <18.5 kg/m^2 also showed a higher in the critical illness than in the non-critical illness patients.

Patients with chronic diseases (diabetes mellitus, hypertension, CKD), cardiovascular diseases (heart failure, chronic stable heart disease), respiratory disorder (asthma, COPD), cancer, and/or dementia presented higher rate of critical illness than those without. No significant difference in severity was seen between patients with chronic liver disease or rheumatic disorder and those without. Among the 271 critically ill patients, 19 survived with invasive ventilation and 11 ECMO, whereas the remaining 241 did not survived.

Figure 2 shows the disease frequency and critical illness ratio according to sex and age. There were some differences between males and females in the distribution of disease and severity according to age. For example, despite the high frequency of COVID-19 in patients in their 20s, no cases of critical illness were found. In addition, the rate of critical illness increased significantly with age, but this characteristic was more prominent in males.

Logistic analyses were performed to evaluate the risk factors for critical and fatal illness (**Table 2**). In the univariate analyses of **Table 2**, all variables were significantly related to both critical and fatal illness except for chronic liver disease and rheumatic disease. Importantly, age was an important risk factor, with those aged <50 years having less risk. Those age ≥70 years had sharply increased ORs. In particular, in patients aged ≥80 years, heart failure, CKD, and dementia had a high OR above 7.0. In the multivariable model 1 in **Table 2**, asthma and COPD lost their significance for critical and fatal illnesses. Heart failure showed a decreased odds ratio as 2.13 (1.12–4.05) for critical illness and lost the significance of 1.94 (0.99–3.77) for fatal illness.

In addition, we performed multivariable analyses with four major cardiovascular risk factors (model 2). The results showed similar ORs with model 1 in **Table 2**. However, ORs of those with age ≥80 was markedly elevated and hypertension lost statistical power of 1.29 (0.94–1.77) for fatal illness.

Model 1 and model 2 showed good performance for prediction of critical illness (original c-statistics, 0.905 and 0.902; optimism-corrected c-statistics, 0.899 and 0.900) and fatal illness (0.917 and 0.912; 0.912 and 0.910). Interestingly, model 2 showed excellent performance similar to model 1. Furthermore, all the values of model 2; bootstrap, original, and corrected, c-statistics showed ≥0.9 for critical and fatal illness.

According to the result of model 2, we calculated risk score with simplified four variables: age ≥60 years, male sex,

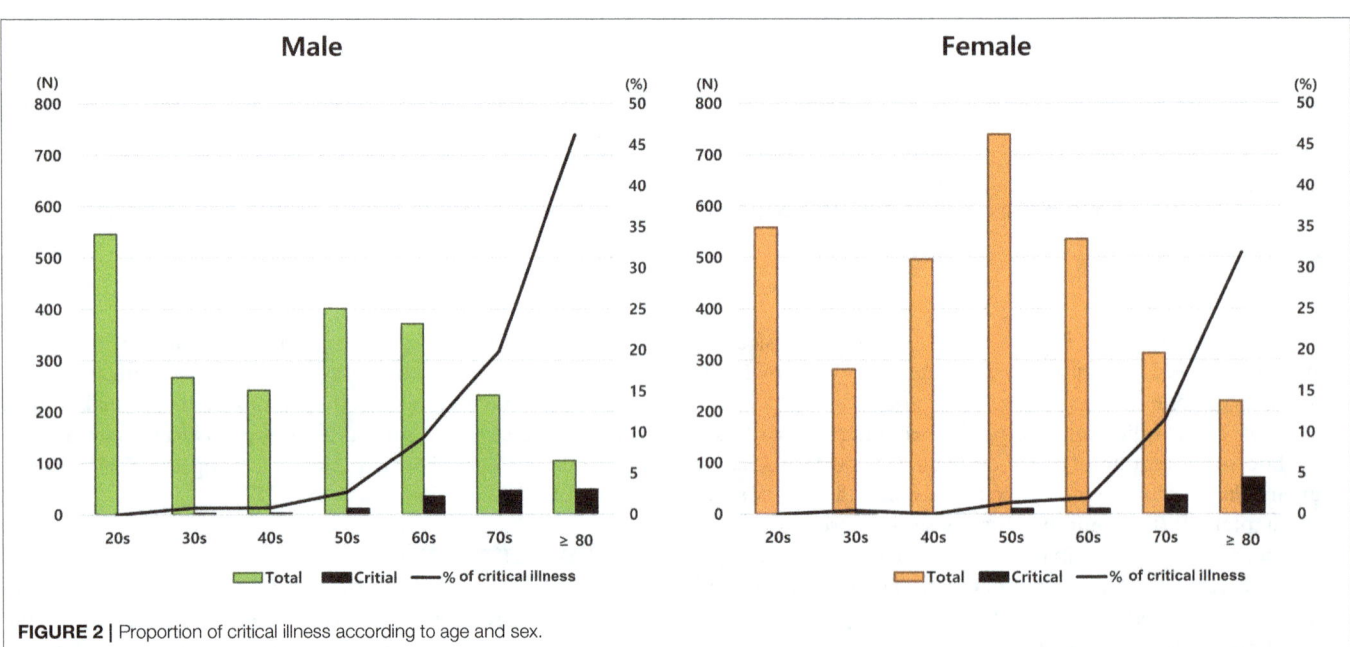

FIGURE 2 | Proportion of critical illness according to age and sex.

TABLE 2 | Logistic analyses and c-statistics for critical and fatal illness.

	Critical illness Odds ratio (95% CI)			Fatal illness Odds ratio (95% CI)		
	Univariate	Multivariable		Univariate	Multivariable	
		Model 1	Model 2		Model 1	Model 2
Age (years)						
<40*	0.04 (0.01–0.11)	0.05 (0.02–0.18)	0.05 (0.01–0.15)	0.03 (0.01–0.13)	0.05 (0.01–0.21)	0.04 (0.01–0.17)
40s	0.05 (0.01–0.22)	0.08 (0.02–0.32)	0.07 (0.02–0.29)	0.07 (0.02–0.29)	0.11 (0.03–0.44)	0.09 (0.02–0.39)
50s	0.36 (0.21–0.61)	0.45 (0.26–4.16)	0.43 (0.25–0.73)	0.34 (0.19–0.63)	0.43 (0.23–0.80)	0.41 (0.22–0.75)
60s	1 (reference)	1 (reference)	1 (reference)	1 (reference)	1 (reference)	1 (reference)
70s	3.39 (2.32–4.96)	2.80 (1.89–4.16)	3.10 (2.11–4.58)	3.97 (2.60–6.05)	3.29 (2.13–5.10)	3.68 (2.39–5.65)
≥80	10.96 (7.53–15.96)	7.18 (4.65–11.07)	11.66 (7.87–17.27)	14.11 (9.35–21.29)	9.40 (5.87–15.05)	15.51 (10.09–23.83)
Male (vs. Female)	1.89 (1.48–2.42)	2.47 (1.85–3.31)	2.35 (1.77–3.11)	1.85 (1.42–2.40)	2.51 (1.84–3.43)	2.34 (1.73–3.16)
Diabetes mellitus	3.80 (2.93–4.92)	1.84 (1.36–2.50)	1.89 (1.40–2.55)	4.02 (3.06–5.28)	2.07 (1.50–2.87)	2.09 (1.52–2.86)
Hypertension	4.35 (3.37–5.6)	1.49 (1.10–2.01)	1.49 (1.11–2.00)	4.14 (3.17–5.41)	1.30 (0.94–1.79)	1.29 (0.94–1.77)
Heart failure	7.96 (4.57–13.85)	2.13 (1.12–4.05)		7.72 (4.36–13.66)	1.94 (0.99–3.77)	
CHD	3.10 (2.04–4.71)	2.13 (1.12–4.05)		3.08 (1.99–4.78)	1.02 (0.60–1.72)	
Asthma	2.01 (1.11–3.64)	1.43 (0.70–2.92)		2.30 (1.27–4.16)	1.71 (0.83–3.53)	
COPD	4.62 (2.17–9.87)	1.23 (0.48–3.16)		4.50 (2.04–9.93)	1.04 (0.38–2.83)	
CKD	7.93 (4.43–14.19)	2.75 (1.33–5.72)		7.54 (4.13–13.77)	2.54 (1.19–5.43)	
Cancer	2.83 (1.77–4.54)	2.41 (1.38–4.20)		3.24 (2.02–5.22)	2.89 (1.64–5.10)	
CLD	1.37 (0.62–3.00)	1.10 (0.46–2.68)		1.55 (0.71–3.42)	1.32 (0.54–3.23)	
Rheumatic disease	1.18 (0.36–3.86)	1.91 (0.52–6.99)		1.34 (0.41–4.39)	2.38 (0.64–8.82)	
Dementia	9.42 (6.90–12.87)	2.32 (1.57–3.42)		10.94 (7.96–15.03)	2.58 (1.74–3.84)	
Bootstrap[†]		0.908 (0.891–0.923)	0.903 (0.886–0.919)		0.920 (0.904–0.934)	0.913 (0.896–0.928)
Original, Corrected[‡]		0.905, 0.899	0.902, 0.900		0.917, 0.912	0.912, 0.910

<40*, 20–39 years; CHD, chronic heart disease; COPD, chronic obstructive lung disease; CKD, chronic kidney disease; CLD, chronic liver disease. [†]Mean of c-statistics (and 95% confidence interval) of bootstrap samples; [‡]C-statistics of original data, the optimism corrected c-statistics.

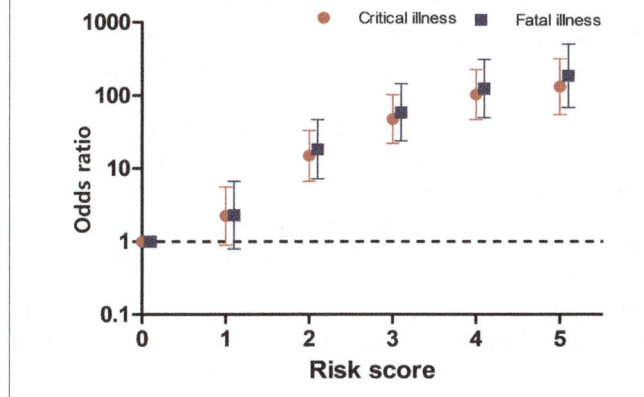

FIGURE 3 | Odds ratios for critical and fatal illness according to the risk score. The scores represent the number of risk factors.

3; 58.4 (36.9–12.8) and 69.2 (27.9–171.8), and 4; 104 (45.6–240.6), and 136.2 (52.3–354.9), respectively. This risk scoring model showed good model fitness (original c = 0.8300 and 0.8321, corrected c = 0.8303 and 0.8324) for critical and fatal illness, respectively.

DISCUSSION

This study demonstrated that cardiovascular risk factors are also significant risk factors for severe COVID-19. In particular, age ≥60 years was shown to be a strong risk factor; the risk of severe COVID-19 significantly increased by 10 times in those aged ≥80 years compared to those in their 60s. Similar to heart disease, male had a higher risk, and more than twice the odds ratio for critical COVID-19 than female. Hypertension was a risk factor for critical illness rather than fatal illness which was same to heart failure. Additionally, dementia and cancer were found to be poor prognostic factors. Respiratory diseases, such as asthma and COPD were not found to be significant risk factors. Regarding the risk score model, the risk of critical or fatal illness increased sharply according to every increase in score compared to those without risk factors (risk score zero). Therefore, the more risk factors a patient has, the greater their likelihood of progressing to severe COVID-19.

diabetes mellitus, and hypertension, which are also known to be cardiovascular risk factors. Each one risk factor was calculated as one point. **Figure 3** shows that the OR for the disease severity increased as the number of risk scores increased relative to the zero point. The ORs (95% confidence interval) for critical and fatal illness were as followings: score 1; 5.1 (2.3–11.5) and 6.4 (2.5–16.3), score 2; 29.9 (13.9–64.7) and 37.2 (15.0–91.9), score

Cardiovascular risk factors are known as smoking, hypertension, diabetes, obesity, physical inactivity, age, male sex (13, 14). However, the data we have only contain diabetes, hypertension, age, sex among the cardiovascular risk factors. Therefore, the risk score was calculated only for the risk factors included in the data. Nonetheless, one interesting thing about this study is that prediction performance of model 2, which included four cardiovascular risk factors (age; six grouped, sex, DM, hypertension), showed as good as that of model 1, which was included 13 variables. When the age groups were simplified as binary group based on the age of 60, the prediction performance was decreased from 0.900 to 0.830 (optimism corrected c) for critical illness. However, which was also good performance. The purpose of this study was to show an association between CV risk factors and the severe COVID-19, rather than developing a new scoring system for predicting severe COVID-19. Through this, we aimed to bring health care providers and patients themselves to have attention of the deleterious effects of multiple CV risk factors in the COVID-19 pandemic era. We intentionally simplified the scoring system as much as possible and included well-known highly prevalence disease.

Previous studies have shown an association between the Middle East respiratory syndrome (MERS) and SARS with acute myocarditis, myocardial infarction, and heart failure as well as a relationship of COVID-19 and myocardial injury (2, 3, 15). These viral infections are all caused by CoV. Furthermore, SARS-CoV-2 has similar pathogenicity to MERS-CoV, which can induce damage to the cardiovascular system, and as a result, can increase the difficulty and complexity of patient treatment (16). There are two implications for this. First is the importance of comorbidities on the prognosis of viral infection. In particular, hypertension and diabetes have been reported as common comorbidities in COVID-19, SARS, and MERS, especially among those with more severe disease (5, 17, 18). In a cohort of 138 hospitalized patients with COVID-19, the reported rate of hypertension was 31% (58% in patients requiring intensive care), and diabetes was 10% (22% in patients requiring intensive care) (5). In the current study, 22.6% had hypertension (60.5% in those with critical illness), 12.9% had diabetes mellitus (39.1% in those with critical illness). Second, it is important to determine whether myocardial damage occurs during viral infection. Data from China showed that elevated level of cardiac biomarker-troponin T was related to increased mortality of patients with COVID-19 regardless of cardiovascular disease (4), and almost 12% of patients without known cardiovascular disease had elevated troponin levels or experienced cardiac arrest during hospitalization (19). We suggest, these results that elevated troponin in other studies is associated with mortality may indirectly explain the mechanism of disease severity and mortality in our study.

Potential mechanisms for the association between acute viral infection and increased myocardial damage are as follows: (1) type 1 myocardial infarction, which is caused by atherosclerotic plaque rupture or coronary thrombosis related acute inflammation; (2) type 2 myocardial infarction, which is related to the mismatch of oxygen demand and supply, and (3) direct effect of the virus and inflammation on the cardiac cells (1, 16, 20). A cardiac metabolic mismatch may be induced by the aggravation of coronary artery stenosis by toxin-mediated vasoconstriction in individuals who already have coronary artery stenosis due to chronic atherosclerotic plaques, particularly in the elderly (1). The current study showed that cardiovascular risk factors are also risk factors for severe COVID-19. However, data regarding cardiac biomarkers, which can evaluate myocardial damage, was not available. Therefore, it can only be presumed that the poor prognosis of patients with multiple cardiovascular risk factors is related to myocardial damage.

Previous studies have shown that elevated cardiac troponin and pro-brain natriuretic peptide are each independently associated with poor outcomes in patients with COVID-19 patients (4, 21). However, there is scarce evidence as to which patients are associated with elevated cardiac biomarkers. The COVID-19 pandemic is still driven by virus mutations, and it is a high possibility that a subsequent global pandemic will be repeated by various respiratory viruses. Therefore, research on COVID-19 and the cardiovascular system should be continued to improve patients' prognoses. Through this study, we identified that patients with multiple CV risk factors are associated with severe COVID-19. Through future follow-up studies, it is important to investigate whether the risk score model/multiple CV risk factors in this study is associated with the proportional increase of cardiac troponin or pro-brain natriuretic peptide or new-onset atrial fibrillation which reflecting cardiac complications and poor outcome of COVID-19 patients.

This study showed that CKD, cancer, and dementia are also risk factors. Dementia is a disease that is more prevalent in older individuals. However, it was still found to be a significant risk factor even after adjusting for age and other comorbid conditions. Several studies have found that CKD is related to an increased risk of mortality from COVID-19 (5, 12). In studies form Europe and America, the mortality of CKD patients was higher than that of the normal group, and inversely proportional to the glomerular filtration rate (11, 22). There are several reasons as to why renal dysfunction worsens COVID-19. First, there is a decrease in immune function in uremic patients (23, 24). A previous study showed that in hemodialysis patients infected with COVID-19, the absolute number of natural killer cells is smaller, and the ratio differs from that in COVID-19 patients without dialysis (25). Second, patients with CKD are known to have a higher risk of cardiovascular disease than patients with normal renal function (26). The mortality rate and risk rate from cardiovascular disease are high, and it is considered to be one of the reasons for the high COVID-19 mortality rate in patients with CKD. In this study, we did not have data on the stage of CKD, and whether patients were undergoing dialysis or had previously had a kidney transplant. We did not include CKD in the risk score model due to heterogeneity and these limitations. However, CKD should be considered an important risk factor for severe COVID-19.

In general, patients with an underlying respiratory disease appear to have a poor prognosis for respiratory infections (27). Previous studies have shown that COPD has a significant effect on the prognosis of COVID-19 pneumonia. As yet, this association has not been confirmed in patients with asthma. In previous meta-analyses, COPD was found to increase the risk of severe COVID-19 with an odds ratio of 4.38 and a relative risk of 1.88, compared to those without COPD (28, 29). However, in the present study, COPD and asthma were not found to affect the criticality and fatality of COVID-19. Since the above studies were meta-analyses, there are methodological differences from the current study. In addition, in this study, only 38 (0.7%) patients had COPD, which might have underpowered the relationship. However, 123 (2.4%) patients had asthma in this study, which also showed no relationship. Hence, further research is needed to determine whether respiratory disease is a risk factor for severe COVID-19.

The current study has some limitations. First, since no cardiac biomarkers were available, such as cardiac troponin or pro-brain natriuretic peptide, that can reflect myocardial damage or heart failure, it is unclear as to whether the disease severity associated with cardiovascular risk factors is directly related to actual heart damage. Second, specific disease condition was not available in this study. For example, we could not know whether the result related to chronic heart disease is due to which of ischemic heart disease, valvular heart disease, and cardiomyopathy. In addition, our data did not include information on atrial fibrillation, which was known to be one of the poor prognostic factors associated with COVID-19 (30). There is no information about the stage of CKD, with the data only indicating whether a patient did or did not have CKD. Third, there was no information about the time or duration for the event (for the critical illness) and censored data. Some variables had missing values and we did not replace the missing values. However, the result of multivariable logistic analysis might not be affected by the missing values. There was no significance difference between the result of multivariable logistic analysis with the limited risk factors which were cardiovascular risk factors and heart diseases (**Table 2**). Further, the missing data did not affect the result of risk score model of **Figure 3**.

This study has a strong point as nation-wide cohort study which minimizing selection bias. The data is based on the unique single-payer, compulsory subscription system of the Republic of Korea and infectious disease control system integrated by the government through KDCA. Hence, the study could be good reference to explore the situation of a single country and elucidate interracial differences for future investigation.

Another novelty of this study is the study population is younger and predominantly females compared to other large series on COVID-19. Since young patients and female patients were included in the analysis, it can be considered to apply to a wider range of populations.

In conclusion, we have described the clinical characteristics and disease severity of hospitalized patients with confirmed COVID-19 in the Republic of Korea, using nationwide data from 5,307 patients. Our results showed that those over 60 years, of the male sex, or those with heart failure, cardiovascular risk factors; hypertension, diabetes mellitus, and CKD have an increased risk of severe COVID-19. Further, the risk scoring model showed the significance of multiple risk factors. Those with four risk factors, old age ($\geq$60 years), male sex, hypertension, and diabetes mellitus, had odds ratio more than 100 of severe COVID-19 than those without these risk factors, although it should be taken into account that it can be statistically exaggerated due to relatively small numbers of patients. In addition, dementia and cancer were also found to be related to severe COVID-19.

AUTHOR CONTRIBUTIONS

KK and IK: conceptualization and data curation. KK: formal analysis. KK, SJ, MY, JP, and IK: investigation and validation. SJ and IK: methodology and writing—original draft. SJ: visualization. KK, SJ, and IK: writing—review and editing. All authors contributed to the article and approved the submitted version.

ACKNOWLEDGMENTS

We acknowledge all the health-care workers involved in the diagnosis and treatment of COVID-19 patients in South Korea. We thank Korea Disease Control and Prevention Agency, National Medical Center and the Health Information Manager in hospitals for their effort in collecting the medical records.

REFERENCES

1. Musher DM, Abers MS, Corrales-Medina VF. Acute infection and myocardial infarction. *N Engl J Med.* (2019) 380:171–6. doi: 10.1056/NEJMra1808137

2. Duan J, Wu Y, Liu C, Yang C, Yang L. Deleterious effects of viral pneumonia on cardiovascular system. *Eur Heart J.* (2020) 41:1833–8. doi: 10.1093/eurheartj/ehaa325

3. Xiong T-Y, Redwood S, Prendergast B, Chen M. Coronaviruses and the cardiovascular system: acute and long-term implications. *Eur Heart J.* (2020) 41:1798–800. doi: 10.1093/eurheartj/ehaa231

4. Tao G, Guo T, Fan Y, Chen M, Wu X, Zhang L, et al. Cardiovascular implications of fatal outcomes of patients with coronavirus disease 2019 (COVID-19). *JAMA Cardiology.* (2020) 5:811–8. doi: 10.1001/jamacardio.2020.1017

5. Wang D, Hu B, Hu C, Zhu F, Liu X, Zhang J, et al. Clinical characteristics of 138 hospitalized patients with 2019 novel coronavirus–infected pneumonia in Wuhan, China. *JAMA.* (2020) 323:1061–9. doi: 10.1001/jama.2020.1585

6. Dahal S, Jenner M, Dinh L, Mizumoto K, Viboud C, Chowell G. Excess mortality patterns during 1918-1921 influenza pandemic

in the state of Arizona, USA. *Ann Epidemiol.* (2018) 28:273–80. doi: 10.1016/j.annepidem.2017.12.005

7. Mehra MR, Desai SS, Kuy S, Henry TD, Patel AN. Cardiovascular disease, drug therapy, and mortality in Covid-19. *N Engl J Med.* (2020) 382:e102. doi: 10.1056/NEJMc2021225

8. Vaduganathan M, Vardeny O, Michel T, McMurray JJV, Pfeffer MA, Solomon SD. Renin–angiotensin–aldosterone system inhibitors in patients with Covid-19. *N Engl J Med.* (2020) 382:1653–9. doi: 10.1056/NEJMsr2005760

9. Kang E, Lee SY, Jung H, Kim MS, Cho B, Kim YS. Operating protocols of a community treatment center for isolation of patients with coronavirus disease, South Korea. *Emerg Infect Dis.* (2020) 26:2329–37. doi: 10.3201/eid2610.201460

10. Bangalore S, Sharma A, Slotwiner A, Yatskar L, Harari R, Shah B, et al. ST-segment elevation in patients with covid-19 — a case series. *N Engl J Med.* (2020) 382:2478–80. doi: 10.1056/NEJMc2009020

11. Henry BM, Lippi G. Chronic kidney disease is associated with severe coronavirus disease 2019 (COVID-19) infection. *Int Urol Nephrol.* (2020) 52:1193–4. doi: 10.1007/s11255-020-02451-9

12. Marshall JC, Murthy S, Diaz J, Adhikari N, Angus DC, Arabi YM, et al. A minimal common outcome measure set for COVID-19 clinical research. *Lancet Infect Dis.* (2020) 20:e192–e7. doi: 10.1016/S1473-3099(20)30483-7

13. Bots SH, Peters SAE, Woodward M. Sex differences in coronary heart disease and stroke mortality: a global assessment of the effect of ageing between 1980 and 2010. *BMJ Glob Health.* (2017) 2:e000298. doi: 10.1136/bmjgh-2017-000298

14. Thomas A. Gaziano DP, Gaziano JM. Global burden of cardiovascular disease. In: Mann DL, Zipes DP, Libby P, Bonow RO, editors. *Braunwald's Heart Disease: A Textbook of Cardiovascular Medicine.* 10th ed. Philadelphia: Elsevier (2014). p 1–20.

15. Tavazzi G, Pellegrini C, Maurelli M, Belliato M, Sciutti F, Bottazzi A, et al. Myocardial localization of coronavirus in COVID-19 cardiogenic shock. *Eur J Heart Fail.* (2020) 22:911–5. doi: 10.1002/ejhf.1828

16. Clerkin KJ, Fried JA, Raikhelkar J, Sayer G, Griffin JM, Masoumi A, et al. COVID-19 and cardiovascular disease. *Circulation.* (2020) 141:1648–55. doi: 10.1161/CIRCULATIONAHA.120.046941

17. Booth CM, Matukas LM, Tomlinson GA, Rachlis AR, Rose DB, Dwosh HA, et al. Clinical features and short-term outcomes of 144 patients with SARS in the Greater Toronto Area. *JAMA.* (2003) 289:2801–9. doi: 10.1001/jama.289.21.JOC30885

18. Badawi A, Ryoo SG. Prevalence of comorbidities in the Middle East respiratory syndrome coronavirus (MERS-CoV): a systematic review and meta-analysis. *Int J Infect Dis.* (2016) 49:129–33. doi: 10.1016/j.ijid.2016.06.015

19. Zheng YY, Ma YT, Zhang JY, Xie X. COVID-19 and the cardiovascular system. *Nat Rev Cardiol.* (2020) 17:259–60. doi: 10.1038/s41569-020-0360-5

20. Thygesen K, Alpert JS, Jaffe AS, Chaitman BR, Bax JJ, Morrow DA, et al. Fourth Universal definition of myocardial infarction. *J Am Coll Card.* (2018) 72:2231–64. doi: 10.1093/eurheartj/ehy655

21. Caro-Codón J, Rey JR, Buño A, Iniesta AM, Rosillo SO, Castrejon-Castrejon S, et al. Characterization of NT-proBNP in a large cohort of COVID-19 patients. *Eur J Heart Fail.* (2021) 23:456–64. doi: 10.1002/ejhf.2095

22. Uribarri A, Núñez-Gil IJ, Aparisi A, Becerra-Muñoz VM, Feltes G, Trabattoni D, et al. Impact of renal function on admission in COVID-19 patients: an analysis of the international HOPE COVID-19 (Health Outcome Predictive Evaluation for COVID 19) Registry. *J Nephrol.* (2020) 33:737–45. doi: 10.1007/s40620-020-00790-5

23. Betjes MGH. Immune cell dysfunction and inflammation in end-stage renal disease. *Nat Rev Nephrol.* (2013) 9:255–65. doi: 10.1038/nrneph.2013.44

24. D'Marco L, Puchades MJ, Romero-Parra M, Gimenez-Civera E, Soler MJ, Ortiz A, et al. Coronavirus disease 2019 in chronic kidney disease. *Clin Kidney J.* (2020) 13:297–306. doi: 10.1093/ckj/sfaa104

25. Arslan H, Musabak U, Ayvazoglu Soy EH, Kurt Azap O, Sayin B, Akcay S, et al. Incidence and immunologic analysis of coronavirus disease (COVID-19) in hemodialysis patients: a single-center experience. *Exp Clin Transplant.* (2020) 18:275–83. doi: 10.6002/ect.2020.0194

26. Major RW, Cheng MRI, Grant RA, Shantikumar S, Xu G, Oozeerally I, et al. Cardiovascular disease risk factors in chronic kidney disease: a systematic review and meta-analysis. *PLoS ONE.* (2018) 13:e0192895. doi: 10.1371/journal.pone.0192895

27. Metlay JP, Waterer GW, Long AC, Anzueto A, Brozek J, Crothers K, et al. Diagnosis and treatment of adults with community-acquired pneumonia. An official clinical practice guideline of the American Thoracic Society and Infectious Diseases Society of America. *Am J Respir Crit Care Med.* (2019) 200:e45–e67. doi: 10.1164/rccm.201908-1581ST

28. Zhao Q, Meng M, Kumar R, Wu Y, Huang J, Lian N, et al. The impact of COPD and smoking history on the severity of COVID-19: a systemic review and meta-analysis. *J Med Virol.* (2020) 92:1915–21. doi: 10.1002/jmv.25889

29. Alqahtani JS, Oyelade T, Aldhahir AM, Alghamdi SM, Almehmadi M, Alqahtani AS, et al. Prevalence, severity and mortality associated with copd and smoking in patients with COVID-19: a rapid systematic review and meta-analysis. *PLoS ONE.* (2020) 15:e0233147. doi: 10.1371/journal.pone.0233147

30. Romiti GF, Corica B, Lip GYH, Proietti M. Prevalence and impact of atrial fibrillation in hospitalized patients with COVID-19: a systematic review and meta-analysis. *J Clin Med.* (2021) 10:2490. doi: 10.3390/jcm10112490

28

High Inflammatory Burden: A Potential Cause of Myocardial Injury in Critically Ill Patients with COVID-19

Yanjun Song[1], Peng Gao[1], Tian Ran[1], Hao Qian[1], Fan Guo[1], Long Chang[2], Wei Wu[1]* and Shuyang Zhang[1]

[1] Department of Cardiology, Chinese Academy of Medical Sciences and Peking Union Medical College, Beijing, China,
[2] Department of Internal Medicine, Chinese Academy of Medical Sciences and Peking Union Medical College, Beijing, China

*Correspondence:
Wei Wu
camsww@163.com

Background: Myocardial injury is a severe complication of novel coronavirus disease (COVID-19), and inflammation has been suggested as a potential cause of myocardial injury. However, the correlation of myocardial injury with inflammation in COVID-19 patients has not been revealed so far.

Method: This retrospective single-center cohort study enrolled 64 critically ill patients with COVID-19. Patients were categorized into two groups by the presence of myocardial injury on admission. Demographic data, clinical characteristics, laboratory tests, treatments, and outcomes were analyzed in this study.

Result: Of these patients, the mean age was 64.8 ± 12.2 years old, and 34 (53.1%) were diagnosed with myocardial injury. Compared with non-myocardial injury patients, myocardial injury patients were older (67.8 ± 10.3 vs. 61.3 ± 13.3 years; $P = 0.033$), had more cardiovascular (CV) risk factors such as smoking (16 [47.06%] vs. 7 [23.33%]; $P = 0.048$) and were more likely to develop CV comorbidities (13 [38.2%] vs. 2 [6.7%]; $P = 0.003$). Scores on the Acute Physiology and Chronic Health Evaluation II (median [interquartile range (IQR)] 19.0 [13.25–25.0] vs. 13.0 [9.25-18.75]; $P = 0.005$) and Sequential Organ Failure Assessment systems (7.0 [5.0–10.0] vs. 4.5 [3.0–6.0]; $P < 0.001$) were significantly higher in the myocardial injury group. In addition, patients with myocardial injury had higher mortality than those without myocardial injury (29 [85.29%] vs. 18 [60.00%]; $P = 0.022$). Cox regression suggested that myocardial injury was an independent risk factor for high mortality during the time from admission to death (hazard ratio [HR], 2.06 [95% confidence interval (CI), 1.10–3.83]; $P = 0.023$). Plasma levels of high-sensitivity C-reactive protein (hs-CRP), interleukin (IL)-1β, interleukin-2 receptor (IL-2R), IL-6, IL-8, IL-10, and tumor necrosis factor-α (TNF-α) exceeded the normal limits, and levels of hs-CRP, IL-2R, IL-6, IL-8, and TNF-α were statistically higher in the myocardial injury group than in the non-myocardial injury group. Multiple-variate logistic regression showed that plasma levels of hs-CRP (odds ratio [OR] 6.23, [95% CI, 1.93–20.12], $P = 0.002$), IL-6 (OR 13.63, [95% CI, 3.33–55.71]; $P < 0.001$) and TNF-α (OR 19.95, [95% CI, 4.93–80.78]; $P < 0.001$) were positively correlated with the incidence of myocardial injury.

Conclusion: Myocardial injury is a common complication that serves as an independent risk factor for a high mortality rate among in-ICU patients with COVID-19. A high inflammatory burden may play a potential role in the occurrence of myocardial injury.

Keywords: COVID-19, critical patients, myocardial injury, inflammation, In-ICU mortality

INTRODUCTION

Coronavirus disease 2019 (COVID-19), a novel coronavirus–infected pneumonia caused by severe acute respiratory syndrome coronavirus 2 (SARS-CoV-2), has currently become a severe global health problem (1, 2). Myocardial injury was suggested to be prevalent in COVID-19 patients, which has contributed to fatal complications and high mortality rates (3–5). However, the mechanism underlying myocardial injury has not yet been confirmed. Recently, several studies revealed that COVID-19 patients were mostly in a high systemic inflammatory status with severe cytokine storms (e.g., high levels of interleukin [IL]-6, IL-8, and tumor necrosis factor-α [TNF-α]), which contributed to fatal complications (6–8). Given that inflammation has been revealed as a great contributor to all forms of myocardial injury (9), COVID-19-induced systemic inflammation was suggested to potentially cause myocardial injury in COVID-19 patients. In this study, we aimed to investigate the association of inflammation with myocardial injury in critically ill patients with COVID-19.

MATERIALS AND METHODS

Study Design and Participants

This single-center, retrospective, observational study was performed in a newly built intensive care unit (ICU) of Tongji Hospital (Sino-French New City Campus), Huazhong University of Science and Technology, Wuhan, China. This ICU was designated to treat critically ill patients with COVID-19. We retrospectively analyzed 64 COVID-19 patients admitted to the ICU in this study. The data cut-off for investigation of survival status was March 26, 2020. All the patients were confirmed as COVID-19 with a positive result on real-time reverse-transcriptase–polymerase-chain-reaction (RT-PCR) assay of throat-swab specimens. The study protocol conformed to the ethical guidelines of the 1975 Declaration of Helsinki and was approved by the Ethics Committee of PUMC Hospital. Written informed consent was waived due to the rapid emergence of this infectious disease. No potentially identifiable human images or data is presented in this study. Plasma levels of inflammatory cytokines test were finished within 24 h when patients were admitted. All the other laboratory tests were finished within 6 h after admission. All the data included in this study were part of routine patient care in ICU.

Data Collection and Study Design

The data collected in this study were extracted from electronic medical records reviewed by the clinical team from Peking Union Medical College Hospital (PUMCH). Patient data included demographics, survival time from ICU admission to death, baseline characteristics (i.e., prior medical illness, cardiovascular risk factors), in-ICU clinical information (i.e., vital signs, complications, and therapeutic measures), laboratory results and outcomes. We also documented patients' Acute Physiology and Chronic Health Evaluation II (APACHE II) and Sequential Organ Failure Assessment (SOFA) scores on admission to the ICU.

Outcome

Patients were categorized into two groups (myocardial injury vs. non-myocardial injury) based on their on-admission high-sensitivity cardiac troponin I (hs-cTnI) levels. The primary outcome was 28-day mortality after ICU admission. myocardial injury was defined as an elevated cardiac troponin value above the 99th percentile of the upper reference limit (34.2 ng/ml) according to the fourth Universal Definition of Myocardial Infarction (10). Prior cardiovascular (CV) disease was defined as coronary artery disease (CAD), myocardial infarction, heart failure or stroke, and in-ICU CV complications were defined as arrythmias (atrial tachycardia, atrial fibrillation, ventricular tachycardia, and/or ventricular fibrillation), cardiac arrest, cardiac shock or myocardial infarction.

Acute respiratory distress syndrome (ARDS) and acute kidney injury (AKI) were diagnosed according to the Berlin Definition and KDIGO clinical practice guidelines, respectively (11, 12).

Statistical Analysis

Categorical variables were presented as counts and percentages. Continuous variables were described as means ± standard deviations (SDs) for normally distributed data and medians (interquartile ranges [IQRs]) for non-normally distributed data. A two-sample T-test was used to assess whether there were significant differences in continuous variables when they were normally distributed; otherwise, the Mann-Whitney U-test was used. The χ^2 test was applied to test the differences in categorical variables, although Fisher's exact test was used for comparisons with small sample sizes. Kaplan-Meier (K-M) plots and Cox proportional hazards regression models were used for survival analysis, which was based on the time from ICU admission to death. The log-rank test was used to confirm the differences between K-M plots. Logistics regression was applied to test the contribution of inflammation to the incidence of myocardial injury. Concretely, we firstly involve single variate into logistics regression, and then put the variates with $P < 0.05$ into regression equation thereby giving the final result. Statistical significance was determined when two-sided α was <0.05. All statistical analyses were performed using SPSS 21.0 software (IBM, Armonk, NY).

RESULTS

General Characteristics of Critically Ill Patients With COVID-19

Night-nine adults admitted to the ICU from February 4 to March 3, 2020, were studied. After excluding 6 patients who were not admitted for COVID-19-related critical illness and 19 patients with incomplete data (1 patient had no troponin result and 18 patients had no inflammatory cytokines), we included 64 in-ICU patients in the final analysis (**Figure 1**).

Of these patients, 42 (65.6%) were men, the mean age was 64.8 ± 12.2 years (range, 26–92 years), and 47 patients reached the primary endpoint during the follow-up time. Prior CV diseases and CV risk factors were common in critical patients, as there were 13 patients (20.3%) with pre-existing CV diseases (CAD: 7 [10.9%]; heart failure: 2 [3.1%]; stroke: 8 [12.5%]) and 43 (67.2%) patients with 1 or more coexisting CV risk factors (hypertension: 35 [54.7%]; diabetes: 15 [23.4%]; smoking: 23 [35.9%]). ARDS was the most common in-ICU complication (62 [96.88%]), followed by AKI (21 [32.8%]) and CV complications (15 [23.4%]). Laboratory results showed that coagulation dysfunction and high inflammatory burden were common in these critical patients, as most coagulation indicators and inflammatory indicators were higher than the normal limits. In addition, plasma levels of N-terminal pro-B-type natriuretic peptide (NT-proBNP) and hs-cTnI were also significantly increased (**Table 2**). Fifty-two (81.3%) patients received invasive mechanical ventilation, and 19 (29.7%) received non-invasive mechanical ventilation. Immune therapies were commonly used in critical patients (glucocorticoids: 54 [84.4%]; tocilizumab: 7 [10.94%]). More detailed information is presented in **Tables 1, 2**.

Differences Between Myocardial Injury Patients and Non-myocardial Injury Patients

In our study, 34 patients (53.1%) were diagnosed with myocardial injury. Compared with non-myocardial injury patients, the myocardial injury patients were significantly older (67.8 ± 10.3 vs. 61.3 ± 13.3 years; $P = 0.033$), more likely to have preexisting cardiovascular diseases (13 [38.2%] vs. 3 [10.0%]; $P = 0.009$), and had more CV risk factors (smoking: 16 [47.1%] vs. 7 [23.3%]; $P = 0.048$) and CV comorbidities (13 [38.2%] vs. 2 [6.7%]; $P = 0.003$) (**Table 1**). Concomitantly, patients with myocardial injury had higher APACHE II (19.0 [13.25–25.0] vs. 13.0 [9.25–18.75]; $P = 0.005$) and SOFA system scores than those of the non-myocardial injury group (7.0 [5.0–10.0] vs. 4.5 [3.0–6.0]; $P < 0.001$).

Regarding laboratory results, myocardial injury patients showed significant increases in the plasma levels of creatinine, blood urea nitrogen, D-dimer, high-sensitivity C-reactive protein (hs-CRP) (155.0 [78.3–210.9] vs. 45.0 [16.0–96.0]

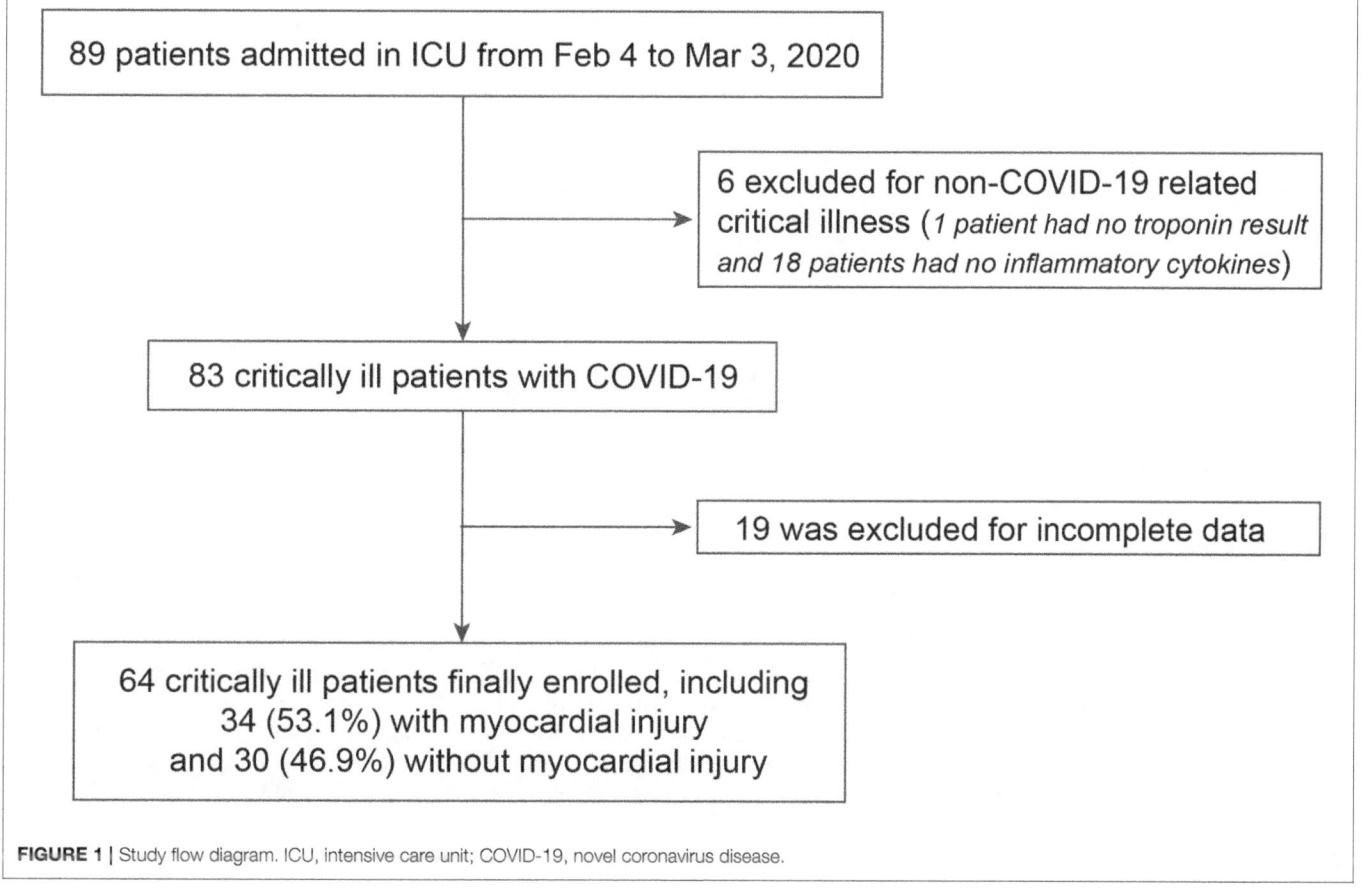

FIGURE 1 | Study flow diagram. ICU, intensive care unit; COVID-19, novel coronavirus disease.

TABLE 1 | Demographics and clinical characteristics of critically ill patients with COVID-19.

	Myocardial injury (n = 34)	Non-myocardial injury (n = 30)	Total (n = 64)	P-value
Age (yrs)	67.8 ± 10.3	61.3 ± 13.3	64.8 ± 12.2	0.033
Male	24 (70.6%)	18 (60.0%)	42 (65.6%)	0.37
Prior CV diseases				
CAD	6 (17.7%)	1 (3.3%)	7 (10.9%)	0.11
Heart failure	2 (5.9%)	0 (0.00%)	2 (3.1%)	0.49
Stroke	6 (17.7%)	2 (6.7%)	8 (12.5%)	0.27
CV risk factors				
Hypertension	22 (64.7%)	13 (43.3%)	35 (54.7%)	0.087
Diabetes	10 (29.4%)	5 (16.7%)	15 (23.4%)	0.23
Smoking	16 (47.1%)	7 (23.3%)	23 (35.9%)	0.048
Vital signs				
Fever	12 (35.3%)	14 (46.7%)	26 (40.6%)	0.36
HR (bpm)	112.9 ± 20.4	106.7 ± 18.5	110.0 ± 19.6	0.21
SBP (mmHg)	124.6 ± 26.3	127.8 ± 20.5	126.1 ± 23.6	0.60
DBP (mmHg)	74.8 ± 14.5	77.7 ± 14.2	76.2 ± 14.4	0.42
RR (times/min)	29.3 ± 8.8	27.5 ± 7.1	28.4 ± 8.0	0.38
Critical score				
APACHE II score*	19.0 (13.3–25.0)	13.0 (9.3–18.8)	15.0 (12.0–22.0)	0.005
SOFA score*	7.0 (5.0–10.0)	4.5 (3.0–6.0)	6.0 (4.0–8.0)	<0.001
Complications				
CV complications	13 (38.2%)	2 (6.7%)	15 (23.4%)	0.003
ARDS	34 (100.0%)	28 (93.3%)	62 (96.9%)	0.22
AKI	13 (38.2%)	8 (26.7%)	21 (32.8%)	0.33
Live dysfunction	6 (17.7%)	10 (33.3%)	16 (25.0%)	0.15
Symptom onset to ICU admission (days)	15.0 (11.0–23.0)	16.5 (9.3–23.5)	15.5 (10.0–23.3)	0.91
In-ICU therapy				
Non-invasive mechanical ventilation	12 (35.3%)	7 (23.3%)	19 (29.7%)	0.30
Invasive mechanical ventilation	26 (76.5%)	26 (86.7%)	52 (81.5%)	0.30
Immunoglobulin	26 (76.5%)	25 (83.3%)	51 (79.7%)	0.50
Glucocorticoids	26 (76.5%)	28 (93.3%)	54 (84.4%)	0.064
Vasoconstrictive agents	24 (70.6%)	18 (60.0%)	42 (65.6%)	0.37
Tocilizumab	2 (5.9%)	5 (16.7%)	7 (10.9%)	0.17
Death				
All-cause death	29 (85.3%)	18 (60.0%)	47 (73.4%)	0.022
Survival time*	7.0 (3.0–13.75)	19.0 (10.0–38.75)	11.5 (5.0–35.0)	0.002

*Continuous variables with non-normal distribution presented as "median (IQR)." CV, cardiovascular; CAD, coronary artery disease; ICU, intensive care unit. HR, heart rate; RR, respiratory rate; SBP, systolic blood pressure; DBP, diastolic blood pressure; APACHE II, Acute Physiology and Chronic Health Evaluation II; SOFA, Sequential Organ Failure Assessment; AKI, acute kidney injury; ARDS, acute respiratory distress syndrome. P-values present the differences between myocardial injury and non-myocardial injury patients.

mg/L; $P < 0.001$), interleukin-2 receptor (IL-2R) (1152.0 [741.0–1679.0] vs. 731.0 [302.0–1224.5] pg/ml; $P = 0.02$), IL-6 (1144.7 ± 1466.7 vs. 204.4 ± 400.3 pg/ml; $P < 0.001$), IL-8 (48.5 [21.1–156.1] vs. 22.7 [14.4–42.9] pg/ml; $P = 0.015$) and TNF-α (19.8 [14.7–40.1] vs. 9.0 [7.1–11.0] pg/ml; $P < 0.001$) (**Table 2**). In addition, the levels of creatinine, blood urea nitrogen and D-dimer were also significantly increased in the myocardial injury group. However, no significant differences were found in the applications of in-ICU therapies between myocardial injury and non-myocardial injury patients (**Table 1**).

In the survival analysis, the mortality rate was much higher in the myocardial injury group than in the non-myocardial injury group (29 [85.29%] vs. 18 [60.00%]; $P = 0.022$). Furthermore, myocardial injury was demonstrated as an independent risk factor for reduced survival time from admission to death (hazard ratio [HR], 2.06 [95% confidence interval (CI), 1.10–3.83]; $P = 0.023$) by a multivariable adjusted Cox proportional hazard regression model adjusting for age, smoking history and pre-existing with CVD. The high mortality in the myocardial injury group was also shown in the K-M survival curves (log-rank test, $P = 0.003$) (**Figure 2**).

TABLE 2 | Laboratory tests between COVID-19 patients with and without myocardial injury.

	Normal range	Myocardial injury (n = 34)	Non-myocardial injury (n = 30)	Total (n = 64)	P-value
White blood count, ×10⁹/L	3.5–9.5	12.5 ± 5.1	11.1 ± 5.7	11.9 ± 5.4	0.30
Neutrophils* (%)	40.0–75.0	91.7 (88.7–95.1)	90.7 (83.2–93.4)	91.1 (85.9–94.0)	0.05
Lymphocytes, ×10⁹/L	1.1–3.2	0.5 ± 0.4	0.7 ± 0.4	0.6 ± 0.4	0.25
Hemoglobin, g/L	130.0–175.0	121.8 ± 21.7	123.0 ± 19.8	122.4 ± 20.7	0.82
Platelets, ×10⁹/L	125.0–350.0	155.0 ± 89.4	197.0 ± 105.6	174.7 ± 98.8	0.09
ALT*, U/L	≤41.0	26.0 (14.0–41.0)	27.5 (22.0–36.8)	29.0 (19.8–42.0)	0.89
Total bilirubin*, μmol/L	≤26.0	13.2 (9.6–21.2)	14.5 (8.0–18.7)	13.7 (8.7–19.0)	0.40
Albumin g/L	35.0–52.0	28.0 ± 4.3	30.5 ± 6.1	29.2 ± 5.3	0.065
Creatinine*, μmol/L	59.0–104.0	88.5 (71.5–124.0)	67.0 (48.5–86.0)	81.0 (58.0–107.8)	0.005
BUN*, mmol/L	3.6–9.5	10.2 (7.1–20.7)	7.1 (5.4–10.3)	7.8 (6.3–14.4)	0.013
Serum potassium, mmol/L	3.5–5.1	4.5 ± 0.8	4.5 ± 1.0	4.5 ± 0.9	0.84
PT*, s	11.5–14.5	17.3 (15.7–18.2)	15.4 (14.7–16.3)	16.15 (15.0–17.6)	0.005
APTT*, s	29.0–42.0	41.8 (38.4–45.3)	41.5 (37.4–45.1)	41.6 (37.5–45.2)	0.68
INR*	0.8–1.2	1.4 (1.2–1.5)	1.2 (1.1–1.3)	1.3 (1.2–1.4)	0.002
Fbg, g/L	2.0–4.0	4.5 ± 3.9	4.6 ± 2.1	4.5 ± 3.2	0.29
D-dimer*, mg/L	<0.5	21.0 (7.5–21.0)	3.7 (1.9–21.0)	14.7 (2.8–21.0)	0.005
hsCRP*, mg/L	<1.0	155.0 (78.3–210.9)	45.0 (16.0–96.0)	86.5 (34.7–194.3)	<0.001
IL1 β, pg/ml	<5.0	6.5 ± 4.4	5.2 ± 0.7	5.9 ± 3.3	0.53
IL2 R*, pg/ml	223.0–710.0	1152.0 (741.0–1679.0)	731.0 (302.0–1224.5)	1041.0 (554.3–1485.3)	0.02
IL-6, pg/ml	<7.0	982.2 ± 1517.9	204.4 ± 400.3	617.6 ± 1197.4	0.008
IL-8*, pg/ml	<62.0	48.5 (21.1–156.1)	22.7 (14.4–42.9)	29.4 (18.1–76.7)	0.015
IL-10*, pg/ml	<9.1	10.7 (6.3–24.0)	10.5 (5.1–15.5)	10.7 (5.5–19.6)	0.30
TNF-α*, pg/ml	<8.1	19.8 (14.7–40.1)	9.0 (7.1–11.0)	13.8 (9.3–23.0)	<0.001
HscTnI*, ng/L	≤34.2	276.1 (139.1–909.7)	12.1 (4.7–18.9)	46.5 (12.1–374.1)	<0.001
NT-proBNP*, ng/L	<241.0	1947.5 (644.8–4393.5)	372.0 (73.8–836.5)	816.5 (254.5–2585.0)	<0.001

*Continuous variables with non-normal distribution presented as "median (IQR)." ALT, alanine aminotransferase; BUN, blood urea nitrogen; hsCRP, high-sensitivity C-reative protein; IL, interleukin; IL-2R, interleukin-2 receptor; TNF-α, tumor necrosis factor α; PT, prothrombin time; APTT, activated partial thromboplastin time; INR, international normalized ratio; Fbg, fibrinogen; hs-cTnI, high-sensitive cardiac troponin I; NT-proBNP, N-terminal pro-B-type natriuretic peptide. P-values present the differences between MI and non-MI patients.

Association of High Inflammatory Burden With the Incidence of Myocardial Injury in Critically Ill Patients With COVID-19

Most inflammatory biomarkers were significantly higher in COVID-19 patients with myocardial injury than in those without myocardial injury (**Table 2**). Consistently patients with higher inflammatory burden (plasma levels of inflammatory cytokines higher than the median levels) were also more likely to develop myocardial injury (**Figure 3**). To investigate the relation between high inflammatory burden with myocardial injury, we set the dependent variable to "myocardial injury" and set independent variables to the high/low inflammatory burden which was divided according to the cut-off of the median levels of inflammatory cytokines. In the univariate logistic regression analysis, we found that high plasma levels (higher than the median levels) of high-sensitivity C-reactive protein (hs-CRP) (odds ratio [OR] 10.80, [95% CI, 1.97–59.15]; $P = 0.006$), IL-6 (OR 9.13, [95% CI, 2.92–28.50]; $P < 0.001$), IL-8 (OR 7.27, [95% CI, 1.35–39.05]; $P = 0.021$) and TNF-α (OR 17.36, [95% CI, 3.04–99.20]; $P = 0.001$) were positively associated with the incidence of myocardial injury. We further entered these biomarkers into the multivariate logistic regression with adjusting variates of age,

smoking history and pre-existing with CVD, and found that high plasma levels of hs-CRP (odds ratio [OR] 6.23, [95% CI, 1.93–20.12], $P = 0.002$), IL-6 (OR 13.63, [95% CI, 3.33–55.71]; $P < 0.001$), and TNF-α (OR 19.95, [95% CI, 4.93–80.78]; $P < 0.001$) were positively correlated with the incidence of myocardial injury (**Table 3**).

DISCUSSION

This study revealed that myocardial injury was associated with a high mortality rate in critically ill patients with COVID-19, and a high inflammatory burden was one of the potential causes of myocardial injury occurrence.

Of 64 in-ICU patients (42 males, 64.8 ± 12.2 years), 52 (81.5%) received invasive mechanical ventilation, and 47 (73.4%) died during the follow-up. A high incidence of COVID-19-induced myocardial injury was suggested by this study, since we found that 34 (53.1%) patients were diagnosed with myocardial injury, which is much higher than the incidence of myocardial injury in non-ICU patients (7.2% to 37.5%) (1, 4, 5). Myocardial injury usually contributes to various CV complications, such as cardiac dysfunction,

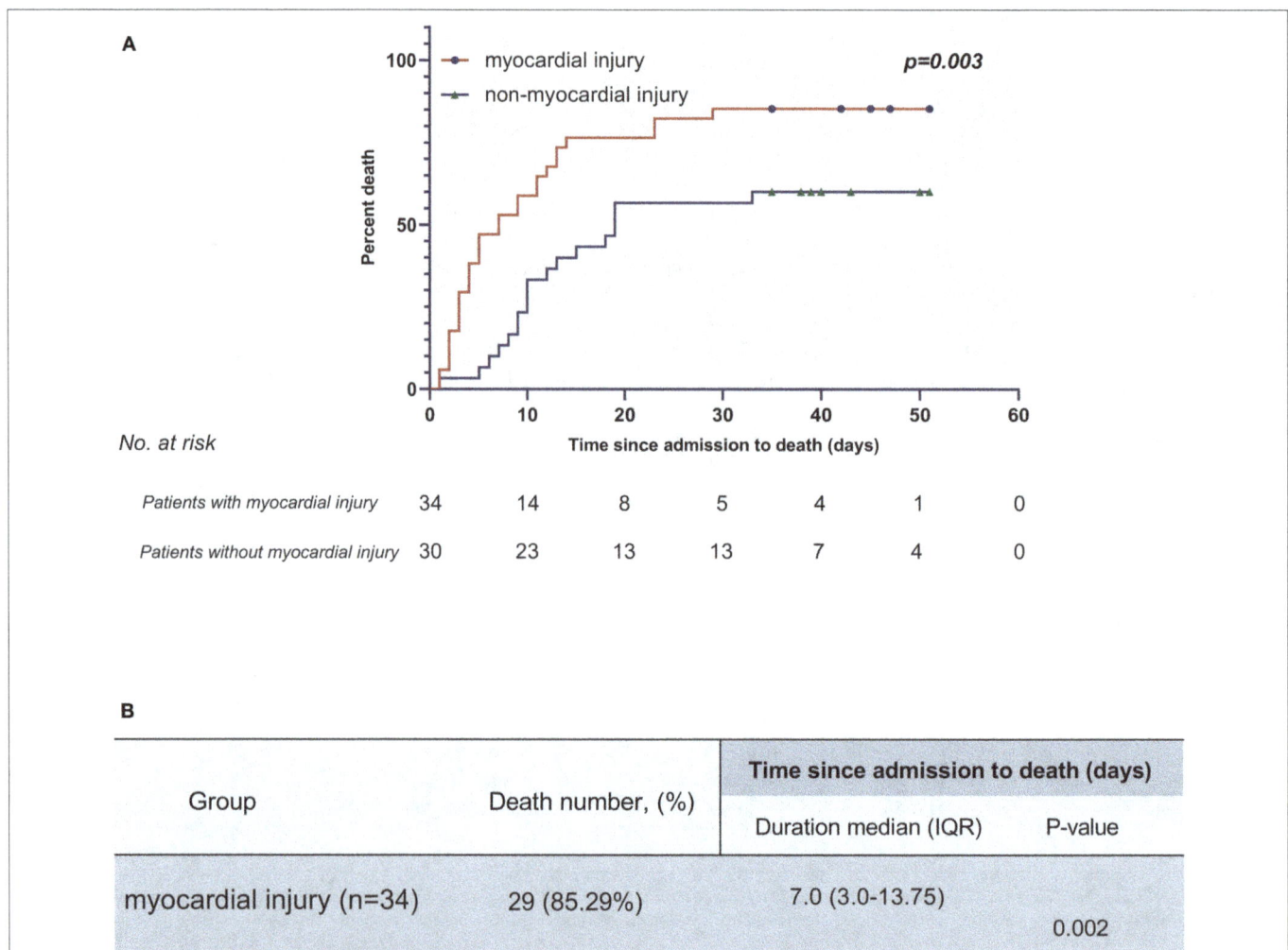

A

B

Group	Death number, (%)	Time since admission to death (days)	
		Duration median (IQR)	P-value
myocardial injury (n=34)	29 (85.29%)	7.0 (3.0-13.75)	0.002
non-myocardial injury (n=30)	18 (60.00%)	19.0 (10.0-38.75)	

FIGURE 2 | (A) K-M plot for patients with myocardial injury and without myocardial injury. **(B)** Comparisons of death number and time since admission to death between myocardial injury group and non-myocardial injury group.

arrhythmias and sudden death in patients with viral infectious diseases, which are associated with adverse events and a high mortality rate (13, 14). Several current studies have demonstrated that myocardial injury is associated with fatal outcomes and high mortality rates in hospitalized patients with COVID-19 (3, 5). In our study, in-ICU patients with myocardial injury were more likely to have preexisting cardiovascular diseases, develop cardiovascular complications, have higher APACHE-II/SOFA scores and have increased in-ICU mortality. In addition, Cox regression analysis suggested that myocardial injury was an independent risk factor for mortality, supporting that myocardial injury was associated with adverse events and high mortality rate in COVID-19 patients with critical illness.

Patients with COVID-19 were revealed to have a high systemic inflammatory status (1, 8). To date, the high systemic inflammation in hospitalized COVID-19 patients has been speculated as one of the potential causes of myocardial injury, as investigators found that hs-CRP levels positively correlated with plasma troponin levels in patients with COVID-19 (4). A similar finding was shown in our study. In addition to plasma hs-CRP, plasma levels of IL-1β, IL-2R, IL-6, IL-8, IL-10, and TNF-α were analyzed in this study, and IL-2R, IL-6, IL-8, and TNF-α were significantly increased in myocardial injury patients (**Table 2**). Moreover, patients with the high inflammatory burden were also shown to more likely develop myocardial injury (**Figure 3**). After univariate and multivariate logistic regression, the levels of hs-CRP, IL-6, and TNF-α were shown to be positively correlated with the incidence of myocardial injury, supporting the hypothesis that a high systemic inflammatory burden might contribute to myocardial injury in COVID-19 patients.

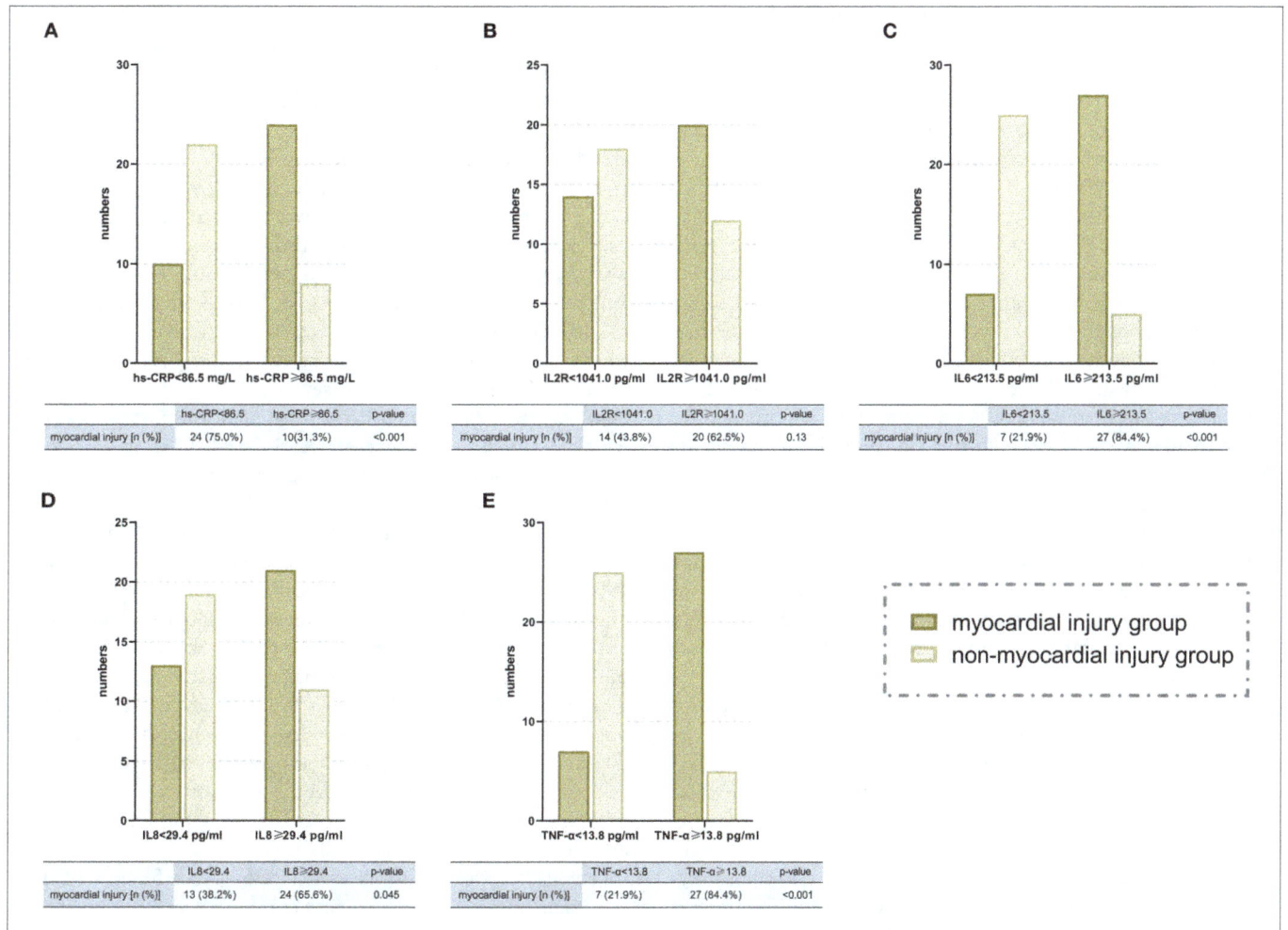

FIGURE 3 | Comparisons of the numbers of patients with myocardial injury in high/low inflammatory burden groups (divided according to the cut-off of median levels of different inflammatory cytokines. **A**, hs-CRP; **B**, IL-2R; **C**, IL-6; **D**, IL-8; **E**, TNF-α). hsCRP, high-sensitivity C-reative protein; IL, interleukin; IL-2R, interleukin-2 receptor; TNF-α, tumor necrosis factor α; OR, odds ratio; CI, confidence interval.

TABLE 3 | Logistics regression for the association of inflammation with myocardial injury.

	Univariate			Multivariate		
	OR	**95% CI**	*P*-value	**OR**	**95% CI**	*P*-value
hs-CRP ≥ 86.5 mg/L	10.80	1.97–59.15	0.006	6.23	1.93–20.12	0.002
IL-2R ≥ 1041.0 pg/ml	3.81	0.86–16.94	0.079	2.23	0.71–7.02	0.17
IL-6 ≥ 703.9 pg/ml	9.13	2.92–28.50	<0.001	13.63	3.33–55.71	<0.001
IL-8 ≥ 29.4 pg/ml	7.27	1.35–39.05	0.021	2.53	0.84–7.58	0.098
TNF-α ≥ 13.8 pg/ml	17.36	3.04–99.20	0.001	19.95	4.93–80.78	<0.001

OR, odds ratio; CI, confidence interval. hsCRP, high-sensitivity C-reative protein; IL, interleukin; IL-2R, interleukin-2 receptor; TNF-α, tumor necrosis factor α. Adjusted variates included age, smoking history, and pre-existing CVD.

Hypoxemia, septic shock, coagulation disorders and cardiac arrhythmias are potentially involved in the process of systemic high inflammatory burden-induced myocardial injury in patients with severe acute respiratory syndrome coronavirus 2 (SARS-CoV-2) infection (15–17). These pathophysiological disorders were further illustrated by our study. In our patients, more than 95% of them developed ARDS with a significantly

rapid heart rate, which caused an imbalance between cardiac metabolic demand and oxygen supply. Moreover, a prevalence of shock or insufficient peripheral perfusion was indicated by the common application of vasoconstrictive agents in our patients. Concomitantly, coagulation disequilibrium (higher D-dimer levels and longer PT) and the incidence of CV complications, including arrythmias, were also widely found in these patients. Myocardial inflammation might be another cause of myocardial injury in coronavirus-infected patients (15). In a study performed with 21 autopsies of SARS-CoV infected patients, Oudit et al. reported increased inflammation in the myocardium of these patients associated with cardiac interstitial fibrosis and hypertrophy (18). For COVID-19, a brief case report suggested the potential occurrence of myocarditis in COVID-19 patients by describing a 53-year-old woman diagnosed with COVID-19 who developed acute myocarditis during hospitalization (19). However, COVID-19-induced viral myocarditis has not been supported by pathological data so far. In current autopsy reports of COVID-19 patients, researchers revealed that there was only a mild infiltration of inflammatory cells without substantial necrosis of cardiomyocytes (20, 21). It seems that systemic inflammation, but not localized myocardial inflammation plays a pivotal role in myocardial injury of COVID-19 patients. A similar conclusion was also given by another retrospective study that enrolled 112 COVID-19 patients, as they revealed that there were no typical signs of myocarditis on echocardiography, such as segmental wall motion abnormality, reduced LVEF or wall thickening, in COVID-19 patients with myocardial injury during hospitalization (5). The roles of myocardial inflammation in myocardial injury still need more investigation.

The mechanisms underlying the activation of inflammation in COVID-19 patients have been recently investigated by Zhang et al. (22). It has been suggested that COVID-19 induced the destruction of alveolar epithelial cells, which led to an increase in cell permeability and the release of virus. This result subsequently activated the innate immune system and induced the overproduction of cytokines (e.g., IL-6 and TNF-a), finally causing a systemic inflammatory response (22, 23). In this process, macrophage recruitment, which has been demonstrated to regulate SARS-CoV-2-induced inflammation (24, 25), was suggested to be one of the potential contributors, as interstitial mononuclear inflammatory infiltrates were observed in both lungs of patients with COVID-19. In addition, the plasma levels of macrophage-produced pro-inflammatory cytokines, such as IL-6 (26) and TNF-α (27), were shown to be significantly increased in patients with COVID-19, further supporting the contribution of macrophages to systemic inflammation in COVID-19 patients. In addition to macrophages, the activation of lymphocytes was also suggested as a factor in systemic inflammation in COVID-19 patients (6). Although decreased blood lymphocyte count of COVID-19 patients has been widely reported (4, 28), lymphocytes were shown to be activated as the increases in the expression of HLA-DR in $CD4^+$ and $CD8^+$ cells, the percentage of $CD4^+$ $CCR4^+$ $CCR6^+$ Th17 cells. The expression of cytotoxic particles (e.g., perforin and granulysin) in CD8 + T cells was demonstrated in an autopsy report of COVID-19 patients (21).

The efficiencies of anti-inflammatory treatments such as glucocorticoids, tocilizumab (TCZ) and anti-TNFα agents in COVID-19 patients were recently investigated by various registered cohort studies (6, 29). In this study, glucocorticoids and TCZ were applied in these patients. Glucocorticoids were widely applied during the outbreaks of several viral infectious diseases, such as SARS-CoV (30), Middle East respiratory syndrome (MERS)-CoV (31) and influenzas (32). However, the benefit derived from corticosteroids in the treatment of these diseases has not been revealed (33). For COVID-19, there are no clinical data indicating the benefits of corticosteroids, and the recommendation for their use is controversial (6, 33). Other investigators held a positive opinion for glucocorticoid usage, as systematic corticosteroid therapy in the first 3–5 days was shown to effectively inhibit severe inflammatory storms and alleviate critical symptoms in ICU patients with MERS (34). Currently, short-term systematic corticosteroid treatment (methylprednisolone, <1–2 mg/kg/d, 3–5 days) is recommended for the treatment of selective severe COVID-19 patients while being cautious of glucocorticoid-mediated immunosuppression, which delays the clearance of SARS-CoV-2 (35). In our study, systemic corticosteroid administration (methylprednisolone, 1–2 mg/kg/d × 5–7 days) was empirically used for patients with high inflammatory status. However, the efficiency is still not confirmed. Elucidating the benefit of glucocorticoids for COVID-19 patients is of immediate clinical importance. In contrast to glucocorticoids, TCZ, a recombinant human IL-6 monoclonal antibody, showed potential therapeutic value for COVID-19 patients. In a current clinical trial (clinical trial registration ID: ChiCTR2000029765), TCZ was administered once to 21 critical patients with COVID-19 at 400 mg intravenously. After a few days, the febrile patients' body temperature returned to normal, and all other symptoms improved significantly, in conjunction with better respiratory function, absorbed pulmonary lesions and lower plasma levels of hs-CRP (36). Moreover, several recent case reports also described the successful use of TCZ treatment in COVID-19 patients combined with other diseases (37, 38). In our study, TCZ was applied in several selective patients with high IL-6 levels. However, due to the insufficiency of related evidence, guidance and specialist consensus for the application of TCZ in COVID-19 patients is still lacking. Studies with larger populations are expected to further confirm the therapeutic value of TCZ against COVID-19 development. TNF-α inhibitors, such as infliximab (Remicade) and adalimumab (Humira), were not applied in our patients due to the lack of related information in COVID-19 patients. However, the therapeutic value of TNF-α for the severe immune-based pulmonary injury caused by SARS coronavirus has been implicated (39). Since high plasma levels of TNF-α have been widely observed in our patients, it is worth investigating the effects and safety of TNF-α inhibitors in the treatment of COVID-19.

This study still has several limitations. First, several pieces of cardiac information, such as echocardiography data and electrocardiography data, were lacking in this study, which limited the evaluation of myocardial injury. Second, plasma levels of certain inflammatory cytokines, such as granulocyte-colony stimulating factor, monocyte chemoattractant protein-1 and macrophage inflammatory protein 1-α (chemokine ligand 3), were not tested in our study. Finally, this study only involved 64 patients, and further studies with larger populations or multicenter study should be performed to confirm our results.

CONCLUSION

This study demonstrated that myocardial injury was a common complication of COVID-19, and myocardial injury was associated with the occurrence of adverse events and a high mortality rate. The positive correlation of high inflammatory burden with the incidence of myocardial injury was further revealed in critically ill patients with COVID-19 in this study.

AUTHOR CONTRIBUTIONS

YS, PG, TR, WW, and SZ: concept and design. YS, PG, TR, HQ, FG, LC, and WW: acquisition, analysis, or interpretation of data. YS, WW, and SZ: drafting of the manuscript. YS, PG, TR, HQ, FG, LC, WW, and SZ: critical revision of the manuscript for important intellectual content. YS and WW: statistical analysis. WW and SZ: administrative, technical, material support, and supervision. All authors contributed to the article and approved the submitted version.

REFERENCES

1. Huang C, Wang Y, Li X, Ren L, Zhao J, Hu Y, et al. Clinical features of patients infected with 2019 novel coronavirus in Wuhan, China. *Lancet.* (2020) 395:497–506. doi: 10.1016/S0140-6736(20)30183-5

2. Guan WJ, Ni ZY, Hu Y, Liang WH, Ou CQ, He JX, et al. Clinical characteristics of Coronavirus Disease 2019 in China. *N Engl J Med.* (2020) 382:1708–20. doi: 10.1101/2020.02.06.20020974

3. Bonow RO, Fonarow GC, O'Gara PT, Yancy CW. Association of Coronavirus Disease 2019 (COVID-19) with myocardial injury and mortality. *JAMA Cardiol.* (2020) doi: 10.1001/jamacardio.2020.1105. [Epub ahead of print].

4. Guo T, Fan Y, Chen M, Wu X, Zhang L, He T, et al. Cardiovascular implications of fatal outcomes of patients with Coronavirus Disease 2019 (COVID-19). *JAMA Cardiol.* (2020) e201017. doi: 10.1001/jamacardio.2020.1017. [Epub ahead of print].

5. Deng Q, Hu B, Zhang Y, Wang H, Zhou X, Hu W, et al. Suspected myocardial injury in patients with COVID-19: Evidence from front-line clinical observation in Wuhan, China. *Int J Cardiol.* (2020) 311:116–21 doi: 10.1016/j.ijcard.2020.03.087

6. Zhang W, Zhao Y, Zhang F, Wang Q, Li T, Liu Z, et al. The use of anti-inflammatory drugs in the treatment of people with severe coronavirus disease 2019 (COVID-19): the perspectives of clinical immunologists from China. *Clin Immunol.* (2020) 214:108393. doi: 10.1016/j.clim.2020.108393

7. Ruan Q, Yang K, Wang W, Jiang L, Song J. Clinical predictors of mortality due to COVID-19 based on an analysis of data of 150 patients from Wuhan, China. *Intens Care Med.* (2020) 46:846–8. doi: 10.1007/s00134-020-06028-z

8. Conti P, Ronconi G, Caraffa A, Gallenga CE, Ross R, Frydas I, et al. Induction of pro-inflammatory cytokines (IL-1 and IL-6) and lung inflammation by Coronavirus-19 (COVI-19 or SARS-CoV-2): anti-inflammatory strategies. *J Biol Regul Homeost Agents.* (2020) 34:1. doi: 10.23812/CONTI-E

9. Trachtenberg BH, Hare JM. Inflammatory cardiomyopathic syndromes. *Circ Res.* (2017) 121:803–18. doi: 10.1161/CIRCRESAHA.117.310221

10. Thygesen K, Alpert JS, Jaffe AS, Chaitman BR, Bax JJ, Morrow DA, et al. Fourth universal definition of myocardial infarction 2018. *J Am Coll Cardiol.* (2018) 72:2231–64. doi: 10.1016/j.jacc.2018.08.1038

11. Ranieri VM, Rubenfeld GD, Thompson BT, Ferguson ND, Caldwell E, Fan E, et al. Acute respiratory distress syndrome: the Berlin definition. *JAMA.* (2012) 307:2526–33. doi: 10.1001/jama.2012.5669

12. Kellum JA, Lameire N. Diagnosis, evaluation, and management of acute kidney injury: a KDIGO summary (Part 1). *Crit Care.* (2013) 17:204. doi: 10.1186/cc11454

13. Paddock CD, Liu L, Denison AM, Bartlett JH, Holman RC, Deleon-Carnes M, et al. Myocardial injury and bacterial pneumonia contribute to the pathogenesis of fatal influenza B virus infection. *J Infect Dis.* (2012) 205:895–905. doi: 10.1093/infdis/jir861

14. Yu CM, Wong RS, Wu EB, Kong SL, Wong J, Yip GW, et al. Cardiovascular complications of severe acute respiratory syndrome. *Postgrad Med.* (2006) 82:140–44. doi: 10.1136/pgmj.2005.037515

15. Madjid M, Safavi-Naeini P, Solomon SD, Vardeny O. Potential effects of coronaviruses on the cardiovascular system: a review. *JAMA Cardiol.* (2020) doi: 10.1001/jamacardio.2020.1286. [Epub ahead of print].

16. Jou C, Shah R, Figueroa A, Patel JK. The role of inflammatory cytokines in cardiac arrest. *J Intens Care Med.* (2020) 35:219–24. doi: 10.1177/0885066618817518

17. Xiong TY, Redwood S, Prendergast B, Chen M. Coronaviruses and the cardiovascular system: acute and long-term implications. *Eur Heart J.* (2020) 41:1798–800. doi: 10.1093/eurheartj/ehaa231

18. Oudit GY, Kassiri Z, Jiang C, Liu PP, Poutanen SM, Penninger JM, et al. SARS-coronavirus modulation of myocardial ACE2 expression and inflammation in patients with SARS. *Eur J Clin Invest.* (2009) 39:618–25. doi: 10.1111/j.1365-2362.2009.02153.x

19. Inciardi RM, Lupi L, Zaccone G, Italia L, Raffo M, Tomasoni D, et al. Cardiac involvement in a patient with Coronavirus Disease 2019 (COVID-19). *JAMA Cardiol.* (2020) doi: 10.1001/jamacardio.2020.1096. [Epub ahead of print].

20. Yao XH, Li TY, He ZC, Ping YF, Liu HW, Yu SC, et al. [A pathological report of three COVID-19 cases by minimally invasive autopsies]. *Zhonghua Bing Li Xue Za Zhi.* (2020) 49:411–17. doi: 10.3760/cma.j.cn112151-2020031 2-00193

21. Xu Z, Shi L, Wang Y, Zhang J, Huang L, Zhang C, et al. Pathological findings of COVID-19 associated with acute respiratory distress syndrome. *Lancet Respir Med.* (2020) 8:420–2. doi: 10.1016/S2213-2600(20)30076-X

22. Zhang C, Wu Z, Li JW, Zhao H, Wang GQ. The cytokine release syndrome (CRS) of severe COVID-19 and Interleukin-6 receptor (IL-6R) antagonist Tocilizumab may be the key to reduce the mortality. *Int J Antimicrob Agents.* (2020) 55:105954. doi: 10.1016/j.ijantimicag.2020.105954

23. Fu Y, Cheng Y, Wu Y. Understanding SARS-CoV-2-mediated inflammatory responses: from mechanisms to potential therapeutic tools. *Virol Sin.* (2020) 1-6. doi: 10.1007/s12250-020-00207-4. [Epub ahead of print].

24. Hwang DM, Chamberlain DW, Poutanen SM, Low DE, Asa SL, Butany J. Pulmonary pathology of severe acute respiratory syndrome in Toronto. *Mod Pathol.* (2005) 18:1–10. doi: 10.1038/modpathol.3800247

25. Cameron MJ, Ran L, Xu L, Danesh A, Bermejo-Martin JF, Cameron CM, et al. Interferon-mediated immunopathological events are associated with atypical innate and adaptive immune responses in patients with severe acute respiratory syndrome. *J Virol.* (2007) 81:8692–706. doi: 10.1128/JVI.00527-07

26. Becker S, Quay J, Soukup J. Cytokine (tumor necrosis factor, IL-6, and IL-8) production by respiratory syncytial virus-infected human alveolar macrophages. *J Immunol.* (1991) 147:4307–12.

27. Gong JH, Sprenger H, Hinder F, Bender A, Schmidt A, Horch S, et al. Influenza A virus infection of macrophages. Enhanced tumor necrosis factor-alpha (TNF-alpha) gene expression and lipopolysaccharide-triggered TNF-alpha release. *J Immunol.* (1991) 147:3507–13.

28. Shi S, Qin M, Shen B, Cai Y, Liu T, Yang F, et al. Association of cardiac injury with mortality in hospitalized patients with COVID-19 in Wuhan, China. *JAMA Cardiol.* (2020) e200950. doi: 10.1001/jamacardio.2020.0950. [Epub ahead of print].

29. Russell B, Moss C, George G, Santaolalla A, Cope A, Papa S, et al. Associations between immune-suppressive and stimulating drugs and novel COVID-19-a systematic review of current evidence. *Ecancermedicalscience.* (2020) 14:1022. doi: 10.3332/ecancer.2020.1022

30. Chen RC, Tang XP, Tan SY, Liang BL, Wan ZY, Fang JQ, et al. Treatment of severe acute respiratory syndrome with glucosteroids: the Guangzhou experience. *Chest.* (2006) 129:1441–52. doi: 10.1378/chest.129.6.1441

31. Arabi YM, Mandourah Y, Al-Hameed F, Sindi AA, Almekhlafi GA, Hussein MA, et al. Corticosteroid therapy for critically ill patients with middle east respiratory syndrome. *Am J Respir Crit Care Med.* (2018) 197:757–67. doi: 10.1164/rccm.201706-1172OC

32. Ni YN, Chen G, Sun J, Liang BM, Liang ZA. The effect of corticosteroids on mortality of patients with influenza pneumonia: a systematic review and meta-analysis. *Crit Care.* (2019) 23:99. doi: 10.1186/s13054-019-2395-8

33. Russell CD, Millar JE, Baillie JK. Clinical evidence does not support corticosteroid treatment for 2019-nCoV lung injury. *Lancet.* (2020) 395:473–5. doi: 10.1016/S0140-6736(20)30317-2

34. Zhou W, Liu Y, Tian D, Wang C, Wang S, Cheng J, et al. Potential benefits of precise corticosteroids therapy for severe 2019-nCoV pneumonia. *Signal Transduct Target Ther.* (2020) 5:18. doi: 10.1038/s41392-020-0127-9

35. National Health Commission of the People's Republic of China. *The 5th Trial Version of Diagnosis and Treatment Scheme for Pneumonitis With 2019-nCoV Infection.* (2020). Available online at: http://www.nhc.gov.cn/yzygj/s7653p/202002/d4b895337e19445f8d728fcaf1e3e13a.shtml (accessed February 8, 2020).

36. Xu XL, Han MF, Li TT, Su W, Wang DS, Fu BQ, et al. *Effective Treatment of Severe COVID-19 Patients With Tocilizuma.* (2020). Available online at: http://chinaxiv.org/abs/202003.00026 (accessed March 11, 2020).

37. Mihai C, Dobrota R, Schroder M, Garaiman A, Jordan S, Becker MO, et al. COVID-19 in a patient with systemic sclerosis treated with tocilizumab for SSc-ILD. *Ann Rheum Dis.* (2020) 79:668–9. doi: 10.1136/annrheumdis-2020-217442

38. Zhang X, Song K, Tong F, Fei M, Guo H, Lu Z, et al. First case of COVID-19 in a patient with multiple myeloma successfully treated with tocilizumab. *Blood Adv.* (2020) 4:1307–10. doi: 10.1182/bloodadvances.2020001907

39. Tobinick E. TNF-alpha inhibition for potential therapeutic modulation of SARS coronavirus infection. *Curr Med Res Opin.* (2004) 20:39–40. doi: 10.1185/030079903125002757

Permissions

The contributors of this book come from diverse backgrounds, making this book a truly international effort. This book will bring forth new frontiers with its revolutionizing research information and detailed analysis of the nascent developments around the world.

We would like to thank all the contributing authors for lending their expertise to make the book truly unique. They have played a crucial role in the development of this book. Without their invaluable contributions this book wouldn't have been possible. They have made vital efforts to compile up to date information on the varied aspects of this subject to make this book a valuable addition to the collection of many professionals and students.

This book was conceptualized with the vision of imparting up-to-date information and advanced data in this field. To ensure the same, a matchless editorial board was set up. Every individual on the board went through rigorous rounds of assessment to prove their worth. After which they invested a large part of their time researching and compiling the most relevant data for our readers.

The editorial board has been involved in producing this book since its inception. They have spent rigorous hours researching and exploring the diverse topics which have resulted in the successful publishing of this book. They have passed on their knowledge of decades through this book. To expedite this challenging task, the publisher supported the team at every step. A small team of assistant editors was also appointed to further simplify the editing procedure and attain best results for the readers.

Apart from the editorial board, the designing team has also invested a significant amount of their time in understanding the subject and creating the most relevant covers. They scrutinized every image to scout for the most suitable representation of the subject and create an appropriate cover for the book.

The publishing team has been an ardent support to the editorial, designing and production team. Their endless efforts to recruit the best for this project, has resulted in the accomplishment of this book. They are a veteran in the field of academics and their pool of knowledge is as vast as their experience in printing. Their expertise and guidance has proved useful at every step. Their uncompromising quality standards have made this book an exceptional effort. Their encouragement from time to time has been an inspiration for everyone.

The publisher and the editorial board hope that this book will prove to be a valuable piece of knowledge for researchers, students, practitioners and scholars across the globe.

List of Contributors

Yonghao Lan
Department of Cardiology, Beijing Jishuitan Hospital, Peking University Fourth Hospital, Beijing, China
Department of Cardiology, Beijing Anzhen Hospital, Capital Medical University, Beijing, China

Wei Liu and Yujie Zhou
Department of Cardiology, Beijing Anzhen Hospital, Capital Medical University, Beijing, China
Beijing Key Laboratory of Precision Medicine of Coronary Atherosclerotic Disease, Clinical Center for Coronary Heart Disease, Beijing Institute of Heart Lung and Blood Vessel Disease, Capital Medical University, Beijing, China

Marijana Tadic
Department of Cardiology, University Hospital "Dr. Dragisa Misovic - Dedinje", Belgrade, Serbia

Sahrai Saeed
Department of Heart Disease, Haukeland University Hospital, Bergen, Norway

Guido Grassi
Department of Cardiology, University of Milan-Bicocca, Milan, Italy

Stefano Taddei
Department of Clinical and Experimental Medicine, University of Pisa, Pisa, Italy

Giuseppe Mancia
University of Milano-Bicocca, Milano and Policlinico di Monza, Monza, Italy

Cesare Cuspidi
Department of Cardiology, University of Milan-Bicocca, Milan, Italy
Department of Cardiology, Istituto Auxologico Italiano, Scientific Institute for Research, Hospitalization and Healthcare, Milan, Italy

Audrey A. Y. Zhang, Nicholas W. S. Chew, Yin Nwe Aye and Kalyar Saw
Department of Cardiology, National University Heart Centre, National University Health System, Singapore, Singapore

Cheng Han Ng, Aaron Mai and Gwyneth Kong
Yong Loo Lin School of Medicine, National University of Singapore, Singapore, Singapore

Raymond C. C. Wong, William K. F. Kong, Kian-Keong Poh, Koo-Hui Chan, Adrian Fatt-Hoe Low, Chi Hang Lee, Mark Yan-Yee Chan, Ping Chai, James Yip, Tiong-Cheng Yeo, Huay-Cheem Tan and Poay Huan Loh
Department of Cardiology, National University Heart Centre, National University Health System, Singapore, Singapore
Yong Loo Lin School of Medicine, National University of Singapore, Singapore, Singapore

Kailun Phua
Department of Medicine, National University Hospital, Singapore

Linna Huang, Xu Huang, Xiaoyang Cui, Ye Tian, Zeyu Zhang, Qingyuan Zhan and Xiaojing Wu
Center for Respiratory Diseases, China-Japan Friendship Hospital, Beijing, China
Department of Pulmonary and Critical Care Medicine, China-Japan Friendship Hospital, Beijing, China
National Clinical Research Center for Respiratory Diseases, Beijing, China

Ziying Chen
Center for Respiratory Diseases, China-Japan Friendship Hospital, Beijing, China
Department of Pulmonary and Critical Care Medicine, China-Japan Friendship Hospital, Beijing, China
National Clinical Research Center for Respiratory Diseases, Beijing, China
Peking University Health Science Center, Beijing, China

Lan Ni
Department of Pulmonary and Critical Care Medicine, Zhongnan Hospital of Wuhan University, Wuhan, China

Lei Chen
Department of Pulmonary and Critical Care Medicine, Tongji Hospital, Tongji Medical College, Huazhong University of Science and Technology, Wuhan, China

Changzhi Zhou
Department of Pulmonary and Critical Care Medicine, The Central Hospital of Wuhan, Wuhan, China

Chang Gao
Department of Critical Care Medicine, The First Affiliated Hospital of Soochow University, Suzhou, China

Lin Hua
School of Biomedical Engineering, Capital Medical University, Beijing, China

Bálint Károly Lakatos, Márton Tokodi, Alexandra Fábián, Zsuzsanna Ladányi, Liliána Szabó, Emese Csulak, Máté Babity, Anna Réka Kiss, Zsófia Gregor, Andrea Szűcs and Attila Kovács
Heart and Vascular Center, Semmelweis University, Budapest, Hungary

Hajnalka Vágó, Nóra Sydó, Orsolya Kiss and Béla Merkely
Heart and Vascular Center, Semmelweis University, Budapest, Hungary
Department of Sports Medicine, Semmelweis University, Budapest, Hungary

Takaharu Asano, Sarvesh Chelvanambi, Julius L. Decano and Mary C. Whelan
Center for Interdisciplinary Cardiovascular Sciences, Cardiovascular Division, Department of Medicine, Brigham and Women's Hospital and Harvard Medical School, Boston, MA, United States

Elena Aikawa
Center for Interdisciplinary Cardiovascular Sciences, Cardiovascular Division, Department of Medicine, Brigham and Women's Hospital and Harvard Medical School, Boston, MA, United States
Center for Excellence in Vascular Biology, Cardiovascular Division, Department of Medicine, Brigham and Women's Hospital and Harvard Medical School, Boston, MA, United States
Department of Human Pathology, I.M. Sechenov First Moscow State Medical University of the Ministry of Health, Moscow, Russia

Masanori Aikawa
Center for Interdisciplinary Cardiovascular Sciences, Cardiovascular Division, Department of Medicine, Brigham and Women's Hospital and Harvard Medical School, Boston, MA, United States
Center for Excellence in Vascular Biology, Cardiovascular Division, Department of Medicine, Brigham and Women's Hospital and Harvard Medical School, Boston, MA, United States
Department of Human Pathology, I.M. Sechenov First Moscow State Medical University of the Ministry of Health, Moscow, Russia
Channing Division of Network Medicine, Department of Medicine, Brigham and Women's Hospital and Harvard Medical School, Boston, MA, United States

Chi Zhang, Ke-Jia Le, Mang-Mang Pan, Zhi-Chun Gu and Hou-Wen Lin
Department of Pharmacy, Renji Hospital, School of Medicine, Shanghai Jiaotong University, Shanghai, China

Long Shen and Ling-Cong Kong
Department of Cardiology, Renji Hospital, School of Medicine, Shanghai Jiaotong University, Shanghai, China

Hang Xu and Wei-Hong Ge
Department of Pharmacy, Nanjing Drum Tower Hospital, The Affiliated Hospital of Nanjing University Medical School, Nanjing, China

Zhen Zhang
Department of Pharmacy, Roswell Park Comprehensive Cancer Center, Buffalo, NY, United States

Regitse Højgaard Christensen
Centre for Physical Activity Research, Rigshospitalet, University of Copenhagen, Copenhagen, Denmark
Department of Cardiology, Rigshospitalet, University of Copenhagen, Copenhagen, Denmark

Ronan M. G. Berg
Centre for Physical Activity Research, Rigshospitalet, University of Copenhagen, Copenhagen, Denmark
Department of Biomedical Sciences, Faculty of Health and Medical Sciences, University of Copenhagen, Copenhagen, Denmark
Department of Clinical Physiology Nuclear Medicine & Positron Emission Tomography (PET), Rigshospitalet, University of Copenhagen, Copenhagen, Denmark
Neurovascular Research Laboratory, Faculty of Life Sciences and Education, University of South Wales, Newport, United Kingdom

Maria-Luiza Luchian, Stijn Lochy, Andreea Motoc, Bram Roosens, Esther Scheirlynck, Sven Boeckstaens, Karen Van den Bussche, Berlinde von Kemp, Xavier Galloo, Clara François, Caroline Weytjens, Steven Droogmans and Bernard Cosyns
Department of Cardiology, University Hospital of Brussels (Centrum voor Hart-en Vaat ziekten, Universitair Ziekenhuis Brussel), Brussels, Belgium

Dries Belsack, Johan de Mey and Kaoru Tanaka
Department of Radiology, University Hospital of Brussels, Brussels, Belgium

Julien Magne
CHU Limoges, Hôpital Dupuytren, Service Cardiologie, Limoges, France
INSERM 1094, Faculté de médecine de Limoges, 2, rue Marcland, Limoges, France

Tom De Potter
Faculty of Medicine and Pharmacy, Vrije Universiteit Brussel, Brussels, Belgium

Audditiya Bandopadhyay and Gyaneshwer Chaubey
Cytogenetics Laboratory, Department of Zoology, Banaras Hindu University, Varanasi, India

Alok Kumar Singh
M.D.D.M. (Cardiology), Senior Intervention Cardiologist, Lifeline Hospital, Varanasi, India

Xiaowei Shi, Jiong Yu, Xinyu Sheng, Qiaoling Pan, Jinfeng Yang, Hongcui Cao and Lanjuan Li
State Key Laboratory for the Diagnosis and Treatment of Infectious Diseases, National Clinical Research Center for Infectious Diseases, The First Affiliated Hospital, Zhejiang University School of Medicine, Hangzhou, China
Collaborative Innovation Center for Diagnosis and Treatment of Infectious Diseases, Hangzhou, China

Jing Ma
State Key Laboratory for the Diagnosis and Treatment of Infectious Diseases, National Clinical Research Center for Infectious Diseases, The First Affiliated Hospital, Zhejiang University School of Medicine, Hangzhou, China
Collaborative Innovation Center for Diagnosis and Treatment of Infectious Diseases, Hangzhou, China
Department of Laboratory Medicine, The First Affiliated Hospital, Zhejiang University School of Medicine, Hangzhou, China

Feifei Lv
Department of Laboratory Medicine, The First Affiliated Hospital, Zhejiang University School of Medicine, Hangzhou, China

Jian Wu
State Key Laboratory for the Diagnosis and Treatment of Infectious Diseases, National Clinical Research Center for Infectious Diseases, The First Affiliated Hospital, Zhejiang University School of Medicine, Hangzhou, China
Department of Laboratory Medicine, The First People's Hospital of Yancheng City, Yancheng, China

Philipp Jud, Paul Gressenberger, Viktoria Muster, Reinhard B. Raggam and Marianne Brodmann
Division of Angiology, Department of Internal Medicine, Medical University of Graz, Graz, Austria

Alexander Avian
Institute for Medical Informatics, Statistics and Documentation, Medical University of Graz, Graz, Austria

Andreas Meinitzer
Clinical Institute of Medical and Chemical Laboratory Diagnostics, Medical University of Graz, Graz, Austria

Heimo Strohmaier
Department Center of Medical Research, Medical University of Graz, Graz, Austria

Harald Sourij
Division of Endocrinology, Department of Internal Medicine, Medical University of Graz, Graz, Austria

Martin Helmut Stradner and Ulrike Demel
Division of Rheumatology and Immunology, Department of Internal Medicine, Medical University of Graz, Graz, Austria

Harald H. Kessler
Diagnostic and Research Institute of Hygiene, Microbiology and Environmental, Medical University of Graz, Graz, Austria

Kathrin Eller
Division of Nephrology, Department of Internal Medicine, Medical University of Graz, Graz, Austria

Heidi S. Lumish and Eunyoung Kim
Division of Cardiology, Columbia University, New York, United States

Caitlin Selvaggi, Tingyi Cao and Andrea S. Foulkes
Biostatistics Center, Massachusetts General Hospital, Boston, MA, United States
Department of Medicine, Harvard Medical School, Boston, MA, United States
Department of Biostatistics, Harvard T. H. Chan School of Public Health, Boston, MA, United States

Aakriti Gupta
Division of Interventional Cardiology, Cedars-Sinai Medical Center, Los Angeles, CA, United States

Muredach P. Reilly
Irving Institute for Clinical and Translational Research, Columbia University, New York, United States

Hiroyuki Futatsugi, Masato Iwabu and Toshimasa Yamauchi
Department of Diabetes and Metabolic Diseases, Graduate School of Medicine, The University of Tokyo, Tokyo, Japan

Miki Okada-Iwabu
Department of Diabetes and Metabolic Diseases, Graduate School of Medicine, The University of Tokyo, Tokyo, Japan
Laboratory for Advanced Research on Pathophysiology of Metabolic Diseases, The University of Tokyo, Tokyo, Japan

Koh Okamoto
Department of Infectious Diseases, The University of Tokyo Hospital, Tokyo, Japan

Yosuke Amano
Department of Respiratory Medicine, The University of Tokyo Hospital, Tokyo, Japan

Yutaka Morizaki
Department of Orthopaedic Surgery, The University of Tokyo Hospital, Tokyo, Japan

Takashi Kadowaki
Department of Diabetes and Metabolic Diseases, Graduate School of Medicine, The University of Tokyo, Tokyo, Japan
Department of Prevention of Diabetes and Life-Style Related Diseases, The University of Tokyo, Tokyo, Japan
Toranomon Hospital, Tokyo, Japan

Arnaud Lyon
School of Medicine, University of Lausanne, Lausanne, Switzerland

Ziyad Gunga, Lars Niclauss and Piergiorgio Tozzi
Service de Chirurgie Cardiaque, Centre Hospitalier Universitaire Vaudois, Lausanne, Switzerland

Valentina Rancati
Département d'anesthésiologie, Hôpital Universitaire de Lausanne (CHUV), Lausanne, Switzerland

Andrea Sonaglioni, Elisabetta Rigamonti and Michele Lombardo
Department of Cardiology, Istituto di Ricovero e Cura a Carattere Scientifico (IRCCS) Multi Medica, Milan, Italy

Adriana Albini
Scientific and Technological Pole, Istituto di Ricovero e Cura a Carattere Scientifico (IRCCS) Multi Medica, Milan, Italy

Gian Luigi Nicolosi
Department of Cardiology, Policlinico San Giorgio, Pordenone, Italy

Douglas M. Noonan
Scientific and Technological Pole, Istituto di Ricovero e Cura a Carattere Scientifico (IRCCS) Multi Medica, Milan, Italy
Department of Biotechnology and Life Sciences, University of Insubria, Varese, Italy

Alexander Carpenter, Aziza El Harchi, Oliver Hanington, Stephen C. Harmer, Jules C. Hancox and Andrew F. James
School of Physiology, Pharmacology and Neuroscience, University of Bristol, Bristol, United Kingdom

Owen J. Chambers
Liverpool Heart and Chest Hospital NHS Foundation Trust, Liverpool, United Kingdom

Richard Bond
Gloucestershire Hospitals NHS Foundation Trust, Gloucester, United Kingdom

Zhi-Yao Wei, Hai-Yan Qian and Wei-Xian Yang
State Key Laboratory of Cardiovascular Disease, Department of Cardiology, Center for Coronary Heart Disease, National Center for Cardiovascular Diseases of China, Fu Wai Hospital, Peking Union Medical College, Chinese Academy of Medical Sciences, Beijing, China

Rui Qiao and Chong-Huai Gu
Department of Cardiology, Anqing Hospital, Anhui Medical University, Anqing, China

Jian Chen
Guangdong Provincial Key Laboratory of Biomedical Imaging, Department of Cardiovascular Medicine, Fifth Affiliated Hospital of Sun Yat-sen University, Zhuhai, China

Ji Huang
Department of Cardiology, Beijing Anzhen Hospital, Capital Medical University, Beijing, China

Wen-Jun Wang
Department of Cardiology, Daye Chinese Medicine Hospital, Daye, China

Hua Yu
Division of Life Sciences and Medicine, Department of Cardiology, The First Affiliated Hospital of University of Science and Technology of China, Hefei, China

Jing Xu
Division of Life Sciences and Medicine, Department of Infectious Diseases, The First Affiliated Hospital of University of Science and Technology of China, Hefei, China

Hui Wu and Jun Yang
Institute of Cardiovascular Disease, China Three Gorges University, Yichang, China
Department of Cardiology, Yichang Central People's Hospital, Yichang, China

Chao Wang
Coronary Care Unit, Baoding No.1 Central Hospital, Baoding, China

Hong-Jiang Li
Sixth Department of Hepatopathy, Baoding People's Hospital, Baoding, China

Mi Li
Department of Gastroenterology, Yingcheng Chinese Medicine Hospital, Yingcheng, China

Cong Liu
Department of Otolaryngology, Daye People's Hospital, Daye, China

Hua-Ming Ding
Department of Radiology, Infection Hospital of Anhui Provincial Hospital (Hefei Infectious Diseases Hospital), Hefei, China

Min-Jie Lu
State Key Laboratory of Cardiovascular Disease, Department of Magnetic Resonance Imaging, National Center for Cardiovascular Diseases of China, Fu Wai Hospital, Peking Union Medical College, Chinese Academy of Medical Sciences, Beijing, China

Wei-Hua Yin
State Key Laboratory of Cardiovascular Disease, Department of Radiology, National Center for Cardiovascular Diseases of China, Fu Wai Hospital, Peking Union Medical College, Chinese Academy of Medical Sciences, Beijing, China

Yang Wang
State Key Laboratory of Cardiovascular Disease, Medical Research and Biometrics Center, National Center for Cardiovascular Diseases of China, Fu Wai Hospital, Peking Union Medical College, Chinese Academy of Medical Sciences, Beijing, China

Kun-Wei Li
Department of Radiology, Fifth Affiliated Hospital of Sun Yat-sen University, Zhuhai, China

Heng-Feng Shi
Department of Radiology, Anqing Hospital, Anhui Medical University, Anqing, China

Yong-Jian Geng
Division of Cardiology, Department of Internal Medicine, The Center for Cardiovascular Biology and Atherosclerosis Research, McGovern Medical School, University of Texas Health Science Center at Houston, Houston, TX, United States

Zhenxing Sun, Ziming Zhang, Jie Liu, Yue Song, Shi Qiao, Yilian Duan, Haiyan Cao, Yuji Xie, Rui Wang, Wen Zhang, Manjie You, Cheng Yu, Li Ji, Chunyan Cao, Jing Wang, Yali Yang, Qing Lv and Mingxing Xie
Department of Ultrasound Medicine, Union Hospital, Tongji Medical College, Huazhong University of Science and Technology, Wuhan, China
Hubei Province Key Laboratory of Molecular Imaging, Wuhan, China

Hongbo Wang
Department of Gynecology and Obstetrics, Union Hospital, Tongji Medical College, Huazhong University of Science and Technology, Wuhan, China

Haotian Gu
British Heart Foundation Centre of Research Excellence, King's College London, London, United Kingdom

Liberato Berrino
Section of Pharmacology "L. Donatelli", Department of Experimental Medicine, University of Campania "Luigi Vanvitelli", Naples, Italy

Annamaria Mascolo, Cristina Scavone, Concetta Rafaniello, Carmen Ferrajolo, Francesco Rossi and Annalisa Capuano
Section of Pharmacology "L. Donatelli", Department of Experimental Medicine, University of Campania "Luigi Vanvitelli", Naples, Italy
Campania Regional Centre for Pharmacovigilance and Pharmacoepidemiology, Naples, Italy

Giorgio Racagni
Department of Pharmacological and Biomolecular Sciences, Università degli Studi di Milano, Milan, Italy

Giuseppe Paolisso
Department of Advanced Medical and Surgical Sciences, University of Campania "Luigi Vanvitelli", Naples, Italy

Renata Moll-Bernardes and Mayara Fraga Santos
D'Or Institute for Research and Education, Rio de Janeiro, Brazil

Andrea Silvestre de Sousa and Fernando A. Bozza
D'Or Institute for Research and Education, Rio de Janeiro, Brazil
Evandro Chagas National Institute of Infectious Disease, Oswaldo Cruz Foundation, Rio de Janeiro, Brazil

Thiago Ceccatto de Paula
Hospital São Luiz Jabaquara, São Paulo, Brazil

Ariane V. S. Macedo
D'Or Institute for Research and Education, Rio de Janeiro, Brazil
Hospital São Luiz Jabaquara, São Paulo, Brazil
Santa Casa de São Paulo, São Paulo, Brazil

Renato D. Lopes
D'Or Institute for Research and Education, Rio de Janeiro, Brazil
Duke Clinical Research Institute, Duke University Medical Center, Durham, NC, United States
Brazilian Clinical Research Institute, São Paulo, Brazil

Narendra Vera, Luciana C. R. Maia and Pedro M. Pimentel-Coelho
Institute of Biophysics Carlos Chagas Filho, Federal University of Rio de Janeiro, Rio de Janeiro, Brazil

André Feldman
D'Or Institute for Research and Education, Rio de Janeiro, Brazil
Hospital São Luiz Anália Franco, São Paulo, Brazil

Vitor A. Loures and Rafael A. M. Domiciano
Hospital São Luiz Anália Franco, São Paulo, Brazil

Guilherme D. A. S. Arruda
Hospital São Luiz São Caetano, São Caetano do Sul, Brazil

Mauro J. C. Castro
Instituto de Microbiologia Paulo de Góes, Federal University of Rio de Janeiro, Rio de Janeiro, Brazil

Denílson C. de Albuquerque
D'Or Institute for Research and Education, Rio de Janeiro, Brazil
Cardiology Department, Rio de Janeiro State University, Rio de Janeiro, Brazil

Thyago A. B. Furquim
Hospital Sino Brasileiro, Osasco, Brazil

Karla G. D. Giusti and Nathália M. de Oliveira
Hospital Villa Lobos, São Paulo, Brazil

Fábio A. De Luca and Marisol D. M. Kotsugai
Hospital São Luiz Morumbi, São Paulo, Brazil

Olga Ferreira de Souza
D'Or Institute for Research and Education, Rio de Janeiro, Brazil
Hospital Copa Star, Rio de Janeiro, Brazil

Ronir Raggio Luiz
D'Or Institute for Research and Education, Rio de Janeiro, Brazil
Institute for Studies in Public Health — IESC, Federal University of Rio de Janeiro, Rio de Janeiro, Brazil

Emiliano Medei
D'Or Institute for Research and Education, Rio de Janeiro, Brazil
Institute of Biophysics Carlos Chagas Filho, Federal University of Rio de Janeiro, Rio de Janeiro, Brazil
National Center for Structural Biology and Bioimaging, Federal University of Rio de Janeiro, Rio de Janeiro, Brazil

Peter Jirak, Moritz Mirna, Bernhard Strohmer, Clemens Seelmaier, Uta C. Hoppe and Lukas J. Motloch
Clinic II for Internal Medicine, University Hospital Salzburg, Paracelsus Medical University, Salzburg, Austria

Zornitsa Shomanova, Jan Sackarnd, Jürgen Sindermann, Holger Reinecke and Rudin Pistulli
Department of Cardiology I — Coronary and Peripheral Vascular Disease, Heart Failure, University Hospital Münster, Münster, Germany

Gerrit Frommeyer
Department of Cardiology II — Electrophysiology, University Hospital Münster, Münster, Germany

Robert Larbig
Department of Cardiology II — Electrophysiology, University Hospital Münster, Münster, Germany
Division of Cardiology, Hospital Maria Hilf Mönchengladbach, Mönchengladbach, Germany

Dominyka Butkiene
Division of Cardiology, Hospital Maria Hilf Mönchengladbach, Mönchengladbach, Germany

Daniel Dankl and Nino Frank
Department of Anesthesiology, Perioperative Care, and Intensive Care Medicine, University Hospital Salzburg, Paracelsurs Medical University, Salzburg, Austria

Flavio D'Ascenzi, Matteo Cameli, Sergio Mondillo and Serafina Valente
Division of Cardiology, Department of Medical Biotechnologies, University of Siena, Siena, Italy

Silvia Forni, Fabrizio Gemmi, Claudia Szasz and Valeria Di Fabrizio
Regional Health Agency of Tuscany, Florence, Italy

Maria Teresa Mechi and Matteo Nocci
Quality of Care and Clinical Networks, Regional Health Department of Tuscany, Florence, Italy

Kristen Kopp, Michael Lichtenauer and Lukas Jaroslaw Motloch
Department of Internal Medicine II, Cardiology, Paracelsus Medical University, Salzburg, Austria

Alexander Egle
Department of Internal Medicine III, Hematology, Medical Oncology, Hemostaseology, Rheumatology and Infectious Diseases, Paracelsus Medical University, Salzburg, Austria

Helmut J. F. Salzer and Bernd Lamprecht
Department of Pulmonology, Kepler University Hospital, Linz, Austria
Medical Faculty, Johannes Kepler University, Linz, Austria

Josef Tomasits
Institute for Medical and Chemical Laboratory Diagnostics, Kepler University Hospital, Linz, Austria

Hannes M. Müller
Department of Cardiac, Vascular, and Thoracic Surgery, Kepler University Hospital, Linz, Austria

Anna Dieplinger
Institute for Nursing and Practice, Paracelsus Medical University, Salzburg, Austria

Sunil Kumar Shambu and Nagaraj Desai
Department of Cardiology, Jagadguru Sri Shivarathreeshwara Medical College and Hospital, Jagadguru Sri Shivarathreeshwara Academy of Higher Education and Research (JSS AHER), Mysore, India

Shyam Prasad Shetty B
Department of Cardiothoracic and Vascular Surgery, Jagadguru Sri Shivarathreeshwara Medical College and Hospital, Jagadguru Sri Shivarathreeshwara Academy of Higher Education and Research (JSS AHER), Mysore, India

Oliver Joel Gona, Ramesh Madhan and Revanth V
Department of Pharmacy Practice, Jagadguru Sri Shivarathreeshwara College of Pharmacy (JSS CPM), Jagadguru Sri Shivarathreeshwara Academy of Higher Education and Research (JSS AHER), Mysore, India

Madhu B
Department of Community Medicine, Jagadguru Sri Shivarathreeshwara Medical College and Hospital, Jagadguru Sri Shivarathreeshwara Academy of Higher Education and Research (JSS AHER), Mysore, India

Randa M. Breikaa
Center for Cardiovascular Research and The Heart Center, Nationwide Children's Hospital, Columbus, OH, United States
Molecular, Cellular and Developmental Biology Program, The Ohio State University, Columbus, OH, United States

Brenda Lilly
Center for Cardiovascular Research and The Heart Center, Nationwide Children's Hospital, Columbus, OH, United States
Department of Pediatrics, The Ohio State University, Columbus, OH, United States

Kyoung Ae Kong
Department of Preventive Medicine, College of Medicine, Ewha Womans University, Seoul, South Korea

Sodam Jung, Junbeom Park and In Sook Kang
Division of Cardiology, Department of Internal Medicine, Ewha Womans University Mokdong Hospital, College of Medicine, Ewha Womans University, Seoul, South Korea

Mina Yu
Division of Nephrology, Department of Internal Medicine, Ewha Womans University Seoul Hospital, College of Medicine, Ewha Womans University, Seoul, South Korea

Yanjun Song, Peng Gao, Tian Ran, Hao Qian, Fan Guo, Wei Wu and Shuyang Zhang
Department of Cardiology, Chinese Academy of Medical Sciences and Peking Union Medical College, Beijing, China

Long Chang
Department of Internal Medicine, Chinese Academy of Medical Sciences and Peking Union Medical College, Beijing, China

Index

www.ingramcontent.com/pod-product-compliance
Lightning Source LLC
Chambersburg PA
CBHW080410190526

45161CB00003B/193